THE EXPERT MEDICAL GUIDEBOOK
WRITTEN ESPECIALLY FOR
HOME USE

"This fine dictionary . . . explains in simple, non-technical language the meanings of medical terms. The several hundred crisp diagrams bring into clear focus many medical conditions which have heretofore been obscure to the average man."

> —Major General Clinton S. Lyter
> United States Army Medical Corps (Ret.)
> Denver, Colorado

Robert E. Rothenberg, M.D., is Emeritus Professor of Surgery at New York Medical College and Consultant Surgeon at the Cabrini Medical Center in New York. He is a fellow at the American College of Surgeons and a Diplomate of the American Board of Surgery. Formerly, he was Attending Surgeon and a member of the Board of Trustees at the French and Polyclinic Medical School and Health Center. From 1954 to 1964, Dr. Rothenberg served on the Board of Directors of the Health Insurance Plan of Greater New York, and from 1960 to 1966, he was Civilian Surgical Consultant to the United States Army Hospital, Fort Jay, New York.

OTHER BOOKS WRITTEN AND/OR
EDITED BY THE AUTHOR

GROUP MEDICINE & HEALTH INSURANCE IN ACTION

UNDERSTANDING SURGERY

THE MEDICAL ENCYCLOPEDIA FOR HOME USE

THE NEW AMERICAN MEDICAL DICTIONARY

REOPERATIVE SURGERY

HEALTH IN THE LATER YEARS

THE CHILD CARE ENCYCLOPEDIA

THE PREMARITAL MEDICAL ADVISER

THE COMPLETE SURGICAL GUIDE

THE FAST DIET BOOK

WHAT EVERY PATIENT WANTS TO KNOW

FIRST AID IN EMERGENCIES

THE NEW ILLUSTRATED MEDICAL ENCYCLOPEDIA
FOR THE HOME

DISNEY'S GROWING UP HEALTHY

THE COMPLETE BOOK OF BREAST CARE

THE PLAIN LANGUAGE LAW DICTIONARY

Robert E. Rothenberg, M.D., F.A.C.S.

The New American Medical Dictionary and Health Manual

NEWLY REVISED AND ENLARGED SEVENTH EDITION

Illustrated by Mary E. Miner
and
Sylvia and Lester V. Bergman

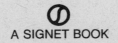

A SIGNET BOOK

SIGNET
Published by New American Library, a division of
Penguin Putnam Inc., 375 Hudson Street,
New York, New York 10014, U.S.A.
Penguin Books Ltd, 27 Wrights Lane,
London W8 5TZ, England
Penguin Books Australia Ltd, Ringwood,
Victoria, Australia
Penguin Books Canada Ltd, 10 Alcorn Avenue,
Toronto, Ontario, Canada M4V 3B2
Penguin Books (N.Z.) Ltd, 182–190 Wairau Road,
Auckland 10, New Zealand

Penguin Books Ltd, Registered Offices:
Harmondsworth, Middlesex, England

First published by Signet, an imprint of New American Library,
a division of Penguin Putnam Inc.

First Printing, February 1962
First Printing (Newly Revised and Enlarged Seventh Edition), April 1999
10   9   8   7   6   5   4

To the loving memory of my mother, Caroline,
whose interest and affection for words and
their meaning caused the dictionary to play an
essential role in the daily life of our home.

ACKNOWLEDGMENTS

Much of the credit for the idea of compiling a medical dictionary for general use goes to the late medical writer Susan Ellis, whose warm friendship I shall always cherish. I am also indebted to the brilliant publisher Fritz Landshoff, whose advice was so important as to the ultimate form the manuscript should take.

The conscientious devotion and industry of my late wife, Eileen, played a significant part in seeing the tedious work completed, and for her efforts I express loving gratitude. I also want to thank Mary A. Herbert for her invaluable help in finalizing this seventh edition of the work.

To the Metropolitan Life Insurance Company, the U.S. Vitamin and Pharmaceutical Corporation, the Technicon Instruments Corporation, the United States Department of Health and Human Services, the American Heart Association, and to the Harry N. Abrams, Inc. publishing company, I wish to extend my thanks for permission to use or adapt charts, tables, and other data which appear in the Manual section of this book.

—R.E.R.

PREFACE

The purpose of this dictionary and manual is twofold: first, to translate medical terms and phrases into language that can be easily understood, and second, to supply medical information in simple form so that it can be interpreted readily by those who are unfamiliar with medical matters. It is our belief that people are entitled to know, as precisely as possible, what physicians mean when they use complicated or esoteric terminology or when they refer to obscure tests and procedures. It is also our conviction that better health will result from increased knowledge and understanding of medical problems. This work hopes to add to such knowledge and thus promote the cause of improved health.

Many of the words defined in the dictionary section are also used in ordinary, nonmedical conversation. The definitions given herein are invariably the *medical* definitions and relate only by coincidence to their usage in everyday conversation. As an example, the word "accommodation" refers to changes in the size of the pupil of the eye, not to "lodgings," or a "favor."

The inclusion in the dictionary of certain trademarked items and patented products does not necessarily constitute their endorsement. Some might be worthy of recommendation; others not. They are included mainly because of the widespread use accorded them by the public.

Repetition is avoided when possible by omitting the recording of the several forms of the same word. Thus, "amputation" is defined while the word "amputate" is not recorded. And since this dictionary is meant primarily for purposes of explanation, information on the pronunciation of medical terms is not included.

—R.E.R.

CONTENTS

Contents

HOW TO USE THIS BOOK

Entries are all alphabetized strictly on letter sequence, regardless of space or hyphen which may occur between entry words.

> Example: Banting, Frederick Grant
> Banti's disease

In some instances, compound entries, such as those consisting of an adjective and a noun, are listed in alphabetical order according to the first word of the expression. Thus, the entry for "absolute alcohol" follows that for "absinthism," that for "chylous cyst" follows that for "chylous ascites," etc.

The table of contents for the Manual appears at the end of the Dictionary. A table of contents for the Medicare Handbook appears on page 557.

A section listing Abbreviations, including Diplomates in Specialties, Fellows of Specialty Colleges, Medical Associations and Societies, and Medical Terms, appears at the end of the Manual.

The New American Medical Dictionary

A

aa An abbreviation used in writing prescriptions, meaning "equal parts of."

abacterial Free of germs.

abasia Lack of motor or muscular coordination in walking.

abatement A decrease in the severity or intensity of a symptom.

abaxial Off center; not on the axis.

abdomen That part of the body occupying the space between the chest and the pelvis.

abdominal cavity That portion of the body extending from beneath the diaphragm down to the pelvis. It contains all the abdominal organs.

abdominal pregnancy A pregnancy rooted in the abdominal cavity rather than in the uterus; a rare occurrence in which the pregnancy does not often proceed to term.

abdominocentesis Tapping the abdominal cavity with a needle, a procedure helpful in making diagnoses of internal bleeding, in noting the presence of malignant cells, or in removing fluid or pus collections.

abdominohysterectomy The surgical procedure which removes the uterus (womb) through an abdominal incision.

abdominohysterotomy A surgical approach to the interior of the uterus (womb) carried out through an incision in the abdomen.

abdominoperineal resection Surgical removal of part or all of the large intestine and the rectum. An operation sometimes carried out for an extensive cancer or ulcerative colitis.

abdominoplasty An operation to remove excess fat from the abdomen.

abducens The sixth cranial nerve. It regulates the muscles which rotate the eyeball away from the midline of the body.

abduct To draw away from the midline of the body; as to raise the arm out sidewards.

abductor A muscle that draws a part of the body away from the midline; the opposite of adductor.

aberrant Straying from the normal. (Aberrant thyroid tissue may occasionally be located in the chest cavity, or in the floor of the mouth.)

aberration Deviation from the normal.

ABG Abbreviation for arterial blood gases, an important set of analyses performed on blood taken from an artery in the arm. The alkalinity or acidity of the blood, the amounts of oxygen and carbon dioxide can be measured by these tests.

abiogenesis The development of living organisms from nonliving matter.

abiology The study of nonliving things.

abiosis Nonliving; the state of not having life.

abiotrophy Degeneration or loss of life or function of tissue.

abirritant A substance or agent which relieves irritation.

ablactation The end of the period when a breast gives milk; weaning.

ablation Surgical removal of a part of the body, such as amputation of a limb.

ablatio placentae Premature separation of the placenta from the wall of the uterus. (This sometimes leads

1

to death of the unborn child.) Also called *abruptio placentae*.

ablephary Partial or total absence of the eyelids; a birth deformity.

ablepsy Absence of sight.

ablution The act of washing the body.

ablutomania A mania for washing the body, or parts of the body.

abnormal Not conforming to type or standard.

abocclusion Failure of the upper and lower teeth to mesh properly; *malocclusion*.

ABO incompatibility A type of blood incompatibility, found rarely. Transfusion reactions may occur as a result of such incompatibility.

abort To miscarry.

abortifacient A drug which tends to bring on an abortion.

abortion A miscarriage. The spontaneous or induced passage of a nonliving embryo during the early stages of development.

criminal The illegal interruption of pregnancy.

habitual The tendency to miscarry during the early months of pregnancy.

incomplete One in which only part of the products of the embryo or fetus have been passed.

induced A miscarriage intentionally brought on. It may be criminally induced or legally induced for sound medical reasons.

spontaneous A miscarriage which takes place unexpectedly and without attempts to induce it.

therapeutic A surgical procedure performed, for reasons of health, to interrupt a pregnancy.

threatened Bleeding from the vagina and abdominal cramps during early pregnancy. It may or may not be followed by the expulsion of the embryo.

abortionist One who performs an abortion.

abortive Coming to an abrupt, premature end; cutting short the duration of a disease.

abrade To rub off, as to *abrade* the skin.

abrasion A scrape or scratch of the skin, mucous membranes or the cornea (covering of the eye).

abrasive A substance which will scrape off the superficial cells of an organ or part of the body.

abreaction A process by which unconscious, forgotten thoughts and feelings are brought to consciousness and relieved. This technique is employed by psychoanalysis.

abruptio placentae Premature separation of the placenta from the wall of the uterus, occurring during the latter part of pregnancy.

abscess A localized collection of pus. It may occur in any organ or part of the body.

abscission Excision. Surgical removal of a part of the body.

absinthism A nervous and mental disorder resulting from the excessive use of the liqueur, absinthe.

absolute alcohol Pure alcohol, containing less than 1 percent of water.

absorb To incorporate within the body; to soak in. (Fluids, food, light rays, can all be absorbed by the body.)

absorbefacient A substance which promotes absorption.

absorbent Able to absorb, such as *absorbent* cotton.

abstemious Resisting excesses, particularly excess drinking or excess expression of lustful desires.

abstinence Self-denial, usually applied to voluntarily abstaining from sex, food, or alcohol.

abstraction The refinement of a drug from its crude, original form. Psychologically, absentmindedness, preoccupation.

abulia A mental state in which the patient is unable to make decisions.

ABVD Abbreviation for a combination of chemotherapy drugs that are frequently utilized, namely, Adriamycin, bleomycin, decarbazine and vinblastine.

a.c. An abbreviation used in writing prescriptions, meaning "before meals."

acalcerosis A condition characterized by deficiency of calcium in the body.

acampsia Inability to bend or extend a joint.

acanthesthesia A feeling of "pins and needles."

acanthocytosis A condition in which there are many deformed red blood cells. Instead of being spherical in shape, the cells contain thornlike projections. (An inherited disorder)

acanthoma A tumor of the skin.

acanthosis A skin condition marked by thickening and warty growths.

    nigricans An uncommon disease characterized by pigmented, wartlike growths on the skin and mouth and, rarely, in internal organs.

acapnia A state in which there is a decreased amount of carbon dioxide in the blood.

acapsular Without a capsule or sheath; a term often applied to certain tumors which have extended out into surrounding tissues.

acardia A deformity in which the fetus is born without a heart.

acariasis Any disease caused by the mite family known as *acarids*.

acarid A tick or mite.

acarophobia A morbid fear of mites and small things or dread of developing an itch.

acatalepsy Deterioration of mental ability.

acatamathesia A mental state in which the person is unable to understand spoken conversation.

acataphasia Inability to speak in orderly sentences.

acathexia Inability to retain bodily secretions and excretions.

acathexis Lack of feeling toward something which is actually very important.

acaudal Without a tail; said of man and ape.

accelerator A nerve or muscle which hastens a function.

accident prone A tendency toward having more than the usual number of accidents; thought to be a neurotic manifestation.

acclimation Adjustment to a new environment.

accommodation Adjustment of the eye to new surroundings, as to the dark when coming in from the daylight.

accouchement Childbirth (French).

accoucheur A French word for an obstetrician.

accrementition A growth process.

accretion Growth by the adding of substance to the outside of a structure. An accumulation.

Accutane A medication used in the treatment of stubborn acne. It acts by decreasing the amount of oily substance secreted by glands in the skin.

acenesthesia Loss of the sense of well-being, or visceral sense, occurring in certain depressed mental states.

acenocoumarol An oral medication whose action prolongs blood clotting; an anticoagulant drug.

acephaly A deformity in which the embryo is born without a head.

aceratosis Absence of nails.

acetabulectomy Removal of the hollow, cuplike portion of the hip joint; carried out in some instances in which the hip socket has been destroyed by disease such as tuberculosis.

acetabuloplasty An operation to reshape the acetabulum to fit the head of the thigh bone (femur).

acetabulum The hollow, cuplike portion of the hip joint; the hip socket.

acetanilid A drug having actions similar to those of aspirin; it relieves pain and lowers the temperature.

acetanilide A pain-relieving and fever-lowering drug, toxic when used over a prolonged period of time.

acetate An acetic acid salt.

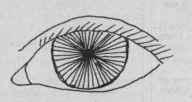

Response to strong light

Response to weak light

Accommodation of the pupil of the eye

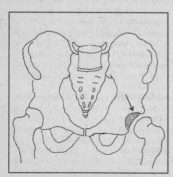

Acetabulum of the hipbone

acetic Sour; relating to vinegar or acetic acid.
acetic acid(Ch_3COOH) The acid

of vinegar. In dilute solution, it is sometimes used as an astringent (contracting) or styptic agent.
acetone A chemical substance often found in large quantities in patients with diabetes. When found in large quantities, it indicates acidosis.
acetonemia The condition in which acetone bodies are present in the blood.
acetonuria Excess acetone in the urine, encountered especially in diabetic acidosis.
acetophenetidin A drug used to reduce fever and to relieve pain. An ingredient of many of the pain-relieving and fever-relieving drugs.
acetylcholine A chemical produced within the body and thought to be the substance released by

nerves to activate muscle contractions. It has been made into a useful drug.

acetylphenylhydrazine A chemical which destroys red blood cells. Used in a condition known as polycythemia in which there is an excess of red cells.

acetylsalicylic acid Aspirin; one of the most popular pain-relieving medications.

achalasia Constriction of the lower portion of the food pipe (esophagus) due to inability of the muscles to relax.

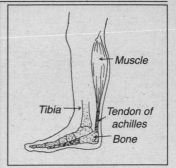

Achilles tendon

is seen in cases of pernicious anemia, in some cases of cancer of the stomach, and in some normal individuals.)

acholia Absence of bile.

acholuria Absence of bile pigments in the urine, occurring in certain types of jaundice.

achondroplasia A birth deformity characterized by imperfect bone formation. It results in dwarfs with normal-sized heads but short arms and legs.

achromacyte A decolorized or pale red blood cell, caused by lack of hemoglobin within the cell.

achromasia Absence or loss of normal skin pigmentation. An "albino" is born with *achromasia*.

achromatic Without color.

achromatosis A condition associated with a lack of normal pigment in the skin.

achromaturia Water-colored urine; seen when the urine is particularly dilute.

achromotrichia Lack of pigment in the hair; graying of the hair.

achromycin Same as tetracycline. An antibiotic effective in the treatment of many infections of the gastrointestinal, urinary, and respiratory systems.

achylia Lack of gastric (stomach) juices.

acid Any chemical containing hy-

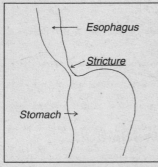

Achalasia

Achievement quotient (A.Q.) The measurement of a child's education in relation to his age.

Achilles tendon The tendon which attaches to the heel and originates from the muscles in the calf (the gastrocnemius and soleus muscles).

achillobursitis Inflammation of the bursa lying around, especially in front of the Achilles tendon.

achillodynia Pain in the region of the Achilles tendon.

achillotenotomy Cutting of the Achilles tendon in such a way as to release a shortening or contracture.

achiria A hysterical condition in which the patient has the sensation he has lost one or both of his hands.

achlorhydria The absence of free hydrochloric acid in the stomach. (It drogen replaceable by a metal to form a salt.

acid alcohol A substance used to take out color.

acid-base balance The equilibrium between alkali and acid in the body, resulting, when normal, in a pH of 7.4.

acidemia Excess acid in the blood.

acid-fast This term refers to certain staining characteristics of bacteria, particularly those germs causing tuberculosis or leprosy.

acidify To make acid.

Acidogen A trade-marked drug which stimulates the liberation of hydrochloric acid in the stomach.

acidophil Acid-staining cells, such as are found in the pituitary gland.

acidophilism Overactivity of the acidophil cells in the pituitary gland located in the base of the skull.

acidophilus milk *See* Milk, acidophilus.

acidosis Acid intoxication due to faulty metabolism and elimination of acid chemicals.

acid phosphatase <3.0 ng/mL Increased quantities may indicate possibility of a cancer of the prostate gland.

acidulate To make acid.

Acidulin A medication, in capsule form, which supplies acid for stomach juices. Useful in those who lack sufficient quantities of hydrochloric acid.

aciduria Acid urine.

acinus The smallest component of a gland; that part of a gland which secretes the product produced by the gland.

acne A pustular condition of the skin, seen most often on the face, chest and back of adolescents and young adults.

acolasia Intemperance or self-indulgence without restraint.

aconuresis Lack of control of urination.

Acosta's disease Mountain sickness; resulting from dwelling at extreme heights.

acoumetry Testing the acuteness of the sense of hearing.

acoustic nerve The eighth cranial nerve, which supplies the organ of hearing (ear).

acousticophobia Morbid fear of sounds.

acoustics The science of sound.

acquired characteristic A trait developed as a result of environment, as opposed to an inherited characteristic.

acquired immune deficiency syndrome *See AIDS.*

acquired immunity Immunity not present at birth but is developed during life.

acrid Irritating.

acritochromacy Color blindness.

acro- A prefix referring to an arm or leg.

acroagnosis Lack of sensation in an arm or leg.

acroanesthesia Loss of sensation in one or more limbs.

acroarthritis Arthritis in the arms or legs.

acrocephaly A pointed head; a birth deformity.

acrocyanosis Blueness of the hands and feet caused by a disturbance in the blood vessels and their ability to contract and expand.

acrodermatitis Skin disease involving the arms or legs.

acrodynia Neuritis affecting the toes or fingers.

acroedema Swelling of the arms and feet.

acrogeria Wrinkling of the skin of the hands and feet, caused by premature aging.

acrohyperhidrosis Excessive sweating of the hands and feet.

acromioscapular The shoulder point and shoulder blade.

acrokeratosis Warty growths on the skin of the hands and feet.

acromania Craziness, madness.

acromastitis Inflammation of the nipple of the breast.

acromegaly A disease caused by excessive function of the pituitary gland. It is characterized by marked distortion of the bones of the face, skull, hands and feet.

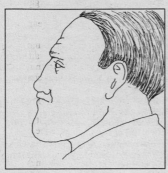

Acromegaly

acromioclavicular separation A common injury to the tendons joining the scapula and the clavicle (collarbone), seen often in baseball and football players.

acromion Part of the scapular bone of the shoulder to which important muscles and ligaments are attached.

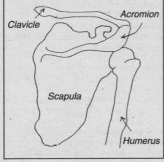

Acromion

acronine An anticancer drug.

acroparesthesia An upset in the functioning of the smaller blood vessels in the hands and feet leading to sensations of tingling, numbness, occasional pallor or redness of the hands or feet, etc. Seen particularly in neurotic women.

acrophobia Morbid fear of great heights.

acrosclerosis Hardening, as within the arteries, in the arms or legs.

acrotic pulse A very weak pulse.

acrotism Absence of a pulse.

acrylics Plastic materials used in making false teeth and dentures.

ACTH See adrenocorticotropic hormone.

acting out Actions which allow an outlet for emotional problems.

actinic Pertaining to light rays or radiant energy.

actinic ray A chemically active ray toward and beyond the violet of the spectrum.

actinocymography X-raying an organ while it is in motion.

actinodermatitis Skin irritation and dermatitis caused by exposure to X rays.

actinogen Any substance that produces radiation, such as radium.

Actinomycin D An anticancer medication found to be especially effective when used in conjunction with radiation in the treatment of Wilm's tumor, a malignant kidney tumor affecting infants.

actinomycosis "Lumpy jaw." Primarily a disease of hogs and cattle, caused by a parasite. It is sometimes transmitted to man, in whom it can produce a chronic infection.

actinoneuritis Inflammation of nerves caused by excessive exposure to X rays and other radioactive substances.

actinotherapy Treatment by use of sunlight, ultraviolet ray, X ray or radium.

action The performance of any bodily function, mental, chemical, or physical.

activator A substance which causes another substance to become active.

active immunity Acquired immunity, derived from the body's production of its own antibodies.

acuity Clearness.

acumen Keen perception.

acupuncture Needling of deep structures in order to relieve pain.

acute Rapid; short; sudden; severe. Not chronic.

acute abdomen A condition in which there has been a rapid onset of symptoms and signs within the abdomen, frequently requiring surgical treatment.

acute yellow atrophy of the liver Destruction of liver tissue, often occurring as the result of poisoning.

Acyclovir A drug being used against the virus causing herpes simplex infections.

ad to (Latin). Used in prescription writing to denote that a sufficient quantity of a substance should be used to arrive at a desired amount.

adacrya Absence of tears, due to a deficiency in the tear glands.

adactylia A birth deformity in which there is an absence of fingers or toes.

adamantine Referring to the enamel of the teeth.

adamantinoma A tumor of a low degree of malignancy, occurring usually in the lower jawbone.

Adam's apple A prominence in the neck formed by the larynx (voice box).

Adams-Stokes disease A slowed heart action caused by heart block, associated with attacks of fainting and convulsions.

adaptation disease Any disease associated with stress and the reactions to stress.

adapter A metal part which enables one instrument to fit into another.

addict Someone who is habituated to alcohol, narcotics or some other drug.

addiction The state of being habituated to a drug.

addictology That branch of medicine dealing with addictions.

Addison's disease A serious disease caused by insufficiency or nonfunction of the adrenal glands.

adducens muscle One of the muscles attached to the eyeball, enabling the eye to turn inward.

adduct To move a part of the body, usually an arm or leg, toward the midline.

adenectomy The surgical removal of a gland.

adenitis Inflammation of a lymph node or gland.

adeno- A combining form denoting an association with glands. An *adeno*carcinoma is a cancer involving gland cells.

adenoacanthoma A slow-growing, not very malignant, type of cancer of the uterus.

adenocarcinoma Cancer originating in a gland, a very common form of cancer.

Adenocystoma A nonmalignant tumor of a gland containing cysts.

adenofibroma A combined nonmalignant tumor consisting of gland tissue and fibrous tissue; seen most often in the breast or uterus.

adenoid Lymph gland located in the throat behind the nose. Enlargement, especially in children, often obstructs nasal breathing.

adenoidectomy Removal of the adenoid glands located in the throat behind the nose.

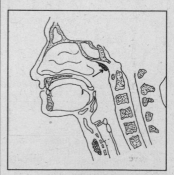

Adenoids

adenoma A tumor in which the cell arrangement resembles a glandlike structure.

adenomatosis A condition in which the entire glandular portion of an organ is overgrown, as in a breast.

adenomyoma A noncancerous tumor composed of gland and muscle tissue; seen most often in the uterus.

adenomyosis A condition in which the gland tissue lining the uterus grows into the muscle wall of the uterus. It is not malignant.

adenopathy Swelling or disease of a lymph gland.

adenosarcoma A malignant tumor containing both gland and connective tissue.

adenosis Any disease of a gland.

adenotonsillectomy Removal of the tonsils and adenoids.

adenovirus A group of viruses thought to be responsible for causing the common cold.

ADH The antidiuretic hormone, vasopressin, that inhibits the excretion of urine.

adhesion A band or fiber. Abdominal adhesions are caused by abnormal bands which bind the organs to one another.

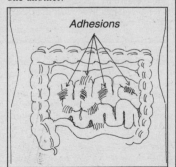

Adhesions

Adhesions

adhesive Sticky, such as *adhesive* tape.

adiadochokinesia Inability to perform rapid, alternating motions, such as rotating the hands quickly.

adiaphoresis Absence of sweat.

Adie's syndrome A condition in which the pupils of the eye fail to react to light and accommodation, and the knee jerks and ankle jerks are not present.

adipose tissue Fat tissue.

adiposis dolorosa A disease in which there are areas of painful fat beneath the skin. Seen in women more often than in men. Also called *Dercum's disease.*

Adjunct A junior member of a staff of a hospital.

adjuvant A medication given to enhance the effect of another medication.

ad lib. Abbreviation of *ad libitum,* a Latin term meaning "as much as desired."

adnexae The fallopian (uterine) tubes and ovaries.

adolescence The period between puberty and maturity.

adolescent nodule A small, rounded, mildly tender lump appearing beneath the nipple. It occurs both in adolescent boys as well as girls.

adrenalectomy Removal of the adrenal glands.

adrenal glands Two glands in the upper posterior part of the abdomen which produce and secrete vital hormones.

    cortex The outer portion of the adrenal gland, responsible for the production of cortisone.

    medulla The central portion of the adrenal gland, responsible for production and secretion of adrenalin.

adrenalin Also known as *epinephrine.* When injected, it may be helpful in restoring heart activity after cardiac arrest; it may control certain hemorrhages, and it can combat severe allergic reactions.

adrenalism Inadequate adrenal gland function, resulting in debility, weakness, and a state of poor health.

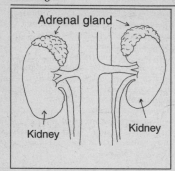

Adrenal gland

adrenergic Referring to sympathetic nerve fibers that produce an adrenalin-like substance.

adrenergic blocking agent A substance that blocks responses to sympathetic nerve activities. *See* sympathetic nerve system.

adrenocorticomimetic Mimicking the functions of the cortex of the adrenal glands.

adrenocorticotropic hormone (ACTH) The glandular secretion of the anterior portion of the pituitary gland, in the base of the brain. This hormone influences the function of the adrenal and other glands of the body.

adrenogenic Arising from the adrenal glands. (The adrenals are located above the kidneys and among other functions, they produce adrenalin and cortisone.)

adrenotropin A hormone produced by the cortex of the adrenal glands.

Adriamycin A powerful anticancer chemical, administered intravenously. (Its use is frequently followed by temporary loss of hair.)

adsorption The process in which a solid substance, such as silica, activated charcoal, etc., attracts and takes up fluids.

adventitia The covering tissue of an organ.

Advil Trade name for an anti-pain medication.

adynamic Lacking muscle or vital power.

Aedes aegypti The mosquito which transmits yellow fever and dengue fever.

Aedes albopictus A mosquito whose bite can cause dengue fever. *See* dengue fever.

aeration The exposure of blood to air and oxygen, such as takes place in the lungs.

Aerobacter A type of bacteria composed of short gram-negative organisms, causing infections that produce gas and acid.

aerobe A germ which requires oxygen for the maintenance of its life.

aerobic exercises Those contrived to stimulate heart action with resulting increases in pulse and breathing rates.

aerobiology The study of substances which are airborne, such as pollens, molds, dusts, etc.

aerobiotic Referring to an organism that lives in an oxygen-containing atmosphere. The opposite of *anaerobic*.

aerodynamics The science which studies gases in motion.

aeroembolism A condition produced by sudden changes in atmospheric pressure, as occur among aviators. Nitrogen bubbles are released in the blood and tissues. Commonly called "the chokes."

aeroemphysema The collection of bubbles of nitrogen in the tissues and bloodstream, resulting from too sudden a return to the surface after deepsea diving or by too quick an ascent to a high altitude. Symptom caused by this condition is known as *the bends*.

Aerohalor An apparatus that gives forth a mist which, when sprayed into the respiratory passage, relieves spasm of the bronchial tubes, particularly useful in asthmatics.

aerogenic Gas-forming.

aeromammography X ray of the

breast after injecting air into the ducts. (A rarely used procedure)

aeromedicine That branch which concerns itself with medical conditions associated with aviation.

aeroneurosis A neurosis seen among aviators in which there is marked restlessness and anxiety.

aero-otitis Inflammation of the middle ear caused by changes in altitude in airplane flights.

aerophagia Air-swallowing, seen often in hysterical patients.

aerophil 1. An organism whose life depends on the presence of air. 2. Someone who loves the open air.

aerophobia Fear of fresh air or drafts.

aeroscope An instrument which measures the purity of air.

aerosol A compressed gas containing particles of a substance to be used in the treatment of a patient. The medication is administered by releasing the compressed gas.

aerospace The earth's atmosphere and the space beyond it.

Aesculapius In Greek mythology, the god of medicine, the son of Apollo.

afebrile Without fever, usually referring to a patient whose temperature is normal.

affection An illness or disease.

afferent Referring to a nerve or blood vessel which carries impulses or blood from the surface of the body inward.

affinity Attraction toward or relationship between atoms, diseases, groups, species, etc.

afibrinogenemia Lack of fibrinogen in the blood, a condition which may cause delayed blood clotting.

Afrin nasal spray A powerful decongestant; not to be used for long periods of time.

afterbirth The placenta and membranes which are discharged from the vagina following the birth of a child.

aftercare Postoperative or convalescent treatment.

afterdamp Poisonous gases often found in coal mines.

aftereffect A delayed reaction to a drug or stimulant.

afterimage The visual impression of a continuation of the image after it has actually disappeared.

afterpains Pains continuing after childbirth.

Ag The chemical symbol for silver.

agalorrhea The stoppage of milk flow from the breast.

agamic Reproducing without sexual union. (A biologic term)

agammaglobulinemia A condition in which there is a reduction in the amount of antibodies circulating in the blood. This is associated with an increased susceptibility to infections.

agamogenesis Reproduction without sex. (Seen only in primitive forms of life)

agar A gelatin-like substance obtained from seaweed. Used extensively as a medium for growing bacteria in bacteriology laboratories.

agenesis Imperfect development, as applied to a part of the body.

agent A substance which causes a reaction.

Agent Orange An herb-killing compound which, when in contact with people, may develop certain cancers.

agglomeration A cluster, a grouping together of cells so as to form a mass.

agglutination The joining together of separate or suspended particles. The formation of clumps.

agglutinin An antibody which causes agglutination. *See also* agglutination.

aggression A psychological term used to describe a hostile attitude associated with a hostile action, often arising out of a sense of insecurity or inferiority.

aglutition Difficulty in swallowing.

agnathia A birth deformity in

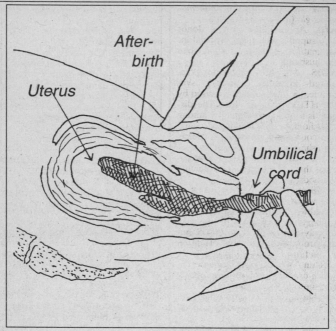

Afterbirth

which there is lack of development of the jaw.

agnosia Loss of ability to recognize persons or things.

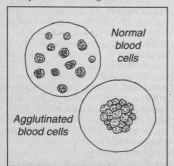

Normal blood cells

Agglutinated blood cells

Agglutination

agonad An individual without sex glands.

agony Extreme pain.

agoraphobia Fear of open spaces.

agranulocytosis An acute, dangerous condition in which there are too few white blood cells in the blood. (This may be brought on by taking poison or by a sensitivity to certain drugs.)

agraphia Loss of ability to write, due to a brain disorder.

agromania An irrational desire to live in isolation or in the open.

ague An outmoded term for malaria.

AHF Abbreviation for *antihemophilic factor*, the substance that combats bleeding and promotes blood clotting in people suffering from hemophilia.

AHG Abbreviation for *antihemophilic globulin*.

AID Abbreviation for a donor who supplies sperm for artificial insemination; someone other than the husband.

AIDS An abbreviation for "acquired" immune deficiency syndrome," a fatal condition caused by the HTLV-III/LAV virus. The disease is found predominantly among male homosexuals who practice anal intercourse and among drug addicts who share intravenous needles.

The virus destroys T-cell lymphocytes that are essential in protecting the body against infections.

AIDS antibodies A blood test to tell whether or not someone is infected with the AIDS virus. If found to carry the virus such people may or may not suffer from AIDS but are prone to develop the condition in the future.

ainhum An African disease in which one or more toes drop off. (It is somewhat like leprosy.)

air blast injury Hemorrhage or rupture of organs caused by proximity to an explosion.

air embolus Air getting into the bloodstream, and interfering with the flow of blood. If it enters in large quantities, it may cause death.

air sickness Symptoms of nausea and vomiting caused by the motion of an airplane. A condition similar to seasickness or car sickness.

air swallowing A hysterical condition in which a patient swallows large quantities of air. This may result in serious distention of the stomach with hiccuping, disturbance in heart function, etc.

airway The maintenance of an unobstructed passageway between the outside and the lungs.

akaryocyte A red blood cell.

akinesthesia Loss of sense of movement, as in a muscle.

Al Symbol for aluminum.

ala A winglike structure.

alalia Loss of speech.

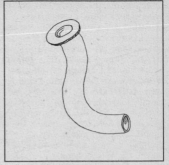
Airway (in anesthesia)

alanine An amino acid found in many proteins.

alastrim A mild form of smallpox. (An old term)

Albee's operation Spinal fusion; placing pieces of bone alongside the vertebrae in order to make the spinal column more stable and rigid.

albinism Lack of pigment in the skin, as in *albinos*.

albumin One of the chief protein components of living animal tissues.

albumin-globulin ratio (A/G r) *See* section on Chemical Analysis. A ratio below 1 indicates insufficient protein in the body.

albuminuria The finding of albumin on urine analysis, which may indicate kidney disease.

    orthostatic albumin in the urine due to standing for long periods.

Albumisol A preparation of albumin, given to patients with abnormally low albumin in the blood.

albuterol A medication that is inhaled in order to relieve spasm of the bronchial tubes of the lungs.

Alcoholics Anonymous A nonprofit organization that helps alcoholics to end their addiction.

alcoholism A disease caused by the repeated ingestion of large quantities of alcohol.

Aldactone (spironolactone) A diuretic medication causing excretion of excess body fluids. Often highly effective in cases of cirrhosis of the liver, heart failure, or nephrosis.

Aldomet A patented drug, effective in lowering blood pressure.

aldosterone A hormone produced by the adrenal gland. It regulates potassium and sodium metabolism.

aldosteronism A condition characterized by excessive loss of potassium from the blood, paralysis, swelling of the extremities and high blood pressure. It is caused by a tumor in the adrenal gland.

alethia A mental condition in which there is difficulty in forgetting. Also, a state in which one dwells excessively upon past events.

aleukemia True leukemia (cancer of the white blood cells) in which the number of white blood cells found in the circulating blood is *not* increased; there may even be less than normal.

alexia Loss of the ability to understand the meaning of printed or written words.

ALG An abbreviation for *antilymphocytic globulin,* a substance which combats the rejection phenomenon seen so often after organ transplantation.

algesic Painful.

algolagnia A perverse sexual act in which one gets pleasure from causing pain to the sexual partner.

Alienist A psychiatrist.

alimentary tract The food tract, beginning with the esophagus (food pipe) and extending for 20 to 25 feet to the rectum and anus. Also called *gastrointestinal tract.*

alimentation

    forced Forced feeding; often carried out by inserting a tube through the nose into the stomach.

    rectal Feeding by giving retention enemas.

aliquot A portion of a substance or a compound.

alkalemia Excess alkalinity of the blood; a state existing when the pH of the blood exceeds the normal 7.4.

alkaline Containing more hydroxyl

than hydrogen ions. The opposite of acid.

alkaline phosphatase *See* phosphatase.

alkaloid Any one of dozens of medications derived from plants, such as morphine, digitalis, etc.

alkatosis A condition in which there is too much bicarbonate in the blood. The opposite of acidosis. It is associated with dizziness and jerky muscular contractions.

alkaptonuria An inherited defect characterized by the passage of exceptionally dark urine.

alkylating agents Chemicals used in chemotherapy to destroy malignant cells.

alkylating drug One which destroys tumor cells by altering their chemical composition.

allantoin A substance extracted from amniotic fluid which surrounds the embryo. It is sometimes used as a local application to promote healing of wounds and infections.

allantois A membrane in the developing embryo. It enters into the formation of the urinary bladder.

Allele A series of two or more genes that occupy the same position on a specific chromosome.

Allerest A patented medication of reduce the congestion and discharge from mucous membranes that occurs in allergies.

allergen Any substance which is able to cause an allergic condition.

allergic rhinitis An inflammation of the membranes of the nasal passages caused by an allergy, such as hay fever.

Allergist A physician who treats conditions of allergic origin.

allergy An altered response to an allergen. Hypersensitivity to certain irritating substances with which one comes in contact.

alloerotism Sexual excitement caused and directed toward someone other than oneself. The opposite of autoerotism.

allograft A graft from one member

of a species to another, as from man to man.

allopathy A method of medical treatment in which an inflammatory reaction is purposely produced in order to cure the afflicting disease.

alloplasty Any plastic operation in which a foreign substance, such as a metal or bone, is used.

allopurinol A medication which suppresses the body's production of uric acid. Effective in controlling gout.

allotransplantation The taking of tissue or an organ from one individual and grafting it into another.

alloy A combination of two or more metals.

aloe An herb used as a laxative.

alopecia A skin disease characterized by loss of hair, partial or total.

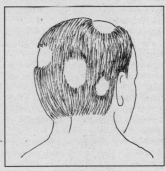

Alopecia areata

ALS Abbreviation for *antilymphocytic serum;* same as antilymphocytic globulin.

alter ego A second self; a bosom friend whom one admires greatly.

Alternaria A fungus or mold which causes a form of hay fever.

altitude sickness Shortness of breath, dizziness, mental and physical fatigue, caused either by a flight to a high altitude or by travel in high altitudes. It is due to low oxygen content of the air.

alum An astringent, or a substance which produces constriction.

aluminum (Al) A chemical found in combination with many other elements. In medicine, it is used in various forms as an antiseptic, a shrinking agent, and as an antiperspirant.

hydroxide A powder or gel used as an antacid in cases of ulcer or excess stomach acidity.

Alupent A patented medication helpful in relieving the spasm of bronchial tubes in asthma.

alveolectomy Removal of a bony socket of a tooth.

alveolus 1. The bony socket of a tooth. 2. An air cell in the lungs. 3. A depression or cavity.

Alzheimer's disease Premature senility in a patient not considered old enough to demonstrate signs of old age.

A.M.A. The American Medical Association.

amastia A rare birth deformity in which one or both breasts are absent.

amaurosis Blindness.

amaurotic familial idiocy An inherited condition in which a child, seeming to develop normally during the first few months of life, stops progressing, shows signs of blindness and metal deterioration, and eventually dies. Also called Tay-Sachs disease.

ambi- A combining form meaning "both."

ambidexterity The ability to use both hands equally well.

ambisexual Feelings and reactions which are neither typically male nor female, but which have traits of both sexes.

ambivalence The coexistence of feelings of both love and hate toward the same person or thing.

ambivert A type of personality supposedly both extrovert and introvert.

amblyopia Partial loss of eyesight.

Ambrosia Ordinary ragweed; the cause of most hay fever.

ambulance chaser An unethical lawyer who runs after accident victims and attempts to promote lawsuits.

ambulation, early Getting out of bed within a short time (hours or days) after an operation or bed-confining illness.

ambulatory Ambulant. Not bed-ridden, able to walk by oneself.

ambulatory cardiac monitoring A recording of heart action around the clock, obtained by attaching the monitoring apparatus to the patient's body.

ambulatory surgery Surgery performed either in a special ambulatory care facility in a hospital or in a doctor's office.

ameba A one-celled organism. (Certain amebae cause dysentery.)

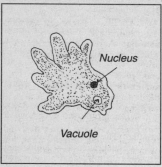

Ameba

amebiasis Infection with the *Endamoeba histolytica*.

amelia The absence of a limb or limbs, present at birth.

amelioration An improvement in the course of a disease.

amenorrhea Failure of menstruation.

amethopterin A chemical used to combat leukemia and other malignant diseases. It is known as a *folic acid antagonist*.

ametropia Poor vision due to failure of the image to focus upon the retina (the portion of the eye which

records light rays and transmits the impulse to the brain).

amicrobic The absence of microbes.

amigen A proteinlike substance given by mouth, or intravenously, as a dietary supplement. Sometimes used in debilitated pre- and post-operative patients.

amino acids A large group of organic compounds, many of which are necessary for the maintenance of life. Their basic formula is NH_2-R-COOH. They represent an end product of protein metabolism. From these amino acids the body rebuilds its proteins. The amino acids essential to life are: arginine, histidine, isoleucine, leucine, lysine, methionine, phenylalanine, threonine, tryptophane and valine.

aminophylline A drug used to dilate blood vessels, lower the blood pressure, relieve asthmatic attacks and stimulate urination.

Aminopterin A patented drug used in the treatment of certain kinds of leukemia.

aminopyrine (Pyramidon) A drug used to lower fever, relieve pain and headache. (Its use has been more or less discontinued, as it may have a dangerous effect upon white blood cells.)

aminuria Amines (ammonialike chemicals) in the urine.

amitosis Reproduction of cells by simple division of the nucleus. Simple fission.

ammoniated A substance containing ammonia, such as the ointment *ammoniated mercury*.

ammoniemia Ammonia intoxication associated with intestinal upset, weakness, liver dysfunction, and possibly coma and death.

ammonium (NH_4) It exists only in combination. It is normally present in small quantities in the blood. When present in excessive quantities it can cause ammonia intoxication. In combination with other chemicals such as acetate, arsenate, benzonate, bromide, carbonate, chloride, mandelate, etc., it has numerous medicinal uses.

ammoniuria Excess ammonia in the urine.

amnesia Loss of memory.

amniocentesis Tapping the womb of a pregnant woman to obtain amniotic fluid; performed to analyze the fluid for abnormal cells which would indicate abnormality of the fetus. Cells obtained from this procedure can predict the sex of the fetus.

amniography An X ray of the pregnant uterus after the injection of an opaque dye; performed only in rare cases.

amnion The membranous sac surrounding the embryo in the womb.

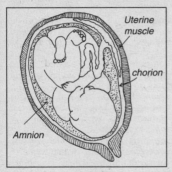

Uterine muscle

chorion

Amnion

Amnion

amniotic fluid The fluid surrounding the embryo in the mother's womb.

amniotomy Rupturing the fetal membranes to accelerate the process of childbirth.

amoeba *See* ameba.

amorphinism The state that results when morphine is withdrawn from an addict.

amorphous Without form or shape.

Amoxicillin An antibiotic effective against many types of bacteria.

amperage The number of amperes in an electrical circuit.

amphetamine A drug used to decrease nasal congestion, to decrease one's appetite, and as a stimulant in tired or depressed states. It often leads to addiction.

amphi- A combining form indicating the involvement of both sides of an organ or body.

amphibious Able to live on land and in water, such as frogs.

Amphojel A patented medicine containing aluminum hydroxide, used as an antacid in patients with excess stomach acidity.

amphoric A sound heard when listening to a chest in which there is a cavity in a lung or in which the lung is collapsed; an empty, hollow sound.

amphoteric Used to describe a substance that can react as an acid or as an alkaline.

amphotericin B A medication used to eradicate fungus infections. Fungizone.

Ampicillin A powerful antibiotic similar in structure and actions to penicillin. (It may cause fewer allergic reactions than ordinary penicillin.)

ampule A sealed glass container for sterile preparations intended for injection.

ampulla The dilated opening of a canal or duct, such as the enlarged segment of a milk duct near its exit at the nipple.

of Vater A dilatation of the ducts (tubes) from the liver and pancreas at the point where they enter the small intestine (duodenum).

amputation The surgical removal of a limb or part of a limb.

amputee One who has undergone amputation of an arm or leg.

amydriasis Contraction of the pupil of the eye.

amylase An enzyme which acts in the digestion of sugar. It is found in exceptionally large quantities in patients with an acute inflammation of the pancreas.

amyl nitrite A drug usually inhaled, which relaxes muscle spasm. Very helpful in cases of angina pectoris (coronary artery spasm).

amyloid degeneration The deposit of amyloid (a protein substance) in tissues and organs which are undergoing degeneration.

amyloidosis The extensive deposit of amyloid in many organs of the body.

amylopsin Pancreatic enzyme, amylase, which aids in digestion by converting starch into simpler sugars.

amyotonia Absence of muscle tone.

amyotrophic lateral sclerosis Muscle degeneration and spinal cord degeneration secondary to long-standing severe diabetes.

Amytal A patented barbituarate, used to control insomnia (sleeplessness).

A.N.A. American Nurses' Association.

anabolism The process by which food is converted into living tissue.

anacidity Total lack of hydrochloric acid in the stomach. Also termed *achlorhydria.*

Anacin A compound given to relieve many painful symptoms such as headaches, backaches, and those associated with the ordinary cold.

anaerobe A germ which can grow and multiply in the absence of air or oxygen.

anal Referring to the anus (the termination of the rectum).

anal character A psychiatric term, referring to one whose anal erotic characteristics persist after childhood.

analepetic drugs Restorative medications, such as are used to stimulate convalescence.

analgesia Pain relief by insensibility production without loss of consciousness.

analgesic drugs Pain-relieving medications (anodynes) such as aspirin.

analogue A structure with a func-

tion similar to that of some other structure.

analysis The examination of the components and nature of a substance, such as urinalysis, blood analysis, etc.

Analyst A popular name for one type of psychiatrist. A *Psychoanalyst* practices psychotherapy by means of the analytic technique.

analyzer An instrument constructed so as to determine various amounts of substances within the body, such as a chemical *analyzer,* a blood gas *analyzer,* etc.

anamnesis The ability to remember.

anaphoresis Lack of function of the sweat glands.

anaphrodisiac A substance that will lower sexual desire.

anaphylaxis A state of shock or hypersensitivity. An extreme allergic reaction, brought on by a substance in which one is extremely sensitive.

anaplasia Regression of fully developed cells toward a more primitive (embryonic) form with increased tendency toward multiplication. (Seen often among cancer cells)

Anaprox An effective, non-narcotic pain-relieving drug.

anasarca Generalized accumulation of fluid (serum) beneath the skin and in the various cavities of the body. Also termed *generalized edema.*

anastomosis The joining together of two or more hollow organs. This is sometimes accomplished through surgical procedures; such as the joining of two loops of bowel after the removal of a segment, or, the surgical suturing of blood vessels.

anatomy The science of structure of the body or its organs.

Ancef A powerful antibiotic of the group known as the cephalosporins. Must be given by injection.

ancillary Secondary; auxiliary.

anconal Referring to the elbow.

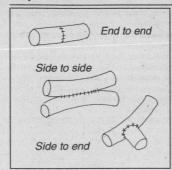

End to end

Side to side

Side to end

Anastomosis

Ancylostoma Hookworm. The parasite causing hookworm disease.

androblastoma A rare tumor of the testicle, sometimes accompanied by changes which give a female appearance to the male.

androgen The male sex hormone responsible for masculine characteristics.

androgyny Having both male and female traits and behavior.

Android A male sex hormone tablet, administered to patients with hormone deficiency, and to some children with undescended testicles.

androphobia Unusual fear of men.

androsterone A steroid found in the urine of both men and women.

Anectine A muscle relaxant for intravenous use during anesthesia.

anemia Insufficiency of red blood cells, either of quality or quantity.

    Addison's *See* anemia, pernicious.

    aplastic Anemia due to bone marrow defects and degenerative changes.

    Cooley's A familial type of anemia found most often in people living near the Mediterranean Sea.

    hemolytic Anemia caused by an agent which destroys red blood cells. (Snake-bite anemia)

    hyperchromic Anemia in which red blood cell deficiency is greater than hemoglobin deficiency.

    hypochromic Anemia associated with red blood cell deficiency and a marked deficiency in hemoglobin.

    idiopathic A form of anemia in which the blood-forming organs themselves fail to function properly.

    lymphatica *See* Hodgkin's disease.

    macrocytic Anemia associated with abnormally large red blood cells. Pernicious anemia and sprue are of this type.

    Mediterranean *See* Cooley's anemia.

    megaloblastic Anemias in which nuclear patterns of megaloblasts are formed in the blood. There are many forms of megaloblastic anemia.

    microcytic Anemia associated with abnormally small red blood cells with hemoglobin deficiency.

    neonatorum Anemia of the newborn.

    normocytic One in which the red blood cells and hemoglobin are of normal size.

    pernicious A serious specific type of anemia associated with lack of hydrochloric acid in the stomach juices and nervous disorders. The administration of vitamin B_{12}, folic acid, liver and stomach extracts have been found effective in control of this condition.

    pregnancy A type of anemia which is associated with pregnancy.

    secondary Anemia which is due to some other disease, such as cancer, tuberculosis, etc., or to loss of blood.

    sickle cell A type of anemia seen mostly among Negroes or dark-skinned persons. Characterized by the sickle shape of the red blood cells.

anencephaly A deformed newborn having no brain. (Such monsters do not survive.)

anergy Lack of energy.

anesthesia Loss of sensation, usually produced in order to permit a painless surgical operation.

caudal The injection of an anesthetic agent, such as Novocain, into the lower caudal (spinal) canal near the end of the vertebral column.

dissociative An anesthesia that doesn't cause complete unconsciousness.

endotracheal General anesthesia administered through a tube, placed through the mouth or nose, directly into the trachea (windpipe).

epidural Produced by the injection of an anesthetic agent, such as Novocain, into the space just outside of the spinal canal.

field block A local anesthesia applied directly to the area to be operated upon.

general Any anesthesia associated with loss of consciousness.

hypotensive An anesthesia given when the blood pressure has been purposely lowered in order to cut down on operative blood loss.

hypothermic An anesthesia given when the body temperature has been purposely lowered.

inhalation Anesthesia produced through the inhalation of gases or vapors.

intravenous The injection of an anesthetic agent, such as Pentothal, into a vein.

peripheral Loss of sensation in the nerves of the skin.

regional Anesthesia restricted to a part of the body.

saddle block Spinal anesthesia given so as to affect only the genital region, buttocks, and thighs.

spinal That produced by the injection of an anesthetic agent, such as Novocain, directly into the spinal fluid within the spinal canal.

topical Application of an anesthetic agent, such as cocaine, on a body surface; as with a spray or a cotton swab.

Anesthesiologist A physician who

specializes in the administration of anesthesia.

anesthetize To put under anesthesia.

aneurysm An abnormal condition characterized by the dilatation of a portion of the wall of an artery. (The aorta is particularly susceptible to aneurysm formation.)

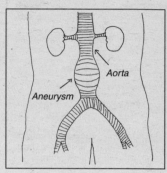

Aorta

Aneurysm

Aneurysm

ruptured One that has hemorrhaged through the wall of an artery into surrounding tissues.

arteriovenous An aneurysm connecting a vein to an artery, thus making a dilatation that will facilitate repeated injections in cases requiring dialysis. *See* dialysis.

dissecting An aneurysm in which the arterial wall has split, allowing blood to escape into surrounding tissues.

aneurysmectomy Removal of an aneurysm of an artery. Usually, following such a procedure, an arterial graft is stitched into place to fill the defect.

angiitis Inflammation of a lymph channel or blood vessel.

angina pectoris Pain in the chest, sometimes radiating to the left arm, caused by a spasm of the coronary artery of the heart.

angio- Pertaining to a lymph or blood vessel.

angioblastoma A malignant tumor composed of blood vessel tissues.

angiocardiography X-ray visualization of the chambers of the heart and the large blood vessels entering or leaving the heart.

angiofibroma A fibrous (connective tissue) tumor containing many tiny blood vessels.

angiography X ray of blood vessels after injection of a radiopaque substance to show their outlines.

angioma A tumor, usually benign, composed of lymph and blood vessels.

angioneuroma (glomus tumor) A small benign growth containing many blood vessels and nerve fibers. It is extremely tender to the touch. A common site is beneath a fingernail.

angioneurotic edema Localized swellings, usually about the face, caused by allergic or emotional factors.

angioplasty Plastic surgery performed upon arteries or veins.

angioradiography Studies of blood vessels and of the heart with X rays, after the intravenous injection of an opaque substance.

angiorrhaphy Surgical repair of a blood vessel.

angiosarcoma A malignant tumor originating from blood vessels.

angiospasm Prolonged, strong contraction of a blood vessel.

Angiostatin and Endostatin Drugs that have been reported to cause eradication of or reduction in size of certain cancers in mice.

angiotelectasia A condition characterized by dilatation and enlargement of groups of capillaries.

angiotensin A body substance whose action results in constriction of blood vessels.

anhidrosis Failure of sweat gland function.

anhydrase An enzyme which stimulates the elimination of water from a chemical compound.

anhydremia Deficiency in the fluid portion of the blood.

anhydrous A chemical term meaning lack of water.

aniline A coal tar derivative.

animus Hostility.

anion An ion carrying negative charges.

anisocytosis Variations in the size of cells which are usually uniform in size.

anisomastia A condition in which the two breasts are of noticeably different sizes.

anisotonic Unequal osmotic pressure.

ankle A joint connecting the leg and the foot.

ankle replacement An operation in which the ankle joint is replaced with a metal prosthesis; an artificial ankle.

ankylodactyly Webbed fingers or toes.

ankylosis Inability of a joint to function, because of stiffness or fusion of the joint surfaces.

ankylostoma Lockjaw.

anlage The embryonal cells which go to form an organ or part of the body.

annular Ring-shaped.

anococcygeal The region between the anus and the coccyx (tail bone).

anode The positive pole of a battery.

anodyne Any medication that relieves pain.

anomaly A deviation from the normal, such as a congenital or birth deformity.

anomia Loss of ability to name people or objects, usually associated with a brain disorder.

Anopheles A genus of mosquitoes which transmits malaria and other diseases such as yellow fever, dengue fever, etc.

anophthalmia A birth defect in which the newborn's eyes are missing.

anoplasty Surgical repair of the anus.

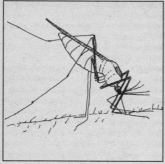

Anopheles mosquito

anopsia   Failure to use one's sight.

anorchidism   Absence of the testicles.

anorectal   Pertaining to the anus and rectum.

anorexia   Lack of desire for food.

     nervosa   A hysterical aversion toward food.

anorgasmy   Failure or inability to reach a climax during sexual intercourse.

anoscope   An instrument used for the examination of the anus and rectum.

anosmesia   Absence of sense of smell.

anotia   A birth defect in which the newborn's ears are missing.

anovular menstruation   Menstruation not associated with ovulation.

anovulatory drugs   Those medications which inhibit and prevent ovulation. (Birth control pills act by preventing ovulation.)

anoxemia   Lack of sufficient oxygen in the blood, seen in heart failure, overdose of anesthesia, etc.

anoxia   Inadequate oxygen supply, with consequent disturbance in body functions.

Antabuse   A drug which causes violent nausea and vomiting when taken along with alcohol. The use of this medication mainly to prevent drinking among alcoholics who fear the use of alcohol after taking an Antabuse tablet.

antacid   A substance which will relieve excess acidity, such as stomach acidity.

antagonist   A drug which neutralizes the effect of another drug.

antecubital   The area in front of the elbow; a favorite site for drawing blood for examination.

anteflexion   Bending forward.

antemortem   Before death.

antenatal   Existing prior to birth.

antepartum   Before childbirth.

anterior   Located in the front; the opposite of posterior.

anterior pituitary gland   The front portion of the pituitary gland located in the base of the skull. It produces important hormones, such as ACTH, growth hormone, etc.

anterior resection operation   A surgical procedure in which the lower sigmoid colon and the upper portion of the rectum are removed because of cancer. The remaining sigmoid colon is then stitched to the remaining portion of the rectum, thus avoiding a colostomy.

anteroposterior   Extending from the front to the back.

anterotic   An avoidance of erotic feelings.

anteverted   Tipped forward, as an anteverted uterus.

anthelmintic   A drug which destroys intestinal worms.

anthracosis   An inflammation of the lungs secondary to the prolonged inhalation of carbon dust, seen often among coal miners.

anthrax   A serious infection in sheep or cattle, which is sometimes transmitted to humans, caused by *Bacillus anthracis*.

anthropogenesis   The evolution of man.

anthropoid   Resembling a human; an ape.

anthropology   The science of man.

anthropomorphic   Having human form or shape.

anthropophagy   Cannibalism.

anti- A prefix signifying "opposed to" or "against."

antiardrenergic drugs Drugs that block the impulses from the sympathetic nerves. *See* sympathetic nerves.

antiallergics The antihistamine drugs used to overcome allergic effects.

antiarthritics Medications used to combat or relieve the distress and pain of arthritis.

antibacterial Stopping the growth and multiplication of germs.

antibiotic drugs Drugs composed of extracts of living organisms, such as molds, which have the ability to destroy other organisms (bacteria).

antibiotic sensitivity test One that tests how sensitive certain bacteria are to certain antibiotics.

antibody A substance produced in the blood of an individual which is capable of producing a specific immunity to a specific germ or virus.

anticancer drug Any one of a large number of chemicals that destroy cancer cells. (To date, none has been found that can permanently destroy cancer and permit the patient to survive.)

anticarcinogen A substance used in the attempt to block cancer development.

anticholinergic Referring to a drug which blocks the passage of impulses through the autonomic nerves. *See also* autonomic nervous system or parasympathetic nervous system.

anticoagulant A substance which prevents blood clotting (coagulation).

anticonvulsive A medication tending to prevent fits or convulsions.

antidepressant medications Those that aid in combating a mentally depressed state.

antidiabetic A substance used to prevent or treat diabetes.

antidote A substance given to counteract poison. *See also* Manual, Antidotes and Emergency Measures for Poisoning.

antiemetic A drug to prevent vomiting.

antifungal A substance which is effective against fungal infections.

antigen Any substance which stimulates the formation of an antibody.

antihelix Part of the external ear.

antihemolytic A substance which prevents hemoglobin liberation or the destruction of blood cells.

Antihemophillic Factor See AHF

antihistamine A medication which tends to counteract an allergic condition.

antihypertensive drugs Medications that lower elevated blood pressure.

anti-inflammatory drugs Any that tend to reduce inflammation.

antiketogenic A substance which reduces acidosis, such as insulin, given to diabetic patients.

Antilymphocytic Globulin (ALG) A substance injected into recipients of organ transplants in order to combat the rejection reaction.

antimalarial drug Any drug used to prevent, suppress, or treat malaria.

antimicrobial Any drug, medication, or agent that acts to destroy bacteria.

antimycin A An antibiotic that is effective in killing fungus, insects, and mites.

antioncogene A gene that tends to suppress the growth of cancer cells.

antiperistalsis Reverse contractions of the intestines and stomach, sometimes resulting in vomiting.

antiphlogistic A substance which counteracts inflammation.

antiplatelet drugs Those that inhibit the formation of platelets, thus decreasing the body's blood coagulation efficiency. Used after an attack of coronary thrombosis.

antiprothrombin A substance that suppresses blood clotting; heparin.

antipruritic A substance which relieves itching.

antipyretic Any drug which tends

to lower the body temperature, such as aspirin or the other salicylate medications.

antiseptic An agent which inhibits or destroys bacteria.

antisocial reacton A reaction in which one acts contrary to the demands of society; as in juvenile delinquency, criminality, etc.

antispasmodic medications Those that help to prevent spasms.

antisudorific A drug which checks the secretion of sweat.

antithrombin A normal component of blood which neutralizes the clotting effect of thrombin. It is a necessary substance to prevent the clotting of circulating blood.

antioxidant Any substance that inhibits oxidation. *See* oxidation.

antitoxin A substance which neutralizes the effects of a toxin (poison released by bacteria).

antitussive drug One that helps to prevent coughing.

antivenin An antitoxin to snake poison.

Antivert A medication used to control nausea and vomiting due to motion sickness (seasickness, airsickness, etc.).

antiviral agent A substance, such as interferon, that attacks viruses.

Antivivisection Opposition to animal experimentation, particularly to operating upon live animals.

antrectomy 1. Surgical removal of the antrum of the stomach; done in conjunction with vagotomy in the treatment of duodenal ulcer. 2. Surgical removal of the antrum of the mastoid antrum.

antrotomy A surgical incision into the maxillary sinus in the face. (This operation is performed by making an incision in the gums above the upper teeth.)

antrum A cavity; referring specifically to the bony cavity which forms the sinus in the cheek (maxillary antrum).

Antuitrin A patented drug com-

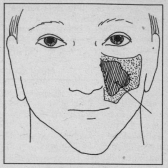

Antrum, maxillary

posed of the growth hormone from the pituitary gland.

anuria Lack of urination, caused by failure of the kidneys to function properly.

anus The outlet of the gastrointestinal tract; the final one or one and one-half inches of the rectum.

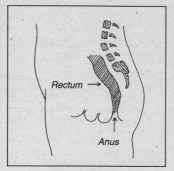

Rectum →

Anus

Anus

anxiety Fear, apprehension.

anxiety neurosis Emotional instability with periods of marked apprehension.

Anusol A rectal suppository helpful in relieving the symptoms of hemorrhoids, fissure-in-ano and other local rectal conditions.

AOA An honorary medical student society; the "Phi Beta Kappa" of medical schools.

aorta The large artery originating from the left ventricle of the heart. Its branches carry blood to all parts of the body.

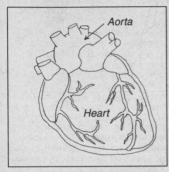

Aorta

aortic insufficiency An aortic heart valve that fails to open and close efficiently; caused by disease of the valve and consequent deformity of its structure.

aortic stenosis A narrowed aortic heart valve, caused either by a birth defect or by acquired disease.

aortocoronary bypass An operation in which grafts from the saphenous vein in the leg are placed from the aorta to a point on the coronary artery beyond an obstruction. Also known as coronary bypass.

aortofemoral bypass A surgical procedure in which a graft is inserted between the abdominal aorta and the femoral arteries in the thigh, performed to improve blood circulation to the legs.

aortogram X ray of the aorta after injection of a radiopaque substance.

aortography A technique enabling one to see the outline of the aorta on X-ray films.

aortorrhaphy Repair of the aorta, as in rectifying an aneurysm by inserting a graft.

apareunia The absence of ability to have sexual intercourse.

apathy Lack of interest or feeling.

APE Anterior pituitary extract.

aperient Any medication producing a natural movement of the bowels.

aperture An opening; an orifice; an entrance to a body cavity.

apex The top; the summit of an organ, as the apex of the lung.

Apgar Score A recording of the physical health of a newborn infant, determined after examination of the adequacy of respiration, heart action, muscle tone and reflexes, etc.

APHA The American Public Health Association.

aphagia Inability to swallow.

aphakia Absence of the lens of the eye.

aphasia Loss of the ability to speak coherently; seen often following a cerebrovascular accident (a stroke).

aphemia Inability to speak in intelligible words or sentences, usually secondary to a brain hemorrhage, blood clot, or tumor.

aphonia Loss of speech due to a condition located in the larynx.

aphrodisiac An agent which stimulates sexual desire.

aphrodisiomania Excessive sexual interest and desire.

aphthous stomatitis Sore throat and sore mouth associated with many small, white blisters. Seen usually in infants and young children.

apical abscess An infection at the root of a tooth.

APL Abbreviation for *anterior pituitarylike hormone;* a hormone of the placenta which is excreted in the urine.

aplasia Failure of a part or an organ to develop; a birth deformity.

aplastic anemia *See* anemia.

apnea A temporary stopping of breathing, usually caused by an excess accumulation of oxygen or an insufficient amount of carbon dioxide in the brain.

apocrine glands Sweat glands.

apomorphine A derivative of morphine used to induce vomiting; particularly useful after one has taken poison.

aponeurosis A tendon which is flattened out and forms a sheetlike membrane.

apoplexy Hemorrhage into the brain. A stroke. It is usually associated with loss of consciousness and paralysis of various parts of the body.

apothecary A druggist.

apparatus Devices designed to aid a patient mechanically, such as a brace or splint.

appendage Anatomically, an appendage is an added or accessory part, such as the external ear, eyelashes, nails, etc.

appendectomy Surgical removal of the appendix.

appendices epiploicae Fatty projections from the outer wall of the large intestines. (They sometimes become inflamed or twisted, usually causing pain and tenderness in the left lower part of the abdomen.)

appendicitis Inflammation of the appendix.

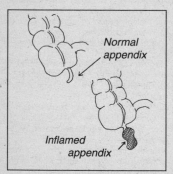

Normal appendix

Inflamed appendix

Appendicitis

appendix The wormlike projection from the cecum (the first portion of the large bowel). It is normally about three to four inches long and has the appearance of an ordinary earthworm.

apperception Relating of new situations to past experiences.

appestat A brain center concerned with control of food intake.

applicator A wooden stick with a cotton tip, used for making a local application. Also, any instrument applied to a body surface.

apposition Fitting together; the act of placing something next to another object.

approach A surgical term referring to the technique of getting to an organ. (The surgical approach to the appendix is through an incision in the lower right part of the abdomen.)

approximate To bring close together.

apraxia Inability to coordinate one's muscles and movements; usually due to a brain condition.

apyrexia Lack of fever.

A.Q. Achievement quotient.

Aq. dest. An abbreviation for distilled water.

Aquaphor A patented ointment which has the ability to absorb water, useful in many skin diseases.

aqueous Watery.

aqueous humor The fluid in the anterior chamber of the eye.

arachnephobia Excessive fear of spiders.

arachnids Scorpions, spiders, ticks, mites.

arachnoid A membrane covering the brain and spinal cord. It is the middle one of three such membranes.

arachnoiditis Inflammation of the arachnoid membrane covering the brain and spinal cord.

Aralen An anti-malaria medication. While effective in most types of malaria, certain very severe types are not helped by this drug.

Aramine A drug used to raise blood pressure and increase the force of heart action in states of shock. A vasopressor drug.

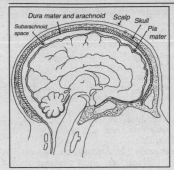

Arachnoid

ARC Abbreviation for AIDS-Related Complex; usually symptoms that occur prior to the onset of full-blown AIDS.

arciform Shaped like a bow.

arcuate Curved or arched.

arcus senilis An opaque ring around the iris (colored portion of the eye), seen most often in elderly people.

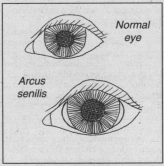

Arcus senilis

ARDS Abbreviation for *acute respiratory distress syndrome*.

areflexia Lack of reflexes.

areola A rim around the central area, such as the mammary areola (the pigmented ring surrounding the nipple).

argentaffin tumors A certain type of tumor, which stains readily with silver impregnation. Also called carcinoid tumors.

arginine An amino acid (product of protein metabolism) essential to life.

Argyll Robertson pupils Pupils of the eye which react to accommodation but not to light. Seen in certain types of syphilis.

argyria A bluish-gray discoloration of the skin seen in people who have been treated with silver preparations over a long period of time. (Not common today)

Aristocort (triamcindone) A cortisonelike, steroid medication which tends to reduce pain and inflammation in cases of rheumatoid arthritis, bursitis, and muscle strains. (Not for prolonged administration)

Arlidin (nylidrin hydrochloride) A drug helpful in producing blood vessel dilatation and combatting arterial spasm. Used in cases of intermittent claudication and arteriosclerosis of blood vessels in the legs.

armamentarium The equipment, including instruments, books, etc., which a doctor uses in treating patients.

aromatic A substance with a spicy odor and taste.

arrest To check or halt the progress of a disease.

arrhenoblastoma A special type of tumor of the ovary, usually associated with masculine changes in the woman so affected.

arrhythmia Lack of rhythm, applied especially to irregularities of heart beat.

arsenic An element which, when combined with bromides, oxides, etc., is a helpful drug. It is used to stimulate blood cell formation. In excess doses, it is a potent poison.

arsenic poisoning A very serious, often fatal, type of poisoning due to an overdose of arsenic. It causes marked destruction of blood cells and degeneration of the liver.

arsphenamine A arsenic preparation formerly used in treating syphilis. It is the famous "606" drug discovered by Paul Ehrlich.

artefact A term applied to an artificial structure or finding, especially one viewed through a microscope.

arterial blood gases Chemical analysis of arterial blood in order to note the adequacy of levels of oxygen and carbon dioxide.

arterialization The formation of new arteries (blood vessels).

arterial system The network of arteries which supplies blood to the various parts of the body.

arteriectomy Surgical removal of an artery or portion of an artery.

arteriography X ray of arteries.

arteriolar sclerosis Hardening of the very small arteries.

arteriole A small artery.

arterioplasty An operation to reconstruct a deformed or damaged artery.

arteriosclerosis Hardening of the arteries.

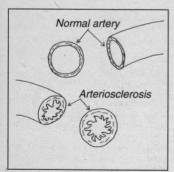

Arteriosclerosis

arteriospasm A spasm of an artery.

arteriovenous Involving both an artery and a vein.

arteriovenous fistula A false communication between an artery and a vein. Often the result of an injury or bullet wound.

arterioventricular block A partial or total interference of the electric stimuli going from the atrium (the upper chamber of the heart) to the ventricle (the lower chamber). *See* heart block.

arteritis Inflammation of an artery.

artery A vessel carrying blood from the heart. *See* Manual for list of Important Arteries.

arthralgia A painful joint.

arthritic One who is afflicted with arthritis.

arthritis Inflammation of a joint.

    acute A joint inflammation which comes on quickly and is associated with pain, heat, redness and swelling.

    allergic Joint inflammation originating from a substance to which the patient is allergic; also, after injection of a serum to which a patient is sensitive.

    chronic Joint inflammation with persists for many months or years.

    degenerative The type seen in older people, accompanied by loss of cartilage about the joint, stiffness, and deformity of the joint.

    gonorrheal Joint inflammation secondary to a severe gonorrhea infection.

    gouty Joint inflammation due to gout, or an upset in uric acid metabolism. Usually affects one joint at a time, such as the toe, knee, etc.

    hemophilic Joint inflammation seen in hemophiliacs secondary to bleeding into a joint.

    menopausal Joint pain seen in women during change of life. Often clears after hormone treatment.

    rheumatoid One of the most common chronic forms of joint inflammation, often affecting many joints simultaneously, such as the fingers, and characterized by pain and limitation of motion. The cause for rheumatoid arthritis is not specifically known, although it is today thought to be infectious in origin.

    tuberculous Joint inflammation secondary to a tuberculosis infection.

arthrocentesis Tapping a joint with a needle.

arthrodesis Fusing the bones which make up a joint; a surgical procedure sometimes performed to obtain more stability in a limb or part of a limb.

arthrography X ray of a joint.

arthroplasty The surgical construction of an artificial joint or the alteration of a stiff joint into a usable one.

arthropod A form of animal life, including those with horny shells on the outside of their bodies, such as crabs, lobsters, insects, etc.

arthroscopy A procedure wherein an orthopedist looks into a joint with a specialty designed, lighted hollow instrument. (Often, a torn knee cartilage can be removed through an arthroscope.)

arthrosis Degeneration of a joint, involving partial or complete incapacity of its use.

arthrotomy Making a surgical incision into a joint.

Arthus phenomenon The inflammation, redness, swelling and pain which comes on secondary to an allergic reaction, usually localized to the site where the irritant (antigen) has been injected or applied.

articulate To speak.

articulation The junction of two or more bones; a joint.

artifact *See* artefact.

artificial insemination A procedure whereby a physician takes the live sperm of a husband, or donor, and places it, by syringe injection, at the entrance to the cervix of the uterus.

artificial joints Joints, made of metal, that substitute for a body's own joint Hips, knees, elbows, shoulders, etc., can now tolerate artificial joints.

artificial respiration To carry out the processes of breathing for one

who has stopped breathing. The artificial forcing of air or oxygen into the lungs. *See also* Manual, First aid.

ARV Abbreviation for AIDs-related virus.

arytenoid cartilage A cartilage in the larynx (the voice box).

asbestos acne Pimples and acne of the skin due to prolonged and repeated exposure to asbestos.

asbestosis A chronic inflammation of the lungs sometimes seen among those who habitually work in areas laden with asbestos dust.

ascariasis Worms in the intestinal tract, particularly round worms.

Ascaris A worm which sometimes infests the intestinal tract of humans.

Aschoff's bodies Characteristic cells seen in the heart muscle of one afflicted with heart disease caused by rheumatic fever.

ascites An abnormal accumulation of fluid in the abdominal cavity, seen often in cirrhosis of the liver.

ascorbic acid Vitamin C. This vitamin is found in citrus fruits, in fresh green vegetables and other edible substances.

asemia A brain condition in which a patient is unable to understand speech or writing.

asepsis A sterile state wherein no germs are present.

aseptic necrosis Death of tissue due to lack of blood supply.

asexual Lack of distinction between male and female. Also, reproduction (among lower forms of animal life) without sexual union.

ASHD An abbreviation for arteriosclerotic heart disease.

Asiatic influenza A respiratory virus infection with rather severe symptoms resembling ordinary "grippe."

asocial Not interested in the people surrounding one or in the activities of one's life.

asparaginase A chemical frequently used in the treatment of certain types of leukemia.

Aspartame A synthetic sweetening agent having many of the same properties as saccharin.

aspergillosis Infection of the organs of the body with the fungus known as *Aspergillus*. (It may involve the brain, lungs, bones, etc.)

aspermia Failure to ejaculate sperm.

asphyxia Suffocation.

fetalis Suffocation of the fetus.

aspidium A substance used in the treatment of tapeworm infestations.

aspiration Sucking out a fluid or solid into the respiratory tract (windpipe or lungs); removal of fluids by suction.

aspirin One of the most reliable pain-relieving (analgesic) medications. Acetylsalicylic acid.

Assistant A junior rank on a hospital staff, usually the rank at which one commences his medical association with a hospital.

Associate An intermediate rank of a physician on a hospital staff; a rank above that of assistant but below that of chief of a medical or surgical service.

association A mental activity wherein two or more events or things are considered together, as in free association.

astasia-abasia A hysterical condition in which a patient is unable to stand or walk.

asthenia Weakness, loss of vigor.

astereognosis Loss of the ability to interpret an object by feeling and touching it.

asthma An allergic condition characterized by wheezing, coughing, mucous sputum and difficulty in exhaling air.

astigmatism An eye condition leading to faulty vision. It is caused by an irregularity in the curvature of the front portion of the eye.

astragalus The ankle bone.

astringent A medication or agent which causes contraction or constriction of tissues.

astroblastoma A malignant brain tumor.

astrocytoma A malignant brain tumor.

asylum An institution constructed to take care of those unable to care for themselves. (A more or less obsolete term for mental institution.)

asymmetry Not symmetrical; lacking equal proportion or size of corresponding parts.

asymptomatic Without symptoms; usually referring to someone who previously did have symptoms.

asynergy Lack of coordination among structures or organs that normally function in harmony,.

asystematic Not localized. Diffuse.

asystole Imperfect or incomplete heart contractions.

A.T. 10 Trademark for a drug used in treating deficiency of the parathyroid gland (tetany).

Atabrine A well-known, time-proven, effective drug in the treatment of malaria. Recently found to be helpful in combating cancer; it has been injected into the chest or abdominal cavities and has delayed the spread of malignancy.

Atarax A patented medication, often effective in relieving tension and anxiety.

atavism The cropping up of primitive traits in a civilized person.

ataxia Lack of muscle coordination.

atelectasis A collapsed or partially collapsed condition of a lung, or portion of a lung.

atenolol *See* beta blockers and sotolol.

atheroma A fatty deposit in the walls of arteries undergoing hardening (arteriosclerosis). The fatty substance deposited is composed of cholesterol.

atherosclerosis Hardening of the inner lining (intima) of arteries.

athetosis Purposeless movements of the limbs, seen most often in children with chorea (St. Vitus' dance).

athlete's foot A fungus infection

(dermatophytosis), most often occurring between the toes.

athlete's heart A misused term, referring to a strained or overworked heart.

Ativan *See* lorazepam.

ATL Abbreviation for T-cell leukemia.

atlas The first vertebra in the neck, upon which the skull rests.

atom The smallest amount of an element which can exist alone.

atonia Absence of tone, especially muscle tone.

atony Lack of tone, as in a muscle.

atopic 1. Relating to an allergy. 2. Misplaced.

atopy Allergy.

atresia Failure of development of an opening in an organ, such as the bile ducts, the rectum, the vagina, the pupil of the eye, etc.

atrial fibrillation Irregularity of the heart beat, originating in the atrium (auricle of the heart).

atrial flutter A very fast heart beat (200–300 beats per minute) originating from a point in the atrial (auricular) muscle.

atrioseptoplasty Surgical repair of a defect in the atrial septum of the heart.

atrioventricular Referring to the auricle and ventricle of the heart.

atrium The upper chamber of the heart which receives blood from the veins (vena cava). The auricle.

atrophy The withering of an organ which had previously been normally developed.

atropine A medication with innumerable usages and effects. Its most noted action is that it paralyzes parasympathetic nerve fibers. It is used in anesthesia to dry up bronchial secretions; in ophthalmology to dilate the pupil; in intestinal conditions to relax colic and bowel spasm, etc.

attack An acute episode of a disease, usually one that is prone to recur intermittently.

Attending physician 1. The chief of a medical, surgical, or specialty service of a hospital. 2. Any physician who attends a patient.

attention span The length of time one can concentrate on a particular subject.

attenuate To reduce the potency of a virus or bacteria.

attitude Anatomically, the position of the body or part thereof.

atypical Not typical, used in referring to a disease; *atypical* pneumonia.

Au The chemical symbol for gold.

audio Pertaining to hearing.

audiogram An instrument which records the acuity of hearing.

audiometer An electrical device to measure the acuity of hearing.

audiovisual presentations A method of teaching, utilizing the senses of hearing and seeing.

auditory Referring to the sense of hearing.

Augmentum A powerful antibiotic composed of penicillin and other ingredients. Can be taken orally.

aura A premonition before a convulsion; a warning sign to an epileptic.

aural Relating to the ear.

auricle The external or visible portion of the ear; also the upper chamber of the heart which receives blood from the veins.

auricular fibrillation An irregularity of the heart caused by lack of transmission of the beat impulse to the ventricle. This is usually associated with poor heart function and disease.

auscultation The study and detection of sounds by use of a stethoscope.

autism Daydreaming.

autism, infantile A form of mental disorder in which the child is completely withdrawn and communicates with no one.

auto- Pertaining to oneself.

autoagglutinin A substance, agglutinin, found occasionally in the blood of individuals suffering from liver or other diseases.

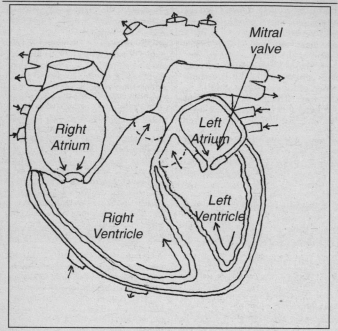

Atrium

autoanalyzer An apparatus that automatically analyses samples of blood, usually for their chemical composition.

autoclave An apparatus used for sterilizing by a steam process.

autodigestion The eating away of a portion of the wall of the stomach or duodenum by the gastric juices, as occurs in peptic ulceration.

autoeroticism Masturbation or self-stimulation and manipulation (self-love).

autogenous vaccine A vaccine manufactured from bacteria taken from the body of the patient.

autograft A graft of tissue from one part of a patient's body to another.

autohemolysis Destruction of one's blood cells brought about by one's own serum.

autohypnosis Self-hypnosis.

autoimmune diseases A group of disease in which the individual produces antibodies that attack his own tissues.

autoimmunization Immunity resulting from a substance developed within the patient's own body.

autointoxication Poisoning brought about by an upset metabolism of some substance within one's own body.

autolysis Self-digestion of tissue (as when the gastric juice creates an ulcer in the lining of the stomach).

automatism Acts not under voluntary control (sleepwalking, etc.)

autonomic imbalance Lack of normal function of the involuntary nervous system, that is, the nerves which supply the internal organs and blood vessels.

autonomic nervous system That portion of the nervous system over which there is no voluntary, conscious control; or, the self-governing portion of the nervous system.

autonomy The ability of an organ or structure to function on its own, without dependence upon other organs.

autophagy Eating one's own flesh; biting oneself.

autopsy Examination of the body after death, usually carried out to determine precisely the cause of death.

autosomal dominant An inherited disorder caused by a dominant abnormal gene on an autosome, as in Huntington's chorea. *See* autosomes.

autosomal recessive disorder An inherited disorder caused by a recessive abnormal gene on an autosome, as in Tay-Sachs disease.

autosomes Chromosomes other than the sex chromosomes found in sperm and ova (eggs). They normally occur within cells in pairs.

autosuggestion Self-suggestion.

autotherapy Self-treatment.

autotransfusion A procedure in which blood lost by the patient is re-injected into his bloodstream; carried out occasionally from blood loss into the abdominal cavity.

A-V Abbreviation for *arteriovenous* or *atrioventricular*.

avascular Bloodless; having very few blood vessels.

avascular necrosis Death of tissue because of lack of blood supply.

avitaminosis A disease brought on by lack of sufficient vitamins.

avoirdupois Weight.

A-V shunt An artificial connection made between an artery and a vein, often performed in the forearm to make dialysis (artificial kidney) more easy to perform.

avulsion The tearing away of a piece of tissue.

axilla The armpit.

axillary dissection Removal of the glands (lymph nodes) in the armpit, often performed for a cancer that has spread from the breast.

axillofemoral bypass When the lower aorta, iliac and upper portion of the femoral arteries have extensive arteriosclerosis, a graft may be inserted extending from the axillary artery in the armpit down beneath the skin of the chest and abdomen down to a healthy portion of the femoral artery in the thigh.

axis An imaginary line passing through the center of the body or through the long diameter of an organ.

axon The extension of a nerve cell (like the cord leading away from an electrical socket).

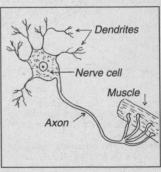

Axon

azidothymidine A medication helping to prolong the lives of patients with AIDS. It is not a cure.

azoospermia Lack of sperm in the semen.

azotemia Uremia (poisoning secondary to disease or poor function of the kidneys).

AZT An abbreviation for the antiviral drug *azidothymidine*.

Azulfidine A sulfonamide drug effective in "sterilizing" the intestinal tract prior to intestinal surgery.

azygos vein A vein coursing along the right side of the vertebral col-umn in the chest, emptying into the superior vena cava.

azygous Unpaired.

B

B. An abbreviation for *Bacillus*, a form of bacteria.

Ba The chemical symbol for barium.

Babinski sign A reflex response of the big toe, seen in cases where there has been a "stroke" or other brain disease. When the sole of the foot is scratched with a pin, the big toe turns up instead of down.

bacillary dysentery A diarrheal disease caused by a specific rod-shaped bacillus. It is contracted by eating infected food or drinking infected water. Food handlers also may be responsible for transmission of the disease.

bacilli Germs shaped like a short rod. They can cause many serious diseases such as typhoid fever, dysentery, whooping cough, etc.

bacilliform Shaped like a bacillus (rod-shaped).

bacilluria Bacilli germs in the urine, a common form of urinary infection. (Cystitis, pyelitis and other urinary infections are often caused by the *Bacillus coli communis*.)

bacitracin A powerful antibiotic drug, especially effective against certain staphylococci, streptococci, etc.

backbone The vertebral column; the spine.

bacteremia Blood poisoning; bacteria circulating in the bloodstream.

bacteria Germs.

bacterial endocarditis An infection of the valves of the heart, usually attacking valves which have already been damaged by rheumatic fever. (Streptococcal germs are particularly active in attacking the heart valves.)

bactericidal Pertaining to something which kills germs. The action of most antiseptics is *bactericidal*.

bacteriogenic Caused by germs (bacteria).

Bacteriologist A professional person who devotes himself to the study of germs (bacteria).

bacteriology The study of germs.

bacteriophage A virus which kills bacteria.

bacteriostasis A situation in which the growth and multiplication of bacteria is halted, either temporarily or permanently. (Many of the antibiotic drugs produce *bacteriostasis*.)

bacteriuria Germs in the urine, denoting a urinary infection. Many bacteria, such as the *Escherichia coli* and the *Bacillus proteus*, can cause bacteriuria.

Bacteroides fragilis A gram-negative anaerobic (does not require oxygen to survive) bacteria that causes infections in man.

Bactrim A drug used with good effect in treating urinary tract infections, ear infections, bronchial infections, and the type of pneumonia often affecting patients with AIDS.

bagassosis A lung disease seen among those who work with sugar cane. (*Bagasse*, the broken sugar cane being processed, contains silica.)

bag of waters The liquid surrounding the fetus in the uterus.

Baker's cyst An inflammation with cyst formation in the back of the knee. Also called *popliteal bursitis*.

BAL British anti-lewisite; a medication often effective in combating the effects of arsenic or mercury poisoning.

balance A state of equilibrium, as "fluid balance" wherein the intake and output of body water is under a state of control.

balanced anesthesia A method in which several different agents are employed, including an intravenous sleep-inducing medication, a pain-relieving anesthetic gas such as nitrous oxide, halothane or cyclopropane, and muscle-relaxing drugs.

balanitis An inflammation of the tip of the penis.

balanopreputial Referring to the head of the penis and the foreskin.

balanus The head (glans) of the penis.

ballistocardiograph An apparatus used to measure the volume of blood pumped by the heart.

balloon An inflatable device to stretch or deflate a constricted artery.

ballottement A French term signifying the sensation that a physician obtains when he feels a tumor, pushes it, and notes its rebound against his examining hand.

balneotherapy Bath treatments, such as one receives at a spa.

balsam of Peru A syrupy substance obtained from a Central American tree, used as a medicine to help expel secretions from the lungs and bronchial tubes.

band An adhesion, usually composed of fibrous tissue.

bandage An elongated material (gauze, flannel, etc.) used to bind various parts of the body or to hold a surgical dressing in place.

    adhesive A bandage, one side of which is composed of a sticking substance.

    circular One wound around a part of the body or limb.

    compression One applied with pressure, in order to control bleeding, oozing of serum, etc.

    elastic One composed of rubber or some other material capable of stretching and constricting.

    Esmarch One composed of rubber, used to force the blood out of a limb. Sometimes used prior to performing a limb amputation.

    figure-of-eight A bandage applied around a part in a crisscross manner so as to form an "8."

    many-tailed One composed of many tails which are so applied as to hold a part in tightly. Often used on abdomens recently operated upon.

    pressure One used to stop hemorrhages.

    reversed A method of applying a bandage to a limb by inverting or half-twisting at each turn so as to make it fit snugly on an arm or leg.

    spica A form of figure-of-eight bandage, often used in applying plaster to a leg, thigh and hip.

    suspensory One to hold up the scrotum and its contents (testicles).

    triangular A sling bandage, usually made out of muslin.

    Velpeau's One which holds the upper arm and forearm against the body, with the forearm at right angles. Often used in cases of shoulder injury.

banding A procedure in which rubber bands are placed around internal hemorrhoids, thus causing them to clot, become gangrenous, and fall off.

bandy legged Bowlegged.

Banthine A medication which blocks the action of the parasympathetic nerves. It cuts down on acid secretion by the stomach and is used in cases of ulcer or excess acidity.

Banting, Frederick Grant (1891–1941) One of the two discoverers of insulin, the substance used in the treatment of diabetes. (A Canadian physician)

Banti's disease A disease associated with an enlarged spleen and liver, anemia, and a tendency toward hemorrhage.

barber's itch Ringworm of the bearded areas of the face and neck.

(Formerly a most stubborn condition; newer drugs such as Fulvicin have now proved effective in its treatment.)

barbital A sleep-producing, sedative drug; the basic one of the barbiturate group of medications.

barbiturates A group of drugs found to be effective in calming nerves and inducing sleep. (May become habit forming)

barbotage Repeating the withdrawal and injection of spinal fluid during the administration of spinal anesthesia.

baresthesia The sensation of pressure or weight.

barium (Ba) An opaque substance which shows up on X-ray films. It is used to demonstrate the lining of the intestinal tract.

    enema The giving of a fluid mixture of barium through the rectum prior to X-raying the large intestine.

    meal Swallowing a chalky fluid containing barium prior to X-raying the intestinal tract.

Barlow's disease Scurvy in children. *See also* scurvy.

barometer The instrument which measures atmospheric pressure.

barosinusitis Inflammation of the sinuses caused by a difference in atmospheric pressure within the sinuses and in the outside air.

barotrauma Injury to the middle ear and/or sinuses caused by marked changes in barometric pressure.

Barr bodies Chromatin bodies, small dots of material seen near the periphery of certain nuclei of cells; their presence denotes the fact that the individual is female.

barren Unable to bear children; infertile, sterile.

barrier An obstruction (an anatomical term).

Bartholin cyst A cystlike swelling of the glands at the entrance to the vagina. They readily become infected and cause abscesses.

Bartholin glands Two small glands located near the entrance to the vagina. They often become infected, especially in patients with gonorrhea.

barylalia Dull, thick speech; also called *baryglossia.*

basal cell tumor A common skin cancer, usually about one-half inch or less in diameter, curable by surgery or X-ray treatment. Also called *rodent ulcer.* They frequently are located on the side of the nose or beneath the eyes.

basal metabolic rate (B.M.R.) The amount of energy expended when a patient is at rest. It is measured by a "breathing test."

base 1. The main component of a chemical substance. 2. The foundation or bottom of a structure or organ. 3. The opposite of acid.

Basedow's disease A disease associated with overactivity of the thyroid gland (hyperthyroidism) and bulging of the eyeballs. Also called *Graves' disease* or *exophthalmic goiter.*

basic life support Resuscitation of a dying person by giving first aid, including cardiopulmonary resuscitation (CPR), the control of hemorrhage, treatment of shock, etc.

basilic vein The large vein running on the inner side of the upper arm.

basiphobia Fear of walking.

basophil A form of white blood cell, so named because it takes a base (opposite of acid) stain.

basophilia A condition in which the red blood cells stain with dark specks, or "stippling"; seen in some cases of leukemia, malaria, lead poisoning, severe anemia, etc.

bassinet An infant's cradle, often made of wicker.

Bassini, Edoardo (1844–1924) An Italian surgeon, famous for devising an operation to repair hernias (in guinal).

Bassini's operation A type of repair for a hernia.

bastard Born out of wedlock.

battered spouse syndrome Physical or psychological injury caused by a husband or wife.

BCG A vaccine given in an attempt to immunize against tuberculosis. (More widely used in Europe than in the United States)

b.d. Twice daily; a term used in writing prescriptions.

beading of ribs A typical "bead-like" feel to the ribs encountered in children suffering from rickets. (Rickets is a condition due to lack of vitamin D.)

bearing-down sensation A heavy feeling in the pelvis, as when a pregnant woman is approaching delivery.

beat Pulsation; throb, such as the heart beat.

bedsore An ulceration, usually located in the lower back, caused by prolonged pressure in bedridden patients. Also called *decubitus*.

bedwetting Involuntary urination during sleep. Enuresis.

behaviorism A psychological theory based upon observations of individual activity and concepts of behavior patterns.

belladonna A most valuable drug, used in many combinations and forms, for the relaxation of spasm and to stop excess secretions of glands.

Bell's palsy Paralysis of one side of the face due to affliction of the facial nerve. Most people recover from the paralysis, although some do not make a complete recovery.

belly The abdomen.

Benadryl A patented antihistaminic medication used to combat allergies, such as hives, hay fever, etc.

Bence Jones protein test A test upon urine which, when positive, may denote the presence of a certain type of bone tumor (myeloma).

Bendectin A patented medicine used in the treatment of the nausea of pregnancy.

bends Caisson disease, a condition characterized by pains in the arms or

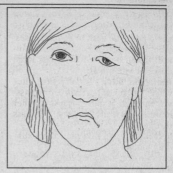

Bell's palsy

legs due to the presence of free nitrogen. It occurs among divers who come to the surface too quickly, and among those who are exposed to too-high altitudes.

Benedict test A chemical test for the presence of sugar in the urine.

Benemid (probenecid) A drug effective in controlling and preventing attacks of gout.

benign Not cancerous; not malignant.

Bentyl A medication that is helpful in relieving bowel symptoms associated with spasm.

Benylin A cough syrup, active in suppressing the cough reflex and helpful in relieving allergies.

Benzedrex A drug to shrink congested mucous membranes; the active ingredient in some nasal inhalers.

benzidine A chemical compound used to test for the presence of blood in the stool.

benzocaine A long-lasting local anesthetic.

benzoin A resin with several uses in medicine, such as an inhalant with steam for bronchitis cases or as a skin protective agent, etc.

Benzamycin A patented medicine used in the treatment of acne.

beriberi A vitamin deficiency disease seen particularly among those who eat large quantities of polished rice. The main deficiency is that of thiamin. Symptoms include weakness, neuritis, and in severe cases, mental disturbance and heart failure. It can be cured by giving large doses of vitamin B.

Berkefeld filter A very fine filter which prevents bacteria from passing through it but permits smaller matter, such as viruses, to pass through.

berserk Being in a mad rage; running amok.

beryllosis A chronic lung infection due to prolonged inhalation of metal dust (beryllium).

Best, Charles Herbert The co-discoverer of insulin, used in the treatment of diabetes. (A Canadian physician)

bestiality Sexual relations between a human and an animal.

beta blockers A large group of drugs that tend to slow the heart rate and the force of heart contractions, and lower the blood pressure. They act by blocking the beta-adrenergic receptors of the autonomic nervous system. *See* autonomic nervous system.

Betadine An iodine preparation used as a skin antiseptic in surgery.

Beta-lactam antibiotics A group of antibiotics especially effective against gram-negative bacteria. (Penicillin is one of the Beta-lactam antibiotics.)

Betalin A preparation of vitamin B complex frequently administered by intramuscular injection.

Betapace See sotolol.

beta rhythm A low voltage brain wave, noted when someone is alert and conscious.

betatron An apparatus generating millions of electron volts; the "beta" rays thus generated are sometimes effective in inhibiting the growth of cancer cells.

bezoar A ball of hair, or other undigested material, found in the stomachs of mentally unbalanced people who have eaten large quantities of such substances.

Bi Chemical symbol for bismuth.

bicarbonate (HCO_3) A salt of carbonic acid. It is present, as part of the alkali reserve, in the blood of all people. Too much bicarbonate is associated with *alkalosis;* too little with *acidosis.*

biceps The powerful muscle in the front of the upper arm. It flexes the forearm.

Bicillin A patented penicillin medication, taken by mouth.

bicornuate Two-horned, or shaped like two horns. A rather common birth deformity is a *bicornuate* uterus.

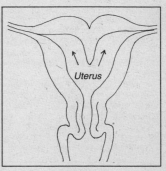

Bicornuate uterus

bicuspid Two cusps; often used in referring to certain teeth; also to the *bicuspid* valve of the heart.

b.i.d. Abbreviation for *twice daily.*

bifid Cleft, or divided into two parts, such as a bifid tongue.

bifocal Spectacles having two parts, one for near and one for far vision.

bifonazole An antifungal ointment, applied locally to the skin.

bifurcation Separation into two branches; such as the aorta which divides or *bifurcates.*

bigeminal Twin; paired.

    pulse One in which two beats

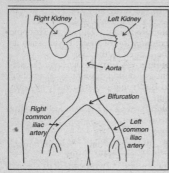

Bifurcation of aorta

occur in rapid succession, followed by a longer interval.

bilateral Pertaining to both sides, as a *bilateral hernia*.

bile The yellow fluid secreted by the liver into the duodenum (intestinal tract). It contains chemicals which aid in digestion, especially of fatty foods.

bile acid An acid formed of bile from the liver. It helps in the digestion of fatty foods in the intestine.

bilharziasis Infestation with a fluke. *See also* Schistosomiasis.

biliary Referring to the bile system, including its ducts (tubes).

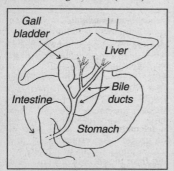

Biliary system

biliary colic Severe pain caused by gallstones, especially when they at-

tempt to pass through the narrow bile ducts.

biliousness A condition associated with a sickish feeling, lack of appetite, indigestion, bad taste in the mouth—commonly thought to be due to a "sluggish liver."

bilirubin Bile pigment.

bilirubinemia Bile pigment in the blood.

biliuria Bile in the urine, seen in patients with jaundice.

biliverdin A bile pigment, formed by the destruction of old red blood cells; often a component of gallstones.

Billroth's operations I and II - Procedures for partial removal of the stomach, frequently performed when an ulcer or cancer is present.

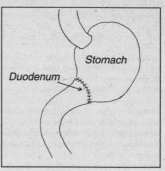

Billroth I operation

bilocular Having two compartments, such as a *bilocular* cyst.

bimanual An examination carried out with two hands, as when performing a pelvic examination upon a female.

binary Referring to something having two compartments.

binaural Pertaining to both ears.

binocular microscope A microscope that has two eyepieces.

bioassay The determination of the strength of a chemical by testing it upon animals, tissues, or germs.

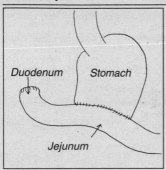

Billroth II operation

biochemistry The chemistry of live tissue.

biodegradable Organic material that will disintegrate naturally on or in the ground.

bioengineering The utilization of engineering knowledge and expertise in handling medical matters and problems.

biofeedback Giving information to an individual, through visual or auditory means, on the state of some of his physiologial responses (such as heart rate, etc.) so that the individual can gain some voluntary control over these processes.

biogenesis The theory which states that living things originate only from living things.

biokinetics The study of movements of living organisms.

biological assay Determination of strength of a drug or chemical by noting its effect upon living things. (Most hormones are first tested by noting their effect upon animals.)

biological clock mechanism The natural rhythmic cycle in a person's life, such as wake-sleep-eat patterns. Abrupt alternations in the rhythm, such as jetlag, can cause upset in body functions and mental activities.

biomedical A reference to the application of the basic sciences in the diagnosis and treatment of patients.

biometals Meals that are inserted into the body and are not rejected, such as metal hip or knee joints.

biomicroscopy The microscopic examination of living tissue, such as the cornea of the eye.

bionics A term to describe the science of biologic functions as applied to electronic devices, such as computers.

biophysics The physics of living processes.

biopsy The surgical removal of tissue in order to determine the exact diagnosis. Tumors are often submitted to biopsy while the patient is on the operating table.

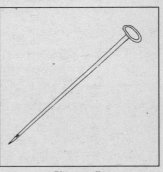

Biopsy needle

bioroentgenography X rays taken while the patient is in motion.

biostatistics The study of vital statistics, including birth statistics, mortality statistics, etc.

biosynthesis The artificial development of a chemical compound by living processes; a process by which living cells make a simple substance into a more complex one.

biotelemetry The transmission of information concerning heart and respiratory functions to a point distant from the site where the patient is located.

biotherapy Treatment with serums, vaccines, or living matter such as bacteria, etc.

biotics The science of life and its activities.

biotin A part of the vitamin B_2 complex; formerly called vitamin H.

biparous Giving birth to twins.

biped Any animal with two feet. (Man is a biped.)

bipolar disorders Mental disorders characterized by periods of manic and depressed behavior.

birth canal The uterus and vagina.

birth control The practice of regulating the time for, or preventing the onset of, pregnancy.

birth defect An abnormality present at birth. It may be genetic (inherited) or it may be acquired during pregnancy or birth; a congenital anomaly.

bisect To cut into two parts.

bisexual Someone who indulges in both homosexual and heterosexual relations.

bismuth (Bi) A chemical with many medical uses. When combined with subcarbonate, it is used as a protective covering for the lining of the stomach and intestines.

bistoury A thin, slender surgical knife, used most often to open an abscess.

bivalent Able to combine with two atoms of hydrogen.

"Black Death" Plague.

Black-Draught A strong laxative containing epsom salts, licorice and senna.

blackhead A plugged sweat gland in the skin.

black lung disease A condition acquired from the repeated inhalation of coal dust; pneumoconiosis. The disease eventually leads to impaired lung function.

blackout Loss of consciousness, usually of short duration, caused by a sudden decrease in the blood flow to the brain.

blackwater fever A colloquial term for a severe form of malaria associated with a dark, bloody urine.

black widow spider A black spider with an hourglass-shaped red color-ing on its abdomen. The bite of this spider causes great pain and swelling in the area, followed by excruciating abdominal pain and a state of shock. Recovery is the general rule.

bladder An organ which acts as a container for fluid, such as the gall bladder or urinary bladder.

blast injury Any injury caused by a nearby explosion. (Injury may be severe and extensive even though there are no external evidences of wounds.)

blastomycosis A disease caused by a yeastlike organism, often producing chronic infection of the skin, bones and other internal organs.

bleb A blister.

bleeder A hemophiliac; one who bleeds excessively even after trivial injuries.

bleeding time The time it takes for bleeding to stop after sticking a finger or earlobe when getting a sample of blood. Normally, it is between 1 and 3 minutes.

blenno A form referring to *mucus*.

bleomycin An antibiotic having inhibitory effects upon certain tumors, especially tumors of lymph glands.

blepharitis Inflammation of the eyelids.

blepharoplasty Plastic repair of an eyelid.

blepharospasm Spasm of the eyelids producing uncontrolled winking.

blighted ovum A fertilized egg that has stopped developing at an early stage.

blind Unable to see.

blind spot The center of the back of the eyeball where the optic nerve enters. This area on the retina does not react to light.

blind study One in which the investigator cannot predict the outcome.

blister A collection of serum or blood just below the most superficial layer of the skin. A *bleb*.

bloat A swollen state, such as puffiness or edema.

Blocadren Trademark for timolol, a medication helpful in preventing recurrent heart attacks.

Block-Aid A patented preparation to block the ultraviolet rays of the sun, thus sparing the individual sunburn.

blocking agent A chemical that inhibits the release of norepinephrine, a hormone present in some nerve endings; also produced by the adrenal glands.

blood The fluid which travels throughout the body in the arteries, veins and capillaries. It is composed of red blood cells, white blood cells, blood platelets and plasma. It brings oxygen and nutriment to all tissues and transports away carbon dioxide and other waste products.

    bank A laboratory which collects donor blood and holds it available for immediate transfusion. (Bank blood may be preserved for several days.)

    coagulation Clotting of the blood.

    compatibility The ability of a donor's blood to mix with a recipient's blood without causing clots to form. (A term referring to blood transfusion reactions.)

    count A microscopic test to determine the number of red and white blood cells in the blood and to find variations from normal.

    donor One who gives his blood to another.

    flow The circulation of blood throughout the body.

    group People's blood fall into four distinct groups O, A, B, AB. These groups depend upon certain sensitivities (antigens) of the red blood cells. If different bloods are mixed, as in an incompatible transfusion, clotting and destruction of red cells will take place.

    -letting Withdrawal of large amounts of blood from a vein. This procedure is performed occasionally in certain heart conditions or other diseased states.

    poisoning Bacteria growing in the bloodstream, *septicemia*.

    pressure The force or pressure exerted by the heart in pumping blood from its chambers. It is measured by a special apparatus placed about the upper arm.

    substitute A substance injected into a patient in place of blood, which may not be immediately available. (This is done frequently in cases of hemorrhage or shock until a blood transfusion can be started.)

    sugar Normally, people have between 80 and 120 milligrams of sugar (glucose) circulating in the bloodstream.

    typing A microscopic test to discover one's blood group.

    vessels The channels through which blood flows; arteries and veins.

    volume The quantity of blood circulating through the blood vessels. In shock, or in markedly debilitated states, blood volume is decreased.

blood gas analyzer An apparatus for determining the amounts of oxygen, carbon dioxide, acid and base, in the blood.

blood gases The pressures of oxygen and carbon dioxide in blood. An important chemical determination. *See* Health Manual section.

blood relative An immediate relative who shares another's genes, such as cousins, aunts, uncles, etc.

Blount's disease An acquired disease of the tibial bone of the leg, seen in young children. It will cause the leg to bow in an outward direction.

blue baby A baby born with various defects in the structure of the heart and major blood vessels. (Many such babies can now be saved through surgery.)

blue pill A laxative pill containing mercury and licorice.

B.M.R. *See* basal metabolic rate.

Boas-Oppler bacillus Harmless,

and probably helpful, bacteria found in the intestinal tract. Also called *Bacillus acidophyllus.*

body snatching Stealing a body from a grave.

Boeck's sarcoid *See* sarcoidosis.

bolus The lump of food in the mouth which is just about to be swallowed.

Bonamine A patented drug helpful in preventing seasickness and airsickness.

bond A force that holds adjacent atoms in place and resists their separation from one another.

bone The calcified tissue which makes up the skeleton. *See* Manual for list of Important Bones.

bone cement A substance placed inside the shaft of a long bone, such as a femur or humerus, to keep a prosthesis (artificial metal joint) from moving. It cements the metal of the prosthesis and binds it firmly.

bone marrow The soft tissue inside long bones. Blood cells are formed in the marrow.

bone marrow transfusion A graft of bone marrow from one person to another, sometimes helpful in treating some leukemias, anemias, or immune-deficient states.

bone scan A process by which tumors in bones can be seen long before they become visible on ordinary X rays. (Small amounts of radioactive drugs are given that settle in the bones and light up and are seen when photographed.)

bone setter Someone who specializes in correcting fractures. An outmoded term referring to nonphysicians who, centuries ago, plied this trade.

bone wax A wax used to stop bleeding from bone during surgical procedures upon these structures.

Bonine A drug effective in the control of nausea and vomiting associated with motion sickness.

booster shots An additional vaccination or inoculation given several weeks, months or years after the original immunization.

borborygmus The rumbling noises caused by gas in the intestines.

boric acid A mildly antiseptic acid used as a compress or as an ointment for inflammations of the skin or superficial membranes.

botulism An often fatal form of food poisoning caused by the specific germ *clostridium botulinum.* Seen most often in improperly canned foods, especially meats.

bougie A long, thin rubber or silk instrument used to probe the various body openings such as the urethra, esophagus, cervix of the uterus, etc.

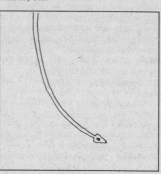

Bougie

bowel The intestine.

bowel ischemia Diminished blood supply to the intestines, frequently caused by arteriosclerosis or a clot in the mesenteric arteries supplying the bowel with blood.

bowel sounds Sounds heard when contractions of the lower intestines propel contents forward.

bowlegs Outward curving of the legs, most often caused by rickets.

B.P. *See* blood pressure.

brace An apparatus constructed to lend support to a part of the body such as the vertebral column or an extremity.

brachial plexus The group of large

nerves in the base of the neck and armpit which supply the arm and shoulder region.

brachium 1. The arm, usually referring to the upper arm. 2. An armlike structure.

brachygnathia Having a particularly small under jaw.

bradycardia Abnormally slow heart beat.

Braille, Louis (1809–1852) The discoverer of the raised alphabet which blind people use to read. (He was a Frenchman.)

brain The origin of the central nervous system, or that part which occupies the inside of the skull.

brain dead A condition in which brain waves, tested by electroencephalography, have ceased. (The heart may still be beating and respiration may continue after brain death has occurred.)

brain stem That part lying between the brain and spinal cord.

brainwashing A process that forces someone to think and act according to another's will rather than one's own.

branchial Referring to the gills (During the early part of the embryo's development, it has gills.)

branchial cysts A deformity in the neck present since birth, caused by failure of the embryo's "gill slits" to close off completely.

brash The belching of burning, sour fluid; secondary to excess stomach acid.

BRCA 1 and BRCA 2 The abbreviations stand for "breast cancer" and refer to mutations (variations) of genes that may be responsible for some types of inherited breasts cancers.

breakbone fever Dengue fever. *See also* dengue fever.

breast A mammary gland. It is made up of cells which, in the female, are capable of manufacturing milk.

breast augmentation An operative procedure to enlarge the contour of the breast, accomplished by the implantation of a plastic sac placed beneath the existing breast tissue.

breastbone The bone in the front of the chest to which the ribs are attached. The sternum.

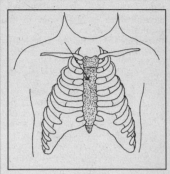

Breastbone

breast pump A suction apparatus applied to the breast for obtaining milk to nurse an infant.

breast reduction An operative procedure to reduce the size of the breast, accomplished by cutting away portions of existing skin and breast tissue.

breast self-examination A procedure in which a woman feels her own breasts in order to discover the presence or absence of lumps. All women should practice self-examination on a monthly basis.

breath Air which is inhaled and exhaled.

breath holding The voluntary stoppage of breathing, usually enacted by an infant or young child.

breath-holding test Normally, one can hold one's breath for 30 seconds. Inability to hold it at least 20 seconds indicates heart and lung insufficiency.

breech delivery Birth, feet first. Whereas breech deliveries may take longer than "head first" deliveries, they nevertheless terminate successfully.

bregma The spot on the skull where the two frontal bones fuse with the parietal bones.

Brethine A drug causing dilatation of the bronchial tubes, especially helpful in those suffering from asthma or spasm of the bronchial tubes associated with pulmonary obstructive disease.

Bricker operation A procedure carried out to cure cancer of the urinary bladder. The bladder is removed and the ureters (tubes leading from the kidneys) are implanted into a segment of small intestine. The isolated segment of small intestine is closed at one end, the other end is stitched to the skin, thus creating an *ileal bladder*.

Bright's disease Inflammation of the kidneys, or chronic nephritis.

Brill's disease Typhus fever.

broad ligament The tissue on either side of the uterus which contains the blood supply of the uterus and which helps to keep the uterus in proper position.

Broca's area An area in the brain which controls speech.

Brodie's abscess A long-standing chronic abscess which probably does not contain growing, active bacteria. Seen following a bone infection or after a tuberculous infection.

bromhidrosis Bad odor to one's sweat. *Body odor.*

bromides Drugs used to calm excess emotional disturbance. They may, on prolonged use, become habit forming.

bromism Poisoning due to an overdose of bromides. It causes foul breath, dizziness, sleepiness and pimples on the skin. (Prolonged use of bromides may produce such a state.)

bromocriptine A substance that inhibits the production of prolactin by the pituitary gland.

Bromo-Seltzer A patented remedy for headache. (May become habit forming.)

Bromsulphalein The trademarked name of a chemical used to test liver function.

bronchial Relating to the bronchial tubes.

bronchial fistula An abnormal communication between a bronchial tube and the chest cavity which surrounds the lung.

bronchiectasis Dilatation of the small bronchial tubes, often associated with chronic inflammation and infection within the lungs.

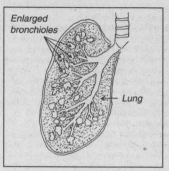

Bronchiectasis

bronchiogenic Originating in a bronchial tube. (Most lung cancer is of such origin.)

bronchioles The small bronchial tubes in the lungs which lead to the air cells.

bronchitis Inflammation of the bronchial tubes.

bronchodilator A medication which dilates a spastic bronchial tube; often prescribed in acute asthma.

bronchogram X ray of the bronchial tubes; usually performed after the patient has inhaled an opaque dye which will light up on the exposed X-ray film.

bronchopheural fistula An abnormal connection (fistula) between a bronchial tube and the cavity surrounding the lungs (pleural cavity). A serious condition often requiring surgical correction.

bronchopneumonia Inflammation of the bronchial tubes and the lungs; a common form of pneumonia usually affecting both lungs.

bronchoscopy Visualization of the bronchial tubes by passage of an instrument (bronchoscope) through the mouth.

bronchospasm Contraction of the passageway of the bronchial tubes due to excessive constriction of the muscles surrounding them. (It is usually only of temporary duration.)

bronchus A bronchial tube.

Brown-Séquard syndrome A nerve disease in which there is paralysis of movement limited to one side of the body and loss of sensation limited to the opposite side.

brow presentation A position of the unborn child in which its brow presents at the vaginal outlet. It is very difficult to deliver a child in this position.

brucellosis Malta fever. A disease caused by a germ transmitted by goats, hogs and cattle. It may be present in their milk. Also called *Mediterranean fever*.

bruit A murmur or sound heard when the stethoscope is placed over the heart or over an artery.

Brunschwig's operation *See* exenteration operation.

bruxism Gnashing the teeth during sleep.

BSP *See* Bromsulphalein.

B.T.U. British thermal unit.

bubo A swelling of a lymph gland; especially one in the groin.

bubonic plague A dangerous, often fatal, highly contagious epidemic disease caused by the bite of infected fleas which have been living on the bodies of rats. High fever, swelling of lymph glands, delirium and death often ensue. (Now controlled by better hygiene and by vaccination)

buccal Referring to the inner surface or membrane of the cheek.

buccolingual Referring to the cheek and tongue.

bucconasal Referring to the cheek and nose.

Bucky's diaphragm An apparatus which improves the quality of X-ray films.

Bucrylate A liquid adhesive substance that when injected into a bleeding varicose vein, will cause clotting. Sometimes used in treating varicosities of the esophagus.

Buerger's disease A chronic inflammatory disease of the arteries and veins of the lower extremities; *thromboangiitis obliterans*. Thought to be most prevalent among heavy smokers.

buffalo neck A protruding neck accentuating the back portion, resembling a buffalo's neck, among some patients who have Cushing's disease. *See* Cushing's disease.

buffer Something which preserves the balance of acidity or alkalinity of a solution.

buggery Anal intercourse.

bulbar poliomyelitis Infantile paralysis affecting the base of the brain and usually accompanied by paralysis of the muscles which enable normal breathing.

bulbous Swollen at the tip; such as a *bulbous nose* in some alcoholics.

bulimia Abnormal, uncontrolled eating, usually occurring in binges. The condition is encountered mainly in females.

bulkage Any one of many substances that will increase the intestinal contents, such as fiber, bran, etc.

bulla A large blister.

BUN Blood urea nitrogen. (An important chemical determination denoting the adequacy of kidney function.)

bundle branch block A disturbance in the transmission of the heart beat impulse from the atrial chamber to the ventricular chamber, due to malfunction in the condition mechanism.

bundle of His Heart muscle fibers that extend from the atrium (auricle) to the ventricle.

bunion A swelling of the bursa on the inner aspect of the big toe.

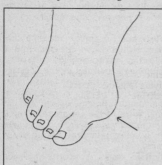

Bunion

burette A glass tube containing markers to measure the quantity of fluids permitted to drip out.

Burkitt's sarcoma A malignant condition seen among African children, thought to originate from a virus. It frequently involves the bones of the face, the ovaries, and lymph nodes within the abdomen. Biting insects are thought to transmit the virus of this disease.

burn First degree: involving only the superficial layers of the skin, as in sunburn. Second degree: involving all but the deepest layer (the corium) of the skin. Third degree: involving all layers of the skin and possibly the tissues beneath the skin.

bursa A small, soft tissue sac located between parts that move upon one another; often lying between bones and muscles.

bursitis Inflammation of a bursa. A favorite site is in the shoulder region.

Buspar (buspirone) A patented medication capable of reducing anxiety.

Butazolidin A patented medicine used in the treatment of arthritis, bursitis, etc.

butterfly eruption A rash over the bridge of the nose and cheeks. *See* lupus erythematosus.

buttock That part of the body behind the hips, upon which one sits.

Butyn sulfate A patented medicine used as an eyedrop to relieve pain and produce a temporary anesthesia of the conjunctiva (eye membrane).

bypass To skirt or shunt, as a blood vessel graft to relieve an obstructed artery.

byssinosis A disease of the lungs caused by inhaling cotton dust over a period of years, seen frequently among textile workers.

C

C The chemical symbol for carbon.

Ca The chemical symbol for calcium.

cachexia An emaciated state caused by a serious, prolonged illness.

cacodylate An arsenic medication used in treating certain skin diseases.

cacophony A loud, harsh noise.

cadaver A dead body.

cadmium sulfide A substance used in treatment of dermatitis of the scalp.

caduceus The insignia of medicine, a staff around which a serpent is coiled. It has been modified by the U.S. Army Medical Corps, with two wings at the top of the staff and two serpents coiled by the remainder. (To be distinguished from the staff of Aesculapius, the official insignia of the A.M.A.)

Cafergot A combination of caffeine and ergot, often helping in allaying migraine attacks.

caffeine A stimulant drug, found in large quantities in coffee and tea.

caisson disease A disease caused by abrupt changes in atmospheric pressure; *the bends.* (Symptoms are produced because nitrogen is released, in the form of bubbles, into the blood.)

caked breasts Breasts hardened and swollen with milk.

calamine lotion A medication composed of zinc oxide and ferric oxide, used as a local application in the treatment of certain skin conditions.

Calan A drug used to allay attacks of angina pectoris by relieving spasm of the coronary artery.

calcaneus The heel bone (os calcis).

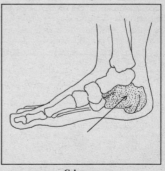
Calcaneus

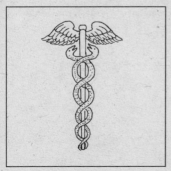
Caduceus

calcareous 1. Containing calcium. 2. Chalky.

49

calcemia Excessive calcium in the blood.

calcification The deposit of calcium in tissues of the body. This process often takes place as one ages, as in hardening of the arteries.

calcinosis Calcium deposits in the skin and subcutaneous tissues, seen in cases of overactivity of the parathyroid glands in the neck.

calcipenia Too little calcium in the tissues.

calcitonin A hormone whose action is opposite to the hormone secreted by the parathyroid gland.

calcium (Ca) A chemical found normally in body tissues, including bone, blood plasma, etc. In combination, it has many valuable usages as a medication.

calcium-45 Radioactive calcium, sometimes used in studies of bone metabolism.

calcium gluconate A drug containing sugar that, when given intravenously, will relieve the symptoms of insulin shock (the shock often results from an overdose of insulin).

calcium lactate Medication given to those suffering from calcium deficiency; often used in treating those with underactivity of the parathyroid glands as a preventive against tetany.

calculus A stone, such as a kidney stone or gall bladder stone.

Caldwell-Luc operation An operation upon a chronically infected maxillary sinus in the cheek. The incision is made in the gums above the upper teeth and the infected lining membrane of the sinus is scraped out.

calf The back of the leg.

calibration The adjustment of an instrument or apparatus so as to ensure its accuracy.

calipers Forcepslike instruments used to measure the thickness of objects.

calisthenics Exercises to develop the use of, and to continue the suppleness of, muscles.

callus 1. Markedly thickened skin. 2. New bone which develops in the area of a fracture.

Calmitol A patented medicine applied to the skin surface to stop itching.

calorie A heat unit. In common usage, it refers to the food value of a particular foodstuff.

calorimeter An instrument which measures the amount of heat given off by the body.

calvarium The top of the skull.

Calvé-Perthes disease *See* osteochondrosis.

calvities Baldness.

calyx A portion of the kidney into which urine is excreted.

camphor A substance, obtained

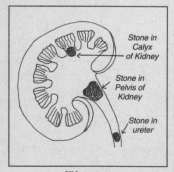

Kidney stone

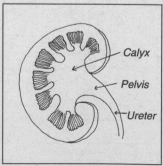

Calyx of kidney

from a plant, used in various combinations as a medication.

canal A channel or duct. (An anatomical term)

of Nuck *See* Nuck's canal.

canaliculus A small canal.

canalization The formation of new channels in tissue, such as the reformation of a passageway in a clotted blood vessel.

cancellous Latticed or spongelike in structure; *cancellous bone.*

cancer A malignant tumor of any type.

cancerocidal An agent that kills cancer cells.

cancerogen A substance which stimulates the formation of cancer, such as petroleum when in contact with the hands of people who work for many years in the petroleum industry.

cancerophobia Fear of cancer.

cancer serum A serum which is supposed to act to stop the growth of cancer. Its effectiveness has not been proved.

cancer smears Cells obtained by swabbing tissues which might contain extruded (detached) cancer cells. Such cells are smeared on a glass slide and examined under a microscope.

Candida albicans A fungus in the monilia group. It can cause thrush and vaginal infections.

canine teeth The sharp teeth located just in front of the premolars.

canities Gray hair.

canker sore An ulceration, often found on the tongue or gums.

cannabis A leaf, which when smoked, may cause symptoms of hallucinations, a sense of exceptional well-being, or other mental effects.

cannibal One who eats humans.

cannula An instrument devised to fit various body channels, such as a cannula for the trachea after performing a tracheotomy.

cantharides Spanish fly; an extract of this specific beetle. When taken

internally, it acts as a potent sex stimulant. In large doses, it is a dangerous poison.

canthoplasty A plastic operation upon the upper eyelid.

canthus The angles formed by the eyelids, either on the inner or outer extremes of the eyes.

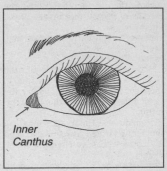

Inner
Canthus

Canthus

capillaries Very small blood vessels. It is from the capillaries that nourishment is fed directly to the tissues.

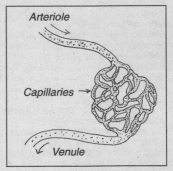

Arteriole

Capillaries →

↙ Venule

Capillaries

capillary permeability The passage of liquids and nutriments through the walls of the smallest blood vessels into the body tissues.

capitate Head-shaped.

capnograph An instrument for monitoring the amount of carbon dioxide in exhaled air, occasionally used during anesthesia.

Capoten An effective medication to lower blood pressure.

capsule A covering or sheath.

capsulotomy Cutting a capsule, such as the capsule of the lens, the capsule of a joint, the capsule of the kidney, etc.

captation The early stage of hypnosis.

caput The head.

    cecum The "head" of the large intestine, that part located in the right lower abdomen where the small intestine enters the large intestine.

    medusae Enlarged veins on the abdomen and lower chest, seen in people who have cirrhosis of the liver.

carbamazepine A medication helpful in relieving the pain of facial neuralgia; also used to stop convulsions.

carbarsone A chemical substance used in the treatment of intestinal parasites.

carbimazole A medication used in treating overactivity of the thyroid gland.

carbohydrate Sugar or starch.

carbolic acid Phenol. A powerful antiseptic agent.

Carbomycin One of the mycin antibiotic drugs.

carbon (C) The most widely distributed element, present in all organic compounds.

    dioxide (CO_2) An end product of respiration (breathing).

    monoxide (CO) A poisonous, odorless gas, capable of killing if inhaled in large quantities over a prolonged period of time.

carbon dioxide snow Dry ice.

carboxyhemoglobin The union of carbon monoxide with the hemoglobin present in red blood cells, often leading to suffocation and death. It is called *carbon monoxide poisoning*.

carbuncle A large boil, usually of the skin and tissues beneath the skin, which discharges pus from several points.

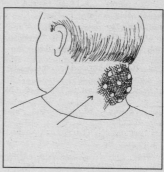

Carbuncle of the neck

carbunculosis A condition in which there are many carbuncles present at the same time.

carbutamide A drug, taken by mouth, that causes lowering of blood sugar.

carcinogen Any substance which stimulates the formation of cancer; *cancerogen.*

carcinoid A cancerlike tumor, not as malignant as true cancer, originating in the appendix or intestines. It tends to grow and spread slowly.

carcinoma Cancer derived from lining cells of organs. It can occur in almost any structure of the body: brain, lungs, liver, pancreas, intestines, kidney, skin, etc.

carcinoma in situ Cancer that has not become invasive of surrounding tissues; the earliest and potentially the most curable type of cancer.

carcinosarcoma A highly malignant tumor of the uterus, involving cancerous changes in both the lining membrane tissues *and* the muscle tissues.

carcinomatosis Cancer widely spread throughout the body.

carcinosis Widely spread cancer.

cardia The upper end of the stomach where the esophagus enters. (It is so called because of its closeness to the heart.)

cardiac   Relating to the heart.

   arrest   Stoppage of the heart. Prompt massage of the heart sometimes restores normal heart action.

   catheterization   This consists of passing and threading a long, narrow, hollow plastic tube into the blood vessel of one of the extremities until it reaches one or more of the chambers of the heart. Pressure recordings are made through the tube, and blood samples are withdrawn. Much can be learned about the working of the heart through catheterization.

   failure   A condition caused by inadequate heart function. (Many cases are curable when treated early and properly.)

   massage   An emergency measure carried out when the heart suddenly stops. The chest is compressed manually, thus squeezing the heart so that it pumps blood and is stimulated to start beating again on its own. *See* closed chest massage.

cardiectomy   Surgical removal of the upper end of the stomach, a procedure sometimes performed for cancer.

cardiodynamics   The mechanism by which the circulation of the body is maintained through the beating of the heart.

Cardiografin   An opaque dye which outlines the chambers of the heart. It is injected into a vein and X rays are taken shortly thereafter.

cardiogram   A recording of the heart's pulsations.

Cardiologist   One who specializes in diseases of the heart.

cardiolysis   An operative procedure for severing adhesions of the heart to its surrounding membrane, the pericardium.

cardiomalacia   Degeneration of heart muscle and replacement with fibrous tissue.

cardiomegaly   Enlargement of the heart.

cardiomentopexy   An operation in which the omentum from the abdomen is stitched to the outer wall of the heart in an attempt to improve circulation. (This procedure is now more or less obsolete.)

cardiomyopathy   Disease of the heart muscle.

cardioneurosis   Pain in the heart, palpitation, and a feeling of suffocation and death, occurring in neurotic people. It is not an organic disease, but is considered a neurotic manifestation.

cardiopulmonary   Referring to the heart and lungs.

cardiopulmonary resuscitation (CPR) A technique of administering simultaneous closed cardiac massage and mouth-to-mouth artificial respiration, performed in cases of cardiac arrest.

cardiorenal   Relating to the heart and kidneys.

cardiorrhaphy   Stitching of the heart after a heart wound.

cardioscope   An instrument that permits inspection of the beating heart.

cardiospasm   A muscular constriction of the lower end of the esophagus and the entrance of the stomach.

cardiovalvulotomy   An open heart operation in which narrowed valves are cut.

cardiovascular   Relating to the heart and blood vessels.

cardioversion   The conversion of an irregular heart rhythm to a normal one, by means of an electric shock. The shock is induced by an apparatus known as a "cardioverter."

carditis   Inflammation of the heart.

Cardizem   Trade name for an antiangina pectoris drug.

Carefate   *See* sucralfate.

caries   Cavities in the teeth.

carminative   A medication used to relieve intestinal gas or colic.

carnivorous   Meat-eating.

carotene A chemical (hydrocarbon) made by plants which goes into the formation of vitamin A. It is found in large quantities in carrots.

carotenemia The presence of carotene in the blood after eating large amounts of carrots. Occasionally, it can cause a yellowish discoloration of the skin resembling a mild jaundice.

carotid arteries The large arteries on either side of the neck which supply blood to the head.

    body tumor A growth within the *carotid body*, a mass of tissue located near the large carotid arteries in the neck.

    gland The same as carotid body. A small group of glandlike cells located in the neck at the site where the large carotid arteries divide.

    sinus syndrome A set of symptoms caused by irritating or over-stimulating the *carotid sinus* in the neck. Dizziness, fainting, convulsions, an abrupt drop in blood pressure and even heart stoppage may result in the occasional cause. Attacks may follow emotional shock, or may be caused by steady finger pressure directly over the carotid sinus.

carpal Referring to the wrist or one of its bones.

carpal tunnel syndrome Numbness, weakness and pain in the hand, especially involving the index, middle and ring fingers, due to compression of the medial nerve at the wrist. The nerve in these cases is compressed by too tight a carpal ligament.

carphologia Picking at the bedclothes, a symptom seen in cases of severe fever such as typhoid.

carpus The wrist.

Carrel, Alexis (1873–1944) Discovered a method for keeping tissues alive outside of the body. Also, the first, with Charles Lindbergh, to construct an artificial heart pump.

carrier A healthy person who harbors or carries germs which can infect and cause disease in another, such as a typhoid *carrier*.

car sickness Headache, nausea and vomiting, caused by riding in automobiles. *See also* Motion sickness.

cartilage Gristle. The elastic semi-hard tissue covering some bones, particularly the joint surfaces. It permits smooth motion and diminishes friction.

cartilagenous calcinosis The replacement of joint cartilage by calcium.

caruncle A reddened, irritated piece of flesh, often seen about the entrance of the female urethra.

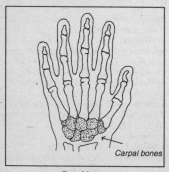

Carpal bones

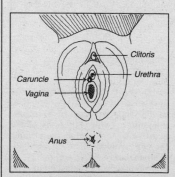

Caruncle of the urethra

cascara A popular laxative used in cases of constipation.

cascarilla A bitter tonic, obtained from the bark of *Croton eluteria*.

case A specific instance of disease or illness; informally, a patient.

caseation The degeneration of tissue into a cheeselike substance, seen as the effect of tuberculosis.

casein The protein found in large quantities in milk.

caseous Having the appearance of cheese.

Casodex An anticancer drug for the treatment of a cancer of the prostate gland.

cassette The holder for unexposed X-ray film.

cast 1. A popular term for crossed eyes (strabismus). 2. Renal casts, found in the urine, denote kidney disease. 3. Plaster cast; a mixture of gypsum and water, used to immobilize parts of the body which are injured.

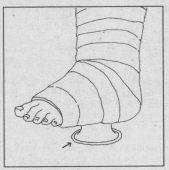
Walking caliper in a cast

castor oil A powerful laxative; the oil is extracted from the plant seed *Ricinus communis*.

castration Removal of the testicles or ovaries.

casualty The victim of an accident.

casuistics The study and reporting of diseases, including statistics.

catabolism The opposite of anabolism; the breaking down of complex compounds during metabolism.

catalase An enzyme active in the process of oxidation.

catalepsy A mentally disturbed state seen in some unbalanced patients, characterized by a trancelike, immobile state with loss of voluntary movement.

catalyst An agent which hastens and stimulates a chemical reaction.

catamenia Menstruation.

cataphasia Repetition of the same word or words over and over again.

cataphoresis Administration of drugs by passage of an electric current into the body.

cataphylaxis The process by which white blood cells are mobilized and migrate to the site of an inflammation.

Catapres A medication to lower elevated blood pressures.

cataract Opacity of the lens of the eye.

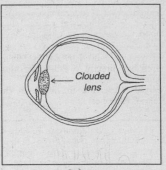
Cataract

cataract extraction The removal of the lens of the eye.

catarrh Irritation of a membrane, particularly of the respiratory tract, accompanied by an excessive secretion of mucus.

catatonia A phase in schizophrenia in which the patient does not talk, move or react.

catecholamine Chemicals that af-

fect the body's responses to stress.
(Some are produced in the medulla
of the adrenal glands; others are
manufactured synthetically.) They
may influence nerve responses,
heart action, muscle activity, etc.

catgut A suture material derived
from sheep's intestine. (It is not derived from cats.) When used on humans, it is eventually absorbed by
the body.

catharsis 1. To purge the intestinal tract, as with a laxative. 2. In
psychiatry, to purge the mind by
permitting the patient to express
verbally all his thoughts, anxieties
and fears.

cathartic A laxative.

catheter 1. A rubber, plastic or
glass tube used to insert into the
bladder in order to withdraw urine.
2. A tube for passage into a structure, for the purpose of injecting or
withdrawing a fluid, such as in cardiac *catheterization*.

catheterization 1. Withdrawal of
urine from the bladder by passage of
a tube. 2. Withdrawal of fluid or
blood for analysis by passage of a
tube.

cathexis The investment of something with mental or emotional energy or psychological significance.

cathode The negative pole in an
electric circuit.

cat's ear A deformity of the external ear.

CAT scan The simultaneous taking of many X rays from many
angles, thus giving a highly defined
set of pictures of an organ or organs.
Also known as *computerized axial
tomography*. Same as CT scan.

cauda equina The "tail" end of the
spinal cord composed of the nerves
which supply the rectal area. (The
nerves somewhat resemble a
horse's tail.)

caudal Toward the tail; downward.

caudal anesthesia One injected
into the spine in the region of the
sacrum and coccyx. It is used in

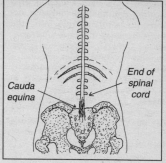

Cauda equina

End of spinal cord

Cauda equina

Cauda equina

childbirth and also when performing
operations upon the rectum.

caul A portion of the fetal membranes. "Born with a caul" means
being born with part of the fetal
membranes still covering the head
of the newborn. (In folklore, a sign
of good luck)

cauliflower ear A deformity of the
external ear, seen often in prize
fighters, due to repeated hemorrhage beneath the skin.

causalgia A burning sensation in
the palms, soles or digits, thought to
be due to irritation or disease in the
nerves supplying these areas.

caustic A substance used to destroy tissue, such as silver nitrate,
potassium hydroxide, etc.

cauterization Burning by application of a caustic, heat or electric
current.

cavernitis An inflammation of the
structures (corpora cavernosa)
which make up the shaft of the
penis.

cavernous Containing a hollow
space.

cavernous hemangioma A large,
benign tumor of veins containing a
great amount of blood; sometimes
seen in the region of the scalp.

cavernous sinus thrombosis Infection and blood clot in the cavernous
sinus lying within the cavernous
sinus lying within the skull, behind

and above the eyes. Infection, arising from the upper lip and nose, occasionally will travel into the cavernous sinus and create this condition. (Unless treated early and strenuously, it may cause death.)

cavitation The formation of a cavity, such as a tuberculous cavity in a lung.

Cavitron A motorized scalpel that cuts through soft tissues but not through blood vessels or ductal tissues. Useful in brain and liver surgery.

cavity A hollow in an organ; such as a cavity in a lung caused by tuberculosis.

cavus Pes cavus, an exceptionally high arch to the sole of the foot.

CBC Abbreviation for complete blood count.

cc. A cubic centimeter, or roughly, fifteen drops of a fluid from an eyedropper.

CCNU Abbreviation for lomustine, a powerful chemotherapeutic drug used in the treatment of Hodgkin's disease, brain tumors, etc.

C.C.U. Abbreviation for Cardiac Care Unit; an intensive care facility for acute cardiac patients.

CDC *See* Centers for Disease Control.

cecitis Inflammation of the cecum, the first portion of the large bowel.

cecostomy A surgical operation in which an opening is made in the cecum and it is brought onto the abdominal wall. Such operations are performed to relieve intestinal obstruction.

cecotomy Incision into the cecum.

cecum The beginning of the large bowel, located in the right lower portion of the abdomen. The small intestine empties into the cecum at the ileocecal value.

Cefadroxil A powerful antibiotic of the cephalosporin group.

Cefamandole An effective antibiotic drug, helpful in treating a wide range of bacterial infections.

cefoxitin sodium An antibiotic

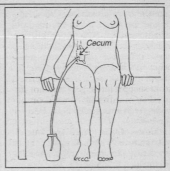

Cecostomy

with a wide range of effectiveness, including activity against the kind of mixed infections that are found in peritonitis.

ceftriaxone A new antibiotic, highly effective in treating gonorrheal infections of the eyes.

celation The attempt to conceal the fact that one is pregnant.

celiac Referring to the abdomen.

celiac disease A disease of infancy associated with intestinal difficulties, malfunction of the pancreas, anemia and inability to grow normally.

celiocolpotomy Entrance into the abdomen through an incision in the vagina.

celiotomy Any operation which opens the abdominal cavity.

cell The unit of protoplasm, containing a nucleus and cytoplasm. All tissue is made up of individual cells. The average cell is so small it can only be seen under the microscope.

cell mass An outgrowth of a group of cells in an embryo.

cellulitis Inflammation of connective tissue, usually the tissues just beneath the skin surface.

cellulose The fibers of plants. Absorbent cotton is derived from this substance.

Celsius The temperature scale in which 0° Centigrade is the point of ice formation and 100° Centigrade is the boiling point.

cement, intercellular The substance in between cells which holds them together. (It is thought that in cancer, the intercellular cement is deficient, thus permitting cancer cells to break away and travel from their original site.)

cementoblastoma A benign tumor originating from the cement-forming cells of a tooth.

cementum The bony substance of the root of teeth.

Cenadase A new drug, beneficial in the treatment of certain cases of Gaucher's disease.

cenesthesia General sensation, such as the feeling of well-being or ill-being, as opposed to specific sensations such as sore throat, pain in a finger, etc.

Centers for Disease Control (CDC) A government agency that specializes in keeping statistics on communicable diseases and disseminates information on how to control them.

centigrade The unit of measure for heat or temperature. In this system, water boils at 100°C. and freezes at 0°C.

centigram (cg.) 1/100 of a gram.

centimeter (cm.) 1/100 of a meter, or roughly 2/5 of an inch.

centrad Toward the center.

central nervous system That part of the nervous system containing the brain, spinal cord and the nerves originating therefrom.

central venous catheter A hollow plastic tube inserted into a vein in the arm or neck and pushed forward until it reaches the vena cava in the chest. It is used for measuring pressure in the central veins, and also to give liquids and medications.

central venous pressure The pressure within the central veins of the vena cava within the chest.

Centrax A tranquilizing drug helpful in the short term control of acutely stressful situations and states of anxiety.

centrifugal Going from the center to the outside; such as *centrifugal*

force which tends to make whirling objects fly away from the center.

centrifuge A machine which whirls things at a rapid pace, exercises centrifugal force, and thus separates substances of varying densities.

centripetal Going from the outside toward the center; such as *centripetal* force; the opposite of centrifugal.

centrosome The material thought to be responsible for the reproductive activity of a cell. It appears as a round dot within the substance of the cell.

Centrum A vitamin and mineral supplement.

cephalad Toward the head of the body.

cephalalgia Headache.

cephalhematoma A collection of blood located beneath one area of the scalp in a newborn child. (It either disappears spontaneously within a few days or it can be tapped and the blood withdrawn.)

cephalic Relating to the head.

    vein A large vein on the outside aspect of the arm.

cephalocaudal Relating to the long axis of the body; from the head downward.

cephaloid Head-shaped.

cephalopathy Any disease of the head.

cephalopelvic Relating to the embryo's head and the mother's pelvis. *Cephalopelvic disproportion* means that the child's head is too large to pass through the pelvis.

cephalosporins A group of antibiotic drugs, effective against many different types of bacteria.

cephalothin An antibiotic of the cephalosporin group, effective particularly against aerobic (oxygen-using) organisms.

cephalotrypesis Boring a hole in the skull; a surgical procedure to aid in diagnosis and treatment of brain conditions.

cera Wax.

cerebellopontine angle tumor A brain tumor involving the acoustic nerve (the eighth cranial nerve supplying the ear). It requires surgical removal.

cerebellospinal Pertaining to the cerebellum and spinal cord.

cerebellum The inferior part of the brain located beneath the cerebrum. It is responsible for muscular coordination.

cerebral Referring to the cerebrum, the brain area containing the higher brain centers.

cerebral edema Excess fluid in the brain.

cerebral malaria A serious type involving high fever and headache, and ending in death in approximately 50 percent of cases.

cerebration The process of thinking.

cerebropontine The cerebrum and the pons (a portion of the lower portion of the brain).

cerebrosclerosis Hardening of brain tissue in the cerebrum.

cerebrospinal fluid Clear, colorless fluid surrounding the brain and spinal cord. It can be withdrawn by performing a spinal puncture.

cerebrovascular accident Apoplexy; a stroke; a hemorrhage or blood clot within a blood vessel in the brain.

cerebrum The higher brain cells; the chief portion of the brain controlling conscious thoughts and actions.

certifiable disease One that must, because of its contagious nature, be reported to the Board of Health. (Diphtheria, smallpox, syphilis, etc.)

certify To place someone in a mental hospital, often against his or her will.

cerumen Wax in the ear canals.

Cerumenex A liquid that dissolves ear wax.

cervical region The neck.

cervical rib One located in the neck above the first rib in the chest. (*Cervical rib* is a birth deformity.)

cervicectomy Surgical removal of the cervix of the uterus; sometimes

performed because of infection or overgrowth (hypertrophy).

cervicitis Inflammation of the cervix of the uterus.

cervicofacial Pertaining to the neck and face.

cervicovaginal Referring to the cervix and vagina.

cervicovaginitis Inflammation of the cervix and vagina.

cervix The entrance and lower portion of the uterus (womb). It protrudes into the vagina and can be readily inspected by the gynecologist.

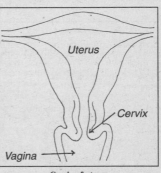

Cervix of uterus

cesarean section Delivery of a newborn child surgically through an abdominal incision; a procedure carried out when delivery through the vagina is inadvisable.

cesium (Cs) An element; its radioactive form is useful in treating certain malignant conditions.

cestode A parasite (worm).

cg Abbreviation for centigram.

chafing Irritating.

Chagas' disease A rare parasitic disease (trypanosomiasis) caused by the *Trypanosoma cruzi*, found mainly in South America. It is characterized by enlarged lymph nodes and irregular episodes of high fever.

chalazion A cyst, usually inflamed, of an eyelid. It usually requires surgery, performed under local anesthesia.

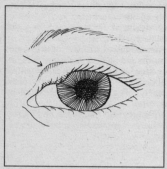

Chalazion

chalicosis Inflammation of the lungs secondary to inhaling the dust of lime.

chalk Calcium carbonate.

chamber 1. A hollow space, such as a chamber of the heart. 2. A room. 3. A "counting chamber" is an area on a slide used for counting blood cells when performing a blood count.

chancre The primary sore of syphilis. It is a small, firm, painless, rounded area about ½ inch in diameter which appears to be raw. It often appears within the area of sexual contact.

chancroid A venereal infection of

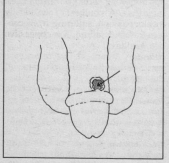

Chancre

the genitals, not syphilis, caused by the specific germ, *Hemophilus ducreyi*. There are frequently several sores present at one time.

change of life Menopause. The time of life when a woman's menstrual periods cease; usually between forty-five and fifty years of age.

channel A canal or passageway.

CHAP An abbreviation for a group of 4 anti-cancer drugs used in the treatment of cancer of the ovaries.

chapped Roughened, cracked skin; usually due to overexposure to wet and coldness.

characteristic A trait. It may be acquired during one's lifetime or may be inherited through one's genes. Some genetic traits are dominant and are inherited frequently; others are recessive and are inherited infrequently.

charcoal, activated A medication to reduce and absorb gas from the stomach and intestines.

Charcot's fever Chills and fever occurring intermittently in patients with a stone in the common bile duct. When the stone causes obstruction of the flow of bile, there is a sudden chill and rise in temperature. When the stone frees the obstruction, symptoms subside.

Charcot's joint A swollen, but painless, joint seen in cases of advanced syphilis.

charlatanism Quackery. The practice of medicine by a quack or charlatan.

charley horse A muscle sprain, associated with tearing of some of the muscle fibers and hemorrhage into the substance of the muscle.

chaulmoogra oil A useful medication for the treatment of leprosy.

CHCL₃ *See* chloroform.

CHD *See* coronary heart disease.

cheek The side of the face.

cheilectomy Surgical removal of part of a lip; usually performed to remove a lip cancer.

cheilitis Inflammation of the lips.

cheilosis Creases, lines and splitting of the skin at the corners of the mouth, usually due to lack of vitamin B$_2$ (riboflavin).

chemistry The study of the composition of matter.

    analytical That branch of chemistry dealing with the qualitative and quantitative analysis of substances.

    biological The chemistry of living things.

    colloid Chemistry of colloids, substances composed of individual particles between 1 and 100 millimicrons in size.

    forensic Chemistry helpful in the detection of crime.

    inorganic That branch of chemistry dealing with noncarbon compounds.

    nuclear That branch dealing with changes within the nucleus of the atom.

    organic That branch dealing with carbon compounds.

    pathological That branch dealing with the chemical changes taking place in disease.

    physiological That branch dealing with the chemical changes in animals and plants.

    synthetic That branch dealing with the production of new compounds.

    toxicological That branch dealing with the detection of poisons.

chemocarcinogenesis The production of cancer through chemical agents.

chemodectoma A benign tumor originating in the carotid body in the neck.

chemolysis Chemical decomposition.

chemonucleolysis Dissolving a herniated disk by injecting it with an enzyme. (The procedure is sometimes a substitute for surgery.)

chemoreceptor A cell that is activated by its chemical environment and, as a result, creates a flow of nerve impulses.

chemosis Swelling of the lining (conjunctiva) of the eyes.

chemosurgery The destruction of tumors with the use of chemicals.

chemotaxis Positive chemotaxis occurs when one substance is attracted toward another, negative chemotaxis is said to take place when one substance is repelled by another.

chemotherapy Treatment of infections or tumors through the use of chemical agents.

chemotropism Attraction of cells due to chemicals.

chenodeoxycholic acid A bile salt which, when given over a period of months or years, sometimes dissolves cholesterol gallstones.

Chenopodium A medication useful in ridding the body of worms, especially roundworms.

Cheracol A patented cough medicine, used in cases of bronchitis.

cherry-red spot An oval red area seen on examination of the retina of the eye in cases of congenital Tay-Sachs disease. *See* Tay-Sachs disease.

chest That part of the body extending from the root of the neck down to the diaphragm.

Cheyne-Stokes breathing Breathing irregularity with long periods of not breathing ending with very deep breathing. A condition seen mostly in older people suffering from congestive heart failure. *See* congestive heart failure.

chiasma Where the two optic (eye) nerves cross; located in the base of the brain.

chicken breasted A pointing of the breastbone (sternum) giving the appearance of a chicken's breast; seen in certain cases of rickets (a vitamin D deficiency disease).

chicken pox (varicella) A highly contagious disease seen mostly in childhood and characterized by pocklike eruptions all over the body. It is caused by a specific virus.

chicken pox vaccine Effective protection results from one injection of the vaccine. Adverse reactions to the vaccine are reported to be rare.

chigger A mite which bites and causes severe itching. Chiggers can be seen as very tiny red insects.

chilblain Swelling and congestion of the skin due to cold; associated with burning and itching. Seen most often on the front of the legs.

child abuse Mistreatment of children, often including severe beatings, long periods of confinement, and withdrawal of the affection parents normally give their offspring.

childbed fever An old term for infection of the uterus secondary to childbirth; *puerperal fever*.

childbirth Giving birth; parturition.

natural An educational program for the expectant mother, designed to adjust her to the ensuing labor and confinement.

chill A cold, shivering sensation, often preceding the onset of an acute infection. It is often associated with an abrupt rise in temperature.

chimney sweeps' carcinoma Cancer of the skin of the scrotum seen among chimney sweeps. It is caused by the long-continued contact and irritation of coal dust on the skin of the scrotum (the sac of the testicles).

chincough Whooping cough.

chiragra Gout of the hand (an old term)

chirapsy An old piece of folklore that a child is marked or blemished in its mother's womb because the mother was frightened, or longed for something, during her pregnancy.

chirology Talking with one's hands, as with deafmutes.

Chiropodist A technician, licensed but not a physician, who treats warts, corns, bunions and other minor conditions affecting the feet.

chirospasm Writer's cramp.

chirurgeon An old term for surgeon.

chirurgery Surgery.

chlamydia infections Those caused by an organism which is an intermediate form between viruses and bacteria. Infections can be transmitted by sexual intercourse causing discharge; it may also cause a conjunctivitis of the eyes.

chloasma Brownish discoloration of the skin, seen often in patches during pregnancy.

chloral hydrate A valuable medication to calm nerves and induce sleep. Also used to combat convulsions in children.

chlorambucil Leukeran. A form of nitrogen mustard used to combat leukemia and Hodgkin's disease.

chloramphenicol (Chloromycetin) A valuable antibiotic drug especially effective in treating certain resistant bacteria.

chlorangiopancreatography X-ray examination of the bile ducts and pancreas.

Chloresium Trademark for many products containing chlorophyll.

chlorhydria Excess stomach acidity.

chloride (Cl-2) The salt of hydrochloric acid, found in large quantities in the human body.

chlorination Disinfecting with the addition of chlorine; used in preparing water for drinking.

chlorine (Cl) A gas with a characteristically strong odor; when combined with water and other liquids, it acts as a strong antiseptic.

chloroform ($CHCl_3$) A chemical which produces anesthesia when inhaled into the lungs.

Chloromycetin A powerful antibiotic particularly effective against resistant germs.

chlorophyll The green substance in plants. It is used, in a purified form, as a deodorant; also to promote the healing of wounds.

Chloropicrin A chemical used in tear gas and as an insect-killing agent.

Chloroptic An antibiotic eyedrop, used in various types of conjunctivitis.

chloroquine A chemical used to treat malaria; also to kill certain parasites which invade the liver.

chlorosis A type of anemia seen most often in young girls or young women.

chlorothiazide A powerful diuretic, especially helpful for patients who are "waterlogged" and are suffering from heart failure.

chlorpromazine (Thorazine) A medication used to combat nausea and vomiting. It has also been used to calm nervous states.

chlorpropamide Diabinase. An orally taken drug to reduce the level of blood sugar. Used in the treatment of diabetes mellitus.

chlorquinaldol A medication effective in overcoming certain fungal and bacterial infections of the skin.

chlortetracycline (Aureomycin) An antibiotic.

chlorthalidone Hygroton. An anti-high blood pressure medication; also helpful in ridding the body of excess fluids, as in pregnancy, obesity, cirrhosis of the liver, etc.

Chlortrimeton A patented medication used to combat various allergies. An antihistaminic drug.

choana The internal back portion of the nasal openings.

chocolate cyst A cyst of the ovary containing blood, often old blood that has turned brown in color.

chokedamp Blackdamp; the gas present in mines.

choked disk Swelling of the retina of the eye at the site where the nerve enters. Seen in cases with increased pressure within the brain.

cholagogue A medication used to increase the flow of bile.

cholangiography X ray of the bile ducts.

cholangitis Inflammation of the bile ducts.

cholangiolitis Inflammation of the smaller bile ducts, located in the liver.

cholecyst The gall bladder.

cholecystectomy An operation for removal of the gall bladder; advocated when this organ contains stones or is the seat of infection.

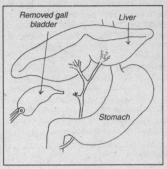

Cholecystectomy

cholecystitis Inflammation of the gall bladder.

cholecystoduodenostomy A surgical procedure uniting the gall bladder and the duodenum (a portion of the small intestine).

cholecystogastrostomy A surgical procedure in which the gall bladder is joined to the stomach.

cholecystography X ray of the gall bladder, after it has been visualized by the oral administration of a dye, or after injection of a dye. (Failure of the gall bladder to be visualized usually indicates that it is diseased.)

cholecystojejunostomy A surgical procedure uniting the gall bladder and jejunum (small intestine); advocated when there is obstruction, by a cancer, to the flow of bile into the intestines.

cholecystostomy A surgical procedure which establishes an opening into the gall bladder in order to drain its contents; performed in some cases of acute infection of the gall bladder where removal of the entire organ would prove dangerous.

choledochitis An inflammation of the common bile duct, usually secondary to gallstones in the bile duct.

choledochoduodenostomy An operation in which the common bile duct is sutured to the duodenum in order to short-circuit biliary obstruction.

choledocholithotomy The surgical removal of stones from the common bile duct.

choledochoscope An instrument to view the passageway of the common bile duct, inserted after making a surgical opening in the duct.

choledochotomy A surgical opening into the common bile duct, performed to remove stones.

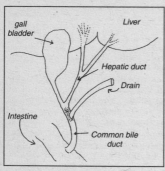

Choledochotomy

choledochus The common bile duct leading into the duodenum.

cholelithiasis The presence of stones in the gall bladder. (It can often be diagnosed by taking special X rays.)

cholemia Bile in the blood. This term is used to characterize a set of symptoms, usually ending fatally, caused by failure of the liver to get rid of its bile and bile products.

cholera A serious infectious disease characterized by vomiting, diarrhea, dehydration, cramps, high fever and collapse. Death ensues in 20 to 50 percent of cases.

choleresis Increased secretion of bile.

choleric Easily disturbed and irascible.

cholesteatoma A tumor containing cholesterol, occurring in the brain, middle ear, and elsewhere.

cholesterase An enzyme which changes cholesterol esters into cholesterol and fatty acids.

cholesteremia Excess cholesterol in the blood; thought to be a forerunner of hardening of the arteries.

cholesterol A chemical component of animal oils and fats. Excessive amounts are deposited in blood vessels and may be a factor in the causation of hardening of the arteries (arteriosclerosis).

cholesterosis Excessive cholesterol deposits in tissues or in an organ, such as *cholesterosis* of the gall bladder ("strawberry gall bladder").

cholinergic Referring to medications which block the action of parasympathetic nerves.

chologogue A medication that stimulates greater flow of bile.

cholografin An opaque dye injected into a vein which will, after X rays are taken, show the interior outline of the gall bladder and bile ducts.

choluria Bile in the urine.

chondral Pertaining to cartilage.

chondral calcinosis Replacement of cartilage within a joint by calcium. It may sometimes cause severe pain in a joint. Also known as pseudogout.

chondritis Inflammation of cartilage.

chondrocarcinoma A mixed tumor of a salivary gland, containing cartilagelike cells as well as other types of cells.

chondrocostal Referring to cartilage and ribs.

chondrocyte A cartilage cell.

chondrodystrophy A birth deformity in which the bones do not grow properly, often resulting in a stunted stature (dwarfism).

chondrofibroma A tumor, not malignant, containing cartilage and fibrous tissue.

chondroma A benign tumor of cartilage.

chondromalacia Softening of a cartilage.

chondromyxoma A tumor composed of cartilage cells and connective tissue cells.

chondrosarcoma A malignant tumor of cartilage.

CHOP An abbreviation for anticancer drugs, frequently used in the treatment of malignancies of the lymph glands (nodes).

chord A ligament, tendon or band of fibrous tissue.

chordae tendinae Strands of tissue attached to the papillary muscles of the ventricles of the heart and extending to the valves which are located in between the atria and the ventricles. They aid in normal heart action and in the smooth functioning of the heart valves.

chordee Curvature of the penis; an unusual condition.

chorditis Inflammation of the spermatic cord which connects with the testicle.

chordoma A rare tumor located at the base of the spine. Although it is malignant, it grows very slowly over a period of years.

chordotomy An operation performed upon the spinal cord to relieve pain, advocated in certain cases of incurable cancer where the pain is excruciating.

chorea A nervous disease characterized by involuntary and irregular movements of the muscles of the limbs and face. It is sometimes associated with rheumatic fever.

choreoathetosis A condition characterized by aimless muscle movements and involuntary motions.

chorioadenoma A tumor within the uterus, potentially malignant.

chorioallantois Membranes sur-

rounding the embryos of birds, used in chicks in the preparation of certain vaccines.

choriocarcinoma A very malignant form of cancer arising from primitive genital tissue, that is, the testicle in the male or the uterus or ovary in the female.

choriomeningitis An inflammation of the membranes covering the brain and spinal cord (the arachnoid and choroid).

chorion A membrane surrounding the fetus (embryo) within the womb (uterus).

chorionepithelioma Choriocarcinoma.

chorioretinitis An inflammatory condition in the back of the eye.

chorioretinopathy Disease of the retina of the eye and the choroid, a membrane of the eyeball.

choristoma A developmental defect in which groups of cells of one organ are located in a nearby organ where they don't belong.

choroid A membrane of the eyeball containing blood vessels.

    plexus A grouping of small blood vessels and covering membranes which project into the ventricles (the hollow space filled with fluid) of the brain.

choroiditis Inflammation of the choroid, a membrane or coat of the eyeball.

chrematophobia Fear of money.

Christian-Schüller disease A rare disease of infants in which there are abnormal deposits of fatty substance. There is softening of the skull and other bones, with marked prominence of the eyeballs, etc.

Christian Science healing A method of bringing about healing through prayer.

Christian-Weber disease A condition in which there is marked inflammation of the subcutaneous fat in patchy areas, often in the abdominal region. It tends to clear up and return frequently.

Christmas disease A hereditary

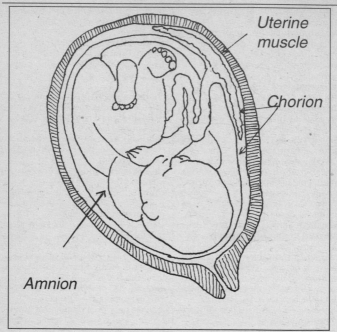

Chorion

disease having many of the characteristics of hemophilia. (Laboratory tests distinguish one from the other.)

chromaffin Cells of the adrenal and other glands and certain nerves which stain deeply with chromium dye.

chromaffinoma A tumor containing chromaffin cells; also referred to as paraganglioma; pheochromocytoma.

chromaphil Cells which take a deep stain when being prepared with chromium salts for microscopic examination.

chromatin The substance within the nucleus of a cell which stains easily when being prepared for microscopic examination.

chromatin body A small dot of stainable material seen near the periphery of a nucleus. It is normally present in females and absent in males. Also called a Barr body.

chromatosis Abnormal pigmentation in the tissues.

chromhidrosis Having colored perspiration; a rare condition.

chromogen A substance which produces color.

chromophobe Cells which do not take stains readily when being prepared for microscopic examination.

chromosome The body within a cell that contains the genes, which are responsible for the child's inheritance of the parents' appearance and traits.

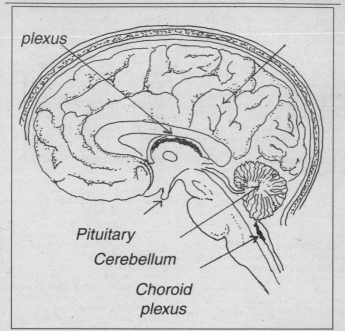

plexus

Pituitary

Cerebellum

Choroid plexus

Choroid plexus

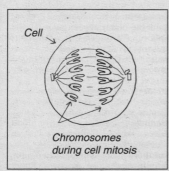

Cell

Chromosomes during cell mitosis

Chromosomes

accessory One that is not paired.

bivalent A temporarily united maternal and paternal chromosome.

dicentric An abnormally constructed chromosome containing two, instead of one, centromeres.

heterotropic Same as accessory chromosome.

Philadelphia (Ph') A tiny abnormal chromosome seen in cells of many patients with chronic leukemia.

sex The pair of chromosomes responsible for sex determination. Males have X and Y sex chromosomes; females have two X sex chromosomes.

X A sex chromosome. If a male sperm containing an X chromosome fertilizes an egg, a female embryo will result.

Y A sex chromosome appearing in half the male sperm. If a male sperm containing a Y sex chromosome fertilizes an egg, a male embryo will result.

chronic Of long duration. Not acute.

chronic cystic mastitis *See* cystic disease of the breasts.

chronic hypertrophic pulmonary osteoarthropathy *See* clubbed fingers.

chrysarobin A local medication for the treatment of eczema, psoriasis, and certain fungal infections of the skin.

chrysotherapy Treatment with gold compounds. Carried out in certain cases of arthritis.

chyle Partially digested fat which is being transported from the intestines through lymph channels.

chylothorax Milky fluid (chyle) in the chest cavity.

chylous ascites A large collection of lymph in the abdominal cavity, sometimes secondary to blockage of the main lymph duct or injury to it.

chylous cyst A sac containing lymph, sometimes located in the abdominal cavity in the region of the small intestines.

chyluria The presence of fat or lymph (a milky fluid) in the urine.

chyme Food which has been acted upon by stomach juices but has not yet been passed on into the intestines.

chymotrypsin An enzyme (chemical) found in the small intestines which aids in the digestion of proteins.

cicatrix A scar or scar tissue.

cicatrization The process of scar formation.

cilia Eyelashes or other hairlike structures found in various bodily tissues.

ciliary body The muscles which dilate and contract the pupil of the eye.

cimetidine A medication that is greatly effective in reducing stomach acidity. (The trade name is Tagamet.)

cinchona The bark of a tree from which quinine is derived; used in the treatment of malaria.

cincophen A chemical used in the treatment of gout and rheumatism. Overdoses are dangerous.

cineangiography The taking of moving pictures to show the passage of an opaque dye through blood vessels.

cinefluorography The taking of moving pictures of organs in motion on a fluoroscopic X-ray screen.

cinematoradiography X rays of organs in motion, such as the heart.

cinephotomicrography The taking of moving pictures of microscopic objects, such as cells that are dividing, bacteria in motion, etc.

cineplastic amputation One in which the muscles and tendons of the amputation stump are arranged so that they can perform movements of the attached artificial limb.

cineroentgenography Motion picture X rays.

Cipro A patented antibacterial drug useful in combating a wide variety of infections of the respiratory, gastrointestinal, and urinary tracts.

ciprofloxacin An antibacterial drug, effective against many bacteria.

circinate Circular or ringlike.

circle of Willis A group of arteries surrounding the base of the brain.

circulation The passage of blood from the heart to all parts of the body and its return from the tissues to the heart.

circulation time The rate of blood flow; a good gauge of heart efficiency.

circumcision Removal of the foreskin of the penis or excision of a circular piece of the prepuce.

circumflex Said of a nerve or blood vessel which winds around a structure.

circumoral Surrounding the mouth, as in the *circumoral* paleness seen in fevers like scarlet fever.

cirrhosis An inflammatory disease of the liver associated with the replacement of liver cells by fibrous tissue. Passage of blood through the liver may eventually be obstructed by the cirrhosis.

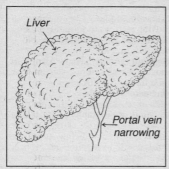

Cirrhosis with portal obstruction

cirsoid Looking like a varicose vein.

cirsoid aneurysm A grouping of dilated undulating small arteries, capillaries, and veins beneath the skin of the scalp. It forms a large soft mass and is most difficult to remove surgically because of the marked bleeding which ensues.

CIS Abbreviation for "carcinoma in situ"; a cancer that has not spread from the local tumor.

Cisplatin A chemotherapy drug, useful in the treatment of advanced cancers of the ovaries, testicles, bladder, and other organs.

cistern A receptacle or reservoir.

cisternal puncture Tapping spinal fluid from a point just beneath the skull in the back of the neck. Performed in certain cases of suspected spinal cord or brain tumors.

citrated Denoting the addition of sodium or potassium citrate to blood, milk, or some other fluid. The addition of citrate to blood to be used for transfusion, will prevent it from clotting.

citric acid The acid found in citrus fruits, such as orange, lemon, grapefruit, etc.

citronella An oil used to repel mosquitoes and other insects.

cittosis An abnormal desire for strange foods, as sometimes occurs during pregnancy; pica.

Cl The chemical symbol for chlorine.

clairvoyance A supposed sixth sense by which one obtains knowledge of events or can discern objects not actually present to the senses.

clamp A surgical instrument used to stop bleeding from cut blood vessels; a hemostat.

clap Slang expression for gonorrhea.

clasmocytoma See reticulum cell sarcoma.

claudication Cramplike pains in the legs due to insufficient arterial blood supply to the muscles. Seen in association with hardening of the arteries of the legs.

claustrophobia Morbid fear of confined or closed-in places.

claustrum An obstruction or barrier. (An anatomical term).

clavicle The collarbone, extending from the sternum (breastbone) to the shoulder tip.

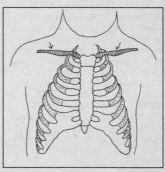

Clavicle

clavus A corn often found on the toes or foot.

clawfoot A foot with an exceptionally high arch: Pes cavus.

clawhand A deformity of the hand

produced by paralysis of nerves to the middle, ring, and little fingers.

clearance test A chemical analysis in which the rate at which a substance passes through the kidney is determined; a test of kidney function.

clearing station In warfare, a point near the battle area where wounded soldiers receive first aid prior to being sent to hospitals to the rear.

cleavage 1. Lines in the skin denoting the direction of underlying fibers. 2. The process of development early in the life of an embryo, when the embryo is a mass of cells.

cleft palate A birth deformity in which the palate (the roof of the mouth) fails to fuse along its midline. It can usually be corrected surgically.

cleido- Pertaining to the collarbone (clavicle).

cleidomastoid muscles The large muscles on either side of the neck running from the back of the skull to the inner portion of the collarbones (clavicles).

Cleocin A patented antibiotic, effective against gram-positive bacteria. A brand of *clindamycin.*

cleptomania An abnormal desire to steal objects which often are useless or unneeded; *kleptomania.*

climacteric The menopause; change of life. It occurs usually from forty-five to fifty years of age.

climatotherapy The treatment of sickness by sending the patient to another more favorable climate, such as sending a hay fever sufferer to a pollen-free region.

climax 1. Orgasm; the peak of the sexual act. 2. The period of peak intensity of a disease.

clindomycin A powerful antibiotic, effective against anaerobic (nonoxygen using) bacteria such as *Bacteroides.* It is also used to combat staphylococcal and streptococcal infections. *See* Cleocin.

clinic An outpatient department of a hospital where patients are treated on an ambulatory basis.

clinical Relating to the course of a disease as observed by the physician.

Clinical assistant The lowest rank on the staff of a hospital, usually awarded to physicians just beginning their hospital affiliation.

Clinician A practitioner of medicine, particularly one who devotes most of his time to practice among patients.

clinicopathological Pertaining to the study of disease in a patient and related changes in the structure and function of tissues and organs.

Clinoril A medication helpful in the treatment of rheumatoid arthritis.

clip A metal appliance, used to hold tissue together, such as a skin *clip,* or to compress a small bleeding vessel.

clitoridectomy Surgical removal of the clitoris.

clitoris Part of the external female genitals, containing erectile tissue and located above the opening which leads from the bladder. (It is the female counterpart of the penis.)

clitoromania Nymphomania. Abnormal sexual desire in a woman.

cloaca A common opening for the intestinal and urinary tracts, present during the early stages of the development of the embryo.

Clomid See clomiphene citrate.

clomiphene citrate A powerful hormone which stimulates ovulation in women who do not ovulate. Its use has been followed in some cases by pregnancies resulting in multiple births (twins, triplets, quadruplets, quintuplets, etc.)

clone A cell derived from a single cell, not from the union of two cells.

clonic Referring to jerky muscle contractions or spasms. Opposite of tonic spasms.

cloning The developing of cells or organisms with identical genes. *See* genes.

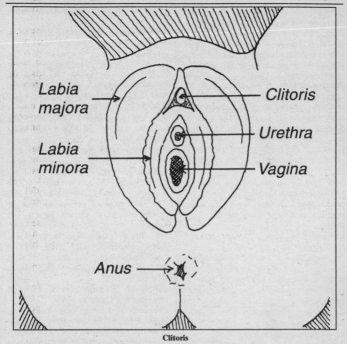

Labia majora

Labia minora

Anus

Clitoris

Urethra

Vagina

Clitoris

closed-chest massage A technique used to revive a heart which has stopped beating; a first-aid measure used upon people who suddenly "drop dead." The palm of the hand is placed upon the breastbone of the patient and rhythmic downward pressure and release of pressure is carried out at the rate of eighty times per minute. The first aider should kneel so as to straddle the patient. The downward pressure should be sufficient to depress the breastbone about 1 inch. Massage should be continued until rigor mortis sets in or the heart beat returns. Mouth to mouth breathing should be carried out simultaneously if another person is available. *See also* artificial respiration in *Manual.*

closed reduction Setting a fracture by manipulation of the bones. The opposite of *open reduction,* in which an operation is performed to place the broken bones in alignment.

clostridium The name of a large group of spore-bearing bacteria which live without oxygen. Many of them can cause severe infections, such as tetanus, lockjaw, gas gangrene, etc.

clostridium perfringens A bacterium that causes gas gangrene.

closure The suturing of a wound.

clot Solidification (coagulation) of blood or lymph.

clotting time The length of time, in minutes, it takes blood to solidify (coagulate) when exposed to air.

Clozapine A medication used in

treating schizophrenic psychosis. Its administration must be closely monitored for unwanted side effects.

clubbed fingers A rounding out of the tips of the fingers, seen in some cases of chronic lung or chronic heart disease. Also called *drumstick fingers.*

clubfoot A birth deformity in which the front portion of the foot is deformed and turned inward. It can be benefited greatly by surgery.

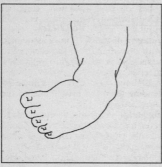
Clubfoot

clumping Cells which group together and adhere to one another. Also referred to as agglutination.

cluster headache A chronic headache condition, also called migrainous neuralgia.

clyster An enema.

cm. Centimeter.

CMA Abbreviation for Certified Medical Assistant.

CMF Abbreviation for cytoxan, methotrexate and 5FU, a combination of chemicals helpful in treating breast cancer that has spread to distant parts of the body.

CMV Abbreviation for cytomegalovirus, encountered often in patients with AIDS.

Co Chemical symbol for cobalt.

CO₂ laser laparoscope A laser beam aimed through a laparoscope to destroy adhesions or harmful implants, such as those found in endometriosis.

coagulation The formation of a clot, as in blood *coagulation.*

coagulopathy A disorder keeping the blood from clotting normally.

coal miner's disease A lung inflammation caused by inhaling coal dust; silicosis. It leads to the formation of fibrous tissue in the lungs.

coal tar derivatives Those chemicals derived from the breakdown and distillation of coal. To name a few: benzene, naptha, phenol, pitch, etc. Many useful drugs are essentially coal tar derivatives.

coarctation A narrowing of the passageway of a blood vessel, such as *coarctation of the aorta,* due to compression of the walls of the vessel.

cobalt (Co) A metal element which, when rendered radioactive, can be used in the same manner as X rays in the treatment of malignant disease.

cobalt-60 Radioactive cobalt used in radiation therapy.

cocaine A strong local anesthetic agent, effective when applied to mucous membrane surface. It can become extremely habit forming when used as an inhalant.

coccidioidosis A disease of the lungs caused by inhaling certain spores of a fungus. Also called *desert fever* or *San Joaquin Valley fever.*

coccus A round-shaped germ, such as the staphylococcus, streptococcus, etc.

coccydynia Pain in the coccyx (tailbone).

coccygectomy Removal of the coccyx bone at the base of the spine; an operation performed when this bone is dislocated and causes continual pain.

coccygeus A muscle in the region of the coccyx.

coccygodynia Pain in the region of the coccyx (the tailbone, located at the base of the spine).

coccyx The last bone of the spinal

column, sometimes referred to as man's vestigial tail.

cochlea The internal ear which harbors the main organ of hearing and is also concerned with the sense of balance (equilibrium).

cochleal implant An experimental operation to relieve deafness.

cocillana An ingredient in medications to help bring up phlegm in cases of bronchitis.

codeine A derivative of opium which is pain relieving to a lesser degree but not as strongly habit forming.

cod-liver oil An oil obtained from the livers of certain fish. It is extremely rich in vitamin D.

coelom The abdominal cavity; the peritoneal cavity.

coenzyme A substance essential to the action of enzymes. Vitamins such as nicotinamide and thiamin are coenzymes.

cognition The process of knowing or being aware.

cohabitation The living together of a man and woman.

coherence 1. Agreement or reasonableness. 2. Sticking together.

cohesion The force which holds together the molecules of a substance.

Cohnheim theory One that postulates that malignant cells originate from embryonic cells that persist in the unborn child's organs.

coin lesion A round shadow seen on X ray, sometimes representing the presence of a cyst, a cancer, or tuberculosis.

coitus Sexual intercourse.

Colace A non-habit-forming stool softener. While it aids bowel evacuation, it is not a laxative.

ColBenemid A combination of colchicine and Benemid, used to prevent attacks of gout and to relieve the pain and swelling associated with an acute attack.

colchicine A medication used in the treatment of gout.

cold The common cold; an inflammation of the mucous membrane of the nose caused by a virus; coryza.

coldsore A crusted sore of the lips seen in people who have had a cold or an illness accompanied by fever.

colectomy Removal of the large bowel, or a portion thereof.

colic Severe abdominal pain.

   renal Excruciating, sudden pain in the kidney region and along the ureter, caused by a kidney stone.

colitis Inflammation of the large bowel (colon). There are many types of this condition, some of minor importance, others very serious.

collagen diseases Those associated with disturbances in the connective tissues, such as that around joints, arteries, etc.

collarbone The clavicle, a bone extending from the breastbone to the shoulder tip.

collateral Secondary; often used to refer to *collateral* circulation (blood vessels which carry the blood when a main blood vessel is blocked).

Colles' fracture The most frequently encountered fracture of the wrist, involving a break in the radius and ulna bones.

collodion "New skin." It is used as a dressing on skin because it has the property of adhering tightly to a skin surface.

colloid A form of matter in which the particles are of such small size that they cannot be seen through a microscope. (A colloid particle measures between 1 and 100 millimicrons in size.)

   degeneration Excessive production of colloid by the thyroid gland (resulting in degeneration of some of the secreting cells within the gland).

   gold test A test for syphilis of the nervous system, performed upon spinal fluid.

collum Neck.

collyrium A popular eye wash.

coloboma A birth deformity of the iris (colored portion) of the eye.

colon   The large bowel, extending from the cecum to the anus. It is approximately five to seven feet in length.

     colonoscopy   Examination of the large bowel through an instrument inserted into the rectum. The instrument is flexible and can be inserted for a distance of several feet.

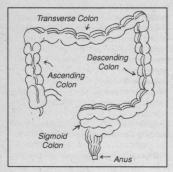

Colon

colony   A growth or cluster of bacteria, a term usually referring to the appearance of bacteria which have been grown in the laboratory.

Colorado tick fever   A virus infection transmitted by the bite of an infected tick. It causes fever for a few days and a lowering of the white blood cell count. Also called *tick fever*.

color-blind   Unable to distinguish colors. This is an inherited characteristic seen only in males. Most colorblindness is present for a limited number of colors, e.g., red-green.

colorectal   The anatomical region consisting of the lower large intestine and the rectum.

colorimeter   An instrument for measuring color. It is used to measure hemoglobin content of blood.

colostomy   An operation in which the large bowel is brought to the abdominal wall and given an opening there. It is often performed to relieve large-bowel obstruction.

colostrum   The first milk from the mother's breast, occurring shortly before or during the first few days after childbirth.

colotomy   A surgical incision into the large intestine (colon).

colpectomy   Surgical removal of the vagina, performed in cases of cancer of this structure.

colpitis   Inflammation of the vagina.

colpolaparoscopy   Viewing the pelvic organs through an instrument passed through the upper portion of the vagina into the abdominal cavity.

colpoplasty   Surgical repair of a tear in the wall of the vagina, a condition common following difficult childbirth.

colporrhaphy   Surgical repair of the vagina; colpoplasty.

colposcopy   Examination of the vagina with a special instrument (speculum).

columella   1. The tissue between the nostrils. 2. The central axis of the cochlea of the ear.

Coly-mycin (colistin)   An antibiotic found to be particularly effective in combating gram-negative urinary infections.

coma   Unconsciousness.

comatose   Being in a state of unconsciousness or coma.

Combid   A medication to control nausea, reduce acid secretion by the stomach, and relieve anxiety.

comedo   A blackhead or clogged pore.

comedocarcinoma   A type of breast cancer in which the malignant cells are in the breast ducts.

Commando procedure   An operation sometimes performed for a cancer of the tongue that involves the lymph glands in the neck. It entails removal of parts of the tongue and lower jaw, and removal of the lymph glands in the neck.

comminuted fracture   One in which the bone is broken into several pieces.

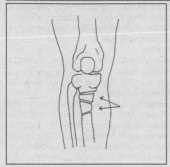

Comminuted fracture

commissure The tissues that bind together opposite but corresponding parts, such as where the eyelids join or where nerve fiber strands unite in the two sides of the brain or spinal cord.

commissurotomy An operation upon the heart in which a deformed heart valve is cut so as to permit a more normal flow of blood.

companionate marriage A "marriage" which has not been legalized but continues by mutual consent.

compatibility 1. The ability of two substances to coexist. 2. In blood grouping, the ability of blood from two different people to mix without clotting. 3. In marriage, two partners who get along well together.

Compazine (prochlorperazine) A drug used to control nausea and vomiting.

compensation To make up for a defect or to counterbalance some deficiency.

compensation case An injury or disease incurred because of the work one performs.

complex In psychology, a group of emotionally important ideas which are related to abnormal thinking or behavior.

complexion Color and appearance of the face.

complication An unforeseen con-

dition occurring during the course of a disease.

compos mentis Of sound mind (a Latin term).

compound Two or more chemicals united chemically into one substance.

compound fracture One in which the skin overlying the bone is lacerated or punctured.

compress A poultice, wet or dry, cold or hot, applied for the purpose of relieving inflammation.

compression Undue pressure; applied to control bleeding.

compulsion An uncontrollable impulse to do something.

compulsive neurosis One in which the person feels compelled to follow a certain behavior pattern, which is repeated over and over again. Such people usually have rigid personalities and are overly conscientious.

computerized axial tomography See CAT scanner.

Computerized Medicine A branch of medicine in which diagnosis and treatment are obtained through computers that have been programmed by a panel of medical experts.

conation The power of the mind as it relates to carrying out a thought or act.

concave Hollowed out; a curved-in surface.

conceive To become pregnant.

concentration 1. The measure of the degree of dilution of a solution. 2. The power to organize one's thoughts and carry out one's aims.

conception Pregnancy.

concha The hollow portion of the outer ear.

concretion A stone, such as a gallstone which is a solidification and concentration of bile.

concussion A blow; a shock; a sudden head injury associated with momentary unconsciousness.

condensation The transformation of a gas into a liquid, as of moisture in the air to form water.

conditioning 1. Getting one's muscles into better shape through graded exercise. 2. Obtaining a new reaction to a familiar stimulus or an old response to a new stimulus; a psychological term.

condom A covering for the penis, used during sexual intercourse to prevent infection or pregnancy.

conduction The passage of an electrical, heat or sound wave along certain tissues, such as nerves, etc.

conductive system of the heart The mechanism by which impulses to contract are transmitted to the muscles of the heart so as to create an orderly rhythmic heart beat.

conductor A body substance which transmits energy in the form of electrical stimuli, sound waves, etc.

condyles The rounded portions of the bones, usually at the joints.

condylitis Inflammation of a bony condyle, usually near a joint.

condyloma Warty growth usually around the orifice of the rectum (anus), or the vulva.

confabulation The giving of plausible answers by a mentally sick patient (thus making the diagnosis of mental disease more difficult).

confidentiality Referring to the fact that physicians must keep information obtained from patients confidential, if that is the wish of the patient.

confinement Giving birth, or the lying-in period.

conflict In psychology or psychoanalysis, the opposition of two or more wishes or desires, causing emotional disturbances.

confluent Running together, such as several boils united to form a carbuncle.

confusion A mental state marked by mingling of ideas and feelings resulting in disorientation and inability to resolve a problem.

congelation Frostbite.

congenital defects Birth deformities; anomalies.

congenital polycystic kidney disease A hereditary disease associated with innumerable cysts in the kidneys. Kidney function tends to fail as the person approaches middle age.

congestion An excessive amount of blood in a body area (hyperemia). Such areas appear pinkish, reddish or reddish-blue.

congestive heart failure Retention of salt and water due to impaired heart function. Symptoms include shortness of breath, swelling of the legs and feet (dropsy), and poor circulation of the blood.

conglomeration Grouped or massed together, such as a *conglomeration* of cells.

Congo red A dye used in tests for mineral acids and in other laboratory tests.

conization Removal of a cone-shaped segment of tissue, as *conization* of the cervix of the uterus (performed for erosion of the cervix).

conjoined anastomosis The stitching of small vessels to one another.

conjugation Fertilization, in lower forms of animal life.

conjunctivitis An inflammation of the covering membrane of the eye. There are many forms of conjunctivitis, depending upon the germ or irritant causing it.

connective tissue Fibrous tissue which connects and holds together cells of an organ. Also, tissues which lie between various structures, such as the tissues between muscles, blood vessels, etc.

Conn's syndrome *See* syndrome, Conn's.

consanguinity Blood relationship.

conscious Mentally aware; awake; not unconscious.

consent 1. Acquiescence or willingness. 2. In legal terms: voluntary authorization for the act in question, such as an operation.

consistency The degree of softness or hardness of a structure.

consolidation The appearance (becoming firm) of a lung involved in pneumonia. A *consolidated* lung is one in which the air cells are filled with fluid, mucus or pus.

constellation A psychiatric term referring to all the factors determining a particular action or reaction.

constipation Difficult bowel evacuation, occurring at prolonged intervals; excessively hardened stool.

constitution The make-up, both physical and psychological, of an individual.

constitutional disease A disease which originates because of the peculiar make-up (constitution) of an individual.

constriction Contraction; narrowing.

Consultant A physician, usually a specialist, called in to see a patient by another physician.

consultation The discussion of a patient by two or more physicians.

consumption An old term for tuberculosis of the lungs.

contact dermatitis An inflammation of the skin due to contact with an irritant, such as a chemical or plant. Poison ivy, detergents, etc., may cause contact dermatitis.

contact lenses Lenses, to aid vision, which fit directly on the anterior surface of the eyeball.

contagion The spreading of disease from one person to another. This may take place by direct contact, as in venereal or other diseases, or it may occur as a result of germs being spread by coughing, by allowing them to get onto dishes, bedclothes, etc.

contamination Soiling; permitting germs or infected material to touch clean surfaces. In an operating room *contamination* occurs when something unsterile touches something sterile.

contiguous Adjacent; bordering upon. Certain localized conditions spread to other body structures because they are *contiguous*.

continence Self-restraint, such as abstinence from sexual intercourse; the ability to retain one's excretions.

continuous positive pressure breathing Mechanically controlled respirations.

continuous wear contact lens A contact lens that can be worn, without removal, for a week or more.

contortion A writhing movement; getting into a distorted position.

contraceptive An agent used to prevent conception (pregnancy).

contractility The ability of tissue to shorten or contract as a result of stimulation, such as a muscle.

contraction A temporary shortening, as of a muscle fiber or muscle.

contract medicine The practice of medicine under prearranged terms of payment, such as is done by a group of physicians who agree to serve a group of people under a prepaid health insurance program.

contracture The shortening of a muscle, tendon or other structure so that it cannot be straightened or readily flexed and extended. Scar tissue often results in *contractures*.

contraindication A condition rendering something else not indicated; not advisable. (A *contraindication* to elective surgery is a cold or bronchitis.)

contralateral Opposite, usually referring to the opposite side of the body.

contrast medium An opaque substance, such as barium, given internally for better visualization of parts of the body on X ray.

contrecoup Injury, by rebound, to a part of the body opposite to that receiving the direct blow; a *contrecoup* injury to the brain.

contrectation The love play which precedes sexual intercourse.

control experiment One carried out to check results and validity of methodology.

controlled drug One which the physician and the druggist must record as having been dispensed. The term applies to drugs that might become addictive or habit-forming.

contusion A bruise; an ecchymosis; hemorrhage into and beneath the skin.

conus A cone-shaped structure, such as the *conus terminalis*, the cone-shaped end of the spinal cord.

convalescence The recovery period after an illness.

conversion 1. A mental protective device whereby an emotional problem is transformed into a physical one. 2. In obstetrics, changing the position of the baby within the uterus so as to aid its delivery.

conversion hysteria A psychoneurosis in which, by an unconscious mental maneuver, a difficult emotional problem is turned into a physical disability, such as hysterical paralysis, hysterical blindness, etc. It is a defense mechanism.

convex Protruding of the surface in a spherical direction; the opposite of concave.

convolution One of the folds of brain tissue in the cerebrum. Each convolution harbors brain tissue concerned with various definite body functions.

convulsion A violent, uncontrolled muscle spasm, or a series of them, sometimes repeated at rapid intervals. Some convulsions are accompanied by unconsciousness.

convulsive disorders Any disease associated with recurring convulsions. Epilepsy is now classified as a *convulsive disorder.*

Cooley's anemia Anemia seen among people who dwell in the Mediterranean area. It is associated with underdevelopment of the body, enlarged spleen, slight jaundice and evidence of destruction of red blood cells.

coordination The proper functioning of organs in relation to each other, such as muscles and nerves, to produce the desired result.

COPD Abbreviation for chronic obstructive pulmonary disease.

copper (Cu) A metal which, when combined with other chemicals, can serve as a useful medication. Often found in preparations for the treatment of anemia.

copremesis The vomiting of feces; often encountered in intestinal obstruction.

coproantibodies Antibodies which grow in the intestinal tract and protect against the development of certain diseases, such as cholera.

coprolalia Using dirty, vulgar speech.

coprophagy The eating of feces, encountered occasionally in infants or in mentally unbalanced patients.

coprophemia Obscene or dirty speech.

coprophilia Excessive interest in feces, as seen in some mentally ill patients.

coprophobia Morbid repugnance to defecation and to feces.

copulation Sexual intercourse.

cor The heart.

coracoacromial Referring to the bones which form the tip of the shoulder.

coracobrachialis A muscle of the upper arm, whose action draws the arm in toward the body.

coracoclavicular Referring to the point where the scapula (wingbone) meets the clavicle (collarbone).

cord A stringlike structure, such as the *umbilical cord* or the *spermatic cord* (to which the testicle is attached).

Cordarone A drug indicated for the treatment of irregularities of the heart, such as fibrillation.

cordotomy An operation to cut certain pain fibers in the spinal cord, employed mainly in cases of extensive cancer to relieve unbearable pain.

cord presentation The appearance of the umbilical cord at the outlet of the vagina during labor. In such instances, rapid delivery is necessary in order to save the child.

Cordran Ointment A cortisone-containing ointment which, when applied to the skin, may reduce inflammation and relieve itching.

corectopia A condition of the eye in which the pupil is not centrally placed.

coreometer An instrument for measuring the size of the pupil of the eye.

coreoplasty An operation to repair a deformed pupil of the eye.

Corgard A drug often effective in the long-term treatment of angina pectoris.

corium The deepest layer of the skin.

Cormax An ointment used on the scalp to relieve irritation; should not be applied for more than a few weeks at a time.

corn A thickening of the skin, located on the toes.

cornea The transparent membrane on the anterior surface of the eyeball. The pupil is located in the center of the cornea.

corneal transplant A transplant of the tissue that covers the pupil and iris (colored portion) of the eye.

cornification A degeneration and thickening of the cells of a skin surface and their hardening into a horny consistency. Also called hornification.

cornu A horn-shaped projection or portion of an organ, such as the portion of the uterus near the entrance of the fallopian tubes.

cornual pregnancy Pregnancy which has implanted in the cornu of the uterus. This can be dangerous because rupture of the uterus may take place as the embryo grows.

coronary arteries Arteries supplying the heart muscle. When these vessels become narrowed with arteriosclerosis, or when a clot forms within them, damage to the heart muscle ensues.

    occlusion Closure (thrombosis) of a coronary artery. It is accompanied by severe pain in the chest, shock, and, in some cases, sudden death. However, the majority of patients survive the initial attack and recover within several weeks' time.

    thrombosis Clotting of a coronary artery in the heart. *See also* coronary occlusion.

coronary bypass operation A heart operation in which a vein graft taken from the leg is used to bypass an obstructed coronary artery. The graft is attached at one end to the aorta, and at the other end to that portion of the coronary artery located beyond the obstruction. Very helpful in the treatment of angina pectoris.

Coronary Care Unit (C.C.U.) An intensive-care unit set aside for those who have had heart attacks.

coronary endarterectomy An operation to ream out arteriosclerotic plaques from the coronary artery. The procedure is in its experimental stage and employed only rarely.

coroner A medical officer whose responsibilities include the investigation of suspicious deaths, or deaths of unknown cause.

corpora cavernosa The spongy tissue making up most of the shaft of the penis. When it fills with blood, an erection ensues.

corpse A dead body.

corpulent Obese; fat.

corpus 1. Body. 2. The main part of an organ.

corpuscle A cell with a rounded shape, as a red blood cell.

corpus cavernosum The lateral portions of the penis. It contains erectile tissue.

corpus delicti The proof and evidence which must be presented in court to establish the commission of a crime.

corpus luteum A small yellow area in an ovary found at the site where an egg has formed and burst from the gland.

corpus spongiosum The middle portion of the penis, through which the urethra passes. It contains erectile tissue.

Corrigan pulse The pounding

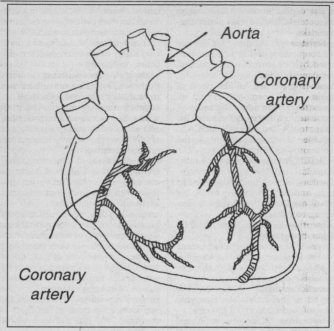

Coronary artery

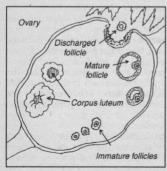

Corpus luteum of the ovary

pulse noted in those who have a diseased incompetent aortic valve
within the heart.

corrosive An agent which destroys
living tissue by chemical action.

Cortate The trademark for an extract of the cortex of the adrenal
gland. It is given to combat shock resulting from insufficient functioning
of the adrenal gland.

Cortef A patented name for hydrocortisone; used as a medication
both locally and internally.

cortex The surface layer of an
organ such as the kidney or adrenal glands.

cortical seizures (Jacksonian) Convulsions limited to one part of the
body, such as an arm or a leg. Such
seizures are usually due to a localized brain tumor or other brain condition.

corticoid Having an action similar

to that of the hormone secreted by the cortex of the adrenal gland; cortisonelike.

corticosteroid A chemical having the properties of the hormone secreted by the cortex (outer layer) of the adrenal gland.

corticotropin *See* ACTH.

Cortin The hormonal extract of the cortex of the adrenal gland.

cortisone A hormone secreted by the cortex of the adrenal gland.

Cortone (cortisone acetate) A steroid (cortisone) medication used in many different conditions, including glandular deficiencies, rheumatic disorders, allergic states, skin diseases, and certain cancers.

Cortril ointment An ointment containing cortisone.

coruscation A sensation of light flashes before the eyes.

coryza The common cold; acute rhinitis. It is thought to be caused by a virus.

cosmesis *See* cosmetic surgery.

cosmetic surgery Surgery performed to beautify or improve the looks of a patient.

cosmic rays Rays of extremely high penetrating power originating beyond the earth's atmosphere.

costal arch The arch formed by the ribs just above the abdomen.

costal cartilage The cartilage which connects the long ribs to the sternum (breastbone).

costochondral Referring to the ribs and the cartilages which join them to the breastbone.

costochondritis Inflammation and pain in the area where the cartilages join the breastbone.

costophrenic angle The angle formed by the diaphragm and the ribs at the lowermost and outermost part of the chest cavity.

costovertebral junction The region in which the ribs meet the spine in the back.

cot, finger A thin rubber covering for the finger; used by physicians during examinations.

cotton wool A material coming from the down which covers cotton seeds. It is sometimes treated and used as a dressing to an injured part.

Coumadin An anticoagulant medication, often used to thin the blood of those who have suffered coronary thrombosis or who show a tendency toward blood clots and phlebitis.

counterirritant A medical agent or substance (such as a mustard plaster) applied to the skin to produce an irritation, in order to counteract a deep inflammation.

countertraction A pull to offset another pull. In cases of fracture, traction and countertraction are employed to bring bones into alignment.

coupled rhythm An irregularity of heartbeat in which each normal beat is followed by a premature contraction. Also called *coupling, bigeminy.*

Courvoisier's law A markedly distended gall bladder in a patient with cancer of the head of the pancreas.

Cowper's glands The glands located at the bulb of the urethra, the outlet from the urinary bladder.

cowpox The reaction caused by vaccination; also called *Vaccinia.* It confers immunity to smallpox.

coxalgia Pain in hip joint.

coxa valga A deformity of the femur (thighbone) in the hip region in which the angle between the neck and the shaft is increased beyond 140°.

coxa vara A deformity of the femur (thighbone) in the hip region in which the angle between the neck and the shaft is too acute; less than 90°.

Coxsackie disease An infectious disease with many of the symptoms of infantile paralysis or meningitis but which clears up without aftereffects within a few days. Thought to be caused by a specific virus.

CPR *See* cardiopulmonary resuscitation.

C-Quens An anovulatory, birth control medication.

crabs A slang expression for pubic lice.

cradle cap A dermatitis of the skin of the scalp seen in infants and characterized by the presence of scaly, crusted yellow patches which feel greasy to the touch. (The condition usually clears within 2 weeks if treated properly.)

cramps Very painful muscle contractions, as those which occur in the calf muscles or those in the uterus during menstruation.

cranial nerves The twelve paired nerves originating from the brain and making their exit via openings in the skull. *See also* Manual, Table of Nerves.

cranial sutures The lines of junction of the various bones composing the skull.

craniocleidodysostosis A birth deformity in which there is improper bone formation of the skull, face, and collarbones.

craniopathy Any disease of the head.

craniopharyngioma A tumor developing in the base of the brain in the vicinity of the pituitary gland.

cranioplasty A plastic operation performed on the bones of the skull.

craniosynostosis Premature hardening of the skull in an infant with closure of the fontanels (soft spots) by bone formation.

craniotabes Thinning of spots and wasting of bones of the skull, often found in an infant having rickets or syphilis.

craniotomy An operation performed upon the skull in which the brain is exposed.

cranium The skull.

crapulous Very drunk or sick from overindulgence in food.

craterization The operation of reaming out a section of bone, as in osteomyelitis.

creatinine A chemical normally found in the blood and excreted into the urine. Excessive amounts may indicate kidney disease.

cremaster The muscle which draws up the testicles. It is located around the spermatic cord originating in the groin.

cremation The burning of a corpse.

crenation A shriveled or scalloped appearance of dead red blood cells seen under a microscope.

crepitation 1. The noise heard when the edges of a broken bone rub together. 2. The sensation one gets upon feeling skin under which there is a collection of gas. 3. Cracking of the joints.

cretinism Severe thyroid deficiency or absent thyroid function occurring at birth or in infancy.

crib death The sudden-death phenomenon seen occasionally in apparently healthy infants. The cause of this tragic condition has not been discovered.

cribriform Sievelike.

cricoarytenoid Cartilages and one of the muscles in the throat.

cricoid cartilage A cartilage of the larynx in the front of the neck.

cricopharyngeus One of the throat muscles.

cricothyroid The muscle which causes the vocal cords to constrict.

crisis The turning point in a severe illness, such as pneumonia.

critical care specialist *See* intensivist.

critical list The list bearing the names of desperately sick hospital patients.

CRNA Abbreviation for Certified Registered Nurse Anesthetist.

Crohn's disease An ulcerative condition of the small and large bowel characterized by areas of granulomas along with the ulcers; also known as "granulomatous enterocolitis."

The disease is to be distinguished from ulcerative colitis, which is strictly limited to the large bowel.

crossmatching The process of mixing a sample of a donor's blood with that of a recipient, in order to make sure that they are compatible and will not cause clotting. This procedure is carried out before giving a blood transfusion.

cross section A slice of tissue to be examined. It is cut in a direction at right angles to the long axis of the part to be examined.

crotch The groin, formed by the junction of the torso and the thighs.

croton oil An extremely powerful and dangerous purgative (laxative).

croup An inflammation of the larynx accompanied by coughing, difficulty in breathing, fever, etc. It usually occurs in young children.

croup kettle A specially devised steam kettle used in the treatment of croup.

cruciate Cross-shaped.

crus Leg-shaped or root-shaped.

crush syndrome Failure of kidney function secondary to an extensive, severe crushing injury to one or more limbs.

crust Scab.

crutch A support to enable an injured person to walk.

cryesthesia Sensitivity to cold.

crymodynia Pain which comes on in damp or cold weather. Arthritic patients appear to have this condition.

cryo- Freezing; cold.

cryoanesthesia Producing anesthesia by the application of intense cold (freezing).

cryobiology That branch of science concerned with the effect of cold upon living matter.

cryoextraction Removal of the lens of the eye by use of the "cold scalpel," an instrument that has been artificially cooled.

cryogenics The science of cold and its uses in treating human ills.

cryohypophysectomy Destruction of the pituitary gland by cold. (A special cold applicator is inserted into the substance of the gland.)

cryoprobe An instrument that produces extreme freezing of a tissue, used in extracting cataracts. Also

used in destroying malignant tissues in bones and other structures.

cryosurgery Surgery using cold to destroy tissue or remove a tumor.

cryothalamectomy An operative procedure to relieve the palsy caused by Parkinson's disease. Intense cold is applied to the thalamus portion of the brain, thus destroying the area from which the palsy originates.

cryotherapy The use of cold in the treatment of disease.

crypt A small cavity or sac, such as the *crypts* in the mucous membrane of the anus.

cryptitis Inflammation of crypts, as occurs in the rectum or in the lining of the penis.

cryptogenic Of unknown origin.

cryptorchidism Failure of one or both testicles to descend.

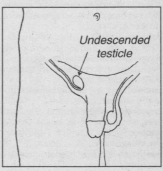

Cryptorchidism

cryptozygous A wide-skulled person with a narrow face.

crystalline lens The lens of the eye.

crystallization The transformation of a substance from a gas to liquid into a solid, thus forming crystals.

crystalloid Having a crystallike structure as opposed to a colloid structure. (This depends upon the size and shape of the individual particles making up the substance.)

crystalluria Crystals, such as urate or phosphate, in the urine.

Crysticillin A patented preparation of penicillin G procaine.

Cs Chemical symbol for cesium.

CSF Abbreviation for *cerebrospinal* fluid, the liquid surrounding the brain and spinal cord.

CT scan Same as CAT scan.

Cu Chemical symbol for copper.

cubital Referring to the forearm or elbow region.

cubitus The forearm.

cuboid An ankle bone.

cul-de-sac A blind pouch or sac, such as that behind the uterus within the abdomen.

culdoscope An instrument inserted through the vagina and into the abdominal cavity for the purpose of visualizing and examining the organs.

Culex A type of mosquito. (Culex tarsalis is thought to play an important role in the transmission of certain types of encephalitis, inflammation of the brain.)

culture Germs artificially grown. This is done in the laboratory in order to identify the bacteria and note their susceptibility to certain antibacterial drugs.

cumulative Accumulating; increasing in amount.

cuneiform Wedge-shaped; specifically, it may refer to bones in the ankle or wrist.

cunnilingus A sex practice in which the external female genitals are licked.

cunnus The external female genitals; the vulva.

cupola Shaped like a dome, as the *cupola* of the lungs.

cupping A method of bloodletting in which many suction cups were applied to the skin surface and blood was supposedly sucked up to the skin surface. This practice is now obsolete.

Cuprex A patented medicine used to get rid of lice.

cupula Any structure shaped like a cup.

curare A poison (used by the Indi-

ans years ago on their arrowheads) which paralyzes nerves and muscles. Modified forms of curare are used extensively today to relax muscles during anesthesia.

curet A scoop-shaped instrument used for scraping tissues.

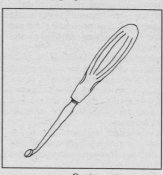

Curet

curettage Scraping the interior surface of an organ with an instrument (curet). Usually, the scraping of the cavity of the uterus.

curvature of the spine A general term applied to many abnormal conditions such as scoliosis, kyphosis, lordosis, etc., in which the spinal column is not in alignment.

Cushing's disease A benign tumor of the pituitary gland.

cusp 1. The pointed part of a tooth. 2. A leaf of a heart valve.

cuspid A canine tooth; having a single cusp.

cutaneous Relating to the skin.

cutdown Surgical dissection and isolation of a vein or, occasionally, an artery, in order to insert a needle for the administration of blood or other fluids.

cuticle That part of the skin adjacent to the finger or toe nails.

cutis The skin.

CVA Abbreviation for *cerebrovascular accident*; a stroke.

CVP Abbreviation for central venous pressure; a method of measuring heart output of blood and blood volume by inserting a polyethylene tube through a vein in the arm or neck. The tube is advanced until it lies within the right atrium (auricle) of the heart.

cyanide poisoning A rapidly fatal type of poisoning resulting from a combination of cyanide with the red blood cells, thus preventing the red cells from carrying oxygen to the tissues.

cyanocobalamine Vitamin B_{12}.

cyanosis Bluish color to the skin and mucous membranes, usually due to poor circulation and insufficient oxygen in the bloodstream.

cybernetics The study of the brain and nervous system through electrical computers, with attempts to explain and control brain actions and reactions through computerized communication.

cycle Bodily changes which occur with regularity and then recede, such as a *menstrual cycle.*

cyclic therapy Hormone treatment carried out intermittently, according to the phases of the menstrual cycle.

cyclitis Inflammation of the ciliary body (around the colored portion) of the eye.

Cyclocort cream and lotion Steroid medications applied to the skin to relieve inflammation.

cyclodialysis An operation to relieve the pressure within the eyeball in glaucoma.

cyclophosphamide A derivative of nitrogen mustard; a chemical compound with considerable anticancer value.

cyclopropane An anesthetic agent formerly used extensively because of its nontoxicity, but now in disfavor because of its explosive potentialities.

cyclops A monster with the two eyes fused into one.

Cyclosporin A A substance used as an immune suppressant to combat rejection reactions after organ transplantation.

cyclotomy A surgical incision through the ciliary body of the eye; performed in cases of glaucoma.

cyclotron A machine which can change stable substances into radioactive substances.

cyesis Pregnancy.

cylindroids Cylinder-shaped bodies sometimes seen on microscopic examination of urine of patients who have kidney disease.

cynophobia Fear of dogs.

cyst A sac containing fluid, blood, sweat gland secretions, etc.

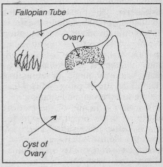

Cysts

cystadenocarcinoma A type of cancer containing many cysts. This type often originates in the ovaries.

cystadenoma A benign tumor which contains many cysts and glandular tissue; seen often in breasts.

cystectomy 1. Excision of a cyst. 2. Surgical removal of the urinary bladder, usually performed for cancer.

cystic Looking like a cyst.

cystic disease of the breast A chronic condition characterized by innumerable small or large cysts of the breast. Also known as chronic cystic mastitis or Schimmelbusch's disease.

cystic duct The duct (tube) connecting the gall bladder to the common bile duct. It is a common site for gallstones to become lodged.

Cysticercus A larval form of tapeworm.

cystic fibrosis A childhood disease, inherited in nature, characterized by the functional failure of the glands that secrete mucus and digestive ferments. It involves the lungs, liver, pancreas, and many other organs. Children so afflicted are especially susceptible to infections. Also known as mucoviscoidosis or viscoidosis. (Formerly called cystic fibrosis of the pancreas)

cystine A component of many proteins.

cystinuria The presence of cystine in the urine, sometimes seen in metabolic disorders present since birth.

cystitis Inflammation of the urinary bladder. It is accompanied by pain and frequency of urination. The diagnosis of this condition can be made by urine examination.

cystocele A hernia of the bladder resulting in its protrusion into the vagina; often the result of a tear following a difficult delivery.

cystogastrostomy An operation to drain a cyst, usually of the pancreas, into the stomach.

cystogram An X ray of the urinary bladder.

cystolithiasis Stones in the urinary bladder.

cystolithotomy The surgical removal of a urinary bladder stone.

cystopyelitis Inflammation or infection of the bladder and kidneys.

cystosarcoma phyllodes A special tumor of the breast characterized by large size, rapid growth, and the presence of both cysts and solid tissue. Most of these tumors are not malignant.

cystoscope An instrument used to examine the interior of the urinary bladder. It is a long metal tube with a light so that the physician can peer into the bladder.

cystosteatoma A sweat-gland cyst located beneath the skin. In the scalp, these cysts are called "wens."

cystotomy An operative incision into the urinary bladder, usually performed when there is obstruction to the outflow of urine from the bladder.

cytoanalyzer A sophisticated electronic device that screens smears suspected of containing malignant cells.

cytobiology That branch of biology which concerns itself with the study of cells.

cytodiagnosis The making of a diagnosis through microscopic examination of tissue cells, such as a Papanicalaou smear for cancer of the uterus.

cytodifferentiators Chemical agents that are sometimes effective in delaying or stopping cancer cells from multiplying.

cytogenetics The science of studying the chromosomes within cells as a means of learning genetic factors.

cytology The science which deals with the nature of cells.

cytolysis Destruction of cells.

cytomegalovirus (CMV) A virus often associated with herpes, AIDS, and other social diseases.

Cytomel A medication containing thyroid hormone, useful in treating patients with underactivity of the thyroid gland.

cytopathology Changes within cells noted through microscopic examination and study; a branch of the science of pathology.

cytoplasm That portion of a cell which does not have the nucleus. The opposite of nucleoplasm.

cytoreductive surgery Surgery to reduce the size of a tumor that cannot be removed completely; done in order to enhance the benefits of chemotherapy or radiotherapy.

cytosine arabinoside A chemotherapeutic drug sometimes used in the treatment of acute leukemia.

cytotoxic drugs Drugs that inhibit the growth and reproduction of cells. Used frequently to inhibit growth of malignancies.

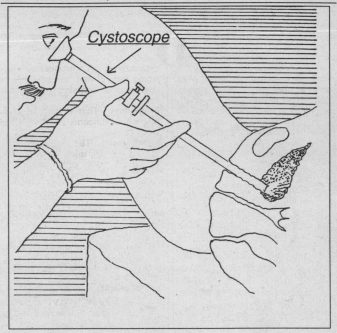

Cystoscope

cytotoxin A chemical used to kill malignant cells, a chemotherapeutic agent.

Cytoxan A powerful chemical, effective in inhibiting growth of some tumors.

D

dacarbazine A chemotherapy drug, useful in treating Hodgkin's disease and melanoma.

dacnomania An insane desire to kill.

Dacron A plastic material used as a blood vessel graft.

dacryoadenitis Inflammation of the tear gland of the eye.

dacryocystitis Inflammation of the tear sac of the eye. It is evidenced by swelling and redness beneath the lower eyelid, and tears. Occurs particularly in young children and elderly people.

dacryocystotomy An operative incision into the tear sac.

dacryolith A stone (calculus) in the tear duct.

dacryorrhea Excessive tear flow.

dacryostenosis An obstruction, due to a constriction, of the tear duct.

dactinomycin An anti-cancer drug useful in treating Wilm's tumor in children, and other malignancies.

dactyl A finger or toe.

dactylomegaly Overgrown toes or fingers; a rather unusual birth deformity.

Dalmane A patented medicine to aid sleeping.

dam A sheet of thin rubber or latex used to drain fluids or pus from a wound.

"D and C" operation Dilatation and curettage; scraping of the interior of the uterus. This operation is often performed as a diagnostic procedure in order to make a diagnosis of cancer of the uterus.

Danazol A medication, hormonal in origin, to relieve cystic disease of the breasts.

dander Scales from the skin of hairy animals, such as dogs, cats, horses, etc. When inhaled by humans, they may produce an allergic reaction.

dandruff Scales from the skin of the scalp, seen in large quantities in cases of (seborrheic) dermatitis.

dark-field examination A microscopic examination especially designed to discover whether the bacteria causing syphilis are present.

dartos The small muscle beneath the skin of the scrotum which enables this structure to contract.

Darvon A non-habit-forming, pain relieving drug, especially helpful to those who are allergic to aspirin and similar medications.

Darwin's theory That higher forms of animal life originate from lower forms, with the "survival of the fittest."

Darwin's tubercle A small projection of cartilage in the upper portion of the outer ear. Darwin thought it an indication that man descended from apes.

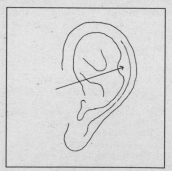

Darwin's tubercle

88

daughter cyst A secondary one, sometimes derived from a previous cyst.

daymare A nightmare occurring during the day.

DBI tablets Phenformin hydrochloride; an oral antidiabetes medication whose action is to lower the level of blood sugar.

DCIS Abbreviation for "ductal carcinoma in situ." This refers to a breast cancer that is localized and has not invaded the surrounding tissues.

D.D.S. A dentist. The degree of *Doctor of Dental Surgery.*

de- A prefix meaning away from, down, etc.

deactivation Loss of radioactivity.

deaf-mute An individual who cannot talk because he has been born deaf.

deafness Inability to hear. This may be caused by a defect in the outer ear, middle ear, inner ear, or by a defect in the nerve of hearing, or in the brain itself.

deamination A biochemical process, carried out within the liver, whereby amino acids are broken down into fatty acids or sugars.

death certificate The recording of a death with the local authorities. This certificate usually requires a doctor's signature.

death instinct The wish to die, prevalent among many people at various times in their lives.

death rate The proportion of deaths each year in the total population.

death rattle A gurgling sound in the throat heard in some people just as they die.

death struggle Convulsions and twitchings just before death.

debility Weakness.

debridement Removal of dead or devitalized tissue around a wound.

debulking operation *See* cytoreductive surgery.

Decadron A synthetic cortisone-like substance, used as an antiinflammatory medication.

Decadron Ointment An ointment containing steroids (cortisone-like substances) helpful in clearing various skin eruptions.

decalcification The process of losing calcium from bone.

decapsulation Surgical removal of the covering (capsule) of an organ, as when the capsule of the kidney is removed in cases of uremia.

decerebration Removal of the brain; carried out on animals in certain experimental work.

dechloridation Removal of salt (chlorides) from the diet. Advocated in some cases of high blood pressure.

deci- One-tenth.

decibel A unit of hearing. Measurement of hearing is calculated in decibels.

decidua The lining cells of the uterus. These are shed each month that a woman menstruates; also after giving birth.

deciduitis An acute inflammation of the lining membrane of the uterus, usually brought on by attempts to induce abortion.

deciduous teeth First teeth; baby teeth.

Declomycin An antibiotic used in the treatment of some gram-negative infections and conditions such as Rocky Mountain spotted fever, typhus fever, etc.

decompensation Failure of the circulation due to poor heart function. It is characterized by shortness of breath, irregular and poor heart beat, and swelling of the ankles (dropsy).

decompression 1. The removal of excess pressure, as in conditions where there is increased pressure within the spinal or cerebrospinal fluid. 2. Reduction of pressure in someone who has been submerged in deep water, as in a *decompression chamber.*

decongestant A medication that

shrinks membranes, such as certain nasal sprays; often composed of epinephrine or substance with similar action.

decontamination Removal of harmful substances or organisms from a body, from clothing, from a building, or from the ground. A word often used when referring to removal of war gases or radioactive substances or to removal of insects or lice from a body surface.

decortication Surgical removal of the cortex or outer portion or covering of an organ or structure; sometimes performed on the lungs after empyema (an infection of the chest cavity).

decrepit Feeble; weak.

decrudescence The subsiding of a disease; abatement of symptoms.

decubitus The act of lying down; the recumbent position.

decubitus ulcer A bedsore, seen in debilitated people who have been lying in bed for several weeks.

decussate To intersect or cross, such as is seen in nerve fibers. The optic nerves to the eyes *decussate* or cross one another within the brain.

dedentition Loss of teeth.

deep sensibility Sense of pressure and movement within the deeper structures of the body such as the bones, joints, muscles, etc. It is responsible for the aches and pains people often feel.

deerfly fever *See* tularemia.

defecation Movement of the bowels; passage of stool; an evacuation.

defect An abnormality or imperfection.

defense mechanism A mental reaction of protecting oneself from blame, shame, sense of guilt, or anxiety.

defervescence The return of fever to normal temperature.

defibrillation A maneuver to stop irregular beating of the heart and to return it to normal rhythm.

defibrillator An electric current passed through the heart, by means of a special apparatus, for the purpose of reestablishing normal heart rhythm.

deficiency disease A disease associated with a lack of vitamins or minerals in the body, such as rickets, scurvy, etc.

defloration The loss of virginity.

deformity A deviation from normal structure.

degeneration Deterioration of tissue with loss of function and eventual destruction of the particular tissue cells.

deglutition Swallowing.

degustation Tasting.

dehiscence The process of ripping open, as the rupturing of a closed surgical wound.

dehydration The loss of water from the body. Such water loss can take place through the kidneys, the lungs, or perspiration.

    fever Elevated temperature due to inadequate fluid intake or loss of large quantities of body fluids; seen mainly in infants.

dehydrocholesterol—7 A sterol chemical normally present in skin. When this sterol is exposed to the ultraviolet rays of sunlight, it becomes transformed into vitamin D. (This process prevents rickets in children.)

déjà vu An impression that a new experience has happened before.

delayed union Failure of the ends of fractured bones to knit in the usual, expected period of time; malunion.

deleterious Harmful; hurtful. Dirt is *deleterious* to an open wound.

delinquency Socially unacceptable behavior, particularly in a minor.

delirium Mental confusion or excitement, as in a severe disease with high fever.

delirium tremens A delirious condition brought on by alcohol poisoning. During this state, there is marked tremor (trembling), hallucinations, ideas of persecution, and ultimate exhaustion.

delivery The act of giving birth.

delouse To remove lice from a person, or his clothing.

delta waves High-voltage brain waves such as those that occur during very deep sleep.

deltoid The broad, flat muscle covering the shoulder. It helps to lift the arm away from the side of the body.

delusion A belief maintained even though it is contrary to the truth.

demarcate To mark; to outline.

dementia Loss of mental coordination to such a degree that one is insane.

dementia precox Schizophrenia. A form of mental illness seen most often among children and young adults.

Demerol A patented medication used as a narcotic. It is a valuable substitute for morphine, since it is not as habit forming.

demi- Half.

demineralization Loss of mineral salts from the body, such as salt loss from excessive exertion and perspiration on a hot day.

demography One of the social sciences, concerned with the study of peoples collectively.

demonomania A form of insanity in which one thinks he is possessed by the devil or demons.

demorphinization The process by which morphine is withdrawn from an addict.

demulcent A medication used to soothe a surface; a medicated ointment.

demyelinization The loss of the sheath tissue which normally covers nerve fibers, seen in certain diseases such as multiple sclerosis.

denarcotize To withhold narcotics from an addict.

denatured alcohol Alcohol which has been altered, so that it may not be drunk.

dendrites Connections and extensions of a nerve cell, which receive impulses and transmit them to the center of the nerve cell.

denervate To cut a nerve going to or from an organ or structure. This is sometimes done surgically to relieve pain.

dengue fever A virus disease transmitted by the bite of the mosquitoes *Aedes aegypti* and *Aedes albopictus*. It is characterized by severe pain in muscles, joints, and bones, and by high fever.

denidation Discharging of the lining cells of the uterus through the vagina.

dentalgia Toothache.

dental implant A false tooth that is implanted into the soft tissues and bones of the jaw.

dentigerous cyst A cyst, in the jaw bones, due to retained, unerupted teeth.

dentistry The science of caring for and treating the teeth, gums and other adjacent tissues.

dentition The teeth; the breaking through the gums by teeth.

denture Artificial teeth, bridgework.

denude To strip bare.

deoxychenic acid A medication sometimes given to help dissolve gallstones. (Its use is in the experimental stage.)

deoxygenation The process of removing oxygen from a substance.

deoxyribonucleic acid (DNA) The fundamental component of living tissue, occurring in the nuclei of all cells. Its structural formula contains the genetic code responsible for the inheritance and transmission of chromosomes and genes.

dependence A situation in which one is dependent upon a certain drug or medication and suffers when it is withdrawn.

depersonalization The sense of loss of one's identity, seen in certain types of mental illness.

depilate To remove hair.

depilatory Any one of many preparations used to remove hair from the body.

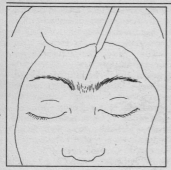

Depilation—electric

depletion Excessive loss of body fluids, chemicals, or tissues.

salt Excessive loss of salt through perspiration or urination.

water Dehydration; excessive depletion, water loss of water from the body through perspiration, urination, or diarrhea.

Depo-heparin A patented medication, containing heparin, injected for the purpose of preventing blood clotting. It is given to patients afflicted with coronary thrombosis.

Depo-provera A long-acting chemical given intramuscularly. It has the same action in promoting menstrual response as Provera. *See* Provera.

depot A place in the body where drugs can be injected and stored for slow release over a period of days or weeks.

Depo-testosterone A long-acting male sex hormone. Given by injection into the muscles of the buttocks.

depressant drug A medication that lowers the functional activity of an organ or organs.

depression Dejection; melancholia.

depressive reaction Melancholia; the depressed phase of a manic-depressive reaction.

depressor An agent or structure which depresses, such as a nerve which causes lowering (depressing) of the blood pressure or heart rate, etc.

Dercum's disease A disease associated with painful areas in the fatty tissue beneath the skin. Also called *adiposis dolorosa.*

derma Skin.

dermabrasion Scraping off the surface layers of the skin with a specially constructed instrument; performed by skin specialists to remove scars due to acne or other skin conditions.

dermatitis Inflammation of the skin. There are many types of dermatitis, each having its own distinguishing characteristics.

dermatitis medicamentosa A drug rash.

dermatofibroma A slow-growing benign tumor of the skin. Also called sclerosing hemangioma or histiocytoma.

Dermatologist A skin specialist.

dermatome A surgical instrument which cuts thin sheets of skin to be used as grafts.

dermatoneurosis A skin rash secondary to emotional upset.

dermatophytosis Athlete's foot; ringworm.

dermographia A condition of the skin, thought to be allergic, wherein the skin becomes red and raised wherever it is irritated or scratched lightly.

dermoid cyst A hollow sac (cyst) whose structure resembles that of skin.

DES Abbreviation for diethylstilbestrol, a chemical having effects similar to estrogen, the female sex hormone.

Desenex ointment A patented medication used to combat certain fungus infections of the skin, such as athlete's foot.

desensitization The process of causing a person to lose his sensitivity to an irritant such as a pollen. This is the basis of most treatment carried out by allergists.

desert fever Valley fever; San Joaquin Valley fever; coccidioidomycosis. A chronic lung infection.

desiccation Drying up; forming into a powdery substance.

desmoid Like a fiber or fibrous tissue, such as a *desmoid tumor* of muscle (seen occasionally in the muscles of the abdomen).

desmology The study of ligaments.

desoxycorticosterone A hormone secreted by the cortex of the adrenal gland. It is administered to keep alive a patient who has inadequate function of the adrenal gland.

Desoxyn A medicine used on a short-term basis in the treatment of hyperactive children. It is used in conjunction with psychotherapy.

desquamate To shed the superficial cells from the surface of a structure or organ. Skin is constantly *desquamating* or shedding superficial cells.

detachment of the retina Separation of the retina from the other layers of the eyeball, seen mainly among those who are markedly nearsighted. This condition may cause partial or total loss of vision in an eye.

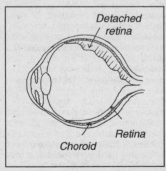

Detachment of the retina

detergent A substance used to cleanse.

detoxication The process of purification or rendering harmful (toxic) substances harmless (non-toxic).

The liver is supposed to serve this function in the human body.

detritus Waste matter.

detumescence The process in which a tumor or swelling becomes smaller or disappears.

devascularize To cut off the blood supply to an organ or part of the body.

deviate One who departs from the usual sex practices of heterosexuals.

deviated septum A crooked or deflected separating wall between the two portions of the nose; often accompanied by inability to breathe through one or both nostrils.

devil's grip Acute pleurodynia. Severe and sudden pain in the chest, aggravated by deep breathing. It is caused by inflammation of the lining of the chest cavity. It lasts a day or two and then disappears.

devitalized Dead.

Dexedrine Amphetamine. A drug with many uses, including that of stimulating mentally and curbing the appetite. It may become toxic or habit forming.

Dexon A synthetic, absorbable suture material, sometimes used as a substitute for silk or catgut sutures.

dextran A substance injected into the veins of people in shock, as a substitute for blood plasma or transfusion.

dextroamphetamine sulfate Dexedrine. A powerful stimulant of the brain and nervous system. Also used to depress appetite.

dextrocardia A heart located more on the right side than on the left. Such a condition is usually a birth deformity.

dextropropoxyphene Darvon; an effective pain-relieving drug. Non-habit-forming.

dextrose A form of sugar found in the blood.

diabetes inspidus A metabolic disease caused by a disorder of the hypothalamus, associated with marked thirst and the passage of huge quan-

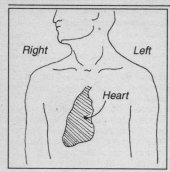

Dextrocardia

tities of urine. Not related to diabetes mellitus.

diabetes mellitus A chronic disease characterized by inability to burn up the sugars (carbohydrates) which have been ingested. It is caused by insufficient production of insulin by the pancreas.

diabetic neuropathy Partial loss of sensation, along with pain and inability to distinguish temperature, especially in the limbs, often seen in aging diabetics.

Diabinase A patented drug which lowers the level of blood sugar; sometimes used in the treatment of diabetes mellitus.

diacritic A condition sufficiently distinctive to permit a diagnosis.

diagnosis The art of discovering the nature of the patient's disease or disorder and the underlying cause or etiology.

Diagnosis Related Group A method of evaluating average hospital stays for various conditions according to their diagnosis. (It is an attempt to cut down on the costs of hospitalization.)

Diagnostician A physician particularly adept at making diagnoses; an internist; a specialist in internal medicine.

dialysis A process by which substances in solution are separated from one another.

Diamox A patented medication which stimulates an increased output of urine; a powerful diuretic.

diapedesis The passage of blood cells out of blood vessels into the surrounding tissues.

diaper rash A rash caused usually by irritation from the diaper or from the soap used in cleansing the diaper.

diaphanography A method of diagnosing breast disease through transillumination. In other words, passing light through the breast and recording the variations in shadows.

diaphoresis Sweating; perspiration.

diaphragm The muscular partition located between the chest cavity and the abdominal cavity. The esophagus, the aorta and the vena cava course through the *diaphragm*.

diaphysis The shaft of a long bone.

diarrhea Increased frequency and liquid consistency of the stools.

diastase An enzyme (chemical agent) of the body which helps in the digestion of starches and sugars.

diastasis 1. Separation of parts which are normally in contact with one another; a dislocation, such as the separation of the abdominal muscles in the midline. 2. Final phase of diastole.

diastole The relaxed phase of heart action. During this period the heart chamber fills with blood. The opposite of *systole*.

diastolic pressure The blood pressure level during the time the heart muscle is relaxed.

diathermy The application of heat to body tissues through the use of a machine which generates an electric current of high frequency. Such heat is capable of deep penetration into the body.

diathesis A tendency toward or a susceptibility to the development of a disease.

diazepam An anti-anxiety drug, also acting as a muscle relaxant. (*See* valium.)

DIC Abbreviation for *dissemin-*

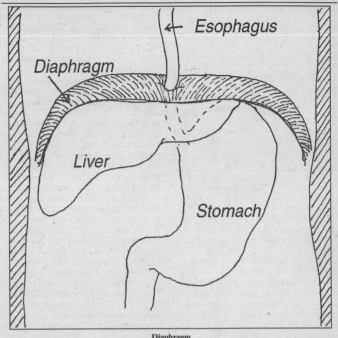

Diaphragm

ated intravascular coagulopathy, an upset in the normal blood-clotting mechanism.

dichotomy Division into two equal parts or branches.

Dick test A test to discover susceptibility to scarlet fever. It is a skin test.

Dicoumarol A patented drug used to prolong the time it takes blood to clot. Used in patients with phlebitis or embolus.

dicrotic Referring to a split pulse beat for every heart contraction.

didelphic A birth deformity in which there is a double uterus.

diencephalon A part of the brain located toward the base of the skull.

Dienestrol An estrogen hormone used in treating various gynecological conditions, such as occur in women after menopause. Also used to stop milk secretion from the breasts after childbearing.

diet An all-inclusive term referring to food regularly eaten and liquids regularly consumed.

Diets *See* Health Manual at rear of dictionary.

dietetics The science of regulating diet in order to preserve health.

diethyistilbestrol Stilbestrol. A synthetic substance possessing estrogenic activity.

Dietl's crisis Excruciating pain in the kidney region and around the flank along the course of the ureter, brought on by a kink, twist or angulation of a ureter (the tube conducting urine from the kidney to the bladder).

differential diagnosis The art of

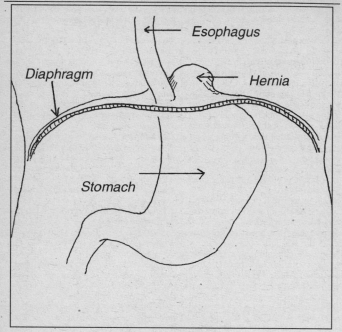

Hernia of the diaphragm

distinguishing one disease from another by comparing symptoms and arriving at a precise diagnosis.

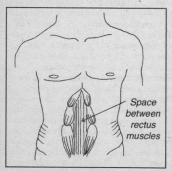

Diastasis of the abdominal muscles

diffuse Spread; not localized.

Diflucan An effective medication to combat fungal infections.

digestant A medication which aids digestion.

digestion The process of breaking down food so that it can be absorbed through the lining of the intestinal tract.

digit A finger or toe.

digitalis A drug helpful in treating heart ailments, particularly those in which the heart muscle is weak. (Used in cases of heart failure, fibrillation, etc.)

digitalization The giving of digitalis to support a failing heart in quantities sufficient to obtain the maximum beneficial effect.

digitoxin The active ingredient in

digitalis, used in treating certain types of heart disease.

digoxin   A form of digitalis.

dihydrostreptomycin   A powerful antibiotic drug, used sparingly because of its toxic effects.

Dilantin   A drug given to prevent epileptic seizures.

dilatation   The state of being distended or stretched, such as the *dilatation* of the stomach with gas.

dilator   A surgical instrument used to stretch (dilate) the opening of an organ such as the anus or cervix of the uterus.

Dilaudid   A patented drug derived from opium, possessing actions similar to morphine.

dildo   An artificial penis, composed of plastic or wood, used by some females for masturbation.

diluent   A liquid used to dilute or reduce the strength of a solution.

dilution   Weakening of a solution; making a solution less concentrated.

Dimetane tablets   Antiallergic drug, prescribed in cases of allergic rhinitis, conjunctivitis, and in certain cases of food allergy.

Dimetapp   A patented anti-allergic medication, distributed both in liquid and tablet form.

dimethyl sulfoxide   (DSMO) A solvent that penetrates the skin; sometimes used to increase the absorption of locally applied medications.

dimpling   A depression in the contour of the skin.

diodoquin   A chemical useful in ridding the intestinal tract of parasites such as intestinal amebas. Used in cases of amebic dysentery.

Diodrast   A patented substance which, when injected into veins, will cast a shadow on X-ray films. It is used to outline the kidneys, blood vessels and other structures.

Dionin   A drug with many of the same actions as codeine, used to relieve pain or reduce the tendency to cough.

dionism   Homosexuality.

diopter   The unit of measurement for the lens of the eye. Nearsightedness or farsightedness can be recorded in *diopters*.

dioptometer   The instrument used for measuring the extent of eye refraction for determining eye defects.

dioxide   Any chemical containing two atoms of oxygen to one atom of another element.

dioxin   A chemical thought to be conducive to the development of malignant lesions.

diphtheria   An acute contagious disease characterized by sore throat, great toxicity and interference with breathing. It can be treated successfully with antitoxin.

diphtheroid   A bacteria resembling the diphtheria germ but having nothing to do with diphtheria itself.

Diphyllobothrium   A kind of tapeworm.

diplegia   Paralysis of two arms, or of two legs.

diplococcus   Round bacteria that occur in groups of two, such as the germs which cause pneumonia (*Diplococcus pneumoniae*).

Diplomate   A physician who has received a diploma, more specifically, the diploma of the American Specialty Boards; a qualified specialist. *See also* Section on Abbreviations, Diplomates in Specialties.

diplopia   Seeing double.

dipsomania   A compulsion to drink excess quantities of alcoholic beverages.

dipsophobia   Morbid fear of drinking.

disarticulation   Amputation of a part (limb) through the joint.

discectomy   *See* diskectomy.

discharge   An emission; a secretion, as of pus or blood.

discission   An operation for cataracts in which the covering of the opaque lens is punctured in several places to stimulate it to become absorbed.

discrete   Separate; not joined together.

disease   A disturbance in the structure or function of an organ or organs. (*See also* under appropriate letter.)

A-B hemolytic A disease of newborns characterized by severe anemia and jaundice, caused by incompatibility between the mother's and fetus's blood.

adaptational A condition caused as a by-product of the body's defense mechanisms, such as high blood pressure resulting from the continued outpouring of excessive quantities of adrenalin.

Addison's Chronic weakness, anemia, low blood pressure resulting from inadequate function of the cortex of the adrenal glands. (Prior to the advent of cortisone, this disease was one hundred percent fatal. Now, it can be controlled indefinitely.)

Albers-Schönberg "Marble-bones," a disease in which the bones become extremely dense.

Aran-Duchenne Muscular atrophy, a progressive condition leading to great wasting.

autoimmune Any disease caused by antibodies acting upon other body cells.

Banti's A chronic disease associated with enlargement of the liver and spleen, anemia, bleeding from the intestinal tract, and episodes of jaundice.

Basedow's Overactivity of the thyroid gland, goiter, and bulging of the eyeballs (exophthalmos).

Boeck-Schaumann *See* sarcoidosis.

Bright's Inflammation of the kidneys; glomeronephritis.

Brill's Typhus fever.

Buerger's A progressive disease characterized by narrowing, inflammation, and obliteration of the passageways of arteries and veins in the legs; thromboangiitis obliterans (TOA).

caisson "The bends." A condition accompanied by great pain in the bones, dizziness, nausea, head-

ache, etc., caused by too-sudden return to normal atmospheric conditions when one has been working under high pressure. (Seen in divers, tunnel workers, etc.)

cat-scratch fever An infection accompanied by swollen lymph nodes, chronic fever, and slow healing wound; caused by the scratch of a cat.

celiac A chronic disease of children due to malabsorption from the intestinal tract. It is characterized by undernourishment, potbelly, large, foul-smelling stools, weakness, and arrested development.

cerebrovascular Any condition of the brain caused by inadequate blood supply or brain hemorrhage or injury.

Chagas' A parasitic disease caused by the trypanosomes, occurring mainly in South America; transmitted through insect bites.

Christensen-Krabbe A disease in infants associated with progressive brain deterioration.

Christmas A form of hemophilia; an inherited condition in which there is poor blood clotting due to deficiency of clotting factor IX.

coal miner's Anthracosis of the lungs due to constant inhalation of coal dust; characterized by chronic cough, shortness of breath, and eventual weakness.

collagen Any disease involving the connective tissues of the body. It is a broad category including such widely diverse conditions as rheumatic fever, lupus, rheumatoid arthritis, serum sickness, etc.

congenital One that is present at birth but does not fall into the category of *inherited*.

constitutional One that is due to an *inborn* defect or tendency.

contagious One caused by bacteria or viruses that can be spread by direct or indirect contact.

Creutzfeldt-Jakob. *See* "Mad cow disease."

Crohn's disease Inflammation of the small and/or large intestine; a chronic ailment associated with ulcer formations.

deficiency Any disease caused by inadequate intake of essential foods, vitamins, or minerals.

deQuervain's An inflammation of the tendon sheath that extends the thumb; characterized by marked pain on bending down the thumb.

Dercum's *See* adiposis dolorosa.

drug Any condition caused by the administration of a drug or medicine.

fibrocystic disease of the pancreas An old term for cystic fibrosis; mucoviscoidosis; viscoidosis.

functional One associated with an upset in function rather than an anatomical defect.

Gaucher's disease A form of anemia occurring in some families. It is associated with enlargement of the liver, spleen, and lymph glands.

Gilbert's An inherited type of jaundice not associated with destruction of red blood cells, usually free of symptoms. Also called *familial nonhemolytic jaundice*.

Graves' disease A goiter associated with overactivity of the thyroid gland.

glycogen storage An inborn disease of infants characterized by an upset in sugar metabolism and an enlarged liver.

Hand-Schüller-Christian A disease of childhood in which an abnormal reaction takes place within the bone marrow. As a consequence, inflammatory changes take place and bone structure is altered. There is also anemia, brain damage, and malfunction of the pituitary gland, the liver, spleen, and lungs.

Hansen's Leprosy.

Hartnup An inherited abnormality in metabolism involving deficient kidney function, intestinal malabsorption, skin rashes, and a staggering gait.

Hashimoto's An inflammatory disease involving the thyroid gland, characterized by goiter.

hemorrhagic disease of the newborn A bleeding tendency in newborn children associated with decreased platelets and increased clotting and bleeding times. It is controlled by administration of large doses of vitamin K.

hereditary One transmitted through the genes from parents to offspring.

Hirschsprung's Megacolon. A congenital disease with enormous enlargement of the bowel secondary to absence of essential nerve fibers. It is characterized by chronic constipation and retarded development. The disease can be cured surgically.

Hodgkin's A malignant disease involving the lymph nodes and, eventually, the spleen and liver.

hyaline membrane. The respiratory distress syndrome. A disease of newborns, especially premature children, caused by a membrane-like layer in the lung's air sacs. The outcome is fatal in a high proportion of cases.

intercurrent One occurring during the course of another disease.

interstitial One involving the connective tissue structure of an organ rather than the functioning tissue.

Kaposi's A tumor of the skin, multiple in nature, associated with marked pigment changes.

laughing Kuru. A very rare, progressive cerebellar degeneration that is invariably fatal. Endemic to the New Guinea Highlands, its most conspicuous symptom is uncontrollable shaking. *Kuru* means *fear*.

Legionnaires' disease An infection associated with influenza and severe pneumonia. Seen frequently in localized epidemics.

Letterer-Siwe Reticulosis. A condition seen in infants due to inflammatory changes within the lymph nodes, liver, spleen, and bone marrow. Sometimes associated with bluish skin rashes and slow mental development.

Little's Progressive paralysis due to degenerative changes within some of the nerves in the spinal cord.

Lyme disease *See* under letter L.

malabsorption Any disease caused by lack of or improper absorption of nutriments, chemicals, vitamins, or minerals through the mucous membrane of the intestinal tract.

maple syrup urine An inherited disease in which the urine of the newborn child has an odor resembling that of maple syrup. The condition, usually fatal, is characterized by faulty protein metabolism.

marble bone A disease in which the structure of the bones becomes extremely dense. Also known as Albers-Schönberg disease.

Marfan's An inherited disease associated with deformities of the fingers, lenses of the eyes, and skin.

Marie-Strümpell A disease involving arthritis of the spine, bulging of the tips of the fingers, an unsteady gait, and changes in function of the pituitary gland.

Mediterranean anemia Cooley's anemia. *See* anemia.

Menétrier's A condition in which the folds of the lining of the stomach are tremendously enlarged and the mucous membrane displays shallow ulcerations.

Meniére's *See* Meniére's disease.

Mikulicz' Swelling of the tear gland and the various salivary glands due to replacement of normal gland tissue by lymphoid tissue.

Milroy's An inherited condition in which there is periodic and chronic swelling of the legs and thighs.

Morquio's A congenital condition associated with bone deformity,

dwarfism, and the development of cataracts.

occupational One resulting from an individual's daily occupation.

organic One associated with anatomical changes in tissues or organs. (The opposite of a functional disease.)

pandemic One that spreads throughout the world. (The Asian flu became a pandemic disease several years ago.)

parrot fever Psittacosis. A serious lung infection caused by a germ affecting parrots, parakeets, and other birds. (Often fatal in humans)

Senear-Usher A form of pemphigus, a grave skin disease involving the head and torso.

serum Fever, hives, enlargement of lymph glands, occurring seven to ten days after receiving an antitoxin containing animal serum. (Recovery is prompt)

silo-filler's A lung condition caused by fresh silage. Constant exposure may lead to a chronic lung condition.

Weber-Christian A disease in which there is an elevation of temperature associated with painful, inflamed areas in the fat beneath the skin. Cause unknown.

Wilson's An inherited disease associated with faulty copper metabolism. Its symptoms include enlargement of the liver and the eventual development of cirrhosis.

disgerminoma A tumor of the ovary composed of primitive cells; if removed, cure usually results.

disk Any circular or flat, rounded structure; commonly referring to the disk of cartilage in between the vertebrae. A "herniated disk" is one which has broken through its normal confines and protrudes from the vertebral column.

diskectomy Surgical removal of a cartilage (disk) in between the vertebrae of the spine.

diskogenic Referring to a condition caused by a slipped disk in the spinal column.

dislocation Out of place; especially a bone that has left its joint.

disomy Having paired chromosomes, a normal state.

disoriented Mentally confused; unaware of one's surroundings.

disparate Unlike.

dispareunia *See* Dyspareunia.

dispensary 1. A place where patients can get free or low cost medical care on an "out-patient" basis; a clinic. 2. Primarily referring to patients who do not require hospital bed care.

dispense To give a prescription to a patient.

dispermy The entrance of two sperm cells into one egg.

dissect To cut tissues in an orderly manner so as to distinguish and separate anatomical parts from one another. Both a surgical and anatomical term.

disseminated sclerosis Multiple sclerosis, a chronic disease of the nervous system.

dissemination The spreading or scattering of disease or disease germs.

dissimulation Making believe one is sick; malingering; feigning illness.

dissociation Separation of actions or ideas which should function as a whole.

dissolution Disintegration or decomposition, as of tissue.

dissolve To break down when put in a solution, as a chemical will *dissolve* in water.

distal Away from the center. Out toward the end. The hand is *distal* to the arm.

distention The condition of being inflated; dilatation.

distillation The process of vaporizing and then condensing a substance; used mainly to separate different liquids from each other.

distortion A deformed state.

Diupres A patented medication whose effect lowers blood pressure and causes excretion of excess body fluids.

diuresis An increased excretion of urine.

diuretic An agent that causes greater quantities of urine to be passed.

Diuril A patented medication effective in increasing the output of urine. Advised in cases of heart failure in which it is necessary to bring about dehydration.

divergence To go in opposite directions, such as *divergence* of the eyes.

diverticulitis An inflammation of a diverticulum of the bowel.

diverticulosis The presence of many diverticula in the large bowel.

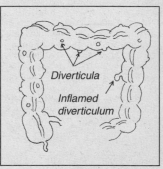

Diverticula

Inflamed diverticulum

Diverticulitis

diverticulum An outpouching or sac arising from the bowel wall. These are sometimes present at birth or may develop in later life. Diverticula only cause disturbance when they become inflamed.

divinyl ether An anesthetic inhaling agent used for short anesthesias.

divulsion The act of ripping or tearing apart.

dizygotic Originating from two fertilized eggs, such as dissimilar twins.

DNA Abbreviation for deoxyribonucleic acid, the fundamental component of living matter.

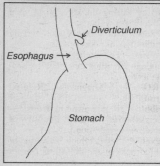

Esophageal diverticulum

DNA fingerprinting A technique used to establish the indentities of particular individuals by precisely designating their DNA patterns.

DNR An abbreviation for "Do not resuscitate." An indication that a terminally ill patient should not be placed on life-prolonging treatment.

D.O.A. Abbreviation for "dead on arrival," a term used by ambulance physicians, police, etc.

Dobell's solution Sodium borate solution, used as a wet dressing for infected areas.

Doctor A licensed practitioner such as a physician, dentist, psychologist, veterinarian, etc.

dolichocephalic One with a long, narrow-shaped head rather than a rounded, broad-shaped head.

Dolobid A patented medicine useful in relieving pain, fever, and inflammation.

dolor Pain (a Latin term).

dominant characteristics Those which have a tendency to be inherited. The opposite of recessive characteristics.

dominant eye The eye which is used most.

donee One who receives transfused blood; also, one who receives grafts of bone, cartilage, skin, etc.

Donnatal A medication which combats spasms of the stomach and intestines.

donor Someone who gives blood (or some other tissue) to a needful patient (recipient or donee).

dopamine An amino acid formed in the body. It is active in the transmission of nerve impulses.

dope fiend A person addicted to the use of a narcotic or other drug.

doppler An instrument that gives out ultrasonic beams into the body. It is very helpful in diagnosing blood vessel and heart disorders.

doraphobia A morbid dread of touching skin or fur of animals.

dorsal Referring to the back, or to the back part of an organ.

dorsalis pedis The artery on the upper surface of the foot. Loss of its pulsation indicates impairment of circulation to the foot.

dorsiflexion Bending the foot toward the upper surface by flexing the ankle.

dorsolumbar Referring to the back of the chest and loins.

dorsum The back of an organ or part.

dosage The appropriate amount of a medication or drug.

dose A slang expression for an attack of acute gonorrhea.

dosimeter An instrument to measure radiation.

Dosimetry The precise determination of the dosage of a medication.

double blind study Wherein neither the investigator nor anyone else can influence the outcome of the study.

double helix The double strand formation that composes the DNA.

douche Cleansing of the vaginal canal by use of a syringe and stream of water. (Also used in referring to cleansing other parts.)

Down's Syndrome An inherited condition caused by the existence of an extra chromosome. Characteristically, there is mental retardation and an Oriental appearance. Also called *Mongolism*.

Doxycycline An antibiotic particularly effective against infections of the intestinal tract associated with diarrhea.

DPT Abbreviation for triple vaccine, containing diphtheria, whooping cough and tetanus vaccines, usually given to a child in one dose.

drain A surgical term usually referring to the removal of pus, blood or other liquid from a diseased area in the body.

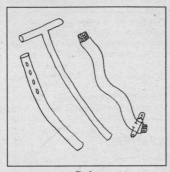

Drains

drainage A method of evoking a discharge, as to obtain drainage from an abscess cavity.

dram(drachm) One eighth of an ounce, as calculated by the druggist.

Dramamine A patented medication used to prevent seasickness, airsickness, and other conditions causing nausea or vomiting.

drape To cover the area around a part to be operated upon or examined. Surgical *drapes* are composed of sterilized cloth.

drastic drug A drug having a violent laxative action, such as croton oil.

draught(draft) A liquid dose of any medication, usually referring to two to four teaspoonfuls.

draw-sheet A sheet placed under the buttocks of a patient which can be removed readily when soiled.

dream Mental activity carried out during sleep.

    day Dreamlike activity occurring during the day, while in a state of wakefulness.

    wet An erotic dream during which orgasm takes place.

dressing The application of gauze, bandage or other materials to protect a wound.

DRG *See* Diagnosis Related Group.

dribble To pass urine in drops, especially after the main quantity of urine has been voided.

drivel 1. Saliva which leaks out of the corners of the mouth. 2. Senseless talk.

drop 1. A small, rounded quantity of fluid which separates from the main body of fluid. 2. The hanging down of a part of the body due to paralysis of a nerve, such as "hand drop," "foot drop," etc.

droplet infection An infection caused by breathing in material coughed or sneezed by someone else, as in "catching a cold."

dropped beat A skipped beat of the heart.

dropsy Swelling of the ankles and legs secondary to heart insufficiency or failure.

drug abuse Incorrect or excessive use of a drug or medication.

drug-fast Bacteria that have become resistant to certain antibiotic medications.

drug interactions Effects that may result from using two or more drugs that don't agree with one another.

drunkometer An instrument used to determine whether or not a person is intoxicated. It measures the alcohol content of breath or of the blood.

dry eye syndrome Dryness of the conjunctiva seen in older people whose tear glands fail to secrete adequately.

duct A tube or channel, such as the bile duct.

ductless glands Endocrine glands, such as the adrenal, pituitary, or thyroid gland, which secrete their hormones into the bloodstream.

ductus arteriosus A blood vessel present in the embryo connecting the pulmonary (lung) artery and the aorta. Normally, the ductus arteriosus closes off by the time the child is born.

Dulcolax A patented laxative.

dumping syndrome Weakness, faintness, sweating, rapid heart beat, and nausea; thought to be caused by the too-rapid entrance and absorption of food from the intestines.

duodenal ulcer Ulcer of the duodenum, that part of the intestine located immediately beyond the stomach. (It is estimated that one out of ten people will develop a duodenal ulcer at some time or other during their lives.)

duodenitis Inflammation of the duodenum; a common condition often associated with excess secretion of acid by the stomach.

duodenojejunostomy An operation which constructs an artificial connection between the duodenum and jejunum (a portion of the small intestine).

duodenoplasty An operation which alters the shape of the duodenum; sometimes performed when there is constriction of the duodenum.

duodenotomy An operative incision into the duodenum.

duodenum The first portion of the small intestine, commencing immediately after the stomach. It receives bile from the liver, food from the stomach, and juices from the pancreas.

Dupuytren's contracture Thickening of the fibrous tissue beneath the

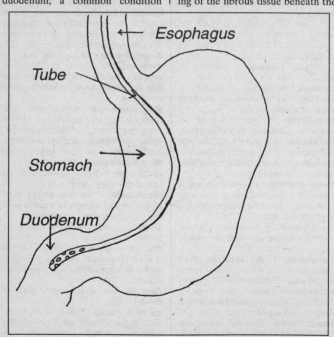

Duodenal drainage

skin of the palm of the hand. It may cause the pulling down and contraction of one or more fingers, usually the little and ring fingers. When advanced, there is inability to straighten the contracted fingers. (Thought to be caused by repeated injury to the palm over a period of years)

Duracillin A patented name for procaine penicillin G.

duralumin An aluminum alloy, particularly useful in orthopedic appliances.

dura mater The outer covering of the brain.

dust count A count of the number of dust particles in the air; done in communities planning to reduce air pollution; also in industry to cut down on occupational lung conditions.

dwarfism A condition in which the person is of smaller than usual size. Often caused by lack of functioning of the pituitary gland.

dynamics The study of motion. In medicine, the study of parts or organs in action.

Dyazide A patented drug to lower elevated blood pressure.

dysarthrosis Disease of a joint.

dysbasia Difficulty in walking.

dyscalculia A learning difficulty in calculating.

dyscrasia An abnormal condition, such as a *blood dyscrasia.*

dysembryoplasia A deformity which develops within the embryo.

dysentery An inflammation of the large bowel associated with pain, cramps and diarrhea. (There are many different types of dysentery, each caused by a specific germ.)

dysfunction Upset function; malfunction.

dysgenesis Defective development within an embryo.

dysgenic The opposite of engenic. (Bad for inheritance.)

dysgerminoma A rare, malignant tumor of the ovary, occurring in teenage girls.

dysgraphia A learning difficulty in writing.

dysinsulinism Upset in insulin metabolism resulting either in excess blood sugar or too little blood sugar.

dyskinesia Poor function of a part which moves or contracts.

dyslalia Impaired power of speech.

dyslexia A learning difficulty in reading.

dysmenorrhea Painful or difficult menstruation.

dysosmia Impaired sense of smell.

dysostosis Impaired bone formation.

dyspareunia Difficult or painful sexual intercourse.

dyspepsia Indigestion. Upset digestion.

dysphagia Impaired swallowing.

dysphasia Impaired speech or comprehension of speech, often caused by a clot or hemorrhage in the brain.

dysphemia Stuttering.

dysphonia Impaired voice.

dyspituitarism Abnormal function of the pituitary gland.

dysplasia Impaired growth processes.

dyspnea Shortness of breath.

dyssomnia An upset of one's sleep pattern.

dysspermatogenic sterility Male infertility due to some abnormality in the production of sperm.

dysspermia Pain on discharge of sperm during orgasm.

dyssynergia Failure of an organ or structure to function in unison with associated organs or structures.

dystocia Impaired labor, often referring to the excessive size of the embryo or to its abnormal position within the uterus.

dystonia Impaired tone, often referring to muscle tone.

dystrophy 1. Abnormal development. 2. Defective nutrition. 3. Degeneration.

dysuria Impaired ability to pass urine; also, painful voiding.

E

ear, external The outer ear, or that part which protrudes from the sides of the head, plus the canal leading down to the eardrum.

inner The part containing the organs of hearing, including the nerve of hearing, and the organ controlling the sense of balance.

middle The ear bones (incus, stapes and malleus), the ear cavity, the eustachian tubes leading to the throat, and the mastoid bone cells. (The middle ear starts on the inner side of the eardrum.)

eardrum The membrane located at the end of the ear canal. It separates the external ear from the middle ear. The *eardrum* is the membrane against which sound waves vibrate.

early ambulation Getting out of bed within a day or two after a surgical operation. (This is done to im-

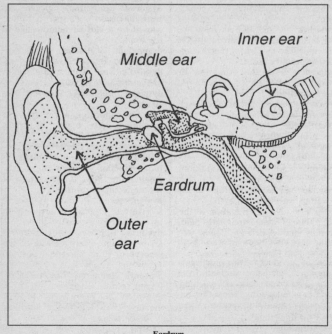

Eardrum

prove circulation and to prevent blood clots.)

early detection Diagnosing disease during its early stages of development.

ear wax cerumen.

Ebola virus A serious hemorragic viral fever. Seen most often in Africa.

Ebstein's disease A birth deformity of the heart associated with displaced heart valves and an abnormal communication between the two sides of the heart.

eccentric Located off center; not in the midline.

ecchymosis Purple discoloration of the skin due to a hemorrhage beneath it; a bruise.

ECG *See* electrocardiography.

echinococcus cyst A cyst caused by infestation with a parasite (worm) often carried by dogs. In man, the liver is the usual favorite site for a cyst to form.

echocardiography A test in which sound waves are directed at the heart. The recordings give important information on the health of the heart muscles and heart function.

echogram *See* sonography.

ECHO virus An upper respiratory virus infection often accompanied by severe headache, stiffness of the neck and other symptoms suggestive of infantile paralysis.

echolalia Repetition of words spoken by other people; seen in certain forms of insanity.

eclampsia A convulsive disorder occurring near the end of pregnancy. It represents a serious toxic condition which endangers the life of both mother and child.

Eclectic A doctor who practices a system of medicine derived from several different schools of teaching, such as homeopathy, allopathy, naturopathy, etc. (Not very prevalent today.)

ecology The study of organisms in relation to the environment in which they live.

Economo's disease Sleeping sickness secondary to an inflammation of the brain. Also called *lethargic encephalitis*.

ECS 1. Abbreviation for electrocerebral silence. Brain dead. 2. *See* electroshock therapy.

ecstasy A trance, accompanied by an extremely pleasurable feeling.

ectasia Dilatation of a part, as a blood vessel or loop of intestine.

ectasia, mammary A breast disease associated with marked dilatation of the milk ducts with deposits of cellular debris.

ectoderm The tissue in the embryo which goes to form skin, the lining of the intestinal tract, the nervous system, etc.

ectogenous Said of bacteria which are able to grow outside their natural hosts.

-ectomy A suffix meaning surgical removal, as in append*ectomy*.

ectopia An abnormally placed organ or part. Usually referring to a birth deformity.

ectopic pregnancy One taking place in the fallopian tube rather than in the uterine cavity. Surgical termination is usually required.

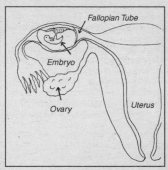

Ectopic pregnancy

ectoplasm The outer layer or "capsule" of a cell.

ectropion The turning out of an

eyelid so that it does not lie close to the surface of the eyeball.

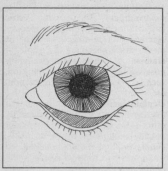

Ectropion

eczema Any inflammatory disease of the skin.

edema Excessive accumulation of fluid in the tissues, thus causing swelling. (Ankle edema, or dropsy, is seen in certain cases of poor heart function.)

edentulous Without teeth.

Edrisal A medication to relieve painful menstruation.

EEA stapler A stapling instrument sometimes used to carry out an end-to-end anastomosis (joining two structures to each other) during surgery, especially of the gastrointestinal tract.

EEG *See* electroencephalography.

effeminate A man who acts like, and has the tastes of, a female.

efferent Leading away from. (*Efferent* nerves are those which arise in the central nervous system and go out toward the organs and superficial tissues.)

effervescent Bubbling, as when gas leaves a liquid.

effluent An outflow.

effluvium Body odor.

effusion The flowing out of liquid from some part of the body.

ego. 1. The self. 2. The conscious realization of oneself.

egocentric 1. Self-centered.

2. Overly concerned with one's own problems.

egomania Excessive belief in and estimation of oneself.

ejaculation An emission, such as takes place during orgasm (the *ejaculation* of semen).

premature Expulsion of semen before consummating the sexual act.

ejaculatory ducts The small tubes (ducts) in the prostate gland through which semen is ejaculated into the urethra when climax is reached. These ducts connect with the tubes from the testicles (vas deferens).

EKG *See* electrocardiogram.

Elase A medication useful in liquefying dead tissues in wounds. Often used as an ointment.

elastic tissue Tissues with the capability of expanding and contracting. Such tissues are found in muscles and blood vessels.

elastoplast An elastic bandage containing an adhesive substance on its inner surface.

Elavil An antidepression drug, helpful in relieving anxiety, but at the same time acting as a sedative.

elbow replacement An operation in which the bones at the elbow joint are replaced by a metal graft.

electrocardiography The recording of the electrical impulses of the heart. Such tracings often give an accurate picture of heart abnormalities and disease.

electrocautery To burn tissue with an electric current by use of a specially designed apparatus.

electrocoagulation The coagulating and destruction of tissue by use of electric current and specially devised apparatus.

electrodesiccation The destruction and drying out of a portion of tissue by use of an electric current and a specially designed instrument.

electroencephalography The recording of brain waves. (Such tracings often give an accurate picture of brain disease.)

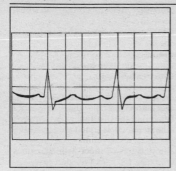

Electrocardiogram (electrocardiographic tracing)

electrolysis Hair removal by use of an electric needle.

electrolyte imbalance A state of acidosis or alkalosis brought about by abnormal balance among the electrolytes chloride, sodium, or potassium.

electrolytes Substances which can, when in solution, convey an electrical impulse. Body electrolytes include such elements as sodium, potassium, chlorides, etc.

electromyograph An instrument which records the electrical impulses that pass through a muscle as it contracts and relaxes.

electronarcosis Unconsciousness produced by electric shock.

electron microscope One that creates tremendous magnification.

electronic fetal monitoring The use of an electronic device to keep track of the unborn child's heart action and pulse, thus giving early warning if the fetus is undergoing dangerous stress.

electrophoresis A method for study of substances in biological mixtures.

electroretinography The study of the electrical responses of the retina of the eye to stimulation by light.

electroshock therapy The giving of convulsions by use of an electroshock machine. (This form of treatment is used by psychiatrists to obtain a remission in certain types of mental illness.)

electrosurgery The use of an electric current for cutting during surgery.

electuary A mixture of a drug or medication and honey or sugar.

element A basic substance composed solely of atoms of one kind, such as oxygen, hydrogen, carbon, etc.

elephantiasis Huge enlargement of the legs, scrotum, and occasionally other parts of the body, due to obstruction of the lymph channels. (This condition is sometimes caused by parasitic infestation of the lymph channels.)

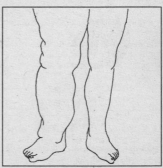

Elephantiasis

elevator Surgical instruments used to lift up parts or to separate them from surrounding tissues.

elixir An alcoholic liquid containing an active medicinal ingredient.

ellipsis Stopping in the middle of an expressed thought or sentence, assuming that the listener will complete it.

emaciation A wasted state, as when someone has lost an excessive amount of weight.

emanation A vapor, gas, or fluid which is emitted by a chemical or other substance. (Radioactive fallout is said to *emanate* from an atomic explosion.)

emasculation Castration; removal of the testicles.

embalm To treat, by injection, a dead body so that it does not decay or putrefy.

embolectomy Surgical removal of a clot (embolus) from an artery in order to reestablish blood flow.

embolism The obstruction of an artery by an embolus, usually a piece clotted blood which breaks away from one part of the circulatory system and travels to another.

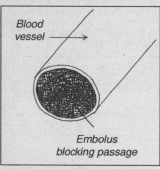

Blood vessel →

Embolus blocking passage

Embolism

embolus Something breaking off from one part of the body and traveling through the bloodstream to another part. (This happens most frequently with a blood clot.)

embryo The developing child during the first few months of pregnancy. (Later during its development, it is called a fetus.)

embryology The study of the embryo and its growth.

embryonal Referring to an embryo; embryonal tissue is that which is growing in the developing embryo.

embryonal cancer A malignant tumor of the testicles.

emesis Vomiting.

emetic A medication which stimulates vomiting; used after a poison has been taken.

emetine A medication given to rid the body of a parasite (ameba).

EMG Abbreviation for electromyogram.

Eminase A drug used in an attempt to dissolve blood clots.

emission The discharge of semen, a *nocturnal emission* taking place during sleep.

emmenagogue A drug used to bring on menstruation.

emollient A skin balm; a soothing ointment.

emotion An intense feeling.

empathy To understand and appreciate the deep feelings of another person.

emphysema A condition in which the air spaces in the lungs are enlarged. This makes breathing more difficult and may eventually damage heart action. (Seen usually in older people)

empirical Referring to conclusions based on practical observations.

Empirin A patented medicine with the same actions as aspirin and other pain-relieving drugs.

empyema The presence of pus in a cavity, as in the chest cavity.

emulsion Particles of one fluid suspended in another fluid; as oil in water.

encanthis A tumor involving the inner corner of the eye.

encapsulation Containing a covering or sheath; having a capsule.

encephalalgia Headache.

encephalitis Inflammation of the brain.

encephalogram A special X-ray technique for seeing the various parts of the brain. (It is carried out by injecting air into the spinal canal or directly into the brain.)

encephalomalacia Loss of brain substance and brain activity, usually caused by hardening of the arteries in the brain.

encephalomeningitis Infection of the brain and its coverings (meninges).

encephalomyelitis Inflammation or

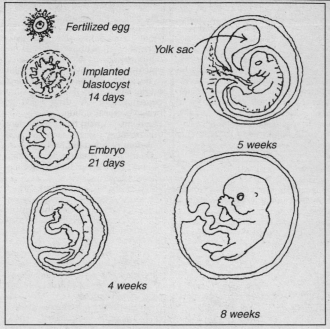

Fertilized egg

Yolk sac

Implanted blastocyst 14 days

Embryo 21 days

5 weeks

4 weeks

8 weeks

Embryo; stages of development

infection of the brain and spinal cord.

encephalon The brain.

encephalopathy Disease of the brain.

encephalosclerosis Hardening of the brain.

encephaloscopy A technique whereby a hole is drilled through the skull and a hollow metal tube (an endoscope) is inserted to inspect the brain.

enchondroma A tumor of cartilage (not malignant).

enchondrosis, multiple Benign tumors of cartilage located within the substance of bones.

encysted Covered by a capsule or sheath.

Endamoeba A parasite, a type of

ameba, which can cause dysentery and other infections in man.

endarterectomy A surgical procedure in which the passageway and inner lining of an artery is reamed out: usually performed to remove a clot or to scrape out the lining of an arteriosclerotic vessel.

endarteritis Inflammation of the inner layer of an artery.

endaural Referring to the inner part of the ear canal.

endemic A disease, usually contagious, which occurs in one locality, such as one town or city.

endo- A prefix meaning within.

endocardiography An electrocardiogram carried out with an electrode that has been inserted directly into the heart.

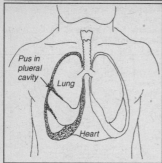

Empyema

endocarditis Inflammation of the valves or lining membrane of the heart.

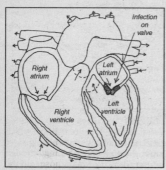

Endocarditis

endocardium The membrane lining the chambers of the heart.

endocervical Referring to the inner lining of the cervix of the uterus.

endocervicitis Inflammation of the membrane lining the cervix of the uterus.

endocrine glands Glands which secrete their hormones into the bloodstream; such as the pituitary, thyroid, and adrenal glands. Also called *ductless glands*.

endocrinology The study of the endocrine glands which secrete their hormones into the bloodstream.

(The pituitary, thyroid, pancreas, adrenal, testicles and ovaries.)

endogenous Something which originates from within the body, as opposed to exogenous.

endometrial cyst A cyst, usually located in or near the ovary, composed of tissue derived from the endometrium (the lining cells of the uterus).

endometriosis The presence of cells which ordinarily line the uterus in unusual places, such as in the bladder or intestinal wall. (This condition may produce irregular or painful menstruation, and sterility.)

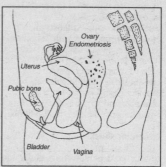

Endometriosis

endometritis Inflammation of the lining of the uterine cavity.

endometrium The mucous membrane lining the uterine cavity.

endomorph One whose bodily constitution tends to be soft, round and fat.

end organ The end (terminal point) of a nerve fiber at the point where it enters the skin, muscle or other structure.

endoscope An instrument used to peer into body cavities and openings, such as a gastroscope for the stomach or a proctoscope for the rectum.

endoscopic retrograde lithotripsy The removal of stones from the ureter by passing a special instrument into the bladder and up into the ureter. It is a form of endourology. *See* endourology.

endoscopist A physician who specializes in endoscopy. *See* endoscopy.

endoscopy That branch of medicine in which interior parts of the body are seen and treated by the passage of an endoscope. The stomach, duodenum, and the entire large intestine can be visualized through an endoscope.

endoskeleton The type of skeleton which supports the body from within, as the skeleton of vertebrates. (The opposite of exoskeleton as found in insects.)

Endostatin *See* Angiostatin.

endothelioma A tumor originating from cells which line blood vessels, lymph channels, etc. It may be benign or may become malignant.

endothelium Cells which form the inner lining of blood vessels, lymph channels and various body cavities.

endothermy Diathermy, or deep heat.

endotoxic shock Rapid pulse, lowered blood pressure, shortness of breath, cold perspiration, chills and fever, etc., brought about by the poisons (toxins) liberated by bacteria and discharged into the bloodstream.

endotoxin A poison formed within bacteria which is not released until the bacterial cell dies.

endotracheal anesthesia Anesthesia given through a rubber tube that is inserted through the mouth into the trachea (windpipe).

endourology A new branch of urology in which stones are removed from the urinary tract either by ESWL (*see* ESWL) or by endoscopic retrograde lithotripsy.

end plate The point at which the nerve ends and transmits its impulse to the organ or structure it serves.

end product The final product; often referring to the breakdown of

a complex chemical into its most basic components.

enema An injection of fluid into the rectum.

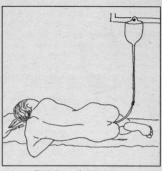

Technique of giving enema

energy The capacity for doing work.

enervation Weakness, loss of energy.

engorge To become filled with blood.

enophthalmos A receded eyeball, as seen in certain afflictions of nerves.

ensiform cartilage The pointed lower tip of the breastbone which points toward the abdomen.

enteral nutrition Feeding through a tube placed down the nose into the stomach. Used for persons who cannot eat or refuse to eat.

enterectomy Surgical removal of part of the intestine.

enteric fever An old term for *typhoid fever.*

enteritis Inflammation of the intestinal tract, either acute or chronic.

Enterobacter A type of bacteria found in feces, which can cause various infections.

enterobiasis Pinworm infestation, usually involving the intestinal tract.

enterococcus A type of streptococcus found in the intestinal tract.

enterocolitis Inflammation of the small and large intestine.

enteroenterostomy A surgical procedure in which an artificial opening is made so as to join two segments of intestine.

enterokinase An enzyme in the intestines which changes trypsinogen into trypsin, an active enzyme important in digesting proteins.

enteroptosis "Dropped" intestines; intestines which are displaced from their usual position so that they occupy the pelvis. (Seen mostly in tall, very thin people)

enterovirus One that infects and enters the body through the intestinal tract, including the virus causing poliomyelitis, Coxsackie virus, etc.

entoderm Primitive tissue found in the embryo. It goes to form the inner lining of the intestinal tract.

entomology The study of insect life.

entomophobia Fear of insects.

entropion A condition in which an eyelid turns in, thus causing eyelashes to rub against and scratch the eyeball.

enucleate To remove an organ surgically. (To *enucleate* an eye)

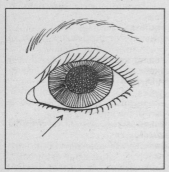

Entropion

enuresis Bedwetting; passage of urine during sleep.

enzyme A substance manufactured by living tissue which stimulates specific chemical changes, such as pancreatic *enzymes* which cause complex food proteins to break down into simpler structures which can be absorbed by the intestines.

enzymolysis The decomposition of a compound through the action of an enzyme.

eonism Transvestitism. The wearing of a woman's clothes and the assumption of a woman's attitude by a male. (Seen among some male homosexuals)

eosinophil A type of white blood cell which has a reddish color when stained and examined under a microscope. (They increase in number when the patient has an allergic condition or when there is an invasion of the body by a parasite.)

eosinophilia An abnormally large number of eosinophils (red staining white blood cells) in the circulating blood. This condition is sometimes found in people with marked allergies or in those infected with a parasite (worms, etc.).

eosinophilic tumor A tumor of the pituitary gland in the base of the skull. When it occurs during childhood, it may result in gigantism, with the child growing to be over 7 feet tall. When it takes place in adulthood, it leads to acromegaly. *See also* acromegaly.

ependyma The innermost lining of the brain and spinal cord cavities.

ependymoma A type of brain tumor, usually one which grows into the ventricle (hollow space) of the brain, arising from the cells which line the brain cavities.

ephedrine A chemical with the same actions as adrenalin. It is used effectively in cases of shock or in conditions such as hay fever, asthma, hives, etc.

ephemeral Fleeting; lasting but a short time.

epicanthus An extra fold of skin covering the inner corner of the eyes, seen among Chinese, Japanese, etc.

epicardia That portion of the esophagus (food pipe) which lies between the diaphragm and the stomach.

epicondyle A protrusion of bone in the region of the condyle near the joint.

epicondylitis Inflammation of an epicondyle.

epicranium The coverings of the skull.

epicrisis A second crisis in the same illness.

epicritic sensation Sensation which can define precisely the stimulus being received, such as the ability to appreciate the sense of pin prick, heat, cold, localized pain, etc.

epidemic A disease which simultaneously affects large numbers of people in a community.

epidemiology The study of the occurrence and prevalence of disease, often applied to the study of the manner of spread of contagious diseases.

epidermal growth factor (EGF) A genetically engineered protein that stimulates rapid healing of skin and the cornea of the eye.

epidermis The outer layer of the skin.

epidermoid tumor One containing elements of skin.

epidermoid carcinoma A cancer originating in the skin or in tissue having the same characteristics as skin. (Almost all of these cancers are curable.)

epidermomycosis Any fungus of the skin, including athlete's foot, etc.

epidermophytosis A fungus infection.

epididymis That portion of the seminal tube immediately attached to the testicle. It collects sperm, from the testicle, which will be transported by the seminal duct.

epididymitis Inflammation of the epididymis, a structure immediately adjacent to the testicle, often caused by gonorrhea.

epidural The space just beyond and around the dura. (The dura is a thick outer covering for the brain

and spinal cord.) Hemorrhage in this area creates great pressure upon the brain and may require surgery.

epidural anesthesia A regional anesthesia in which the anesthetic agent is injected into the epidural space surrounding the spinal canal. (The needle does not penetrate, nor is the anesthetic injected into, the spinal canal.)

epigastric Referring to the epigastrium, or the space in the abdomen just below the ribs in the midline. Sometimes referred to as "the pit of the stomach."

epiglottis The cartilage in the throat which guards the entrance to the trachea (windpipe) and prevents fluid or food from entering it when one swallows.

epikeratophakia An operation in which the cornea of the eye is reshaped to overcome a defect in its contour. Sometimes used to correct keratoconus or nearsightedness. *See* keratoconus.

epilation The removal of hair.

epilepsy A brain disorder accompanied by periodic convulsions and loss of consciousness. It can be caused by many different underlying conditions.

epileptic One who is subject to convulsive seizures ("fits"). (Newer medications are able to prevent such convulsions in the great majority of instances.)

epimysium The thin tissue covering or sheath surrounding a muscle.

epinephric gland The adrenal gland.

epinephrine The hormone secreted by the inner portion of the adrenal gland; also called *adrenalin*. (One of its main actions is to constrict blood vessels and raise blood pressure.)

epineurium The connective tissue sheath surrounding individual nerve fibers. Through the epineurium travel the blood vessels which supply nerve trunks.

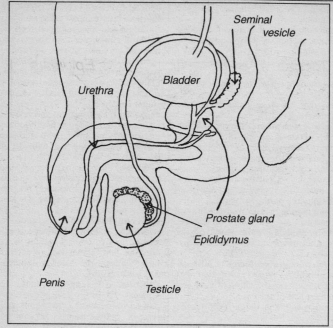

Epididymis

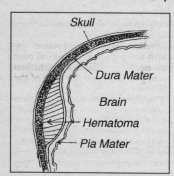

Epidural hematoma

epiphora Excess tearing; occasionally due to blockage of the tear ducts.

epiphysiodesis Premature fusion of the growth plates in bones. (When epiphysiodesis takes place, growth stops.)

epiphysis That portion of bone between the main portion and the cartilage. (It is thought to be the main point of bone growth.)

epiphysitis Inflammation of that portion of bone (epiphysis) located between the cartilage and the main shaft of bone.

epiploectomy Removal of the omentum (the large pad of fat hanging down from the transverse colon and covering the intestines).

epiploon The great omentum; the pad of fat which covers the intestines like an apron.

episcleritis Inflammation of the

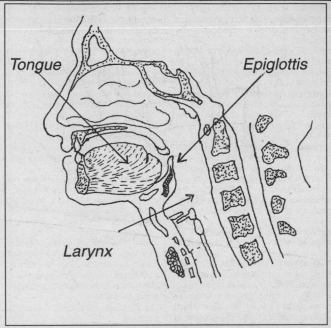

Tongue

Epiglottis

Larynx

Epiglottis

sclera, the white of the eye, and the tissue between it and the overlying membrane (conjunctiva).

episiotomy An incision made from the vaginal outlet toward the anus during childbirth, to avoid undue tearing as the baby's head passes through.

episode An attack of an illness which tends to recur at intervals, such as an epileptic seizure, etc.

epispadias A birth deformity in which the urethra ends short of the tip of the penis and opens somewhere along its shaft.

epistaxis Nosebleed.

epithelioma A tumor of the skin.

epithelium The tissue cells composing the skin; also, the cells lining all the passages of the hollow organs of the respiratory, digestive and urinary systems.

epithelialization The process by which a raw surface is covered over with new skin. The new epithelium (skin) grows in from the sides of the raw space.

epitrochlear lymph node A lymph gland located just above the inner aspect of the elbow. Frequently enlarged in advanced cases of syphilis.

epituberculosis A type of tuberculosis of the lung seen in children. It often resembles pneumonia and usually goes on to recovery.

epizoic Pertaining to parasites which dwell on the skin.

eponychium The cuticle of the nails.

eponym The name of an illness or

disorder derived from the name of the physician who first described it, as Bright's disease, Addison's disease, etc.

epsom salts Magnesium sulfate; used as a laxative and, when dissolved in water, frequently as a wet dressing.

Epstein-Barr virus A virus causing infectious mononucleosis ("mono").

epulis A tumor of the jaw bones which appears as a lump beneath the gums.

Equanil A widely used tranquilizer; meprobamate.

equilibrium Balance. It is maintained through organs of balance in the inner ear.

equinocavus A foot deformity accompanied by an abnormally high arch.

equinovarus A foot deformity associated with a turning inward of the forefoot.

eradication Getting rid of something, as in exterminating a disease.

erasion Scraping away tissue.

ERBF Abbreviation for effective renal blood flow, or that flow which is concerned with the production of urine from constituents originating in the bloodstream.

Erb's palsy A paralysis of the nerves supplying the arm (brachial plexus) as a result of injury during childbirth. (This paralysis may be permanent, if severe.)

ERCP An abbreviation for *endoscopic retrograde choledochopancreatography*. The procedure involves the passage of a flexible instrument down the throat, through the stomach into the duodenum and up the common bile duct. An opaque dye is then injected into the duct and X-ray films are taken.

erectile tissue Tissue which is capable of becoming firm and erect, such as the skin of the nipples of the breasts.

erection The enlarging and hardening of the male organ as it becomes engorged with blood.

erg A unit of work.

ergograph An instrument which measures the amount of work being performed by a muscle.

ergophobia Fear of work.

ergosterol A chemical which, when exposed to ultraviolet light, turns into vitamin D.

ergot A fungus which, when purified and used as a medication, causes strong contractions of the uterus. Often used to stop hemorrhage from the uterus.

ergotamine tartrate A derivative of ergot, especially helpful in relieving migraine headaches.

ergotism Poisoning from the overuse or prolonged use of ergot. In rare instances, it has caused gangrene of the fingers or toes.

erogenous Increasing or stimulating sexual desire.

eros The instinct to live. Libido.

erosion The eating away of a surface of a structure as the result of inflammation, such as an *erosion* of the lining of the stomach resulting in ulcer formation.

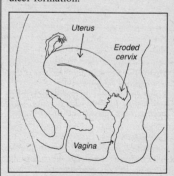

Erosion of the cervix

erotic Pertaining to sexual desire.

eroticism Sexual desire or excitement. In psychoanalysis, the manifestation of sexual instinct.

erotomania Excessive thoughts and activities of sexual nature.

eructate To belch.

eruption To break out, as in a rash.

erysipelas A streptococcus infection of the skin and tissues beneath the skin giving a characteristic reddened, sharply outlined appearance. It is accompanied by high fever and a marked toxic reaction.

erythema A patch of redness of the skin.

multiforme A red, slightly raised rash that appears on the body and limbs secondary to an allergy or to a drug sensitivity. It can be mild or extremely severe, and in all cases it represents an external manifestation of a systemic reaction.

nodosum Painful, rounded areas associated with a red rash, appearing on the front of the legs. It is seen frequently in rheumatic fever and also in patients who have drug allergies.

erythremia A disease in which there is an overproduction of red blood cells; as in polycythemia.

erythroblast A primitive red blood cell.

erythroblastosis An anemia of the newborn occurring when a mother is Rh negative and develops antibodies against her unborn child who is Rh positive. (This condition is responsible for some stillbirths and for infants who die shortly after birth.)

erythrocyte A red blood cell. (Normally, humans have 4,500,000 to 5,000,000 red blood cells per cubic millimeter of blood.)

erythrolysis Destruction of red blood cells.

Erythromycin A powerful antibiotic drug, especially effective against the staphylococcus germ.

erythropoietin A kidney hormone that tends to increase the number of red blood cells and cut down the need for blood transfusions in cases of chronic anemia.

escape mechanism A psychological term used to describe a mental maneuver by which one escapes from a sense of responsibility or a sense of guilt.

eschar A hard crust over a raw surface, as the material covering a deep burn.

Escherichia coli Gram-negative bacteria found in feces; frequently causing inflammation of the bowel, peritonitis, or cystitis. Also called *E. coli.*

escutcheon The formation of hair in the pubic region creating a pattern, such as a *male escutcheon* or a *female escutcheon.*

Esidrix Brand name for a powerful diuretic used in the treatment of high blood pressure.

esophagectomy Removal of the esophagus (food pipe), carried out in some cases of cancer of the esophagus.

esophagitis Inflammation of the esophagus (food pipe).

esophagogastrectomy The surgical removal of a portion of the esophagus and stomach. (Performed in cases where the upper end of the stomach and the lower end of the esophagus are invaded by cancer.)

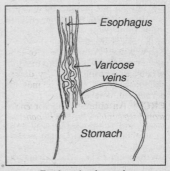

Esophageal varicose veins

esophagogastrostomy A surgical operation in which a new communication is fashioned between the esophagus (food pipe) and the stomach. (Sometimes done when there is a narrowing of the terminal end of the esophagus)

esophagogram An X ray of the esophagus.

esophagomyotomy An operative procedure in which the muscle fibers of the lower end of the esophagus are severed but the mucous membrane lining is left intact; the so-called Heller operation to relieve achalasia (a chronic spasm of the lower end of the esophagus).

esophagoscopy The examination of the esophagus by passage of a specially designed instrument through the mouth.

esophagospasm Contraction and spasm of a portion of the esophagus.

esophagus The food pipe. It extends from the back of the throat down through the chest and diaphragm to the stomach. (It measures about 12 inches in length by about 1 inch in diameter.)

esotropia A form of crossed eyes in which one eye turns inward.

ESP *See* extrasensory perception.

espundia A serious infection caused by the organism *Leishmania*. It is thought to be transmitted through the bite of an insect. (Occurs in America, particularly in heavily wooded regions)

ESR Abbreviation for red blood cell sedimentation rate, a test performed to denote the presence or absence of an infection.

essence The undiluted active ingredient of a solution.

essential hypertension High blood pressure of unknown origin.

ester Any compound formed from an alcohol and an acid, such as cholesterol.

esterification The transformation of an acid or an alcohol into an ester.

esthetic Relating to the senses.

Estinyl A patented drug composed of an extract of the female sex hormone (estrogen).

estival Relating to the summer.

estradiol The female sex hormone.

estrogen The female sex hormone, manufactured by the ovaries.

estrogen receptor test A test to discover the influence of the female sex hormone (estrogen) upon the growth of a breast cancer cell. (Positive receptors in postmenopausal women indicate the administration of the anti-estrogen substance known as tamoxifen.)

estrone An estrogenic steroid.

estrus The animal mating period; "in heat."

ESWL Abbreviation for *endoscopic shock wave lithotripsy*, a procedure in which stones are broken up and eventually are washed out of the kidneys by use of shock waves rather than invasive surgery.

ethambutol An effective antituberculosis medication.

ethanol Ethyl alcohol (the type that goes into alcoholic beverages).

ether A chemical whose vapor is a most widely used anesthetic agent.

Ethicist Someone who specializes in the ethical aspects of practicing a particular profession.

ethics The study of right and wrong.

ethisterone A hormone medication containing the corpus luteum secretion of the ovary; *progesterone.* (Given in certain cases to prevent miscarriage)

ethmoidectomy Surgical removal of the ethmoid cells because of infection. The ethmoid cells are sinus cells back of the nose.

ethmoiditis Inflammation of the ethmoid sinuses.

ethmoid sinus A sinus or cavity in the bones of the base of the skull located behind the bridge of the nose.

ethnic Relating to peoples and races.

Ethrane An inhalation anesthetic agent; enflurane.

ethyl alcohol The type of alcohol in whiskey, wine, etc.

ethyl chloride A highly volatile (vaporizes easily) chemical, used as a local anesthetic. It freezes tissue with which it comes in contact.

ethylene A gas used as an anesthetic.

ethylestrenol A steroid medication helpful in building tissues and combating tissue deterioration.

ethylnorepinephrine A drug used in combating an attack of asthma.

etiology The study of the cause of disease.

eu A prefix meaning *normal*, well, good. (Someone whose thyroid functions normally is said to be euthyroid.)

eucalyptol One of the components of oil of eucalyptus, used occasionally in cases of bronchitis.

eugenics The science of improving the species or race.

Eulexin A medicine used in combination with Lupron for the control of prostate cancer. It is most helpful when the cancer has spread from the confines of the prostate. (Same as flutamide.)

eunuch A male without testicles.

euphoria An exaggerated state of well-being.

eustachian tube The auditory tube leading from the back of the throat to the ear.

euthanasia The putting to death of people who are hopelessly ill (an illegal procedure).

euthenics The science of improving mankind and his offspring by improving the conditions under which he lives.

Euthroid A patented medication of thyroid substance, used to replace the thyroid hormone in cases of thyroid insufficiency.

euthyroid Denoting a state of normal thyroid function.

evacuate To empty, such as the pus from an abscess cavity.

evacuation Commonly referring to the emptying of the bowel.

evagination Bulging out of tissue.

evanescent Transitory; fleeting.

eventration The bulging of intestines through a rupture in the wall of the abdomen.

eversion Turning outward of a part or structure.

evil eye The superstition that when certain people cast their gaze upon someone, he will become ill or die.

eviscerate 1. The accidental splitting open of an abdominal surgical wound with spillage of intestines onto the abdominal wall. 2. A surgical procedure in which the abdomen is opened and the intestines are intentionally lifted out of the abdominal cavity.

Evista An estrogen-like hormone that has been helpful in staving off or treating osteoporosis (thinning of the bones) in women. *See* raloxifene.

evolution The process by which complex animal life has developed from more primitive and simpler forms.

Ewing's tumor A sarcoma (cancerlike malignant tumor) of the shaft of a long bone such as the thighbone, arm bone, etc.

exacerbation Flare-up of a condition; relapse of a disease.

exaltation A sense of great joy.

exanthem subitum A mild noncontagious childhood disease characterized by a rose-colored eruption and fever. It lasts a few days and disappears spontaneously.

exanthropic A condition or disorder originating outside of the body.

excavation A hole or depression in contour or an organ or part.

Excedrin P.M. A pain-relieving medication combined with a mild sleeping agent.

exchange transfusion A transfusion method used to save the lives of newborns having erythroblastosis. It attempts, in stages, to remove most of the child's own blood and to substitute transfused donor blood. (This condition is the result of Rh sensitivity.)

excision To cut out surgically.

excitant Any drug which stimulates the activity of an organ.

excoriation A deep scratch in the skin.

excrement Feces; stool.

excrescence Anything which protrudes or grows out of a flat surface.

excrete To expel or discharge waste matter.

excursion The extent of movement of a part, as the *excursion* of the chest during inhalation and exhalation.

exdural hemorrhage Bleeding originating just beneath the skull, but outside the main covering of the brain (the dura).

exemia Any condition in which most of the blood leaves the major vessels in which it normally travels, as, for instance, in states of shock.

exenteration operation An operation performed upon patients with far advanced cancer in an attempt to prolong life. It often involves removal of many organs, including the bladder and rectum.

exfoliation The shedding or peeling of tissue, as the *exfoliation* of the superficial layers of the skin, which takes place constantly.

exhale To breath out.

exhaustion Fatigue of an extreme degree.

exhibitionism An abnormal desire to expose one's body, particularly the genitals.

exhume To dig out a buried body.

exitus Death.

exocrine glands Glands which secrete onto a surface rather than into the blood (the opposite of endocrine glands). The salivary glands fall into this category.

exodontia The specialty which deals with tooth extraction.

exogenous Arising from a source outside the body. (The opposite of endogenous.)

exomphalos A hernia of the navel through which abdominal organs (usually intestines) protrude.

exophthalmos Bulging of the eyeballs from their sockets, as seen in certain cases of overactivity of the thyroid gland (exophthalmic goiter).

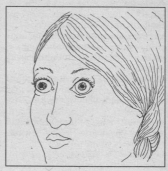

Exophthalmos

exoskeleton A form of animal life in which the skeleton is on the outside of the body, as in insects, crabs, lobsters, etc.

exostosis A tumor of bone characterized by a bulging at one or more sites. (Not malignant)

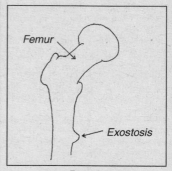

Femur

Exostosis

Exostosis

exoteric Referring to a condition which is of external origin; not arising from within the body.

exotoxin The poison excreted by living germs.

exotropia A form of crossed eyes in which one eye turns outward.

expectorant A medication given to

promote expectoration of secretions in the lungs or bronchial tubes.

expiration Breathing out. Exhalation.

exploration Commonly applied to an operation performed for the purpose of making a diagnosis. (The exploration is usually followed by a remedial procedure.)

exsanguination The loss of huge quantities of blood.

extended radical mastectomy Removal of the breast, including the internal mammary glands located beneath the junction of the ribs and the breastbone.

exstrophy of the bladder A birth deformity of the urinary bladder in which the anterior wall of the bladder is missing and the urine empties onto the abdominal wall.

extended care Care given in an institution especially designed to serve the chronically or terminally ill, or to give prolonged care, such as rehabilitation.

extended wear contact lens Lenses that can be worn 24 hours a day for up to 30 days.

extension The stretching or straightening of a limb which is contracted, dislocated or fractured.

extensor muscles Those which straighten a limb or part. (The opposite of flexor muscles)

exteriorize To bring an organ out onto the surface of the body, as during surgery.

Extern An intern who lives outside of the hospital.

extirpation The surgical removal of an organ or part; excision.

extracapsular Outside a capsule, as a growth which has extended beyond its capsule.

extracellular Outside of a cell, such as *extracellular* fluid.

extracorporeal Outside of the body, such as *extracorporeal circulation* used during open heart operations. (The blood passes through a mechanical pump which connects to the body.)

extracorporeal shock wave lithotrypsy A procedure for breaking up kidney stones by subjecting them to pressure waves generated by electric shocks.

extract 1. In pharmacy, it is the process by which certain ingredients are withdrawn from a drug. 2. In surgery, to remove.

extradural Located outside the dura. (The dura is the outer covering of the brain and spinal cord.)

extrahepatic Referring to a condition that is outside of—though close to—the liver, such as extrahepatic biliary obstruction due to a stone in a bile duct.

extramural Outside the wall of an organ or part; the opposite of intramural.

extrasensory perception Mental telepathy; also clairvoyance. There is considerable scientific doubt as to its existence.

extrasystole A heart beat occurring before its normal time. *Extrasystoles* create an irregular rhythm. Commonly referred to as a "skipped beat."

extrauterine pregnancy A pregnancy which takes place outside the uterus, such as an ectopic pregnancy (tubal pregnancy), or an abdominal pregnancy.

extravasation A condition in which blood, urine, or some other body fluid, leaves its normal channel and flows out into the tissues, as when a blood vessel ruptures.

extremis On the point of dying.

extremity A limb, an arm or leg.

extrinsic Coming from outside, as opposed to intrinsic.

extrophy Deformity of an organ, as *extrophy* of the urinary bladder.

extrovert One whose personality displays great interest in others, rather than in oneself. The opposite of introvert.

extrusion Casting out; expelling.

extubation The removal of a tube, especially a rubber tube placed into the larynx and trachea during anesthesia.

exudate Inflammatory fluid (pus, serum, etc.) which bathes the tissues in the vicinity of an infection.

eye The organ of sight.

  bank A laboratory that stores corneas for future transplantation. (The whole eye is not used for transplantation.)

  grounds The retina or back of the inside of the eye. This can be seen and studied by use of the ophthalmoscope.

  strain Pain in the eyes, redness, tearing, headache, dizziness; secondary to misuse of the eyes, or to fatigue, or to improper glasses, etc.

  teeth The sharp canine teeth in the upper jaw.

  wash A solution used to bathe inflamed eyes.

F

face-lift See rhytidectomy.

face presentation A position of the unborn child during labor in which the face appears at the outlet of the vagina. (Delivery may be very difficult when the child assumes this position.)

facet A smooth, flat area, as on the surface of a bone or on the surface of a gallstone.

facial artery The main artery to the face, originating from the large carotid artery in the neck.

facial nerve The seventh cranial nerve, supplying the muscles and surfaces of the face, tongue, ear, etc. (It is sometimes injured when performing a mastoid operation; other times it may have to be cut when removing a malignant tumor of the parotid gland. Occasionally, it becomes paralyzed, resulting in facial paralysis.)

facies The appearance of the face. (There are characteristic facial expressions for certain diseases, such as the *ulcer facies* with its pinched, hollow cheeks.)

facioplasty A plastic surgical procedure on the skin and subcutaneous tissues of the face.

F.A.C.O.G. Fellow of the American College of Obstetricians and Gynecologists.

F.A.C.P. Fellow of the American College of Physicians.

F.A.C.R. Fellow of the American College of Radiologists.

F.A.C.S. Fellow of the American College of Surgeons.

factor A circumstance which contributes toward bringing about a given result. A fact. (The *Rh factor* is responsible for certain diseases of a newborn child.)

facultative Optional. The ability to do or not to do something.

Fahrenheit A temperature scale commonly used in the United States and Great Britain. In this scale, water freezes at 32° F; water boils 212° F; normal human temperature is 98.6° F.

fainting A momentary loss of consciousness. Swooning. (Fainting is thought to be caused by transient insufficient blood supply to the brain.)

faith healing Healing or "treatment" of illness solely through prayer, practiced by some Christian Scientists.

falciform Sickle-shaped, such as the *falciform* ligament which attaches the liver to the diaphragm.

fallen womb The protrusion of the uterus downward into the vagina usually caused by stretched or torn ligaments which ordinarily hold the uterus in its proper place.

falling sickness Epilepsy.

fallopian tube The uterine tubes, one on either side of the uterus. These structures have a passageway through which the egg is conveyed from the ovary to the uterus.

Fallot's tetralogy A birth deformity of the heart involving defects in the blood vessels and walls of the heart chambers. In certain cases, this condition can be corrected through surgery.

false-negative A test that shows no evidence of disease when disease is actually present.

false pains Contractions of the uterus resembling labor pains, often felt within a few weeks prior to the onset of true labor.

false-positive   A test that shows evidence of disease when disease is not actually present.

familial disease   A disease occurring in several members of the same family. Most familial diseases, such as hemophilia, are inherited. (This term does not refer to contagious diseases.)

familial polyposis   An inherited disease in which the large intestine is the site of hundreds or thousands of growths known as polyps. Surgery is usually necessary to prevent the ultimate development of cancer in some of the polyps.

familial tendency   A tendency for a disease or condition to occur in the same family, among members of several generations. (Diabetes, obesity, etc. are examples of conditions which tend to affect certain families more than others.)

Family doctor   A general practitioner; a general physician who is trained to treat the great majority of illnesses, except those requiring specialized skills.

Fansidar   A new, potent antimalarial drug, to be used cautiously because of possible side effects.

fantasy   Imagination. The mental process by which one constructs fanciful images of things which have not actually occurred.

faradic current   Alternating current, occasionally used in treating nerve paralysis and to stimulate muscles to function.

farcy   *See* glanders.

farsightedness   A condition in which the eyeball is abnormally short, thus causing light rays to focus behind the retina. In farsightedness, one sees distant objects better than near objects.

fascia   Connective tissue located in various places throughout the body, such as beneath the skin, in between muscles, around blood vessels or nerves, etc.

fascicular   Referring to tissue that is arranged in the shape of a bundle, as connective tissue fibers.

fasciitis   Inflammation of fascia (fibrous connective tissue).

fasciotomy   A surgical incision into fascia, sometimes performed to release tension or contractures about joints.

fat   Chemically, fats are esters of certain acids, such as oleic, stearic, or palmitic acid. Fat is one of the three most important sources of calories in food.

fatality rate   1. The number of people who die per 100,000 population. 2. The percentage of people who die from any particular disease.

fatigue   Tiredness; weariness; exhaustion.

fat necrosis   Death of fat tissue, sometimes occurring in breasts or in other tissues composed mainly of fat cells.

fatty acid   An acid originating from hydrocarbons, such as oleic, stearic, or palmitic acid.

fatty degeneration   Degeneration of an organ with replacement of its normal structure by fat. (This occurs in the liver during early stages of cirrhosis or other liver diseases.)

fauces   The area between the back of the mouth and the beginning of the throat.

favism   An acute upset following the eating of a certain type of bean, grown mainly in Italy.

favus   A parasitic disease of the scalp characterized by the formation of yellow crusts. It is caused by the fungus *Microsporum gypseum.*

F.C.A.P.   Fellow of the College of American Pathologists.

FDA   Abbreviation for *Food and Drug Administration,* a federal agency overseeing food and drug approval and sales to the public.

Fe   Chemical symbol for iron.

fear reaction   A neurotic state brought on by reluctance to face danger. It is characterized by anxiety, palpitation of the heart, sweating, faintness, nausea, dizziness, etc.

febrile Feverish; relating to an elevation in body temperature above 98.6° F.

fecal impaction Hard stools in the rectum and large bowel, making normal evacuation difficult or impossible.

fecalith A hardened ball of feces (stool) within the bowel or appendix.

fecaloid Resembling fecal material.

feces The material excreted by the large intestines (stool).

fecundation Fertilization.

fecundity Fertility. The ability to produce offspring.

feeblemindedness A mental state of development below normal but above that of the idiot or imbecile; moronic.

fee splitting The unethical practice of dividing a medical or surgical fee between two doctors without the consent and knowledge of the patient; a secret kickback.

Feldine An anti-inflammatory drug, also causing relief of pain and lowering of temperature. To be used cautiously because of its high incidence of adverse reactions.

fellatio The sex practice in which the male organ is taken into the mouth.

fallator A male who takes the male organ of another into the mouth.

fellatrice A female who takes the male organ into the mouth.

Fellow of the American College of Physicians Membership in this organization signifies that a physician is a qualified medical specialist.

Fellow of the American College of Surgeons Membership in this organization signifies that the member physician is a qualified surgical specialist.

felon An abscess of the palmar surface of the fingertip. If untreated, such infections may involve the bone of the fingertip and cause osteomyelitis.

female Woman; girl. The symbol for female is: ♀

feminism The appearance of female traits, either emotional or physical, in a male.

feminizing tumor A tumor of the ovary which results in the exaggeration of the female sex characteristics. If it occurs in a female child, she may develop breasts and start to menstruate. If it occurs after change of life, it may cause vaginal bleeding and regrowth of breast tissue. Also called *granulosa cell tumor* of the ovary.

femoral Referring to the upper part of the thigh near the groin. (A femoral hernia is one located just beneath the crease of the groin.)

femoral artery The main artery supplying the thigh and leg. (Its pulsation can be felt just below the crease of the groin.)

femoral nerve One of the main nerves supplying the lower extremity. (It lies alongside the femoral artery in the groin.)

femoral-popliteal bypass An operative procedure in which a graft is placed alongside the femoral artery in the thigh down to the tibial artery below the knee. The procedure is done to improve blood circulation to the leg and foot.

femur The thighbone, originating in the hip and extending down to the knee.

fenestration operation An operation performed to relieve deafness in cases where there has been disease and damage to the bones of hearing (the incus, stapes, and malleus) in the middle ear. (A hole is drilled in the bone within the ear canal, permitting sound waves to bypass the damaged middle ear and to reach the inner ear.)

Feosol A patented medication used in treating certain types of anemia. It contains iron as its most active ingredient.

fermentation The breaking down of complex molecules into simple molecules under the influence of enzymes.

ferric Containing iron. (Many such compounds are used as medications for treating anemia.)

Ferro-Sequels A tablet containing iron; given in certain cases of anemia.

ferrous Containing iron.

fertile period The period during the month when a woman is capable of becoming pregnant.

fertility The ability to bear children.

fertilization The entrance of the male sperm into the female egg.

fester To form an abscess; to discharge pus.

fetal Referring to the unborn child.

fetal adenoma A benign tumor of the thyroid gland containing cells of a primitive (fetal) nature.

fetal alcoholic syndrome Children of alcoholic mothers have a tendency to be smaller and underweight at birth. They learn to talk much later, have lower than normal intelligence and have difficulty getting along with other children.

fetal distress Impaired heart action of an unborn child. It may lead to death of the fetus if not relieved promptly.

fetal rickets Rickets having its onset before birth. (*See also* rickets.)

fetal surgery Operations upon the fetus while still in its mother's womb.

fetation Pregnancy.

feticide To kill the fetus (unborn child) while it is in the uterus.

fetid Foul smelling.

fetishism A sexual peculiarity in which one derives gratification from touching or viewing a particular part of a woman's body or merely by handling articles of women's apparel.

fetological surgery Surgery upon the unborn child. By opening the pregnant uterus, the child is partially withdrawn, operated upon, and placed back into the uterus. Several abnormalities can be corrected by this technique.

fetology That branch of medicine which concerns itself with the fetus while it is developing in the uterus.

fetometry To measure the size of the fetus while in the uterus. (The dimensions of its head are most important, in order to evaluate the possibility of delivery through the vagina.)

fetor oris Bad breath.

fetus The unborn child during the later part of pregnancy. (Prior to the third month, it is termed *embryo*.)

fever Elevation of body temperature above the normal of 98.6° F. (Normal rectal temperature may be up to one half degree higher.)

fever blister A sore, usually on the upper lip, sometimes associated with the common cold; other times due to heat sensitivity or unknown causes. Also known as *Herpes simplex.*

fiber Any threadlike structure or tissue; a filament. A general term used to describe muscle or nerve cells.

fiber optics The conduction of light through a conduit composed of pliable plastic fibers. This permits viewing the passageways of the respiratory or intestinal tract through a flexible instrument that can go around curves. Gastroscopes and colonoscopes utilize fiber optics.

fiberscope An instrument used to examine the bronchial tubes, stomach or large bowel, employing fiber optics.

fibrillation An irregular heart action due to abnormal spread of impulses from one portion of the heart to another. *Fibrillation* usually indicates a failing heart which requires support.

    atrial (auricular) Irregular heart action due to abnormal spread of impulses originating in the atrium.

    ventricular Irregular heart action due to abnormal spread of impulses originating in the ventricle. (Continued fibrillation of this type is often fatal.)

fibrin The substance which enmeshes blood corpuscles in the bloodclotting mechanism. *Fibrin* is a body protein which hardens when blood leaves its usual channels.

fibrinogen A protein present in blood plasma. It becomes fibrin during the blood-clotting process.

fibrinolysis The process which takes place when a blood clot dissolves. (The fibrin in the clot dissolves.)

fibroadenoma A benign, noncancerous tumor composed of fibrous and glandular tissue. It is one of the most frequently encountered tumors of the breast.

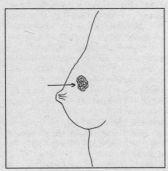

Fibroadenoma of breast

fibroblast A connective tissue cell. (These cells form fibrous and scar tissue.)

fibrocystic disease Tissue which has become cystic and fibrous.

   of bone Cyst formation in bones due to overactivity of the parathyroid glands in the neck (hyperparathyroidism). Bones so affected are exceptionally susceptible to fracture.

   breast A glandular upset resulting in the formation of many cysts in the breasts of women ap-

proaching change of life. These cysts are sometimes associated with the replacement of the normal gland tissue by firm fibrous tissue.

fibroid tumor A benign (noncancerous) tumor of the uterus composed largely of fibrous and muscle tissue. Also known as *fibromyoma* or *leiomyoma*.

fibroleiomyoma Fibroids of the uterus. These tumors are benign and are made up of muscle and fibrous tissue. They constitute the most common tumor of the uterus.

fibrolipoma A noncancerous tumor composed of fibrous and fat tissue. (Most frequently located in the tissues directly beneath the skin.)

fibroma A nonmalignant tumor composed of fibrous tissue. The tissues just beneath the skin are particularly prone to develop such growths.

fibromuscular tissue Tissue composed of fibrous and muscular elements, such as fibroid tumors of the womb.

fibromyositis Inflammation of muscle with the formation of fibrous tissue which often interferes with normal muscle function. (A common condition following a severe muscle injury.)

fibromyxosarcoma A malignant tumor composed of the various elements of connective tissue. (A rather rare tumor affecting tissues of the arms and legs.)

fibroplasia The process in which fibrous tissue grows into a wound, and promotes healing.

   retrolental Blindness in newborns, brought on by excessive oxygen administration.

fibrosarcoma A malignant tumor originating from connective tissue and fibrous tissue cells. Also called *spindle cell sarcoma*.

fibrosis Replacement of the normal components of a structure by fibrous tissue. This process is seen to take place as an organ or structure ages.

fibrositis. The overgrowth of fibrous tissue due to an injury or inflammation in the area, such as that which takes place about a shoulder involved in bursitis. Such a condition often interferes with normal motion and may be very painful.

fibrous   Containing fibers.

fibula   The thinner of the two leg bones, extending from the outer side of the knee to the outer side of the ankle. (It bears relatively little of the body's weight.)

figure   The contour of a structure.

filament   A tiny, threadlike piece of tissue.

filariasis   An infection caused by a parasite, often resulting in elephantiasis, a condition associated with huge swelling. Seen most often in Asia, Africa, and tropical countries.

filiform   Thread-shaped.

filling   The material used to repair a cavity in a tooth.

filter   To separate one substance from another by passing it through a membrane (filter). This process usually results in solids remaining in the filter while the liquids pass through.

filtrate   The fluid which has passed through a filter.

filtration   The process of filtering or straining a fluid mixture.

filum   A thread or threadlike structure.

fimbriated   Fringe-shaped, such as the open end of the fallopian tube.

fine needle biopsy   Obtaining tissue for microscopic examination by passage of a fine needle into an organ or structure, such as the thyroid gland.

finger

baseball   Dislocation of the tip of a finger in a backward direction with the tendons tightening and holding it in its dislocated position.

cot   A rubber sheath for a finger. Used by physicians in examining various openings of the body such as the mouth, the rectum, etc.

clubbed   A bulging and abnor-

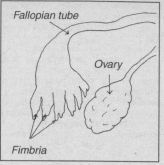

Fimbria of the fallopian tube

mal rounding out of the tips of the fingers, seen in certain kinds of chronic lung disease.

hammer   (mallet) A bending down of the tip of a finger with inability to straighten it; resulting from detachment of the tendon responsible for extending the joint.

trigger   Faulty tendon action resulting in a jerky, halting flexion or extension of a finger. (Often requires surgical correction)

Fiorinal   A pain-relieving drug, especially effective in relieving tension headache.

first aid   Any medical care given in an emergency before professional help arrives. *See* First Aid in Manual.

fission   The process of dividing, as the splitting of a cell or the splitting of an atom.

fissure   A crack or cleft, such as a fissure-in-ano (a crack in the lining membrane of the anal outlet).

-in-ano   A split or ulceration in the mucous membrane lining of the anus, resulting in pain on evacuating the bowels.

fistula   An abnormal canal or tract, often occurring in or about the anus. Such fistulas lead from the lining of the rectal wall out on to the skin alongside the anus. They discharge pus and cause considerable discomfort. They are surgically corrected.

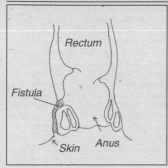

Fistula (rectal)

fistula-in-ano A channel extending from the inside of the anus to the surrounding skin. (A very common type of fistula.)

fistulectomy The surgical removal of a fistula.

fistulization The formation of a fistula. In the rectal region, this may follow an abscess or infection along the rectal or anal wall.

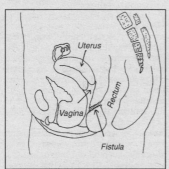

Fistula (rectovaginal)

fit A convulsion; a seizure, as in epilepsy. There is loss of consciousness and spastic contractions and jerkings of muscles. Frothing at the mouth is usually seen in epileptic *fits*.

5-FU An abbreviation for *fluoruracil*, a powerful anti-cancer drug.

fixation 1. Binding down of a part or organ of the body; to make immovable and firm, as fixation of fragments of a broken bone. 2. A situation in which a person or thing is excessively attached to another person or thing.

fixative A substance used to preserve tissues, as for microscopic study. (Applied mainly to tissues removed from the body.)

fixed idea One that is fixed in one's mind even though it has proven to be untrue; a type of delusion.

flaccid Soft and flabby.

flagellate To whip; to beat.

flagellation Whipping as a form of perverse sexual gratification.

Flagyl A medication highly effective against trichomonas infections of the vagina or penis. Also effective against amebic infections and against anaerobic infections caused by the Bacteroides species. (Used in some cases of peritonitis along with other drugs.)

flail chest A loss of stability of the chest cage resulting from multiple rib fractures or a fracture of the breastbone.

flail joint A false joint which occasionally forms at the site where the ends of a broken bone have failed to unite.

flank The loin; the area on the side of the body extending from the lowermost rib to the hipbone.

flap A pedicle graft containing skin, subcutaneous fat, muscle, blood vessels and nerves. *See* myocutaneous flap.

flaps Segments of tissue, usually including skin, subcutaneous fat, muscle, nerves, arteries and veins. Such flaps are used as grafts and are attached to their new sites by utilizing microsurgical techniques. (*See* microsurgery.)

flash, hot A heat wave, frequently followed by profuse perspiration, affecting women who are in menopause (change of life).

flat feet A flattening out of the

normal arch of the foot. Pesplanus. (Some people have great pain from this condition; others are free of symptoms.)

flatulence Excessive gas in the stomach or bowels.

flatus Gas in the lower intestinal tract.

flatworm Tapeworms and flukes belong in this category of worms.

flaxseed poultice Linseed oil extract used as a liniment for application to skin surfaces

Fleet enema A patented preparation containing a chemical which stimulates bowel evacuation. A nozzle is inserted into the rectum and the preparation is squeezed into the bowel. Evacuation takes place in ten to twenty minutes.

Fleming, Sir Alexander (1881–1955) The codiscoverer of "penicillin" and its effects upon bacteria.

flesh, proud Granulation tissue red, spongy tissue seen in ulcerations or in wounds prior to being filled in and healed with skin.

flexible That which may be bent without breaking; pliable.

flexion A bending motion; *flexion* of the arm, leg, etc.

flexor A muscle that bends a limb or part of a limb.

flexure An angle or fold, such as a flexure of the colon.

floaters Floating spots behind the lens of the eye, usually harmless and frequently not visible when exercising normal visual activities.

floating kidney One that moves from its natural position because of slackness in its attachments. Also referred to as a "dropped kidney."

floccillation Picking at the bedsheets and blankets during delirium.

flocculate To have fine particles join together in a fluid so as to precipitate out into a solid or semisolid, such as the curd in milk.

flora, intestinal The bacteria that grow in the small and large bowel. (Normally, bacteria are present and aid in the digestive processes.)

Floraquin A patented medication used in the treatment of inflammations of the vagina.

Florey, Howard W. The codiscoverer of "penicillin" and its effects upon bacteria.

florid A bright red color, often referring to skin color.

flow A discharge of fluids from the body, such as the *menstrual flow*. Also the movement of a fluid within the body, such as the *blood flow*.

flu La grippe. A virus respiratory infection usually accompanied by inflammation of the nose, throat, and bronchial tubes. It is associated with muscles aches, elevation of temperature, and a feeling of weakness.

fluctuate 1. To waver, as when an examining hand or fingers press upon a part of the body containing confined fluid or pus. 2. To be variable, not stable.

Fluid balance The balance between intake and output. (To maintain good health, it is essential that fluid intake and output maintain a fairly equal balance.)

    dram Approximately one teaspoonful.

    level A horizontal line, seen on an X-ray film, separating a layer of fluid from a layer of gas. (*Fluid levels* are often noted in intestinal obstruction, when the X rays are taken with the patient in an upright position.)

    ounce Approximately 30 cc., or 8 fluid drams.

Fluke A worm of the *Trematoda* group. Various forms cause disease in organs such as the intestines, the liver, the lungs, and the bloodstream.

fluorescence The ability to give forth light of longer wavelength after exposure to light.

fluorescin A dye that, when injected intravenously, will light up the retina of the eye. It is used to denote abnormalities of the structure.

fluoridation The adding of fluorine

to drinking water in an attempt to cut down on tooth cavities.

fluorometer A device utilizing ultraviolet light as its power source.

fluoroscopy X-raying a part of the body and recording the rays on a fluorescent screen. This is carried out in order to view various organs in motion.

fluorosis Mottling of the enamel of the teeth secondary to an excessive intake of fluorine. (A rare condition)

fluoruracil The technical name for 5-FU, an effective anticancer chemical.

Fluothane An anesthetic agent; halothane.

fluoxymesterone (Halotestin) A potent male sex hormone, given in tablet form.

flush 1. To blush; to become red. 2. To cleanse a wound by dousing it with water or salt solution.

flutamide A medication that helps to inhibit the progress of prostate cancer.

flutter Extremely rapid contractions of the atria (auricles) of the heart. It can be diagnosed by listening to the heart with a stethoscope or by taking an electrocardiogram.

flux Abnormally large discharge of excretions.

focus The main site of a disease process, such as when a diseased sinus is acting as a *focus* of generalized infection.

foetus Same as fetus.

fold A doubling of a membrane or other part of the body.

Foley catheter A specially de-

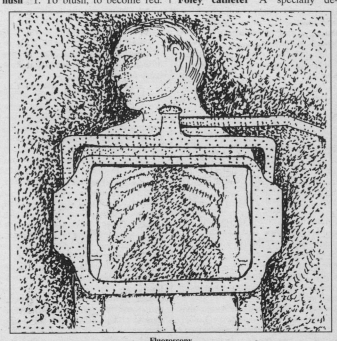

Fluoroscopy

signed rubber tube which is inserted through the urethra into the urinary bladder. It is kept in place by inflating a small balloon which surrounds the catheter.

folic acid A normal chemical constituent of the body necessary for growth and maintenance of health. As a medication, it is useful in treating certain types of anemia.

follicle A small gland or cavity from which secretions arise, such as a *graafian follicle* which secretes an egg from the ovary.

folliculitis Inflammation of hair follicles in the skin. This is easily diagnosed from the formation of small reddish, raised areas.

follow-up study Wherein final results of the study will become obvious only after the passage of time, such as after months, years, etc.

fomentation A hot poultice applied to an inflamed area.

fomes Something, such as an item of clothing, that harbors bacteria or viruses harmful to humans.

fontanel The soft space in between the bones of the skull, found in newborns and infants only. These areas fill in with bone during the first two years of life.

fontanelle Same as fontanel.

food allergy Sensitivity to a food that has been eaten. Such allergies may manifest themselves by nausea, vomiting, diarrhea, or by breaking out in a skin rash or hives.

food poisoning Intestinal upset caused by toxins or bacteria in ingested foods. (Nausea, vomiting, abdominal cramps, and diarrhea are characteristic symptoms and signs of *food poisoning*.)

foot-and-mouth disease A contagious virus disease of animals which is sometimes transmitted to man.

foot drop A falling foot due to paralysis of the muscles which flex the foot.

foramen An opening, such as is found in the bones of the skull, which permits nerves or blood vessels to exit.

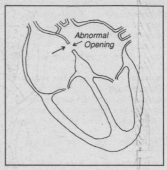

Foramen ovale of the heart

    ovale A birth deformity in which the left and right atria (auricles) of the heart are connected by an opening. This results in mixture of unoxygenated blood (blood which has not passed through the lungs for new oxygen supply) with oxygenated blood.

    of Winslow The entrance to the hollow abdominal space which lies between and beneath the stomach and the transverse portion of the large intestine.

forced feeding *See* enteral nutrition.

forceps delivery Childbirth aided by the application of an instrument (forceps) to the sides of the child's head. (The obstetrician gently lifts the head out of the vagina.)

forearm That part of the arm from the elbow down to the wrist.

foreconscious That part of the mind which stores memories and under certain conditions, brings them to consciousness.

forefinger The index finger.

forefoot The front portion, including the toes.

foregut That part of the embryo which goes to form the esophagus (food pipe), stomach, pancreas, liver, and part of the small intestines.

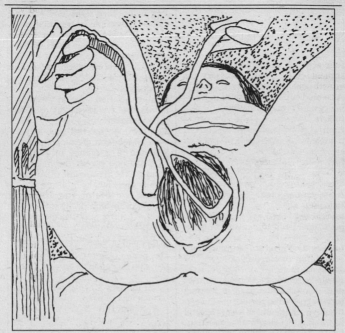

Forceps delivery

forehead That portion of the face between the eyes and the hairline of the scalp.

forensic medicine Legal medicine.

forepleasure The sexual sensations preceding and leading to climax (orgasm).

foreskin The skin over the head of the penis. The prepuce. It is this portion which is removed in circumcision.

formaldehyde An antiseptic used in cleansing and disinfecting rooms. In certain forms it is used as a preservative of tissues which have been removed.

formative The early stage of development; forming.

forme fruste A limited or incompletely developed form of a condition or disease. (A French term not widely used in American medicine.)

formication A sensation that worms or insects are crawling upon or in the skin.

formites The clothes, possessions and articles in the room of a patient afflicted with a contagious or infectious disease.

formula A prescription; a recipe.

formulary A pamphlet or book containing prescriptions for medications.

fornicate To have sexual intercourse. (Often applied to unmarried partners to adultery.)

fornix A concavity or vaultlike structure, such as the *fornix* of the vagina.

fossa A shallow depression in the

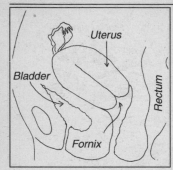

Fornix of the vagina

contour of an organ, bone, or other structure.

fourchette The back part of the female genitals at the entrance to the vagina.

foveation Pitted scar formation, as seen after acne, chickenpox or smallpox, etc.

Fowler's solution Potassium arsenite. A medication used in treating certain types of anemia.

foxglove Digitalis, a drug helpful in treating heart ailments, is manufactured from the common foxglove.

fractional Dividing into parts or frac tions. (*Fractional* urinalysis is carried out in diabetics by examining urine specimens every few hours.)

fracture Any break in a bone.

Fragile X Syndrome A form of inherited mental retardation caused by a recently isolated defective gene.

fragility The quality of being easily broken. (In certain diseases the red blood cells show increased *fragility* and, as a consequence, are easily destroyed.)

fragmentation Breaking into pieces, such as *fragmentation* of bone in a severe fracture.

frambesia *See* yaws.

fraternal twins Non-identical twins, resulting from fertilization of two separate eggs rather than the split-

ting of one egg. One boy and one girl is an example of fraternal twins.

F.R.C.P. Abbreviation for Fellow of the Royal College of Physicians. (British)

F.R.C.S. Abbreviation for Fellow of the Royal College of Surgeons. (British)

free association Saying whatever comes to mind, an activity used during psychoanalysis.

Frei test A skin test used to diagnose lymphogranuloma inguinale.

fremitus The feeling of vibration, as when one places the flat of his hand on the bare chest of someone who is speaking.

frenum A fold of skin or mucous membrane which limits the motion of a structure, such as the *frenum* beneath the tongue.

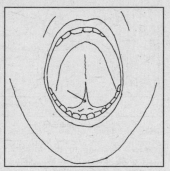

Frenum of the tongue

frequency Commonly referring to the passage of urine at excessively frequent intervals.

Freud, Sigmund (1856–1939) A Viennese psychiatrist; the founder of the branch of psychiatry known as psychoanalysis. He is also credited with being the discoverer of the meaning of the unconscious.

Freudian One who adheres to the teachings of Sigmund Freud.

friable Easily destroyed; fragile.

friction The process of rubbing two things together.

Friderichsen-Waterhouse syndrome
Blood poisoning associated with a meningitis infection. It leads to hemorrhage in the adrenal glands, collapse and death. It is a rare condition affecting children.

Friedreich's ataxia A hereditary disease in which there is paralysis of the lower limbs, speech defects, and marked curvature of the spine.

frigidity Absence of sexual desire in women.

Froehlich's syndrome A lack of function of the pituitary gland in children resulting in marked obesity and underdevelopment of the genitals.

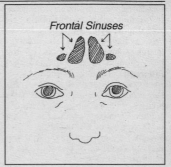

Frontal Sinuses

Frontal sinuses

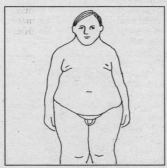

Froehlich's syndrome

frontal Relating to the forehead; the *frontal* bones of the skull occupy the area of the forehead.

frontal bones The bones making up the forehead.

frontal sinuses The sinuses (air spaces) in the skull directly above the eyes.

frostbite A burn resulting from extreme cold. It most often affects the fingers, toes, ears, and the tip of the nose. Severe cases may result in gangrene.

frozen section A technique whereby tissue removed at surgery is subjected to microscopic examination within a few minutes after its removal. The tissue is frozen, cut into thin slices, stained, and then examined.

fructosuria A congenital abnormality of metabolism in which fruit sugar (fructose) is excreted in the urine rather than utilized by the body.

frustration The situation resulting when a strong urge or desire is blocked. A sense of lack of completion.

fulguration Destruction of a segment of tissue or a tumor by use of an electric current.

full-thickness graft One made up of all the layers of the skin, as opposed to a split-thickness graft which contains only part of all the skin layers.

fulminating A severe rapidly progressing illness. One which reaches its full severity within a few hours or days.

Fulvicin A medication, taken by mouth, helpful in clearing up fungus infections such as athlete's foot, ringworm, etc.

functional disease One associated with an upset in function rather than a change in structure, such as migraine headaches, mucous colitis, etc.

functional disorder A disorder caused by upset in function, not by actual organic disease processes.

functional heart murmur One not

associated with any heart condition; an insignificant physical finding.

fundal plication An operation to cure a hiatus hernia. It involves wrapping the upper part of the stomach (the fundus) around that part of the esophagus which has entered the abdominal cavity, thus plugging the opening into the chest cavity.

fundus The base of an organ, such as the *fundus* of the uterus.

fungate To grow rapidly like a fungus, characteristic of certain types of malignant tumors.

fungicide A substance which destroys a fungus.

Fungizone ointment A medication helpful in clearing up fungus infections.

fungus A form of plant life sometimes causing infections in humans such as athlete's foot and trichomoniasis vaginalis.

funiculitis Inflammation of the cord (spermatic cord) leading from the testicle.

funis The umbilical cord.

funnel chest A deformity (depression) of the breastbone (sternum) due to rickets.

funny bone The inner aspect of the elbow where the ulnar nerve is located.

FUO Abbreviation for fever of unknown origin.

Furacin A patented antibiotic drug useful in certain types of urinary and bowel infections.

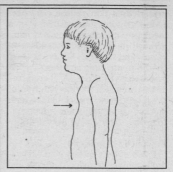

Funnel chest in rickets

Furadantin An antibacterial medication, especially helpful in controlling infections of the kidneys and bladder.

furosemide (Lasix) A potent diuretic, resulting in the excretion of large amounts of urine in a short period of time.

furry tongue A fur-like appearance of the tongue sometimes seen after taking antibiotics. Also called *black tongue* or *hairy tongue*.

furuncle A boil or abscess.

furunculosis A condition in which several crops of boils appear on various parts of the body over a prolonged period.

fusiform Shaped like a spindle.

fusion The act of union, such as of atoms, molecules, metals, etc.

G

g. *See* gram.

gag To choke; to retch; an apparatus for keeping the mouth open during certain surgical procedures.

gage A measuring apparatus. A gauge.

gait The way one walks.

galactocele A milk cyst in a breast, seen occasionally after the nursing period has ended.

galactogogue A medication that increases the flow of milk.

galactography Injecting the milk ducts of the breasts, followed by a mammograph X ray, in order to note deformity or presence of a duct tumor.

galactorrhea Excessive discharge of milk from the breast.

galactose A substance derived from lactose (the sugar in milk from the breast).

galactosemia An inborn disturbance in the metabolism of milk sugar resulting in larger than normal amounts appearing in the bloodstream. Infants with this condition are mentally retarded, physically underdeveloped, have large spleens and livers and cataracts in their eyes.

galactosuria The excretion of milk sugar (galactose) in the urine.

galacturia Milk-colored urine; chyluria.

galea aponeurotica The sheet of fibrous connective tissue lying on top of the skull and extending from the muscles in the forehead to those in back of the head.

gall Bile; the material secreted by the liver and stored in the gall bladder.

Gallamine A muscle relaxant used

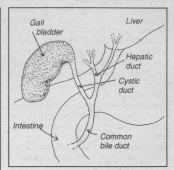

Gall bladder and bile ducts

during inhalation anesthesia. (It is injected, not inhaled.)

gall bladder A hollow, pear-shaped organ located beneath the liver in the right upper portion of the abdomen. It stores and concentrates bile.

Gallium scan A test for the presence of an area of inflammation or tumor formation, performed by injecting a patient with the radioisotope of Gallium and then placing the patient under a scanner to note concentration of the Gallium in the area of inflammation or tumor formation.

gallop rhythm A heart beat which has three rather than the usual two components. (It sounds something like the gait of a galloping horse.)

gallstones Stones in the gall bladder. They vary from the size of a small seed to that of a lemon.

galvanic current Direct electrical current, used in treating muscles which have been paralyzed by disease of their nerves.

gamete An egg or a sperm; the sex cells which unite to form an embryo.

gamma globulin A substance containing antibodies. It is sometimes injected into children who have been exposed to measles or other infections, in order to make the course of the disease milder.

gamma ray A form of radiation, used in treating certain malignant tumors.

gamophobia Fear of getting married.

ganciclovir An anti-virus medicine particularly valuable in treating some infections in patients who have AIDS.

ganglioma A tumor of nerve cells of a ganglion (a nerve center in the sympathetic nervous system). *See also* sympathetic nerves.

ganglion 1. A group of nerve cells located alongside the spinal cord. 2. A cyst of the sheath of a tendon, frequently appearing about the wrist.

ganglionectomy The surgical removal of a ganglion (sympathectomy), sometimes carried out to improve circulation or to lower the blood pressure.

gangrene Death of tissue, usually caused by lack of blood supply, as in *gangrene* of a toe or foot.

Gantanol Trade name of a sulfa drug used to overcome acute or chronic infections of the urinary tract.

Gantrisin A patented sulfa drug, used as a treatment against infections. It is particularly effective in infections of the urinary tract.

Garamycin (Gentamycin) A powerful antibiotic, effective in the treatment of many of the most serious infections. It should only be taken under medical supervision.

Garamycin Ophthalmic Antibiotic eyedrops used for eye infections.

gargle To rinse the mouth and throat.

gargoylism Deformity of a newborn; dwarfed, misshapen, and with a particularly ugly head and face.

gas gangrene A highly dangerous form of gangrene caused by a specific gas-forming germ. Immediate surgical treatment as well as the giving of gas gangrene serum and antibiotics is necessary to save life in these infections.

gasserian ganglion A nerve center from which the fifth cranial nerve (the trigeminal nerve) originates. This nerve sends three branches to the face.

gastrectomy Surgical removal of the stomach, or a portion thereof. This operation is performed for an ulcer of the stomach or duodenum or for a tumor of the stomach.

gastric analysis Examination of the secretions of the stomach, performed by the passage of a tube into the stomach. The presence of blood, hydrochloric acid, lactic acid and other substances is determined in this way.

gastric lavage Washing out of the stomach. This may be done to empty the stomach of tainted foods or poisons. Also, it is often carried out prior to surgery upon the stomach.

gastrin A hormone manufactured by the pyloric portion of the stomach which is thought to stimulate secretion by the glands in the upper portion of the stomach (the fundus).

gastrinoma A gastrin-secreting tumor of the pancreas, often associated with the Zollinger-Ellison syndrome. *See* syndrome, Zollinger-Ellison.

gastritis Inflammation of the lining of the stomach. The acute form may come from eating tainted foods; the chronic form may come from excess acidity, alcoholism, etc.

gastrocnemius muscle The main calf muscle in the back of the leg. Its action bends the foot downward.

gastrocolic fistula An opening (fistula) between the stomach and transverse colon (large bowel). This is usually caused by an ulcer or tumor which perforates from one organ into the other.

gastrocolic reflex Stimulation of activity within the large bowel resulting from food entering the stomach. The desire to evacuate the bowels shortly after eating.

gastroduodenal Referring to the stomach and duodenum.

gastroduodenitis Inflammation of the stomach and duodenum (the first portion of the small intestine).

gastroduodenoscopy A procedure in which an endoscope (gastroduodenoscope) is inserted through the mouth down into the stomach and duodenum.

gastroenteritis Inflammation, usually acute, of the stomach and intestines; cramps and diarrhea are characteristic symptoms.

Gastroenterologist A physician who specializes in diseases of the stomach and intestinal tract.

gastroenterostomy The surgical construction of an opening between the stomach and small intestine; a procedure sometimes carried out for an ulcer of the duodenum.

gastroepiploic Referring to the stomach and its attached omentum (the fatty apron arising from the lower border of the stomach).

gastroesophagostomy *See* esophagogastrostomy.

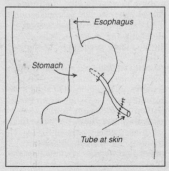

Gastrostomy

Gastrografin A water-soluble opaque dye which, when taken orally, will outline the gastrointestinal tract; sometimes used instead of barium.

gastrohepatic ligament The tissue which extends from the stomach toward the liver. Through it travels most of the blood supply to the stomach.

gastrointestinal Relating to the stomach and intestines.

gastrojejunal anastomosis A surgical operation in which an opening is constructed between the stomach and small intestine (jejunum).

gastrojejunostomy Gastrojejunal anastomosis.

gastrolavage The process of washing out the stomach by use of a rubber tube.

gastromegaly Enlargement of the stomach.

gastrophrenic Referring to the stomach and diaphragm.

gastroplication The folding of the stomach so that it prevents herniation through the diaphragm, used in cases of hiatus hernia (the Nissen operation).

gastroptosis A "dropped stomach" or one which is low in the abdominal cavity. This condition rarely produces any discomfort.

gastroscope An instrument which is passed through the mouth and esophagus into the stomach to permit the examination of the stomach lining.

gastrosplenic Pertaining to the stomach and spleen.

gastrostomy An operation to establish an artificial opening of the stomach on the abdominal wall; performed occasionally when feeding through the mouth is not possible.

gastrula The embryo in the stage following the blastula; an early stage in embryonic development.

Gaucher's disease A chronic disease, often seen in several members of a family, in which there is anemia and enlargement of the spleen and liver. Characteristic Gaucher cells are seen on examination of the tissues.

gauze Material, usually cheese-cloth, used to cover surgical wounds or to sponge wounds during operations.

gavage Artificial feeding through a stomach tube, carried out upon patients who are unwilling or unable to take food in the normal manner.

gay A homosexual.

Geiger counter An instrument used to detect radioactive particles. Placed over the thyroid region, it can detect the presence of radioactive iodine which has been administered to a patient.

gel A mixture of liquid and solid which forms a semisolid substance.

Gelfoam A patented gelatinlike material, impregnated with thrombin, which is applied to bleeding surfaces in order to promote blood clot formation.

Gelusil An effective antacid, used in excess stomach acidity and in the treatment of peptic ulcer.

gemellology The study of twins.

geminate To double; paired.

gemmation Reproduction by budding, seen mostly in plant life.

gene mutation A change in the ordinary configuration of a gene. *See* mutation.

geneology The study of one's heredity (ancestry).

Generalist A family doctor; a general practitioner.

generalized Involving an entire body system or organ.

generation 1. The process of reproduction. 2. The interval between the birth of a child and the birth of the child's child.

generic-named drug One that is sold under its technical name; a nonpatented drug. (Generic drugs are usually much less costly than trade-named drugs.)

genes The units responsible for inheritance; they are present in the sperm cells of the male and the egg cells of the female.

autosomal Genes located on any chromosome other than an X-sex or a Y-sex chromosome.

crossing over The exchange of genetic material between paired chromosomes.

lethal Those that cause death. (Embryos with lethal genes do not survive.)

recessive *See* recessive characteristics.

sex-linked Those located on sex chromosomes.

genesis Origin.

gene splicing The altering of genes so that the organism receiving those genes can perform work helpful to man. As an example, genes from the human pituitary gland have been implanted in bacteria, resulting in those bacteria producing the human growth hormone.

gene therapy Treatment directed toward correcting or eliminating faulty genes in order to overcome disease.

genetic counseling It is a service that physicians trained in genetic medicine give to people who fear that their offspring might inherit certain diseases or defects.

genetic engineering Altering genes so that new forms of bacterial or animal life may be created. The present aim of genetic engineering is to alter the DNA (*See* DNA and deoxyribonucleic acid) in living cells to get those cells to perform tasks that are valuable to humans.

genetic testing A study of one's DNA.

genetics The science dealing with heredity.

genicular Referring to the knee.

geniculate ganglion A nerve center in the face.

genio- Referring to the chin.

geniohyoid muscle A muscle under the chin.

genioplasty A plastic operation upon the chin.

genital herpes *See* herpes genitalis.

genitalia The organs of reproduction. In the male: the penis, testicles, and prostate. In the female: the vulva, vagina, uterus, fallopian tubes, and ovaries.

genitocrural Referring to the genitals and the leg.

genitourinary Referring to the sex organs and the urinary system, including the kidneys, ureters, bladder, prostate, etc.

genius Exceptional mentality, in one or more directions.

genocide Killing a race of people.

genome All the hereditary factors (genes) present in the chromosomes of a person's cells.

genophobia Morbid fear of sex.

genotype The genetic makeup of an individual.

Gentamycin A powerful antibiotic drug, especially efficacious in infections of the urinary tract.

gentian violet A dye used to stain cells prior to examining them under a microscope.

genu The knee.

genucubital position On the knees and elbows.

genupectoral position *See* knee-chest position.

genus A kind or a group, in the classification of living things.

geographic tongue One with raised areas due to thickening of the surface cells, giving the appearance of a map.

geomedicine The branch of medicine which deals with the effect of climate upon health and disease.

geophagy The practice of eating dirt or earth.

geriatric Gerontic; referring to old age.

Geriatrician One who specializes in diseases of old age.

geriatrics The study of conditions affecting old people.

germ Bacteria of microorganisms capable of producing disease.

German measles vaccine A potent vaccine which imparts immunity to German measles.

germ cells The reproductive cells; sperm in the male, ova in the female.

germicide A germ-killing agent.

germinate To grow from a cell or seed into a mature form.

germinoma A tumor of the testicle.

gerontology The study of the aged; geriatrics.

gerontophobia Abnormal fear of old age.

gestalt psychology A theory of psychology which regards behavior as dependent upon the individual's total insight, and not on experience only.

gestation Pregnancy.

gestational age The length of time that an embryo or fetus has been developing.

Ghon tubercle The primary tuberculosis infection in the lung of children visible as a shadow on X ray. While it denotes the presence of the germ of tuberculosis in the body, it is usually not associated with active infection.

giant cell A very large cell containing several nuclei. Seen as a reaction surrounding a foreign body in the tissues, and also in *giant-cell tumors* of bones.

tumor A benign bone tumor which, on microscopic examination shows the presence of many giant cells.

giantism Abnormally large size. In man, height in excess of 6 feet, 6 inches; gigantism.

gibbosity The condition of having a humped back; hunchback.

giddy Dizzy.

gigantism Same as giantism.

gill 1. One quarter of a pint. 2. Breathing organ in fish.

gingiva The gums; the tissue surrounding the teeth.

gingivectomy Surgical removal of a portion of the gums. (Usually, a procedure carried out by an oral surgeon)

gingivitis Inflammation of the gums.

"G.I.'s" A slang expression for an

attack of diarrhea; the term originated during World War II among soldiers and sailors.

ginseng A Chinese root, used as a medicine for many ailments (not used often in Western countries).

glabella The bony prominence located just above the bridge of the nose.

gland An organ which manufactures a chemical which will be utilized elsewhere. If the secretion goes into the blood stream, the gland belongs to the *endocrine* system; if it secretes through a duct (tube) to surrounding tissues it is an *exocrine* gland

> **accessory** An additional gland, not usually found in most bodies, such as an accessory spleen, thyroid, or parathyroid gland.

> **acinous** One that secretes, such as a salivary gland or a milk gland.

> **apocrine** One that sheds part of its substance in the secretion, such as an apocrine gland in the breast.

> **Bartholin** One located alongside the entrance to the vagina. It excretes mucus.

> **Cowper's** One located within the urethra. It excretes mucus.

> **ductless** The endocrine glands, such as the pituitary, thyroid, adrenals, etc. They secrete hormones directly into the bloodstream.

> **endocrine** Glands that secrete hormones into the bloodstream. Also called ductless glands.

> **exocrine** Those whose secretions emerge through ducts, such as sweat glands.

> **mammary** The breast.

> **Meibomian** The tiny glands on the inner surface of the eyelids.

> **Montgomery** The small glands in the outer portion of the nipples.

> **parathyroid** An endocrine gland lying behind the thyroid in the neck. Its hormone controls calcium metabolism.

> **parotid** The salivary gland at the angle of the jaw.

> **pineal** A small gland located within the brain. Its function has not been determined.

> **pituitary** The endocrine gland lying beneath the brain. Its hormones influence all other hormone secretions by other glands.

> **prostate** The gland surrounding the outlet of the bladder in males. When it enlarges as one ages, it may obstruct the passage of urine.

> **salivary** Those that secrete saliva, such as the parotid, submaxillary and sublingual glands.

> **sebaceous** Glands located in the skin which secrete sebum, an oily substance which prevents drying out of the skin.

> **sublingual** A salivary gland located beneath the tongue.

> **submaxillary** A salivary gland located beneath the jaw.

> **suprarenal** The adrenal gland.

> **sweat** A gland in the skin which excretes sweat. Also known as a sudoriferous gland.

> **thymus** A gland composed of a special type of lymphoid tissue, located beneath the breastbone. It shrinks and becomes inactive early in childhood.

> **thyroid** The endocrine gland in the front of the neck which controls body metabolism.

glanders A contagious disease found in horses, but which is occasionally transmitted to humans. It is characterized by high fever, swelling of glands in the neck, and eventual death.

glandular fever Infectious mononucleosis (IM); a subacute infectious disease characterized by sore throat, swollen glands, weakness, and atypical blood count. Recovery ensues in three to eight weeks.

glans The head of the penis.

glaucoma An eye disease associated with increased pressure within the eyeball. If untreated, it may lead to blindness.

gleet Pus discharge from the penis, found in those who have a chronic inflammation of the urethra (lining of the penis).

glenoid cavity The joint surface of the scapula (wing bone) where it meets the humerus (upper arm bone) in the shoulder region.

glioblastoma A common type of brain tumor.

glioma A tumor originating from the tissue which surrounds the brain and spinal cord.

gliosis Overgrowth of the connective tissue elements in the brain, often brought on by chronic inflammation.

Glisson's capsule A membrane covering the liver.

globule A small drop; a droplet. (A *globule* of liquid fat.)

globulin A protein found throughout body tissues in various forms, such as gamma *globulin*, serum *globulin*, alpha and beta *globulin*, etc.

globus hystericus A "lump in the throat" and a choking sensation of hysterical origin. Seen often in women who are passing through change of life (menopause).

glomerate Forming a ball-like structure.

glomerulonephritis An inflammation of the kidneys, often secondary to a severe infection elsewhere in the body.

glomerulus A structure consisting of a tuft of capillary loops extending into the capsule of the tubules. It is within the *glomeruli* that waste materials are separated from the blood and are passed out as urine.

glomus tumor A vessel and nerve tumor, usually no larger than a pea, located beneath the skin or nails of the fingers or toes and extremely painful to touch.

glossa The tongue.

glossalgia Pain in the tongue.

glossectomy Surgical removal of the tongue or major portion thereof; performed for cancer of the tongue.

glossitis Inflammation of the tongue.

glossolabial Pertaining to the tongue and lips.

glossolalia Babbling; jabbering.

glossopalatine Referring to the tongue and palate.

glossopharyngeal nerve The main nerve supplying the tongue and throat; the ninth cranial nerve.

glottis The vocal cords and opening between them.

glucagon A hormone produced by the alpha cells of the islets of Langerhans of the pancreas. It is secreted in response to too little sugar in the blood.

glucokinase An enzyme in the liver active in sugar metabolism.

glucose One form of sugar. Also called d-glucose or dextroglucose.

   tolerance test A blood test performed to determine the ability of the body to metabolize, utilize, and store sugar. A specific test for diabetes mellitus.

glucoside A compound which may be altered so as to become a sugar. It is now more commonly referred to as *glycoside*.

glucosuria The excretion of sugar in the urine.

glucotrol A medicine that reduces the level of blood sugar, used with certain cases of diabetes.

glue-sniffing Sniffing fumes from certain solvents, giving an individual a sense of well-being followed by a sense of depression.

glutamic acid An amino acid which is sometimes used as a medication to release acid in the stomach and for treating muscular dystrophies.

glutathione An amino acid said to inhibit the growth of the HIV virus, which causes AIDS.

gluten A protein found in some grains, including wheat. Children with celiac disease and nontropical sprue are thought to be allergic to gluten and therefore should avoid it.

gluten bread Bread baked with a

sugarless flour, often recommended for diabetic patients.

gluteus muscles The muscles of the buttocks; there are three.

gluttony Excessive eating.

glycemia The presence of sugar in the blood. (All people normally have a certain amount of sugar in their blood.)

glycerin A thick, syrupy substance derived from the breakdown of certain fats. It is used in suppositories, as a skin balm, etc.

glycine A liver enzyme active in nitrogen metabolism and other metabolic processes.

glycogen Sugar as it is stored in the liver and held ready for release to other parts of the body.

glycogenesis The formation of sugar in the liver.

glycolysis The breakdown of sugar in the tissues as a result of the expenditure of energy. The sugar is "burned," resulting in the waste products, lactic acid and pyruvic acid.

glycoproteins Combinations of sugar and protein, naturally occurring in humans. They are contained in mucus secreted by many organs.

glycoside A compound which can be broken down to yield sugar. Also called *glucoside*.

glycosuria Sugar in the urine. This is abnormal and is frequently evidence of diabetes.

gm. *See* gram.

gnatho- Relating to the jaw.

gnosia The mental ability to perceive the nature of animate and inanimate objects.

goblet cell A cell lining the intestinal tract, so called because of its shape.

goiter An enlargement of the thyroid gland. It may involve the entire gland or only parts of it.

    colloid A smooth enlargement of the thyroid gland, not associated with overactivity; seen often

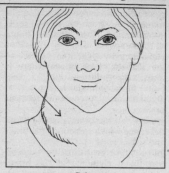

Goiter

in areas where there is an iodine deficiency in drinking water.

    nodular An irregular enlargement of the thyroid gland, sometimes associated with excess activity.

    toxic An enlargement of the thyroid gland associated with overactivity of the gland and with increased basal metabolic rate.

gold salts Chemical compounds containing gold which are used in the treatment of certain types of arthritis. They often cause severe toxic reactions, and only rarely have a lasting beneficial effect.

gonad A sex gland; the ovary or testicle.

gonadotropin A hormone which stimulates the sex glands; it originates in the pituitary gland in the base of the skull.

gonagra Gout affecting the knee joint.

goniopuncture An operation to relieve glaucoma by puncturing the anterior chamber of the eye.

goniotomy Same as *goniopuncture*.

gonococcemia Blood poisoning caused by the germ which causes gonorrhea.

gonococcus The germ *neisseria gonorrhoeae* which causes gonorrhea.

gonorrhea A venereal infection of the lining of the penis (urethra). It is accompanied by swelling, pain on voiding, and discharge of pus.

gooseflesh A roughened appearance to the skin due to contraction of the tiny muscles surrounding hair follicles, occurring especially in extreme cold or during fright.

Gore-tex Trade name for a synthetic material used as an arterial graft.

gouge A chisel used in cutting out portions of bone.

gout A type of arthritis or inflammation about a joint caused by excess uric acid in the blood. Attacks occur suddenly and are accompanied by great pain. The big toe is a frequent site.

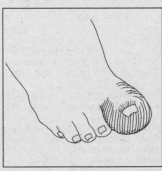

Gout

gr. *See* grain.

graafian follicle The small fluid sac (follicle) in the ovary which contains the mature egg ready to be discharged.

gracilis muscle A thin, long muscle extending from the groin down to the inner side of the knee.

graduate A glass container for measuring liquids. It is marked with lines denoting various fluid quantities.

graft Tissue taken from one part of the body to replace a defect in another part.

    autograft One taken from another part of the patient's own body.

    corneal A graft of the thin,

colorless membrane over the pupil of the eye. (Corneal grafts are obtained from people other than the patient, the so-called eye donors.)

    fascial A graft of fibrous tissue used in hernia operations to strengthen the repair. (These may be obtained either from the patient himself or from treated tissues obtained from animal sources.)

    free One that is separated completely from its former attachments.

    full thickness One that contains all the layers of the skin.

    heterograft One taken from the body of an animal and transferred to a human, such as a kidney from a chimpanzee or cartilage from a cow.

    homograft One that is derived from the body of another person.

    pedicle One that is grafted from one part of the body to another while a portion of its original attachments remain intact.

    pinch A small piece of skin, usually no more than ¼ inch in diameter, that is snipped from one part of the body and is placed as a full-thickness free graft over a raw area in another part of the body. Usually, many grafts are transplanted at the same time to cover a widely denuded region.

    split thickness One that contains only some of the layers of skin. The donor site retains the deepest layers and thus grows new skin.

grain (gr.) A unit of weight; 480 grains equals 1 ounce in the troy weight system.

gram (g. or gm.) The basic unit of weight in the metric system. Equivalent to approximately 1 cc. (15 drops).

Gram-negative bacteria Those that look pink when treated with the Gram stain.

Gram-negative sepsis Blood poisoning caused by a so-called Gram-negative bacteria, such as the colon bacillus, etc. (Patients so afflicted are dangerously sick and may go into irreversible shock unless treated promptly and adequately.)

Gram-positive bacteria Those that look purple when treated with the Gram stain.

Gram's stain The staining of bacteria to distinguish those that stain pink under microscopic viewing (Gram-negative) from those that stain purple (Gram-positive).

grandiose delusions A fantasy that one is rich, famous or powerful when such is not the case.

grand mal An epileptic convulsion of major proportions.

granulated eyelids Crusts on the eyelids due to a chronic inflammation (blepharitis).

granulation tissue Newly formed tissue composed of small capillaries and connective tissue, seen in the process of healing.

granule A very small particle.

granulocyte A white blood cell (polymorphonuclear leukocytes fall into this category).

granulocytopenia A marked decrease in the number of white blood cells, seen in certain conditions where the blood has been affected by poisons or drugs.

granuloma An area of chronic inflammation in which granulation tissue is present. Parasites, fungi, and certain bacteria can induce the formation of a *granuloma*.

granuloma inguinale A veneral infection characterized by chronic ulcerations of the skin and subcutaneous tissues of the genitals or groin.

granulomatous colitis An inflammation of the large bowel associated with ulcer formation and the formation of granulomas (tumor-like masses of an inflammatory nature).

granulosa-cell tumor A special type of tumor of the ovary containing primitive cells.

graph Lines drawn on specially designed paper to illustrate statistics.

graphology The study of handwriting.

gravel "Sand" in the kidneys which is sometimes passed in the urine. The "sand" is composed of minute particles of kidney stones.

Graves' disease Overactivity of the thyroid gland associated with bulging of the eyeballs; also called *exophthalmic goiter.*

gravid Pregnant.

gravity The pull of the earth; the force which holds things down.

Greenfield filter A filter usually placed in the vena cava to prevent thrombi (fragments of blood clots) from traveling through the bloodstream to the lungs or other organs.

greenstick fracture A break, in an oblique direction, which does not go all the way through a bone. It occurs most often in children.

grippe Mild influenza. An upper respiratory infection caused by a virus. Associated with running nose, sore throat and cough, temperature elevation and aches and pains throughout the body.

griseofulvin Fulvicin. A highly effective drug to combat fungus infections.

groin The line of division, a skin crease, between the thigh and the abdomen; often referred to as the *inguinal region.*

group psychotherapy *See* group therapy.

group therapy A form of psychotherapy in which several members of a group are treated simultaneously. Their reactions toward one another constitute an important part of the therapy.

growing pains Aching sensations in the limbs of adolescent children. They are not thought to indicate presence of disease.

growth factors Substances that help wound healing by stimulating the growth of connective tissue cells, skin cells, and cells making up small blood vessels.

growth hormone The hormone secreted by the anterior portion of the pituitary gland in the base of the skull.

grumous fluid Thick fluid sometimes containing solid particles.

gt. An abbreviation meaning one drop.

GU Abbreviation for *genitourinary.*

guaiacol A chemical with several medicinal uses, as in bronchitis, inflammation of the bladder, etc.

guaiac test A test for the presence of blood, usually performed upon a stool specimen thought to contain small quantities of blood.

guarding The voluntary or involuntary tightening or spasm of muscles, in order to minimize pain from underlying organs or structures.

gubernaculum testis In the embryo, the cordlike structure which guides the testicle in its descent from the abdomen into the scrotum.

Guillain-Barre syndrome *See* syndrome.

guillotine amputation A straight cut across a limb without any attempt to close the skin over the amputation stump. Performed in badly infected cases of gangrene.

guinea-pig inoculation An injection of a specimen taken from a patient's sputum or urine into a guinea pig in order to determine the presence of tuberculosis.

gullet The esophagus (food pipe).

gumboil An abscess at the root of a decayed or decaying tooth.

gumma A localized mass denoting the late stages of syphilis. *Gummas* may be found in almost any organ of the body.

gums The mucous membrane surrounding the teeth. Gingiva.

gustatory Referring to the sense of taste.

gut The intestine.

Guthrie Test A blood test denoting the presence or absence of PKU disease in a newborn. (*See* phenylketonuria.)

gynatresia Occlusion due to lack of development of the vagina or of other parts of the female sex organs.

gyne- A combining form referring to the word, *woman.*

Gynecologist A physician specializing in diseases of women, especially those of the reproductive organs.

gynecology That branch of medicine dealing with diseases of the female reproductive organs.

gynecomastia Enlargement of the male breast, usually due to overgrowth of breast tissue. It has no known connection with glandular disturbance.

gynephobia Morbid fear of being with women.

Gynergen A patented medication, containing ergot, used to combat an attack of migraine headache.

gyno- Referring to woman.

gyration A circular movement.

gyrus A portion of brain; a brain convolution or fold of tissue located in the cerebrum.

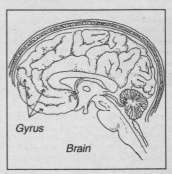

Gyrus

Brain

Gyrus

H

H The chemical symbol for hydrogen.

habit 1. Fixed behavior produced by repetition. 2. The kind of body structure one possesses, such as a tall, thin person or a short, stout person.

habitat The natural living place of an animal.

habituation Acquired tolerance of or addiction to, as with a narcotic drug.

habitus Appearance; nature. A thin, hollow-cheeked, nervous person may be said to have an ulcer *habitus*.

hacking cough A dry cough which does not bring up much phlegm (sputum). Seen during the early stages of bronchitis.

Hadfield-Clarke syndrome A condition present from birth in which the pancreatic gland fails to develop fully or to function normally. *See also* pancreas.

Hagedorn needle A specially designed surgical needle with a cutting edge. It is used to sew up skin and to prick the finger when taking blood.

hair follicle The tiny sac out of which a hair emerges.

Halcion A sleeping tablet most helpful for people having difficulty falling asleep. Not to be taken during pregnancy.

Haldol A drug for people suffering from mental illness, particularly those who require long-term treatment. The drug must be administered repeatedly by injection at intervals of 3 weeks or more.

half-life The time it takes for any radioactive substance to lose half its activity. (All radioactive substances disintegrate, although some may take hundreds of years to lose their activity.)

halfway house An institution for individuals requiring hospital residence, or a stay in a place where they need supervision before leaving to live on their own.

halitosis Bad breath.

Haliver oil Trademarked name of oil from the liver of the halibut. It has much the same properties as cod-liver oil, being rich in vitamin D.

hallucination Imagined or false sense perception, seen among mentally ill people. Also seen occasionally during the delirium accompanying severe illness with high temperatures.

hallucinatory drugs Medications that cause hallucinations such as feelings of grandeur, exquisite senses of pleasure, and freedom from problems, etc. (LSD and hashish are two such drugs.)

hallucinosis A state in which the patient has continuous hallucinations.

hallux The big toe; the great toe.

hallux valgus The bending of the first toe toward the outside of the foot, a condition often associated with bunions.

halogen An element which forms a salt by direct union with a metal; such as iodine, bromine, fluorine, chlorine, etc.

Halotestin An orally effective male sex hormone.

halothane Fluothane. A widely used anesthetic agent, given by inhalation.

Halsted's operations 1. Surgery to correct an inguinal hernia. 2. A radical removal of the breast, including

150

neighboring lymph glands and underlying muscles.

hamartoma A growth which is not made up of true tumor tissue but of the excess growth of normal tissue cells.

hammer toe A toe which is bent and cannot be extended or straightened. Such toes sometimes require surgical correction if they produce pain or interfere with normal walking.

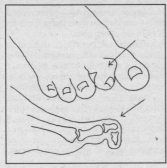

Hammer toe

hamstring muscles The powerful thigh muscles in the back of the thigh. They bend the knee.

hamular Hook-shaped.

hand That part of the upper limb which extends from the wrist to the fingertips.

handedness The dominance of one hand over another, i.e. right-handedness or left-handedness.

handicap A reduction of usefulness of one or more organs or structures.

Hand-Schüller-Christian disease *See* xanthomatosis.

hangnail A piece of loose skin near the base of the fingernail.

Hanot's disease A form of cirrhosis of the liver, associated with marked enlargement of the liver and inflammation of the smaller bile ducts; *cholangiolitic cirrhosis*.

Hansen's disease Leprosy.

haptenes Incomplete antigens. They may neutralize existing antibodies but they are incapable of causing production of new antibodies.

haptic Referring to the sense of touch.

harelip A birth deformity in which there is a cleft in the upper lip. Today, it can be corrected surgically.

Harrington rods Long metal rods that are sutured into the back and retained for several months or years. (Used in the surgical treatment of scoliosis)

Hartmann's pouch A saclike enlargement of the gall bladder near its neck.

Hashimoto's disease A rare inflammatory disease of the thyroid gland resulting in a smooth enlargement of the gland and degeneration of the tissue which secretes thyroid hormone.

hashish A substance obtained from the *Cannabis sativa* plant. It acts as a drug, giving a sense of exhilaration and some loss of a sense of space and time. When taken often, it is habit-forming. *See also* marijuana.

haustra Normal pouchlike bulges in the wall of the colon (large bowel).

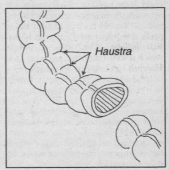

Haustra

Haustra of colon

HAV Abbreviation for hepatitis A virus.

hay fever An allergic condition of the upper respiratory tract caused by sensitivity to the pollen of ragweed. Symptoms are congestion of the mucous membranes, stuffed nose, sneezing and red eyes.

Hb. *See* hemoglobin.

HBV Abbreviation for hepatitis B virus.

HCl *See* hydrochloric acid.

healer A general term for an unlicensed practitioner who attempts to cure illness by prayer, suggestion or other unorthodox methods.

healing by primary union Healing that occurs when the wound edges are stitched together and no infection sets in; normal healing.

secondary union Healing that occurs when a wound is left open and no attempt is made to stitch its edges together. Infected wounds heal in this manner.

Health-Care Proxy A person given the right to make a decision for a patient who is so ill that he/she cannot make a decision for himself or herself. Such right should be given in writing.

health education The art or science of teaching people to improve or maintain their state of good health.

health insurance Arranging through an insurance plan for the payment of medical bills or for the rendering of medical services on a prepaid basis.

comprehensive That type which defrays the whole, or greater share, of the costs of medical care.

indemnity That type in which the insurance company pays a specific amount for a specific type of medical service. It may or may not cover the entire cost of the medical service.

prepaid That type in which the premium covers the costs of medical care.

hearing The process which occurs when sound waves enter the ear and hit the eardrum. They are transmitted through the middle to the inner ear where the impulses are carried to the brain by the acoustic nerve.

heart The hollow muscular organ in the chest which pumps blood throughout the body. *See also* cardiac.

beat The rhythmic contraction and relaxation of the heart as it pumps blood. The beat creates a characteristic sound.

block A disorder of transmission of the heart beat from the atrium to the ventricle.

burn Indigestion associated with a burning pain in the upper abdomen or lower chest.

failure A general term used to define inadequate function of the heart as a pump. Shortness of breath and swelling of the ankles are two common symptoms of heart failure.

rate The rate calculated by counting the number of heart muscle contractions per minute. Normal adult rates vary from 60 to 80 per minute, when the subject is at rest or engaged in average physical activities.

sounds The sounds heard and the impulses felt when heart muscle contracts and relaxes. On listening with a stethoscope, normal heart sounds are heard as "flub-dubb, flub-dubb."

heart-lung machine An apparatus that keeps circulation and respiration going during open-heart surgery.

heart-lung transplant An operation in which the heart and lungs of a person who has just died are transplanted into another's chest.

heart transplant The transplantation of a heart from one individual to another. (With improved cell-matching and suppression of the rejection phenomenon the operation is proving more successful.)

heat cramps Severe muscle cramps occurring in people who have perspired profusely, have lost salt from their bodies and have been overexposed to heat.

heat edema Swelling, usually

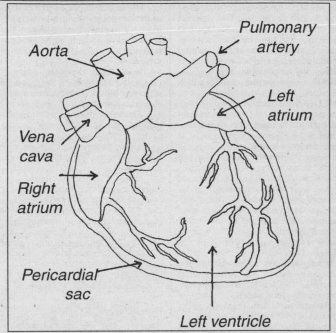

Aorta

Pulmonary artery

Left atrium

Vena cava

Right atrium

Pericardial sac

Left ventricle

Heart

of the ankles, seen when outside temperatures are extremely high.

heat prostration Heat exhaustion; a condition characterized by elevated temperature, poor heart action, and a shocklike state. It is caused by prolonged exposure to high temperature.

rash Small pink and red spots on the skin, usually more pronounced in skin folds, and due to inflammation of the sweat glands. It occurs particularly in children who have perspired profusely in intensely hot weather.

stroke Sunstroke. Similar to heat prostration, caused by excessive exposure to the sun and high temperatures.

hebephrenia A form of insanity in

which the patient's actions are silly and capricious. Seen in schizophrenia of certain types.

Heberden nodes Swellings about the joints of the fingers in people who have osteoarthritis.

hedonism Excessive concentration on the things in life which bring pleasure. "Pleasure-mad."

heel The hind part of the foot.

hegemony The control by one part of the body over the function of other parts. "Mind over body" represents the exercise of *hegemony* by the brain.

Heimlich maneuver A technique for dislodging material on which one has choked. The victim is raised to his feet and the first-aider stands behind him and places both arms about the victim's waist at a level just below the rib cage. The right fist of the first-aider is firmly grasped with the left hand, and with a sudden upward and inward thrust, the grip on the victim is tightened as forcefully as possible. This maneuver will cause the material on which one is choking to be forced out of the windpipe. (*See* chapter on First Aid.)

heliation therapy Treatment of disease by exposure to the sun.

helicobacter pylori The bacteria which are thought to be the cause of most ulcers of the pyloric portion of the stomach. Control of these bacteria with antibiotics may result in the cure of many stomach ulcers.

helio- Referring to the sun.

heliophobia Morbid fear of being out in the sun.

helix The rounded portion of the external ear.

Heller operation A procedure for cutting some of the muscles that constrict the lower portion of the esophagus (food pipe).

helminthiasis Any disease caused by worms.

helosis The condition of having many corns on the feet.

helotomy Cutting of a corn, as on a toe.

hemagglutination The clumping together of red blood cells.

hemangiectasia Dilatation of blood vessels, usually small capillaries in the skin or in the lining of the intestines.

hemangioma A nonmalignant blood vessel tumor. Such tumors appear on the skin as red marks or reddish elevations. Beneath the skin, they have a bluish hue.

hemangiosarcoma A malignant tumor originating from a blood vessel or vessels.

hemapoiesis The production of red blood cells, such as the process which takes place in the bone marrow.

hemarthrosis Blood in a joint, or hemorrhage into a joint cavity; often caused by injury or, in a hemophiliac, by spontaneous bleeding.

hematemesis Vomiting of blood.

hematin The iron constituent of hemoglobin; formerly called, "heme."

hematinic Any medication given to increase the amount of hemoglobin in the blood.

hemato- A prefix referring to *blood*.

hematocele A mass or tumor formed by a collection of blood which has been formed by an internal hemorrhage.

hematocolpos A collection of blood within the vagina, particularly in females whose vaginal outlet is blocked by an intact hymen (maidenhead).

hematocrit test A test on blood to determine the relative proportion of blood cells to plasma. In anemia the proportion of plasma to red cells is increased.

hematogenous Blood-borne, such as an infection that spreads through the bloodstream.

Hematologist A physician who specializes in diseases of the blood and blood-forming organs.

hematolysis Destruction of red blood cells and releasing the hemoglobin from the cells.

hematoma Hemorrhage under the skin with the formation of a blood clot; usually secondary to an injury such as is caused by a direct blow.

hematometra A collection and retention of menstrual blood within the uterus.

hematopoiesis The formation of blood. Much of this process takes place within the marrow of bones.

hematoporphyrinuria Blackish urine due to the presence of porphyrin; it is caused by the breakdown of red blood cells and the release and decomposition of hemoglobin.

hematosalpinx A collection of blood in the fallopian tube, often associated with an ectopic pregnancy.

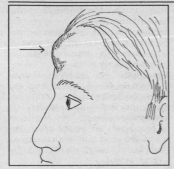

Hematoma

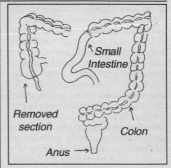

Hemicolectomy

hematospermia The discharge of blood with the ejaculation of semen.

hematoxylin A standard stain for tissues which are to be subjected to microscopic examination.

hematuria Blood in the urine. It may be caused by an infection or may be secondary to a tumor somewhere in the urinary tract.

heme The iron constituent of hemoglobin.

hemi- Half.

hemianopsia Blindness in one half of the visual field of an eye.

hemiatrophy Degeneration limited to one side of the body or one portion of an organ.

hemic Pertaining to blood.

hemicolectomy Removal of one part (roughly one half) the large bowel.

hemicorporectomy The surgical removal of the lower half of the body, performed for extensive malignancy.

hemicrania Headache on one side only, as in migraine.

hemigastrectomy A surgical operation for peptic ulcer in which approximately half the stomach is removed, usually done in conjunction with vagotomy.

hemiglossectomy Surgical removal of half the tongue; usually performed for a malignant tumor of the tongue.

hemihypertrophy Overgrowth of one side or one part of the body.

hemilaryngectomy Surgical removal of half the larynx (voice box); usually done in cases of cancer.

hemiparesis Paralysis of one side of the body; most often secondary to a hemorrhage or blood clot within the brain.

hemipelvectomy A radical cancer operation in which an entire lower limb and part of the pelvis are removed.

hemiplegia Paralysis affecting only one side of the body.

hemisphere One half of the brain (the right or left side).

hemispherectomy Surgical removal of one side (hemisphere) of the brain.

hemithyroidectomy Surgical removal of one half of the thyroid gland in the neck; usually carried out when a goiter affects one side only.

hemizygous Having unpaired genes. As an example: Males are hemizygous for genes on the X chromosome.

hemo- Referring to blood.

hemoagglutinin An antibody in the serum that causes clotting of an individual's own red blood cells.

hemochromatosis A serious disease in which there are skin color changes, cirrhosis of the liver, diabetes, and deposition of iron pigments in various tissues throughout the body.

hemoconcentration Concentration of the blood as a result of loss of body fluid or plasma. Large burned areas may lead to marked loss of blood plasma and *hemoconcentration*.

hemocytometer An apparatus used to determine the number of red blood cells.

hemodialysis A process whereby waste matter normally removed by the kidneys is removed from the blood by use of a special machine. Used in cases of kidney failure.

hemodialyzer An artificial kidney; an apparatus that removes waste products from the bloodstream which, under normal circumstances, would have been eliminated by the kidneys.

hemodilution The opposite of hemoconcentration; the condition in which there is an increase in the proportion of plasma to red cells in the blood.

hemodynamics The study of blood flow, volume and pressure.

hemoglobin The pigment in the red blood cells. It is the substance which carries oxygen to the tissues.

hemoglobinemia 1. A type of anemia in which, although there are sufficient red blood cells, the cells are deficient in hemoglobin. 2. The presence of hemoglobin in the blood plasma.

hemoglobinometer An instrument to measure the amount of hemoglobin in the blood. (It can detect anemia.)

hemoglobinuria Hemoglobin in the urine.

hemolysin A substance that causes destruction of red blood cells.

hemolysis Destruction of red blood cells and escape of the hemoglobin within the bloodstream.

hemolytic anemia An anemia caused by the destruction of red blood cells.

hemopericardium A collection of

blood in the sac surrounding the heart (pericardium).

hemoperitoneum Blood in the abdominal cavity (peritoneal cavity), often caused by rupture of an ectopic pregnancy.

hemophilia An inherited disease in which the blood clots improperly. Hemophiliacs are almost invariably males; they are called "bleeders."

hemopneumothorax A collection of blood and air in the space between the lung and the chest wall (the pleural cavity), often caused by a chest wound.

hemopoiesis The process whereby the various types of blood cells are formed. (Much of this process takes place within the bone marrow.)

hemoptysis The coughing up of blood.

hemorrhage Escape of blood from the blood vessels. It may result in either external or internal loss of blood.

hemorrhoidal banding *See* banding.

hemorrhoidectomy Surgical removal of hemorrhoids (piles).

hemorrhoids Piles. Varicose veins of the rectum or anus. Some protrude from the anal opening (external hemorrhoids); others are within the anal canal (internal hemorrhoids).

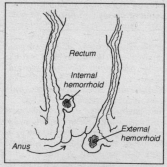

Rectum

Internal hemorrhoid

External hemorrhoid

Anus

Hemorrhoids

hemosiderin A substance found in the tissues which is rich in iron and probably supplies iron to the blood when needed.

hemospermia Blood in the semen, noted on ejaculation.

hemostasis A surgical term denoting the fact that bleeding has been stopped. The act of clamping and tying off bleeding blood vessels.

hemostat An instrument for clamping a bleeding artery or vein.

hemostatic An agent which stops hemorrhage.

hemothorax A collection of blood in the space between the lungs and chest wall (the pleural cavity).

hemotoxin A poison which destroys red blood cells, such as the venom of a poisonous snake.

Henoch's purpura A disease in children, characterized by bleeding into the tissues of the body, particularly beneath the skin. Spontaneous appearance of "black and blue" patches usually occurs.

hepar The liver.

    lobatum Syphilis of the liver.

heparin An anticoagulant given to prolong blood-clotting time and to decrease the clotting tendency. It is used in cases of thrombosis.

heparinize To anticoagulate the blood by administering heparin.

Heparin Lock Heparin (a substance that helps to prevent blood clots and blood clotting) given by injection of a specified dose.

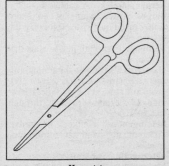

Hemostat

hepatectomy Surgical removal of the liver, with subsequent implantation of a healthy liver secured from a cadaver-donor.

hepatic Referring to the liver.

    artery The blood vessel supplying the liver with arterial blood.

    duct The tube (duct) leading bile from the liver toward the intestine. It joins the cystic duct from the gall bladder to form the *common bile duct.*

    veins The many veins draining the liver and conveying blood to the vena cava and then to the heart.

hepatic transplantation The transplantation of a liver from a recently dead person to a living one.

hepatitis Inflammation of the liver.

hepatitis A Liver inflammation caused by a virus. It can be contracted through contaminated food, by receiving a transfusion of infected blood, or other causes. A vaccine against the disease is available.

hepatitis B Viral inflammation of the liver caused by people injecting themselves with illicit drugs via infected needles, by people who have multiple sex partners, by people with hemophilia, or those undergoing hemodialysis, etc. There is an effective vaccine against the disease.

hepatitis C Liver inflammation caused by a virus, thought to be contracted through receiving an infected blood product.

hepatitis D A form of infection of the liver caused by the "delta virus." The condition frequently becomes chronic.

hepatobiliary Referring to the liver, gall bladder, and bile ducts.

hepatocellular cancer A malignant tumor of the liver.

hepatolithiasis Stones in the liver. These are the same type of stones which form in the gall bladder and bile ducts.

hepatoma A malignant tumor of the liver, seen mostly in children.

hepatomegaly Enlargement of the liver.

hepatonecrosis A condition which involves death of some liver cells.

hepatorenal syndrome Failure of liver and kidney function following surgery; a condition usually terminating in death.

hepatosplenomegaly Enlargement of the liver and spleen, as in diseases such as Gaucher's disease, etc.

hepatotoxic Referring to any substance that is damaging to the liver.

Herceptin A drug that may shrink some breast cancers, particularly in patients with a family history of the disease.

herd instinct The desire of people to group together and to identify with one another.

heredity The passage of bodily characteristics or disease from parent to offspring.

hermaphrodites People born with structures of both sexes; usually these organs are underdeveloped and unable to function normally.

hermetically sealed Airtight.

hernia A rupture. A weakness in the musculature allowing protrusion of tissues normally contained within the abdominal cavity.

herniate To rupture.

herniated disk *See* disk.

hernioplasty An operation to repair a hernia.

herniorrhaphy An operation to repair a hernia.

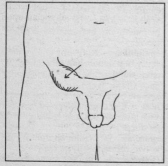

Hernia

herniotomy Opening of the sac of a hernia prior to its surgical repair.

heroin A powerful narcotic closely related to morphine; it is not used medically because addictions to it are readily formed.

herpes Acute inflammation of the skin, caused by a virus, characterized by the formation of small pustular areas.

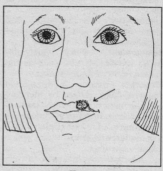

Herpes

herpes genitalis A form of herpes simplex caused by the type 2 virus. It is usually transmitted through sexual contact and is characterized by painful, pustular eruptions on the genitals, and occasionally with fever and lymph gland swelling in the groin.

herpes simplex A cold sore.

herpes zoster Shingles; an eruption, caused by a virus, following the course of a nerve.

hesitancy An inability to start urination.

Hesselbach's triangle An anatomical area (triangle) just above the groin and toward the midline. Direct inguinal hernias protrude through this triangle.

heterogenous Unlike; dissimilar; different; not from same source or species.

heterograft *See* graft.

heterometropia A defect in vision

characterized by different errors of refraction in each eye.

heterophil A white blood cell, recognized by granules in its nucleus.

    test A blood test which, when positive, indicates the presence of infectious mononucleosis (glandular fever).

heterosexuality Sexual feelings for one of the opposite sex.

heterotoxin A poison, or toxin, originating outside the body.

heterotransplant An organ or tissue transplanted from one species of animal to another.

heterotropia Cross-eye, squint, and other conditions in which muscle defects result in lack of alignment of the eyes.

heterozygous Hybrid; heterozygous individuals may resemble the dominant characteristics of their parents but they transmit recessive characteristics to half their children.

hexachlorophene A powerful germicide; used particularly in soaps employed in surgical scrubs.

hexadactylism Six fingers or toes per limb.

Hexadrol (dexamethasone) A cortisonelike drug used against inflammatory conditions and certain allergic states.

Hg chemical symbol for mercury.

hiatus An opening, such as in a hiatus hernia.

    hernia A hernia of the diaphragm taking place through the opening where the esophagus passes.

Hib-Immune Vaccine Trade name for a vaccine that protects children against certain types of meningitis.

hiccup (hiccough) A sudden spasm of the diaphragm.

HIDA scan A procedure performed to light up the gall bladder, thus permitting one to see the presence of a diseased condition of the organ. It may also show how well the gall bladder is functioning.

hidradenitis Abscesses of the

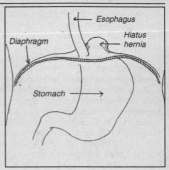

Hiatus hernia

sweat glands, especially those of the armpit.

hidrosis Excessive perspiration.

highly selective vagotomy *See* parietal cell vagotomy.

hilar lymph nodes The lymph glands at the root of the lungs. They are enlarged in cases of inflammation or tumor of the lungs.

hilus The root of an organ, where the nerves and blood vessels enter and leave.

hindgut That part of the embryo which forms the lower bowel and rectum.

hip The joint where the upper end of the thighbone and the pelvic bones meet.

Hippocrates (460–377 B.C.) "The father of medicine" and the supposed author of the Hippocratic oath taken by every physician upon graduation from medical college. He lived in Greece.

Hippocratic oath *"I swear by Apollo the physician, and Aesculapius, Hygeia, and Panacea, and I take to witness all the gods and goddesses that, according to my ability and judgment, I will keep this Oath and this stipulation: To reckon him who taught me this Art equally dear to me as my parents, to share my substance with him, and relieve his necessities if required; to look upon his offspring in the same footing as my own broth-*

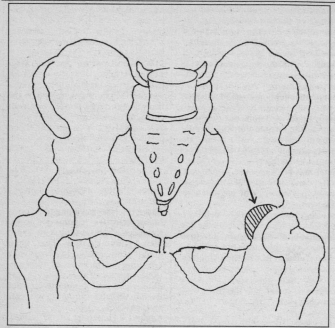

Hip joint

ers, and to teach them this Art if they shall wish to learn it, without fee or stipulation; and that by precept, lecture, and every other mode of instruction, I will impart a knowledge of the Art to my own sons, and those of my teachers, and to disciples bound by a stipulation and oath according to the law of Medicine, but to none others.

"I will follow that system of regimen which, according to my ability and judgment, I consider for the benefit of my patients, and abstain from whatever is deleterious and mischievous. I will give no deadly medicine to any one if asked, nor suggest any such counsel; and in like manner I will not give to a woman a pessary to produce abortion. With purity and

with holiness I will pass my life and practice my Art.

"I will not cut persons laboring under the stone, but will leave this to be done by men who are practitioners of this work. Into whatever houses I enter, I will go into them for the benefit of the sick, and will abstain from every voluntary act of mischief and corruption; and further, from the seduction of females or males, of freemen and slaves.

"Whatever, in connection with my professional practice, or not in connection with it, I see or hear in the life of men, which ought not to be spoken of abroad, I will not divulge, as reckoning that all such should be kept secret. While I continue to keep this Oath unviolated, may it be

*granted to me to enjoy life and the
practice of the Art, respected by all
men, in all times. But should I tres-
pass and violate this Oath, may the
reverse be my lot."*

hippus A jerky movement of the
pupil of the eye.

hip replacement An operation in
which the hipbone (head of the
femur) is replaced by a metal prosthesis, performed upon patients who
have an irreparably damaged hip
joint.

Hirschsprung's disease Megacolon.
Dilatation of the large bowel, present at birth, caused by constriction
of the large bowel in the region of
the rectum. Most cases require surgical correction.

hirsutism Excessive growth of
hair.

histamine A breakdown product
of protein metabolism. It has many
actions within the body, including
the stimulation of secretion of gastric juice, the stimulation of secretions from glands and the dilatation
of small blood vessels.

histidine One of the essential
amino acids.

histiocyte A cell found in connective tissue, thought to have the ability of destroying bacteria and debris
from dead tissue.

histiocytoma A benign skin tumor;
also called a *sclerosing hemangioma*
or a *dermatofibroma*.

histiocytosis An increase in the
number of histiocytes, especially in
the lymph glands.

histocompatibility An immunological term, referring to a state of similarity of tissues permitting a
successful graft from one person to
another.

histogram A graph showing the
comparabilities of various numbers.

histology The study of cells and organs by microscopic examination.

histoplasmosis A serious disease,
usually ending fatally, caused by a
fungus, *Histoplasma capsulatum*. It

causes high fever, emaciation and
anemia.

history The record of symptoms
and the sequence of events in an
illness.

HIV Abbreviation for the virus
causing AIDS.

hives Urticaria. An allergic condition of the skin characterized by the
formation of large blotches or welts
which itch intensely.

HIV negative A blood test showing that an individual does *not* har-
bor the virus that can cause AIDS.
See AIDS.

HIV positive A blood test showing
that an individual harbors the virus
that can cause AIDS. *See* AIDS.

H.L.A. Test Abbreviation for
human leukocyte antigen test, an extremely accurate test to determine
the paternity of a child. Samples of
the mother's, child's, and alleged father's blood are matched to make
the determination.

HMO Abbreviation for a Health
Maintenance Organization. *See*
Managed Care.

HNO₃ Nitric acid.

H₂O Water.

H₂O₂ Hydrogen dioxide or peroxide.

hobnail liver A form of cirrhosis,
giving the liver the appearance of
being covered by numerous hobnails
(knoblike projections.)

Hodgkin's disease A malignant
disease of the lymph nodes and
glands, terminating fatally within a
period of years.

holistic medicine That type which
considers the individual as a whole,
and places responsibility for maintenance of health upon the individual
himself.

hologram A three-dimensional
image.

homatropine A drug used to dilate
the pupil of the eye; ophthalmolo-
gists usually put homatropine drops
into the eyes before examining
them.

homeopathy A branch of medicine, popular at the turn of the century, characterized by the treatment of illness with small doses of drugs that produce, in a healthy person, symptoms like those of the illness being treated.

homeostasis Stability of all body functions at normal levels.

homo 1. Name of the genus of which man is a member. 2. Combining form meaning "the same."

homogeneous Similar in structure because of common ancestry.

homograft A graft of tissue taken from the body of another person.

homolateral On the same side of the body.

homologous Corresponding to the same type.

homologous serum jaundice Inflammation of the liver (hepatitis) with jaundice (yellow discoloration of the skin), following such procedures as blood transfusion, plasma injections, certain serum injections. It usually takes two to four months to appear and may last two to three months before subsiding.

homosexuality Love and physical attraction for members of one's own sex.

homotransplantation A graft from one human being to another.

homozygous The antithesis of heterozygous; pure-bred rather than hybrid; produced from chromosomes containing similar genes insofar as dominant characteristics are concerned.

homunculus A dwarf or little man whose body is well proportioned.

hookworm disease A parasitic disease caused by the hookworm, a nematode parasite. The hookworm penetrates the skin of the feet, enters the circulation and eventually fastens itself to the lining of the intestine. It sucks blood and ultimately causes severe anemia. This disease is sometimes seen in the South among barefoot children and adults.

hordeolum Sty. An abscess or boil on the eyelid.

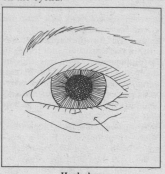

Hordeolum

hormone A chemical produced by a gland, secreted into the bloodstream, and affecting the function of distant cells or organs.

Horner's syndrome A depression of the eyeball, drooping of the eyelid, contraction of the pupil, and flushing of the face, seen in persons who have had sympathetic nerve destruction in the neck.

hornification Callus formation of the skin; cornification.

horripilation Gooseflesh.

horseshoe kidney A birth deformity in which the two kidneys are fused, usually at their lower poles, thus assuming the shape of a horseshoe.

hospice A hospital unit that provides an organized program of relief of symptoms for dying patients. It also renders advice and help to the family of the patient.

hospital An institution for the care of sick people.

    general One that is equipped to take care of most types of conditions.

    private A proprietary institution, usually operated for profit, offering little or no assistance to indigent patients.

    teaching A hospital that emphasizes the teaching of young physicians (interns and residents). It is often affiliated with a medical school.

    voluntary One that has provisions both for paying, private patients and for the indigent. Such institutions are usually not for profit.

hospital ranks Physicians and surgeons on staffs of hospitals are often given ranks. From the lowest to highest they usually are: Clinical Assistant, Assistant, Adjunct, Associate, Attending (Chief).

host The patient who harbors a germ, a parasite or a growth.

hot flashes A feeling of warmth, often followed by profuse perspiration, coming on abruptly in women who are having change of life.

hourglass gall bladder One which is constricted in its midsection, thus assuming the shape of an hourglass.

    stomach One which is constricted in its midsection, thus assuming the shape of an hourglass.

housemaid's knee A swelling just below the knee caused by inflammation and fluid collection in the bursa. It is found occasionally in housemaids who spend long periods on their knees.

House physician An intern or a physician who lives in a building and serves its residents.

House staff The interns and residents of a hospital.

House surgeon The intern who cares for surgical cases in a hospital and who lives in the hospital. Today, *resident surgeons* have largely replaced *house surgeons*.

HTLV Abbreviation for the virus that is thought to be associated with T-cell lymphomas, including certain types of leukemia.

Huggin's operation Castration, as a treatment for cancer of the prostate gland.

Huhner test A test for sterility, whereby sperm from the vagina is examined one hour after intercourse. Normally, some sperm would still be alive.

human antihemophilic factor *See* AHF.

human leukocyte antigen test A paternity test. *See* H.L.A. Test.

Humatin A medication effective against amebic infections of the intestinal tract.

humerus The bone of the upper arm.

humor A body fluid, such as the humor within the eyeball.

humpback A deformity in which the vertebral column is bent, causing a protrusion of the back in the shape of a hump.

Humulin A synthetic insulin manufactured through use of recombinant DNA and genetic engineering techniques, using bacteria. It is identical to insulin produced by the human pancreas. *See* recombinant DNA.

hunchback Same as humpback.

hunger pains A gnawing feeling in the upper abdomen when one is hungry, thought to be due to contractions of the stomach.

Huntington's chorea An inherited disease in which there are purposeless muscle movements of the face, arms and legs, along with speech defects and progressive degeneration of brain tissue, leading to idiocy.

Hürthle-cell tumor A rather rare growth within the thyroid gland. While most of these adenomas are benign, some do appear to become malignant.

Hutchinson-Boeck disease *See* sarcoidosis.

Hutchinson's teeth Teeth with notches in them, seen frequently in congenital (existing at birth) syphilis.

hyaline membrane disease Acute respiratory distress syndrome; a condition seen most often in newborn children. A membranous layer covers the air sacs in the lungs with resultant difficulty in breathing. (Many children succumb to this condition.)

hyalinization The replacement of a

functioning tissue by a firm, amorphous, inert material. It is a degenerative process.

hyaluronic acid A substance found in cementing or protective tissues and in certain bacteria.

hyaluronidase An enzyme which breaks down hyaluronic acid; also an enzymatic substance used to increase the penetrative qualities of certain injected medications.

hybrid A mixed type; the opposite of thoroughbred.

Hycodan A patented cough medicine.

hydatid cyst 1. A cyst originating from the remnants of embryonic tissue. 2. A cyst caused by *Echinococcus granulosus* (dog tapeworm).

hydatid of Morgagni A cyst occurring just above the testicle in the male and near the ovary in the female. It usually is the size of a dime, nickel or quarter. It is a benign condition.

hydralazine A drug used to dilate blood vessels and, in so doing, help to lower blood pressure. Trade name: Apresoline.

hydramnios A condition in which excess fluid surrounds the unborn child.

hydrargyria Poisoning caused by mercury. Seen formerly when syphilis was treated with various mercury compounds.

hydrarthrosis Fluid in a joint, as in "water on the knee." It is a sign of inflammation or injury to a joint.

hydrases Enzymes that withdraw water from a compound.

hydrate 1. To add water. 2. A chemical containing water in combination with other chemicals.

hydremia Excessive fluid content of the blood.

hydro- Referring to water.

hydrobromide A medication used to calm the nerves.

hydrocele A collection of fluid in a sac surrounding the testicle. Surgery may be necessary if the fluid is not absorbed or recurs after withdrawal.

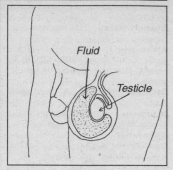
Fluid

Testicle

Hydrocele

hydrocelectomy Surgical removal of a hydrocele.

hydrocephalus A condition coming on shortly after birth in which the head enlarges as a result of accumulation of fluid around the brain. Giant head.

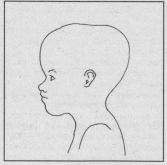

Hydrocephalus

hydrochloric acid (HCl) Hydrogen chloride, an acid secreted by the cells lining the stomach. This acid is helpful in the digestion of foods.

hydrochlorothiazide *See* Esidrix.

hydrocortisone A cortisone medication. *See* cortisone.

hydrocyanic acid Prussic acid. One of the most deadly of all poisons.

Hydrodiuril A patented diuretic

indication having the same action as Diuril.

hydrodynamics The mechanics of liquids.

hydrogen (H) An element which is present in practically all living things. It is the lightest of all elements.

hydrogen peroxide A mild antiseptic.

hydrolysis A breakdown or a chemical reaction with water.

hydrometer An instrument which measures the specific gravity of a fluid.

hydronephrosis A condition in which there is obstruction of the outflow of urine from the kidney. It ultimately results in destruction of kidney tissue.

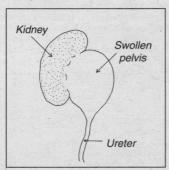

Kidney

Swollen pelvis

Ureter

Hydronephrosis

hydrophobia Rabies, a disease fatal to humans and animals which is caused by the bite of an infected animal, such as a dog, cat, rabbit, squirrel, etc.

hydropic Having "dropsy."

hydropneumothorax A condition in which fluid and air occur in the space between the lung and the chest wall.

Hydropres A patented medicine which brings about lowering of blood pressure and elimination of excess body fluids.

hydrops of the gall bladder An obstruction of the gall bladder with a ballooning out of the sac due to a collection of fluid within it.

hydrosalpinx A collection of fluid within a fallopian tube, the end state of an infection.

hydrotherapy Treatment of muscles, bones, or tendons by the application of water, as in whirlpool baths.

hydroureter A dilatation and enlargement of a ureter (the tube leading from the kidney to the bladder), caused by obstruction of free flow of urine. (Such a ureter may contain large quantities of urine.)

hydroxyphenyluria Faulty metabolism of the protein tyrosine; frequently seen in premature infants.

hydruria The passage of urine in large quantities.

hygiene Observation and practice of health standards.

hygroma A cyst formed out of lymph channels. (Cystic *hygroma* is a condition sometimes seen in the neck region of children.)

hygroscopic Pertaining to a substance which readily absorbs moisture.

Hygroton (chlorthalidone) An effective diuretic medication.

Hykinone A vitamin K preparation, essential in maintaining the normal blood-clotting mechanism.

hymen The maidenhead. The membrane covering the entrance to the vagina.

hymenotomy Cutting the maidenhead (hymen).

hyoid bone The bone located beneath the chin in the upper part of the neck. It is the bone to which the tongue muscles are attached.

hyoscine Scopolamine, the socalled "truth serum." Large doses produce a narcotic effect.

hypalgesia Decreased sensation to pain.

Hypaque The trademark for a substance which, when injected or instilled into the body, is opaque to X rays. It thus helps to outline organs and body cavities and sinuses.

hyper- Prefix meaning "excessive," "above."

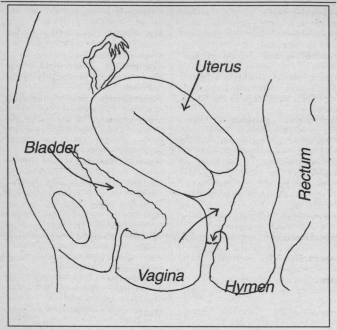

Hymen

hyperacidity Excess acid, as too much acid in the stomach.

hyperactive child One who has a short attention span, is easily distracted, displays impulsiveness and whose physical movements are excessive.

hyperacusis Exceptionally acute hearing.

hyperadrenalism Overactivity and oversecretion by the adrenal gland. It may lead to overactivity of thyroid function, diabetes, etc.

hyperaldosteronism Conn's syndrome; a disorder of the adrenal gland associated with muscular weakness, high blood pressure, increased thirst and increased frequency of urination, caused by excessive secretion of aldosterone.

hyperalgesia Extreme sensitivity to pain. *Hyperalgesia* of the skin may be manifested by great pain even on light pinching.

hyperalimentation *See* total parenteral nutrition (TPN).

hyperbaric chamber A specially devised room in which the oxygen content is greater than under ordinary atmospheric conditions.

hyperbilirubinemia Excess bile pigment in the blood, as seen in jaundice.

hypercalcemia Excess calcium in the blood.

hypercapnia Excess carbon dioxide in the blood.

hypercathexis Attributing unusual sexual connotations to something.

hyperchloremia Excess chloride in the blood.

hyperchlorhydria Excess hydrochloric acid in the gastric juice.

hypercholesteremia Excess cholesterol in the blood.

hyperchromatism Excess pigmentation.

hypercyesis A condition in which there are an abnormally large number of red blood cells in the bloodstream.

hyperemesis gravidarum Excessive vomiting during pregnancy. (This may lead to serious loss of fluid and minerals, requiring replacement by intravenous injection.)

hyperemia An increased amount of blood in an organ or other part of the body, as seen in an area of inflammation.

hyperesthesia Excess sensitivity, such as to touch or pinprick.

hyperextension To overstraighten, as to overextend an arm or a leg.

hyperflexion To overbend, as to overflex a joint.

hyperglycemia Excessive sugar in the blood, found frequently in diabetes mellitus.

hypergonadism Excessive secretion of hormones by the ovaries or testicles.

hypergynecomasia Precocious development of adult female characteristics in a child.

hyperhidrosis Excessive sweating.

hyperimmune Having a large number of antibodies, often resulting from repeated immunizations.

hyperinsulinism Too much insulin, often resulting in too little sugar in the blood (hypoglycemia). This may result from excessive secretion by the pancreas or an overdose of insulin.

hyperkalemia Excessive amounts of potassium in the blood.

hyperkeratosis 1. Overgrowth of the tissue covering the pupil of the eye (cornea). 2. Overgrowth of the horny layer of the skin.

hyperkinetic Excess movement of muscles.

hyperlipemia Excess fat in the blood.

hypermastia Overgrowth of the breasts.

hypermetropia Farsightedness.

hypermotility Overactivity, usually referring to overactivity of the intestines.

hypernatremia Excessive amounts of sodium in the blood.

hypernephroma A tumor of the kidney. (Often, the first symptom is the passage of blood in the urine.)

hyperopia Farsightedness.

hyperparathyroidism Excessive secretion of the parathyroid glands, producing a disease characterized by loss of calcium from the bones, cyst formation within the bones, kidney stones, etc.

hyperperistalsis Overactivity of the contractions of the intestines, leading to diarrhea.

hyperpiesis High blood pressure; hypertension.

hyperpituitarism Overactivity of the pituitary gland, leading to gigantism or to acromegaly.

hyperplasia Overgrowth of a tissue or organ.

hyperpnea Rapid and exceptionally deep breathing.

hyperpotassemia Excess potassium in the blood.

hyperprolactinemia Excess prolactin in the blood, often causing sterility and discharge of milk from the breasts.

hyperpyrexia High fever.

hypersalivation The secretion of excessive amounts of saliva.

hypersensitivity Excessively sensitive, as in an allergic condition.

hypersplenism A set of diseases associated with excess activity and enlargement of the spleen.

hypertension High blood pressure.

Hyper-Tet Tetanus antitoxin, not made from horse serum; especially valuable for those who are allergic.

hyperthermy The treatment of a condition by artificially producing a high fever; formerly, a common method of treating the late stages of syphilis.

hyperthyroidism Overactivity of the thyroid gland. This condition is usually associated with a goiter.

hypertonic 1. Increased tension. 2. In chemistry, said of a solution with greater osmotic pressure than that of another fluid.

hypertrichosis Excess growth of hair, as on a woman's face and body.

hypertrophy Increase in the size of an organ.

hyperuricemia Excess uric acid in the blood, as in gout.

hyperventilation Excessive deep breathing with the washing out of the system of too much carbon dioxide and the taking in of too much oxygen. This may lead to buzzing noises in the head and fainting.

hypervitaminosis Any condition caused by intake of too much vitamin, such as the toxic effects from excessive amounts of vitamin D.

hypervolemia Excess circulating blood and serum; plethora.

hypesthesia Decreased sensitivity, as lessened appreciation of the sense of pain or touch.

hyphemia 1. A hemorrhage in the eyeball. 2. Deficiency of blood, also called oligemia.

hypnoanalysis Psychiatric treatment of the analytic type carried out while the patient is under the influence of hypnosis.

hypnology The science of hypnosis.

hypnophobia Abnormal fear of falling asleep.

hypnosis A trance induced by the repeated suggestions of a hypnotist. A sleeplike state is produced during which the subject retains awareness of the presence of the hypnotist and often responds to his questions and instructions.

hypnotherapy Hypnotism as a means of treatment of an illness.

hypnotic A medication which produces sleep.

hypnotize To bring about hypnosis.

hypo- A prefix signifying that something is below the average.

hypoacidity Too little or a deficiency of acid.

hypoadrenalism An exhausted, depressed, low blood pressure and low metabolism condition caused by inadequate function and secretion of the adrenal glands.

hypo-allergenic A substance that is least likely to evoke an allergic response.

hypobaric Referring to a solution with less specific gravity than that of a body fluid.

hypobarism Decompression sickness, occasionally affecting divers and others, due to sudden changes in barometric pressure.

hypocalcemia Too little calcium in the blood.

hypocapnia Too little carbon dioxide in the blood (Acapnia).

hypochlorhydria Too little hydrochloric acid in the gastric (stomach) juice.

hypocholesterolemia Less than normal amount of cholesterol in the blood.

hypochondriac One who thinks he is afflicted with diseases which are not present. Excessive concern about one's health.

hypochromia An anemia in which there is less than the normal amount of hemoglobin in the red blood cells.

hypodermic Beneath the skin. (A *hypodermic* injection is one made into the tissues beneath the skin.

hypodermoclysis Injection of fluids, usually saline (salt solution) beneath the skin. This method of supplying fluids has been replaced largely by the intravenous route.

hypofibrinogenemia Too little blood-clotting factor in the circulation. (Patients with hypofibrinogenemia show bleeding tendencies.)

hypofunction Lessened function.

hypogammaglobulinemia Too little gamma globulin in the body. (Children with hypogammaglobuli-

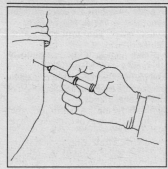

Hypodermic

nemia have extremely poor resistance to infections.)

hypogastrium That region of the abdomen extending down from the navel to the pubic bone.

hypogenitalism Underdevelopment of the sex organs.

hypoglossal Beneath the tongue.

hypoglycemia Too little sugar in the blood.

hypognathous An overdeveloped chin or a marked protrusion of the lower jaw.

hypogonadism Lessened or diminished function of the sex glands.

hypokalemia Too little potassium in the blood.

hypomania An upset bordering upon a maniacal form of insanity but not quite bad enough to be labeled as a true mania.

hyponatremia Too little sodium in the blood. (Excessive loss of salt through vomiting, perspiration, or diarrhea will cause hyponatremia.)

hypoparathyroidism Inadequate function of the parathyroid glands.

hypopharynx The area below the back of the throat and just above the larynx (voice box).

hypophysectomy Surgical removal of the pituitary gland; carried out for tumor, or in some cases of widespread cancer in order to inhibit the growth of the cancer.

hypophysis The pituitary gland located in the base of the skull.

hypopituitarism Insufficient secretion of pituitary hormones. This may cause any number of serious conditions, such as adrenal gland failure, lack of menstruation, sterility or impotence, lowering of metabolic rate, etc.

hypoplasia Underdevelopment of an organ or tissue.

hypopotassemia Too little potassium in the blood.

hypoproteinemia Too little protein in the blood. It may lead to weakness, poor healing of tissues, swelling of the ankles, etc.

hyporeflexia Diminished reflexes.

hyposensitization To reduce sensitivity to an allergen, as in injections for hay fever.

hyposmia Diminished sense of smell.

hypospadias A birth deformity in which the urethra ends before it reaches the tip of the penis.

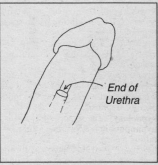

End of Urethra

Hypospadias

hypostasis The settling of a substance, such as the accumulation of secretions at the base of the lungs in *hypostatic pneumonia.*

hypotension Low blood pressure.

hypothalamus A part of the brain below the cerebrum (higher brain center).

hypothenar The fleshy part of the

palm of the hand in the region of the ring and little fingers.

hypothermia A lower than normal body temperature. This is sometimes produced artificially to slow bodily processes during operations upon the heart.

hypothesis A theory.

hypothrombinemia Too little thrombin in the circulating blood, frequently leading to a bleeding tendency.

hypothyroidism Underactivity of the thyroid gland.

hypotonia Lessened muscle tone.

hypotonic solution A solution which has less tension or is less concentrated than another.

hypoventilation Less air and oxygen in the lungs than the normal requirements.

hypovitaminosis A deficiency of vitamins.

hypovolemia Reduced blood volume.

hypoxia Inadequate oxygen in the lungs and in the blood.

hysterectomy Surgical removal of the uterus.

hysteria An extremely emotional state, seen among neurotics.

hysterical blindness A loss of sight, usually temporary, occasioned by a severe shock.

hysterogram An X ray of the uterus.

hysterosalpingogram An X ray of the uterus and fallopian tubes.

hysteroscopic metroplasty An operation upon the uterus performed vaginally by inserting an instrument, a hysteroscope, through the cervix into the uterine cavity.

hysterotomy Surgical incision into the uterus.

hysterotrachelectomy Surgical removal of the cervix of the uterus.

Hytrin A patented drug helpful in reducing high blood pressure and which helps to reduce urinary frequency.

I

I The symbol for iodine.

iatro- Relating to physicians, or medicine in general.

iatrogenic Caused by a physician.

Ibuprofen A patented pain-relieving medication.

I.C.C.U. Abbreviation for intensive cardiac care unit.

ichnogram A footprint.

icteric Referring or pertaining to jaundice (yellow discoloration of the skin).

icterogenic Producing jaundice.

icterus *See* jaundice.

icterus index A calculation of the amount of bilirubin in the blood; an excess causes jaundice.

icterus neonatorium Jaundice of the newborn.

icthyoid Fishlike.

icthyosis Scaly skin, giving the appearance of fish scales. Some types of this condition are inherited.

I.C.U. Abbreviation for intensive care unit.

id In psychoanalysis, the unconscious force which is responsible for the instinctive impulses of self-preservation and reproduction; said to be dominated by the pleasure principle.

IDDM Abbreviation for insulin dependent diabetes mellitus.

idea A belief or thought.

idealization The process by which one gives excessive values to a loved object; the act of idolizing.

ideation The mental process resulting in thoughts and ideas.

identification 1. The process of recognizing a person or thing by its characteristics. 2. In psychology, the unconscious assumption of the traits or characteristics of another person.

ideology The science of ideas and the theory of their origin.

idiocy The condition in which mental development is restricted to less than that of a three-year-old child. Idiots have an I.Q. of less than 25.

idioglossia The jabbering of an infant before he is old enough to talk.

idiopathic Of unknown cause.

idiopathic thrombocytopenia (ITP) An illness characterized by hemorrhages from mucous membranes and multiple bruises on the skin, resulting from low platelet cells in the blood. The disease affects children as well as adults. *See* purpura.

idiosyncrasy 1. A peculiarity in personality differing from normal or usual behavior. 2. An unusual reaction to a drug or treatment.

idiot A mentally defective individual whose development is under that of a three-year-old child.

    mongolian A child born with an extra chromosome in his cells, who looks mongoloid and whose mental development is markedly retarded.

    savant An individual with a less than average intellect who nevertheless displays unusual faculties in one sphere of mental activity.

ileal bladder A urinary outlet constructed by suturing the ureters from the kidneys to a loop of small intestine, which is then brought out onto the abdomen as an ileostomy; performed in cases where the urinary bladder has been removed because of cancer.

ileitis Inflammation of the lower portion of the small bowel, often chronic and requiring surgery to produce a cure.

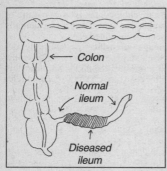

Ileitis

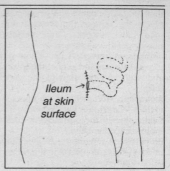

Ileum at skin surface

Ileostomy

ileoanal anastomosis An operation that sutures the small intestine to the anus after removal of the large bowel; performed in some cases of severe ulcerative colitis. The operation preserves function of the anus.

ileocecal valve The muscular mechanism at the junction of the small and large intestine. It regulates the flow of intestinal contents from the ileum into the cecum.

ileocolic Referring to the ileum (last few feet of the small intestine), and the colon (large intestine).

ileocolitis Inflammation of both small and large intestine.

ileoproctostomy The surgical procedure in which the ileum (small intestine) is sutured (stitched) to the rectum.

ileosigmoidostomy An operation in which the ileum of the small bowel is sutured to the sigmoid colon of the large bowel. (This procedure is sometimes done to bypass an obstruction in the large bowel.)

ileostomy A surgical procedure in which the ileum (small bowel) is brought out onto the abdominal wall. Usually performed after the removal of a diseased large bowel.

ileotransverse colostomy An operation in which the ileum of the small intestine is connected to the transverse colon of the large bowel. (This procedure is done when there is an inflammation of the small intestine—regional enteritis—or when there is a tumor of the right side of the large bowel.)

Iletin A patented product containing insulin, used in the treatment of diabetes.

ileum The lower portion of the small intestine, terminating in the cecum (large intestine) in the right lower portion of the abdomen.

ileus Obstruction of the small intestine due either to paralysis of the normal mechanism which pushes intestinal contents onward, or due to mechanical obstruction to the passage of intestinal contents.

meconium A rare disease of the newborn in which the fecal contents of the small intestine cause obstruction. It requires surgery and the thorough cleaning out of the obstructed intestine.

iliac Referring to the ilium, the winglike portion of the hip bones. The flank.

iliococcygeus A muscle in the pelvis which is instrumental in controlling the rectum and anus.

iliofemoral Referring to the iliac bone and the femur (thigh bone).

iliohypogastric nerve A nerve supplying the skin of the lower abdomen and buttocks, and certain muscles of the abdomen.

ilioinguinal nerve A nerve supplying the muscles and skin of the lower abdomen and the skin of the genitals.

iliolumbar Referring to the muscles in the mid and lower back regions. (Inflammation of these muscles is commonly called lumbago.)

iliopectineal ligament A ligament in the groin often useful in the repair of hernias (ruptures).

iliopsoas muscle A strong muscle running in a longitudinal direction on the posterior portion of the abdomen and pelvis.

ilium The flank. The upper portion of the hipbone.

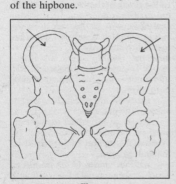

Ilium

illegitimate Born out of wedlock.

illumination, dark field A method of demonstrating germs through a microscope. By darkening the field, light rays and the objects to be seen are reflected vertically through the microscope.

illusion A false impression; the erroneous interpretation of something which has been viewed or perceived.

Ilosone (Erythromycin) An antibiotic especially effective against streptococcal, staphylococcal, and many other potent bacteria.

I.M. or **i.m.** 1. An abbreviation for infectious mononucleosis. 2. An abbreviation for intramuscular.

image 1. The picture which is recorded by the retina of the eye. 2. In psychology, the mental picture of something which has been actually seen or imagined.

image intensifier A specially devised viewing screen in fluoroscopy. It intensifies the image and transfers it to a surface quite similar to a television screen.

imaging The creation of an image by sonography, X ray, tomography, etc.

imbalance Upset, out of balance; lack of proper function.

imbecility A state of mental development in which the I.Q. is between 25 and 50; a condition one grade above that of idiocy.

imbibe To drink.

imbricate To close a structure with overlapping layers of tissue, as in the surgical repair of a hernia (rupture).

Imferon An iron-containing medication, useful in treating certain types of anemia.

immature cataract One that has not become very opaque, and is probably not yet ready to be operated upon.

immersion foot A condition due to prolonged exposure to cold, damp and wet. The foot becomes blue, the blood vessels contract, and ulcerations may form. Sometimes seen among army and navy personnel.

immersion oil Cedar oil, used in high-magnification microscopic work to increase the effect.

immiscible Substances which cannot be mixed; as oil which cannot be mixed with water.

immobilize To render a part immovable, as by applying a splint or plaster cast and weights to a fractured arm or leg.

immortality Living forever.

immune Protected against a disease.

immune globulin A drug given

into the muscles or intravenously to bolster the body's immune system. Used in cases of agammaglobinemia and in some cases of purpura to initiate greater production of antibodies.

immune system The body mechanism that protects against harmful invaders, including the production of antibodies. (The bone marrow, the thymus gland, and lymph tissue are prominent in activating the immune system.)

immunity

 acquired (active) That type resulting from having recovered from a disease or from having been given an immunizing vaccine or toxoid.

 inherent (innate) That type with which one is born.

 local Some tissues, areas, or organs of the body display an immunity against infection. (The intestinal tract is immune to infection from many of the bacteria that live and grow within it.)

 natural That type resulting from recovery from an illness or from innate resistance to a particular kind of bacteria or virus.

immunization The process of making one immune to a disease; protection against susceptibility to a contagious disease.

immunoassay *See* radioimmunoassay.

immunochemistry That branch of chemistry concerned with allergic responses, especially chemical reactions of allergens and antibodies.

immunochemotherapy Combined treatment of a malignancy through use of immunology and chemotherapy.

immunodeficiency Inadequacy of the body's immune system, frequently resulting in overwhelming infections or uncontrolled growth of malignant tumors.

immunoglobulins Antibodies produced in the lymphatic cells to combat infections or other invading substances. Also known as *immune serum globulins.*

immunohematology A branch of medicine which deals both with blood cells and the antibodies and antigens in the blood.

Immunologist A physician who specializes in the study of immunity.

immunosuppression The suppression of immunological responses, often done after performance of an organ transplant. Chemicals are sometimes used to do this; also, substances such as *antilymphocytic globulin* (ALG) are employed.

immunotherapy It is the treatment of disease through the production of immunity.

immunotransfusion A blood transfusion from a donor who is immune to the disease from which the recipient is suffering.

Imodium An antidiarrheal medication effective in slowing down intestinal overactivity.

impacted Firmly lodged or wedged, as one fragment of a fractured bone into another; or, an *impacted* wisdom tooth.

 cerumen Wax which has hardened in the ear canals.

 feces Stool which has hardened in the rectum and cannot be evacuated without an enema or manual removal.

 wisdom tooth A third molar which is lying on its side, pressing against the second molar and only partially erupted through the gum. (Most such teeth should be removed.)

impalpable Not able to be felt with the hands, such as a tumor.

imperforate Not perforated. Lacking a normal opening, such as an *imperforate* hymen or anus.

impermeable Not allowing anything to pass through, such as an *impermeable* membrane.

impetigo A pustular inflammatory disease of the skin, highly contagious, seen often in infants and young children.

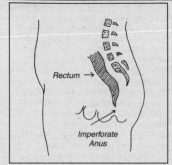

Rectum →

Imperforate
Anus

Imperforate anus

implant A fragment of tissue which grows in an area other than its usual one, such as an *implant* of a tendon from one region to another.

impotence Inability to have sexual intercourse. Unable to have and maintain an erection.

impregnate To make pregnant.

impulse An urge.

impulsive Referring to an emotional rather than a reasoned action or reaction.

imputability A state of legal sanity.

Imuran A drug used to suppress the body's defense mechanisms during the period following transplantation of an organ. (Such suppression is necessary to overcome rejection of the grafted organ.)

inacidity Lack of hydrochloric acid in the stomach juice. Although most people do have acid in their stomach juice, others may lead perfectly normal lives without it.

inanimate Without life.

inanition The physical condition resulting from starvation.

inarticulate Not capable of being understood; unable to express one's self satisfactorily.

inassimilable A substance which cannot be absorbed, especially by the intestinal tract.

inborn Inherited; congenital.

incarcerated Hemmed in; stuck; imprisoned. (An *incarcerated hernia*

is one in which the herniated parts are stuck in the hernia sac.)

incest Intercourse between two members of the same immediate family, as a sister and brother, or a parent and child.

incidence Occurrence, such as the *incidence* of a disease; often used to denote the frequency of occurrence of a condition.

incipient Early, beginning, as *incipient* pneumonia.

incise To cut surgically.

incision A surgical cut.

incisional hernia A rupture occurring through the site of a previous operative incision.

incisor teeth The front, cutting teeth.

incisura A notch or slitlike depression in an organ, such as the *incisura* of the stomach.

inclination The tilt of an organ, such as the *inclination* of the pelvis.

inclusion cyst One which is composed of skin and which lies beneath the normal surface of the skin. It is sometimes secondary to a cut with a piece of skin being driven into the subcutaneous tissues.

incoherent Confused; not intelligible.

incompatible 1. Not capable of living or existing together in a harmonious state. 2. Drugs which cannot be mixed with one another.

incompetent 1. Not functioning adequately, as an *incompetent* heart valve. 2. Legally, one not able to manage his affairs.

incomplete fracture A partial break in a bone.

incontinence Involuntary voiding or involuntary passage of stool.

incoordination Lack of coordination; inability to control muscle activity so as to perform properly.

increment An increase of value.

incrustation Scab formation over a raw surface.

incubation period The interval between exposure to a disease and its appearance; the length of time required for a disease to develop.

incubator 1. A heated and humidified container for a newborn, often premature, child. 2. An apparatus in which bacteria are grown in order to study and identify them.

incubus A nightmare.

incus The "anvil" bone in the middle ear. One of the three bones of hearing.

indentation A depression or notch in the contour of a part or organ.

Inderal Trade name for propanolol, a beta-blocking agent helpful in the treatment of angina pectoris, high blood pressure, and certain other heart ailments.

index Something which points out.

indicant Something which points the way; an indicator.

indicanuria Excessive indican in the urine. (Indican is a product of protein putrefaction.)

indication Something pertaining to a disease which points the way toward treating it. Pus may be an *indication* for surgical incision and drainage.

indicator In chemistry, a substance which shows (usually by its color) that a certain chemical reaction has occurred.

indigenous Originating in the region where it is found. (Yellow fever was *indigenous* to the jungles of Panama.)

indigestion Dyspepsia. Disturbed digestion.

Indinavir A protease inhibitor; a new drug that is most helpful when used with other drugs in treating AIDS. (Similar medications are now being utilized.)

Indocin A nonsteroid drug (contains no cortisone) helpful in relieving pain and swelling in arthritis.

indole A product of intestinal putrefaction. It gives feces part of their characteristic odor.

indolent Inactive; not progressing. An *indolent ulcer* is one that shows little or no signs of healing.

induction 1. The act or process of causing something to happen. 2. The beginning stages of anesthesia before the patient is completely asleep.

induration Thickening, such as might be felt about the edges of an inflamed wound.

indwelling catheter One that is left in place for prolonged periods of time. *See* catheter.

inebriation Drunkenness.

inertia Lack of activity; failure to move or contract, such as *uterine inertia* during labor.

in extremis Denoting that a person is on the point of dying (a Latin term).

infant Any child below the age of two years.

infanticide The killing of an infant.

infantile paralysis Poliomyelitis. A virus disease, often occurring in epidemics, affecting the central nervous system and musculature.

infantile uterus An underdeveloped womb in an adult. This condition is often caused by an upset in glandular function.

infantilism A condition in which an adult retains childish characteristics.

infarct An area of tissue deprived of its blood supply because of a clot within the artery, such as a kidney or spleen *infarct* or an *infarct* in a lung. The *infarcted* area usually undergoes degeneration and is replaced by scar tissue. A massive *infarct* in the lungs or heart may cause sudden death.

Infatabs (Dilantin) A medication helpful in preventing convulsive seizures.

infection The presence and growth of bacteria, viruses or parasites within the body.

  airborne The spread of bacteria from one person to another by coughing or sneezing (droplet infection).

  concurrent Two separate infections that occur at the same time in one individual.

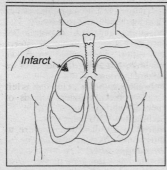

Infarct

cross One occurring in a hospital as the result of transmission from another patient.

focal An infection localized to certain tissues from which bacteria may spread throughout the body.

mixed One in which two or more bacteria are involved.

secondary An infection superimposed upon another infection caused by a different microorganism.

infectious disease A disease caused by or transmitted by bacteria, fungi, or protozoa.

infectious hepatitis An inflammation of the liver caused by a virus. Recovery usually takes place in several weeks to three to four months.

infectious mononucleosis Glandular fever. An infectious disease characterized by sore throat, swollen glands, weakness and the presence of an abnormal blood count, seen especially among adolescents and young adults. It may last for several weeks before recovery takes place.

inferiority complex A term formerly applied to the condition of one who feels inadequate and inferior to others, considered a form of neurotic behavior. Now a colloquial usage.

infertility Sterility; inability to bear offspring.

infestation Invasion of the body by ticks, mites, insects, worms, etc.

infiltration The passage of cells or fluid into tissue spaces usually free of such elements.

infirmary A hospital or nursing home.

infirmity A condition resulting in weakness.

inflammation The reaction of tissues to injury, manifested by pain, heat, swelling, and redness.

inflammatory carcinoma A highly malignant form of cancer, seen not infrequently in the breast.

influenza Grippe. Flu. Asiatic influenza. A virus infection of the upper respiratory system.

Influenza vaccine, Bivalent The vaccine is reportedly effective, for a short few weeks, in protecting against the influenza A and B viruses.

informed consent Permission from a patient to perform an operation, procedure, or test, after having been told all the risks and dangers involved. Informed consent is now mandatory, according to law.

infra- Prefix meaning under, below, beneath.

infraclavicular region The region below the collarbone.

infracostal The region below the ribs.

infradiaphragmatic Pertaining to the area beneath the diaphragm.

inframammary incision A surgical incision beneath the breast; frequently used when operating for a benign tumor in order to hide the scar.

infraorbital region The area below or beneath the orbit floor of the eye.

infrapatellar The region beneath the kneecap.

infrared rays Nonvisible rays of exceptionally long wave length. An infrared-ray apparatus is used to give deep heat to an injured part.

infrascapular Beneath the scapula (wingbone).

infundibulum A stalk or funnelshaped structure.

Infusaid pump An apparatus for the continuous administration of chemotherapy, used sometimes in cases of cancer that has spread to the liver.

infusion The injection of a solution into a vein or beneath the skin, such as a glucose and water infusion.

    reaction Fever and chills following the administration of fluids and medication into a vein. (Most such reactions last but a few hours and then disappear.)

ingest To eat.

ingredient A component of a substance or compound.

ingrown toenail A nail that has grown into the nailfold, often resulting in a painful infection which may require minor surgery.

inguinal region The groin.

inhalant A medication which is administered by inhalation.

inhalation The act of breathing in.

    burn A burn of the respiratory passages and lungs caused by inhaling steam or an irritating gas which is capable of burning the delicate mucous membranes of the trachea, bronchial tubes and lung cells.

inhalation anesthesia Anesthesia obtained by inhaling one or more of the anesthetic agents, such as nitrous oxide, ether, halothane, etc. Also termed *general anesthesia.*

inhalation pneumonia Inflammation or infection of the lungs secondary to inhaling or aspirating an irritating or infecting agent.

inherent Inborn.

inherited Handed down from the parents by genetic transmission of characteristics such as eye color, etc.

inhibition Restraint of a process or action.

inhibitor A substance which offsets or stops the effectiveness of another substance or prevents a chemical reaction from taking place.

injectable A medication that is

specially suited for injection, rather than being administered orally.

injection The act of forcing a liquid medication or other substance into a part of the body by *injection* with a needle and syringe.

inlay 1. A bone graft to fill a defect. 2. In dentistry, a mold set into a cavity defect in a tooth.

innervation The nerve supply to an organ or part.

innocent Not harmful.

innocuous Not harmful.

innominate artery A large artery arising from the arch of the aorta and supplying the right side of the neck, head, shoulder region and right arm.

inoculation The act of injecting a vaccine or other substance for the purpose of inducing immunity to a disease.

inoperable A term referring to a condition so far advanced that it cannot be helped by surgery.

inorganic Not organic; not containing matter originating from plant or animal life.

inositol Part of the vitamin B complex.

inquest A legal inquiry in the presence of a coroner into the cause of a death.

insanity 1. A legal term referring to an individual who is unable to control his life, unable to practice socially acceptable conduct and unable to distinguish right from wrong. 2. Any mental illness in which there is loss of insight. 3. A psychosis.

inseminate To ejaculate sperm into the vagina.

insensible Lacking in sensation; incapable of feeling.

insidious disease One that starts gradually, often without early symptoms or signs.

insight The ability to comprehend.

in situ In place; in its natural position.

insoluble Not capable of being put into solution; incapable of being dissolved.

insomnia Sleeplessness; usually referring to sleeplessness of unknown origin, not that due to illness or disease.

inspection Examination with the eyes, such as the visual *inspection* of a rash.

inspiration The breathing in of air into the lungs; inhalation.

inspiratory capacity The amount of air that can be breathed in after completely breathing out; a guide to lung efficiency.

inspissated Thickened; hardened as a result of being dried out, as wax in the ears.

instability Emotional unbalance; lack of stability.

instep The arch of the foot.

instill To introduce a liquid, such as the *instillation* of drops into an eye.

instinct The primitive, unconscious driving forces, such as the instinct to live, the instinct to reproduce, etc.

instrumentation Treatment by use of instruments.

insufficiency The condition of being inadequate for a given function, e.g., cardiac *insufficiency*.

insufflate To blow a vapor or powder into a part of the body, such as the *insufflation* of powder into the vagina in the treatment of certain vaginal inflammations.

insulate To protect against.

insulin A hormone produced in the cells of the pancreas. When secreted into the bloodstream, it permits the metabolism and utilization of sugar. An insufficient secretion of insulin causes diabetes mellitus. Too much insulin secretion or intake causes hypoglycemia (too little sugar in the blood).

insulinoma A tumor of the insulin producing cells of the pancreas. This leads to too much insulin secretion.

insulin shock A state of shock, often with a convulsion and unconsciousness, brought about by too much insulin; also known as *hypoglycemic shock*.

insult Damage to an organ or part. Trauma.

insusceptibility Immunity.

integration The process by which various functions are coordinated so as to result in a well-organized whole.

integument Skin; the covering of an organ.

intellect The reasoning faculty; the mind.

intelligence quotient (I.Q.) The ratio of a person's mental age to his chronological age, determined by giving psychological tests. I.Q. levels include the genius, the highly intelligent, the normally intelligent, the below average intellect, the moron, the imbecile, the idiot, etc.

intemperance Excessive drinking; overindulgence in food or alcohol.

intensity 1. The degree of power or strength of a process, such as the *intensity* of a light ray. 2. Feeling something or somebody very strongly. 3. Degree of reaction.

Intensive Care Unit (ICU) A separate area in the hospital where extremely sick patients are cared for. The ICUs are manned 24 hours a day by physicians and specially trained nurses. They also are equipped with life-support apparatus.

intensivist A physician who specializes in caring for the critically ill, such as patients who are in Intensive Care Units.

intention tremor A palsy or shaking of the hands on attempting to perform some purposeful movement, such as writing.

inter- A prefix signifying between.

interaction The result when two or more ingredients combine to cause one action.

interarticular Between two joints.

interatrial Between the two atria (auricles) of the heart.

intercellular tissue The area between the cells.

intercondylar Between the condyles, the notched space at the end of bones such as the thighbone (femur).

intercostal Between the ribs, such as *intercostal* spaces.

intercourse Communication between people, as in *social intercourse, sexual intercourse,* etc.

intercurrent cholecystitis An inflammation of the gall bladder occurring during the course of an unrelated condition.

intercurrent disease A disease occurring during the existence of another disease.

interdiction 1. To prohibit a patient from doing something. 2. In legal medicine to prohibit someone, because of mental incapacity, from managing his own affairs.

interdigitate To dovetail; to lock one's fingers.

interdiscipline The overlapping of various branches of medicine.

interferon A substance released by cells that may have an inhibitory effect upon the growth and spread of malignancy.

inteferon-A A substance in white blood cells that exerts antiviral activity.

interferon therapy Treatment of malignancy by cells (lymphocytes) that have already been invaded by a virus. This type of therapy is presently in an experimental stage.

interlabial Between the lips.

interleukin-2 (IL-2) A protein that acts as a natural immune system booster, now being used experimentally in the treatment of certain advanced cancers. Its action tends to increase the number of T-cell lymphocytes circulating throughout the bloodstream.

interlobar Between the lobes of the lungs.

intermarriage 1. Marriage between people of different races. 2. Marriage to a close relative.

intermenstrual pain That which takes place in between periods.

interment Burial.

intermittent Starting and stopping; alternation of activity and nonactivity.

intermittent positive pressure breathing (IPPB) Breathing conducted mechanically, in which there is alternating positive and negative pressure.

intermural Between the walls of a structure.

intermuscular Located between muscles.

intern(e) A medical graduate serving in a hospital in order to receive training by treating patients under the supervision of the medical staff.

internal Within the deep structures of the body, as *internal* organs (lungs, heart, liver, pancreas, etc.).

internal fixation An operation to stabilize a compound fracture of a bone or bones by binding the broken part together with wire or screws or plates, etc.

Internist A physician who specializes in internal medicine and in the diagnosis of medical diseases.

interosseous muscles Small muscles located between the bones of the hand.

interpersonal relations Those existing between individuals.

interphalangeal Between two joints of the fingers or toes.

interposition operation A surgical procedure such as the utilization of the vaginal tract in an attempt to correct a rectocele (a hernia of the rectum).

intersex Someone with a developmental defect of sex differentiation; hermaphrodite.

intersexuality A state in which a person's genitals do not conform clearly to either the male or female sex, such as in hermaphrodites or pseudohermaphrodites.

interspace A space between two similar organs or structures, as that between the ribs.

interestitial Relating to small gaps or intervals in the interspace of tissues or structures.

intertrigo A skin inflammation which takes place in the folds of the skin, as in the crook of the elbow or where the breast contacts the skin below it.

intervention The act of changing the course of a disease or disorder.

interventricular Between the two ventricles of the heart, such as the *interventricular* membrane.

intervertebral Between the vertebrae such as the *intervertebral* discs.

intestinal bypass An operation for obesity in which the major portion of the small intestine is bypassed so that food does not pass through it. Thus, the patient loses great amounts of weight.

intestinal flora The bacteria within the intestinal tract. They are necessary for normal intestinal function, especially the bacteria within the large bowel.

intestinal flu *See* gastroenteritis. (The term *intestinal flu* is a popular, not a medical, term.)

intestinal ischemia Impaired blood supply to the intestines due to arteriosclerosis of vessels supplying the intestines.

intestinal obstruction Blockage of the intestines. It may be located in the small or in the large bowel. (If complete, intestinal obstruction must be relieved surgically.)

intestine That part of the digestive system which extends from the exit of the stomach to the termination of the rectum (anus).

intima The inner lining of a blood vessel.

Intocostrin A patented curarelike substance used to promote relaxation of muscles, particularly during anesthesia.

intoeing The condition of being pigeon-toed.

intolerance Inability to take a medicine because of sensitivity.

intoxication A poisoned state brought on by taking a drug, alcohol, etc.

intra- Prefix meaning inside; within.

intra-abdominal Within the abdominal (peritoneal) cavity.

intra-arterial Within the passageway of the artery. (Occasionally, an injection is given *intra-arterially*.)

intra-atrial Within an atrium (auricle) of the heart.

intracapsular Within the capsule of a joint.

intracardiac Within the heart.

intracardiac catheter One that is pushed forward from the vena cava and on into the heart itself. It can be used to measure venous pressure; to insert material that, on X ray, will show the inner workings of the heart; and to withdraw samples of blood from the heart.

intracath Same as intracatheter.

intracatheter A tube made of plastic, inserted into a vein for the purpose of supplying fluids or medications, or to monitor circulatory function. Also called *intracath*.

intracellular Located within the cells.

intracranial Within the skull.

intractable Incurable; impossible to control.

intracutaneous Within the skin, as an *intracutaneous* injection.

intradermal Within the dermal layer of the skin.

intraductal papilloma A benign growth within a milk duct of the breast, sometimes accompanied by a bloody or yellowish discharge from the nipple.

intrahepatic Within the liver.

intraluminary Within a hollow structure, as within the intestine or within a blood vessel.

intramedullary Within the bone marrow. (The site where blood cells are formed.)

intramural Within the wall of an organ.

intramuscular Within a muscle, as an *intramuscular* injection.

intranasal Within the nose.

intraocular implant A plastic lens inserted into the eye to replace the natural lens removed because of a cataract.

intraocular pressure The pressure within the eyeball. (It is increased in such conditions as glaucoma.)

intraoperative The period during an operative procedure.

intraoral Within the mouth.

intraorbital Within the eye.

intraperitoneal Within the abdominal cavity.

intrapleural Within the chest cavity.

intraspinal Within the spinal canal.

intrathecal injection One given into the spinal canal, as a spinal anesthesia.

intrauterine Within the cavity of the uterus.

intrauterine device See I.U.D.

intrauterine transfusion One in which the blood is injected directly into the fetus, through the mother's abdominal wall and uterus. It is used to combat Rh factor disease.

intravenous Within a vein. (An *intravenous* medication is one injected into a vein.)

intravenous cholangiography A technique for showing stones within the bile ducts. A dye is injected into a vein in the arm and X-ray films are taken immediately thereafter.

intravenous pyelography (IVP) The visualization (lighting up) of the kidneys and uterus, as seen on X rays after the injection of a dye into a vein in the arm.

intraventricular block A break in the normal progress of impulses within the ventricle of the heart, which may seriously impair heart action.

intrinsic Basic; inherent.

intrinsic factor A substance normally secreted by the stomach, essential for the absorption of vitamin B_{12}. Lack of the intrinsic factor may lead to the development of pernicious anemia.

introitus The entrance to the vagina.

introjection A psychological term,

referring to the assimilation into the mind of an external event.

intromission The act of inserting the penis into the vaginal canal.

introspection The examination of one's own thoughts and emotions.

introvert A person whose thoughts dwell upon himself and his problems. The opposite of extrovert.

intubation The passage of a tube, such as the introduction of a rubber tube into the larynx to keep the air passages open in various abnormal conditions.

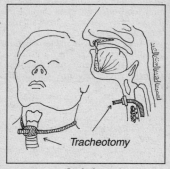

Tracheotomy

Intubation

intumescence An enlargement or swelling of an organ or part.

intussusception The telescoping of one loop of intestine into another. If the condition does not spontaneously correct itself, surgery must be performed.

inunction An ointment which is rubbed into the skin.

in utero Unborn; within the uterus.

invagination The process of folding in tissue so as to form a hollow space.

invalid One whose illness interferes with his ability to take care of himself.

invasive Referring to a localized infection or tumor which moves or grows and invades other parts of the body.

inversion 1. The state of being up-

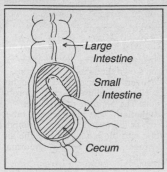

Large Intestine

Small Intestine

Cecum

Intussusception

side down or inside out, such as an *inverted* or tipped uterus. 2. Homosexuality.

invertebrate Animals not having vertebral columns, such as clams, oysters, lobsters, etc.

investment A covering of an organ or structure.

Invirase *See* protease inhibitor.

in vitro Within a test tube.

in-vitro fertilization A technique in which an egg is taken from a woman's ovary, is fertilized by a man's sperm in a laboratory, and then is transplanted into the mother's womb. Same as "laboratory fertilization."

in vivo Within a living organism. The opposite of *in vitro*.

involucrum New bone which forms around dead bone after a bone infection (osteomyelitis).

involuntary Not controlled by the conscious mind, as in an automatic muscle reflex.

involution The process of deterioration which takes place in an organ after it has fulfilled its usefulness or as one advances into old age; *involution* of the uterus occurs after childbirth and after change of life.

involutional psychosis Mental illness taking place at or beyond the menopause (change of life), or in men, after middle life. It is charac-

terized by depression and feelings of persecution, guilt, worry, etc.

iodides Medications composed of the negative ion of iodine.

iodine (I) An element found normally in small quantities in the blood. Its metabolism is intimately associated with thyroid function.

    radioactive Iodine which, having been exposed to radiation, emits beta and gamma rays. (Used in determining thyroid function and, in larger doses, as a method of treating overactivity of the thyroid and certain types of thyroid tumors)

iodoform gauze A surgical dressing impregnated with iodine.

iodotherapy Treatment with iodine, usually in cases of thyroid disease.

IOL An abbreviation for *intraocular lens*, inserted into the eye surgically to replace a lens removed because of a cataract.

ion An atom having a positive or negative electrical charge.

ionization A process in which electrically charged ions are produced.

iontophoresis A technique whereby electrically charged ions are passed into mucous membranes or skin in an attempt to treat certain local conditions.

Iopax A patented iodine-containing substance which is opaque to X rays and is thereby helpful in demonstrating the outlines of certain structures.

ipecac A widely used medication which increases secretions and thus promotes production of phlegm. It is also used to stimulate vomiting when such is desirable.

IPPB Abbreviation for *intermittent positive pressure breathing*. It is carried out by employing a specially designed respirator.

iproniazid An anti-tuberculosis drug.

ipsilateral On the same side of the body. (The opposite of contralateral.)

I.Q. Intelligence quotient.

iridectomy The surgical removal of part of the iris.

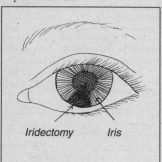

Iridectomy   Iris

Iridectomy

iridencleisis An operative procedure for glaucoma in which a portion of iris is placed in the incision in the cornea. This aids exit of fluids from the anterior chamber of the eye.

iridocapsulotomy A surgical incision into the iris (colored portion of the eye) in order to form a new pupil.

iridochoroiditis Inflammation of the iris (the colored portion) and choroid of the eyes.

iridocyclitis Inflammation of the iris and ciliary body of the eye.

iridocystectomy An operation to construct a new pupil, performed when the natural pupillary region is not normal or has been damaged.

iridokinesis The enlarging or contracting of the pupil by the iris.

iridotomy A surgical incision into the iris.

iris The colored portion of the eye.

iritis Inflammation of the iris.

iron (Fe) An element found normally in the blood in the oxygen-carrying hemoglobin of the red blood cells. Iron, in many forms, has been given as a medication to treat various types of anemia.

iron-deficiency anemia Lack of sufficient iron to produce adequate amounts of hemoglobin.

iron-55; iron-59 Radioactive irons used as tracers in the study of iron metabolism.

iron lung A respirator; used in patients who have paralysis of the muscles of breathing (polio).

iron storage diseases Conditions, such as hemosiderosis or hemachromatosis, caused by the storage of excessive iron in the body.

irradiation Treatment of a disease with radiation, or with radioactive substances, which emit radiation.

irrational Unreasonable.

irreducible hernia One in which the contents of the hernia sac cannot be replaced in their normal position.

irreversible A condition or state which cannot be remedied, such as *irreversible* shock.

irrigate To flush out, as in the case of an infected wound, or to wash out, as in *irrigation* of the bowels.

irritable bowel syndrome One in which there are intermittent periods of abdominal cramps and diarrhea, often associated with mucus in the stool. Also called *mucous colitis*. It occurs most often in young adults who handle stress poorly.

irritant A substance administered for the purpose of producing an irritation, such as a mustard plaster.

ischemia Lack of blood supply to an organ or part due to a spasm or shutting down of the artery which supplies it. Coronary artery spasm causes temporary *ischemia* of heart muscle.

ischialgia Sciatica. Inflammation or pain in the sciatic nerve which originates in the back part of the hip region and courses down the back of the thigh and leg.

ischiopubic bones The bones in which the ischial and pubic bones are joined. These are the bones upon which humans sit.

ischiorectal area The region between the rectum and the bones upon which one sits.

ischium The bone upon which one places his weight when sitting.

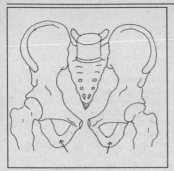

Ischial bones

island A group of cells which is isolated from other similar cells, as in certain glands in the body.

islet-cell tumor A tumor of those cells within the pancreas which secrete insulin. It leads to hyperinsulinism and hypoglycemia.

islets of Langerhans The cells in the pancreas which secrete insulin.

iso- A prefix indicating equal.

isoagglutinin An agglutinin acting upon cells of the same species.

isogenic Relating to those who are genetically similar.

isograft A graft from one identical twin to another. (These have a tendency to take much more often than most grafts from one individual to another.)

isoimmunization The process of immunizing a species with antigens derived from the same species.

isolation The confinement and separation of a patient from others, usually carried out in cases of contagious disease.

isomeric Referring to substances that have the same percentage composition but differ in physical properties.

isometric Of equal proportions.

isometropia Two eyes that are alike, as contrasted to eyes that have varying refraction errors.

isoniazid An antituberculosis drug which has proved effective, particularly in combination with streptomycin and paraaminosalicylic acid.

isopia Equal vision in both eyes.

isopropyl alcohol A type of alcohol used mainly for external application.

Isordil A patented medication to relax spasm of arteries, especially helpful for those who have angina pectoris.

isotonic solution A solution which is compatible with body tissues and one in which red blood cells can be placed without causing them to shrivel or burst.

isotope A substance having the same atomic number as another substance but a different atomic weight. Radioactive isotopes have the property of spontaneous decomposition, during which they give off rays.

isthmus A narrowed part of an organ or structure, such as the isthmus of the thyroid gland.

Isuprel An effective medication to relieve spasm in bronchial asthma.

-itis A suffix meaning "inflammation of."

ITP Abbreviation for idiopathic thrombocytopenic purpura.

I.U.D. Abbreviation for intrauterine device. (Plastic materials placed in the cavity of the uterus as a means of preventing conception)

I.V. Abbreviation for intravenous.

IVDA Abbreviation for intravenous drug abuse.

IVP Abbreviation for *intravenous pyelogram. See* pyelograms.

J

Jacksonian seizure A form of epilepsy which may be limited to one side of body, marked by periods of progressively more intense muscular spasm alternating with periods of relaxation. Consciousness, as a rule, is retained during an attack.

Jackson's membrane A thin sheet or film of tissue, occurring in some people, which binds the appendix and first portion of the large intestine to the posterior wall of the abdomen. Bowel obstruction or mild symptoms of appendicitis may occasionally be caused by the pressure of this membrane on a distended cecum.

jail fever A slang expression for *typhus fever*.

jargon Slang talk; babbling.

jaundice Yellow discoloration of the skin and eyes due to bile pigments in the blood. There are many causes of this condition but most fall into one of two categories, namely jaundice due to obstruction of the flow of bile from the liver to the intestines, and jaundice due to disease within the substance of the liver itself.

    catarrhal Infectious hepatitis, an inflammation of the liver, with jaundice, thought to be caused by a virus.

    congenital hemolytic Jaundice of inherited origin, associated with anemia, enlarged spleen, and extraordinarily fragile red blood cells.

    familial nonhemolytic A mild form of inherited jaundice due to a defect in the body's ability to rid itself of bilirubin (bile pigments resulting from the normal dying out of red blood cells and hemoglobin elements).

    hematogenous Jaundice brought on by an abnormal destruction of red blood cells by a poison or toxin.

    hemolytic Any jaundice caused by inordinate destruction of red blood cells with release of large amounts of hemoglobin.

    hepatocellular Jaundice due to injury, destruction, or lack of function of liver cells.

    infectious Jaundice caused by an infectious agent attacking the liver.

    obstructive That which is caused by blockage of the flow of bile into the intestines. (Stones in the bile ducts or a tumor of the bile passages or pancreas is the most frequent cause of *obstructive jaundice*.)

    painless Often caused by a cancer of the pancreas.

    regurgitation Jaundice due to obstruction of the flow of bile from the liver to the intestinal tract. (Stones in the bile ducts or a tumor obstructing the bile ducts will result in this type of jaundice.)

jaws The bones forming the mouth. The upper jaw is the maxilla; the lower jaw is the mandible.

Jeghers-Peutz disease An inherited condition associated with wartlike (polypoid) tumors of the intestines, brownish discoloration of the skin, bleeding from mucous membranes, and anemia.

jejunitis Inflammation of the jejunum (the portion of small intestine beyond the duodenum which extends for approximately seven to eight feet downward).

jejunoileal bypass An operation in

which the upper end of the small intestine is stitched to the lower end, thus diverting food from most of the small intestines. The operation is done to cause weight loss in pathological obesity.

jejunoileitis Inflammation of the jejunum and ileum, or all of the small intestine except the first 10 to 12 inches, which is called the duodenum.

jejunojejunostomy The surgical creation of a passage between two loops of jejunum, sometimes performed after removal of part of the stomach in order to relieve back pressures.

jejunostomy Surgical creation of an opening through the abdominal wall into the jejunum, sometimes performed to relieve intestinal obstruction or to institute temporary artificial feeding.

jejunum The upper portion of the small intestine, about 8 feet in length, extending from the duodenum to the ileum.

jerk A muscle reflex, such as a knee jerk or ankle jerk. Failure of this response to follow stimulation by the physician may indicate disease within the brain or spinal cord.

jet lag A feeling of lassitude and upset occurring among some people who take long air trips in an East-West or West-East direction.

jockstrap An elastic support for the male genitals; worn during participation in athletics or exercise.

joint The place in which two or more connecting bones are joined; joints such as the shoulder, elbow, and knee joints.

  Charcot's Arthritis of a joint, often the knee, with swelling and loss of pain sensation, secondary to syphilis of the spinal cord.

  flail One that has lost its function because of its inability to remain stable.

  fusion A surgical procedure performed for the purpose of joining (fusing) bones which make up a joint. This operation is sometimes

carried out to improve stability in an other wise poorly functioning joint, as in some cases of polio. Also called *arthrodesis*.

  mouse A loose, calcified, pea-sized body found floating in a joint. It usually arises from a chronically inflamed joint lining (synovitis) and often is seen in large numbers.

  replacement The insertion of a metal device to replace an irreparably damaged joint. Such procedures now involve the finger, elbow, shoulder, ankle, knee and hip joints.

  temporomandibular The joint connecting the lower jaw to the main portion of the skull.

jugular vein The large veins in the neck which drain the blood from the head down to the large veins emptying into the heart.

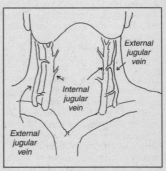

Jugular vein

juice The secretions of the stomach (gastric juice), intestines (intestinal juice), and pancreas (pancreatic juice). These juices contain enzymes which digest food.

junction The point where two or more structures come together.

junction nevus A mole located between the superficial and the deep layers of the skin.

jungle rot Any skin condition originating from a sojourn in a tropical land. Most often associated with a fungus infection.

jurisprudence, medical Legal medicine.

juvenile diabetes Diabetes that makes itself evident during childhood.

juxtaposition The condition in which two structures are situated next to each other; a close anatomical relationship.

K

K Chemical symbol for potassium.

Kahler's disease A widespread disease of the bone marrow in which there is an overgrowth of certain types of primitive white blood cells (plasma cells). This is a tumor condition, also called *multiple myeloma*.

Kahn test 1. A test for syphilis, performed upon blood removed from a vein. 2. A test for cancer based on measurement of the amount of a certain constituent of the blood.

kala-azar A parasitic disease found in China, India, Brazil and around the Mediterranean area. It is characterized by fever, enlargement of the liver and spleen, marked weight loss and anemia.

kalemia Presence of potassium in the blood.

Kanamycin A powerful antibiotic medication, effective against many different types of germs. (May be toxic to the kidneys and occasionally causes impaired hearing)

kangaroo tendon A suture material used occasionally in hernia repair, obtained from the tail of the kangaroo.

Kantrex An oral antibiotic (kanomycin) highly effective against bacteria in the intestinal tract.

kaolin A fine-particle dusting powder often applied to draining wounds and fistulas to absorb moisture from the secretions.

Kaomagma A patented medication given to stop diarrhea and to solidify the feces.

Kaopectate A patented medication given in certain cases of diarrhea to solidify the feces.

Kaposi's sarcoma A malignancy in the skin, often located on the legs, seen frequently in patients who have AIDS.

karyocyte An immature red blood cell; normoblast.

karyogamy A process in which the nuclei of two cells fuse, seen when a sperm fertilizes an egg.

karyokinesis A form of cell division. Mitosis.

karyotype The chromosomal characteristics of an individual. (Karyotype charts are arranged so that chromosomes are paired and are placed in order, from the largest to the smallest.) By studying karyotypes under a high power microscope, cytologists can spot chromosomal defects and can diagnose the presence of such diseases as Mongolism, Turner's syndrome, Klinefelter's syndrome, etc.

karyotyping Analysis of chromosomes.

Kawasaki disease A disease of unknown origin, occurring predominantly in children. It is characterized by fever, joint pain, inflammation of the mouth, and sometimes accompanied by pneumonia, meningitis, and heart involvement.

Keflex Same as Keflin.

Keflin A powerful antibiotic drug, valuable in treating most types of bacterial infection.

keloid An overgrowth of a scar; cause unknown. Surgical removal of keloids is not always successful and may be followed by recurrence.

keratectomy Surgical removal of the cornea of the eye, carried out in some cases of extensive scarring pre-

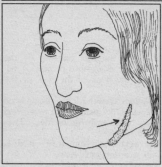

Keloid

paratory to the placement of a corneal graft.

keratin The main component of tissues such as hair, nails, horns, etc.

keratinization A process in which a portion of skin takes on a horny consistency, such as the formation of "corns" on the feet.

keratinocytes Cells of the epidermis of the skin. Recently, they have been grown in cultures and used successfully to help grow new skin over badly burned areas.

keratitis Inflammation of the cornea of the eye, the tissue covering the pupil and iris.

keratoacanthoma A skin tumor composed largely of hard keratin substance; occasionally becomes malignant but can be cured by surgical excision.

keratoconjunctivitis An inflammation of the membrane covering the eye located near the cornea (that portion containing the iris and pupil).

keratoconus A protrusion of the cornea of the eye, which may markedly distort vision.

keratodermatitis Skin inflammation accompanied by overgrowth of the outer, horny layers of cells.

keratoiritis Inflammation of the cornea and the iris.

keratoma A tumor of the outer horny layers of the skin; callus.

keratomileusis An operation involving a change in the curve of the cornea, devised to improve nearsightedness or farsightedness.

keratoplasty An operation for the transplantation of part of the cornea, performed in cases of blindness due to scarring of the cornea.

keratoscleritis Inflammation of the membranes of both the white (sclera) and colored (cornea and iris) portions of the eye.

keratosis A skin condition characterized by an overgrowth of the horny layers and by thickening of the skin.

keratotomy A surgical incision of the cornea.

kernicterus The discoloration and degeneration of the brain and other nerve structures seen in newborns suffering from a certain type of jaundice (erythroblastosis fetalis).

Ketochol A patented medicine composed of bile acids; given to people with gall bladder disease or sluggish liver function in order to stimulate the flow of bile.

ketogenesis The process of forming acetone (ketone) bodies. Excess acetone produces a toxic condition known as acidosis, which is seen in poorly controlled cases of diabetes.

ketolysis The destruction of ketone bodies.

ketone body An acetone body, occurring in body fluids and tissues involved in acidosis.

ketonuria The presence of ketone (acetone) bodies in the urine, which is evidence of acidosis.

ketosis Acidosis, seen sometimes in severe diabetes.

kidney The organ lying in the upper posterior portion of the abdomen which removes waste products and water from the blood stream and excretes them as urine. *See* calculus.

    arteriosclerotic One in which there is hardening of the blood vessels supplying kidney substance.

(Function of such a gland may be markedly impaired.)

artificial An apparatus specially designed to remove waste products. Blood is circulated outside the body through the apparatus and after the waste products are filtered out, the blood is returned to the patient's circulation. (Useful in cases of uremia and drug poisoning)

"floating" A kidney that has loose attachments to surrounding supportive tissues, thus permitting it to drop to a lower anatomical location; an exceptionally moveable kidney.

horseshoe Fusion of the right and left kidney so as to give the appearance of one large, horseshoe-shaped organ; a birth deformity.

pelvic (ectopic) A birth deformity in which a kidney is located low down in the pelvis rather than high up in the back.

polycystic A congenital malformation of a kidney with many cysts scattered throughout. (A kidney so involved has impaired function.)

kidney transplant A whole kidney transplanted from one individual to another, or from an animal to a human.

kilo A prefix meaning thousand.

kilogram One thousand grams; about 2.2 pounds.

kilowatt A unit of electricity equal to 1000 watts.

kineplasty A surgical procedure carried out in certain amputations in which the muscles and tendons in the amputated stump are fashioned in such a way that they can be connected to an artificial limb.

kinescope An apparatus for testing the image-forming capability of the eye.

kinesia Airsickness, seasickness.

kinesitherapy The treatment of conditions through exercise.

kinesthesia The sensation of muscle movements; the knowledge of the position of one's own limbs.

kinetics The science of motion.

kineto- Prefix indicating relationship to motion.

kinetography The recording of muscle or organ movements.

kiotomy Surgical removal of the uvula, the downward-projecting tissue in the back of the roof of the mouth.

Kirschner wires Metal wires placed through holes drilled in bones, used in traction to bring broken bones into alignment.

klebsiella A group of gram-negative, rod-shaped bacteria which frequently cause infections in the respiratory, intestinal and urinary tracts.

pneumoniae The so-called Friedlander's bacillus, the cause of a very serious type of pneumonia.

kleptomania An uncontrollable desire to steal, often directed toward objects which are not needed and have little value; usually a neurotic symptom.

kleptophobia A fear of becoming a thief or kleptomaniac or of being stolen from.

Klinefelter's syndrome *See* syndrome.

Kline test A valuable test for syphilis, performed upon blood withdrawn from a vein.

knee The joint between the thigh and the calf.

housemaid's "Water on the knee"; an inflammation of the bursa beneath the kneecap, often accompanied by a collection of fluid.

knock Bending inward of the bones of the legs so that the inner sides of the knees rub against one another when walking.

locked Inability to fully extend a knee joint because a torn cartilage (semilunar cartilage) protrudes into the joint; football knee.

kneecap The patella, the oval bone covering the knee joint.

knee-chest position One that permits excellent views of the anus, rectum, and large bowel, in addition to permitting examination of the prostate gland.

knee jerk The muscle movement normally found when the tendon below the knee is struck sharply.

knee replacement The operative insertion of a metal substitute for a knee joint that has been irreparably damaged.

knit To heal, as when a fractured bone heals.

knob A rounded protrusion of a structure.

"knockout" drops Chloral hydrate, a liquid sedative that may be given undetected in drinks.

knot The manner in which surgical suture material is secured. There are many different types of surgical knots.

knuckle The joints of the hand, particularly when a fist is formed.

Koch, Robert (1843–1910) A German bacteriologist. One of the pioneers in the formation of the germ theory of infections. In 1882, he discovered the germ which causes tuberculosis.

Kock's continent reservoir ileostomy A surgical procedure in which the ileum of the small bowel is brought out to the surface of the skin in such a manner that it empties only when a catheter (tube) is inserted into it.

Kondoleon operation A procedure in which strips of skin, subcutaneous tissue, and fibrous connective tissue are removed from the legs in the treatment of elephantiasis.

Koplick spots Spots in the mouth which herald the onset of measles.

Koromex foam A contraceptive medication inserted in the vagina prior to intercourse.

Korsakoff's psychosis A mental disease often caused by chronic alcoholism and characterized by loss of memory and development of elaborate systems for justifying untruths. It is usually accompanied by severe neuritis.

koumiss Fermented cow's or mare's milk.

Kraske's operation A surgical procedure for cancer of the rectum in which the rectum, part of the sacrum, and coccyx are removed.

kraurosis A loss of elastic tissue and shriveling of the skin, seen particularly in old people.

kraurosis vulvae Shrinkage of the lining of the vagina.

krebiozen A drug that is supposed to have anticancer properties, not accredited by the United States Food and Drug Administration.

Krukenberg tumor Cancer of the ovaries and pelvic organs as a result of a spread from the stomach or some other abdominal organ.

Kupfer cells Cells within the liver that help destroy worn-out blood cells, foreign particles, and bacteria.

kuru A fatal disease, seen almost exclusively in New Guinea, associated with nerve degeneration. Cause unknown.

Kussmaul breathing The exceptionally deep breathing one encounters in a patient with acidosis. *See* acidosis.

KV Kilovolt.

Kviem test A skin test for the presence of a disease known as *sarcoidosis*.

KW Kilowatt.

K-Y jelly A patented lubricating jelly used in performing examinations.

kyllosis Clubfoot, a birth deformity.

kymograph An apparatus which records physiological reactions on a revolving drum. It is used in many experiments.

kyphoscoliosis Curvature of the spine in two planes, that is, from side to side and from back to forward.

kyphosis Humpback; curvature of the spine in an anterior-posterior direction.

L

labia majora The major lips, or folds of skin, of the female external genitals. They are on either side of the entrance to the vagina.

labia minora The two smaller lips of the female genitals.

labile Referring to a substance or thing which is unstable or fluctuating. (A *labile blood pressure* is one that fluctuates markedly.)

labor Childbirth.

   false The onset of contractions of the uterus several days before real labor. Such labor pains are usually irregular and not severe.

   induced Labor brought on by the physician by the giving of medications or by instrumentation (breaking the bag of waters or dilating the cervix of the uterus).

   instrumental Delivery of the child with forceps. (The instruments are applied to either side of the child's head to help draw the child from the vagina.)

   missed A situation in which a dead embryo is retained within the uterus and labor does not come on at the normal time. In such cases, it is necessary to bring on labor artificially.

   pains The periodic abdominal pains caused by the powerful contractions of the uterus. The nearer delivery, the stronger the pains and the shorter the interval between them.

   precipitate Labor and childbirth that come on suddenly, usually before the mother can receive medical assistance.

   premature Childbirth taking place before the usual period of 9 months (280 days) has elapsed.

   spontaneous Normal childbirth without the use of instruments (forceps) or other medical procedures.

laboratory The place where clinical tests and experiments are performed. Blood, urine, stool, sputum and tissues are examined in the laboratory of a hospital or medical office.

laboratory fertilization The fertilization by sperm of an egg that has been removed from an ovary and placed in a special medium in a laboratory. Such fertilized egg is then inserted into the uterus in the hope that it will implant and grow.

labyrinth The communicating channels that compose the inner ear.

labyrinthitis Inflammation of the inner ear, otitis interna. Such conditions may be accompanied by dizziness and upset in the sense of balance.

lac Milk.

laceration A cut or wound.

lachrymal glands Tear sacs, located beneath the upper eyelids.

lacrimal punctum The opening in the inner corner of the lower eyelid for the exit of tears into the duct leading to the nose (nasolacrimal duct).

lacrimation Crying; weeping.

lactalbumin Protein contained in milk.

lactase An enzyme (chemical) which digests the sugar found in milk.

lactation The secretion of milk from a mother's breast.

lacteals The lymph channels originating in the intestines which carry chyle (the fat which is absorbed from the partially digested food in the intestine).

lactic acid 1. A hydrogen-carbon-oxygen compound which helps in the digestion of milk and is therefore occasionally added to baby feeding formulas. 2. In the body, an acid formed as an end-product of sugar metabolism.

lactobaccillus A species of helpful bacteria, found in the intestinal tract, which produce lactic acid by their action upon carbohydrates in milk. Acidophilus milk contains large numbers of these bacteria.

lactogen A hormone, produced by the placenta, which stimulates milk production by the breast.

lactose Milk sugar.

lactosuria The presence of milk sugar in the urine.

lacuna An anatomical term referring to a small open space, such as the *lacunar* spaces in cartilage.

Laennec's cirrhosis Cirrhosis of the liver with replacement of liver cells by fibrous tissue. There is also obstruction of the flow of blood through the liver, resulting in the accumulation of fluid in the abdomen and the formation of large varicose veins in the region of the esophagus. Fatal hemorrhage is not uncommon. This type of cirrhosis is seen frequently among chronic alcoholics.

la grippe Influenza; an upper respiratory infection with fever, running nose, sore throat, cough, headache, and pains and aches in muscles throughout the body.

laity All people outside of a profession. In medicine, those who are not doctors, nurses, medical technicians, etc.

lallation The gibberish, or unintelligible sounds of infants.

lalorrhea Excessive talking.

Lamaze natural childbirth The method includes instructions to the pregnant woman on how to relax, concentrate, breathe, and use exercises to ease and control labor.

lambda The L-shaped area in the back of the skull where the bones come together.

lame Having a limping gait.

lamella A thin plate of bone.

lamina A layer or thin covering.

propria mucosae The connective-tissue portion of a mucous membrane lining. This layer of tissue gives strength to mucous membranes such as the lining of the intestines.

lamination Arrangement in layers; a layered structure.

laminectomy An operation for the removal of the vertebral arch. Usually done in order to approach the spinal cord for removal of a tumor.

lance To incise; to cut into, as to lance a boil.

lancet A knife used surgically to puncture. It has a sharp, pointed tip.

lancinating pain A shooting, knifelike, sudden, severe pain.

Landry's paralysis An acute infection of the spinal cord with paralysis starting in the legs and ascending to the trunk and upper extremities.

Landsteiner, Karl (1868–1943) An American pathologist, co-discoverer (with Alexander S. Wiener) of the Rh factor.

Langerhans, Paul (1847–1888) A German physician, discoverer of the cells in the pancreas (called the islets of Langerhans) which manufacture and secrete insulin.

Lanoxin A patented medicine containing digitalis.

lanugo The fine, downy hair found on newborns. This is replaced as the child grows older.

laparoscopic appendectomy Removal of the appendix through a laparoscope. *See* laparoscopy.

laparoscopic cholecystectomy Removal of the gall bladder through a laparoscope. *See* laparoscopy.

laparoscopic surgery Surgery performed through small incisions utilizing the insertion of a laparoscope.

laparoscopic vagotomy Cutting the vagus nerves through a laparoscope.

laparoscopy The examination of the abdominal cavity by insertion of a lighted, hollow metal instrument.

laparotomy Any operation in which the incision is made through the abdominal wall and into the abdominal cavity.

laparotomy pads Gauze pads placed in the abdominal cavity to better view the organs to be operated upon.

lapsus linguae A slip of the tongue.

memoriae A slip of the memory.

larkspur A medicine applied to various parts of the body to kill lice, used particularly against lice in the pubic hair.

larval 1. An immature stage of development of an insect or animal. 2. The stage of incomplete development of a disease.

larvicides Substances which destroy the larvae of insects.

laryngectomy Surgical removal of the larynx (voice box), performed for cancer of the larynx.

laryngismus Severe spasm of the larynx.

laryngitis Inflammation of the larynx (vocal cords and voice box). It is characterized by temporary loss of the ability to speak, and by pain in the throat.

laryngopharyngeal Referring to both the throat (pharynx) and the larynx.

laryngoscope An instrument for the examination of the larynx. It is a hollow metal tube which is lighted so as to afford direct vision.

laryngospasm Severe spasm and closure of the larynx. This occasionally occurs during anesthesia and requires immediate correction to prevent suffocation.

laryngotracheal Referring to both the larynx and the trachea (windpipe) lying immediately beyond the larynx.

larynx The voice box, situated between the base of the tongue and the windpipe.

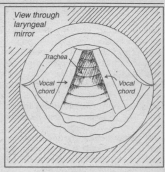

Laryngoscopy

laser An instrument, containing a synthetic ruby, in which atoms stimulated by focused light waves concentrate and amplify these waves and emit them in an intense, small beam. Heat emanating from the laser is the strongest known to man and can destroy all forms of matter. (The laser has been harnessed for surgical use and can be aimed at tumor masses, which it will destroy. It has also been found useful in the treatment of detachment of the retina.)

laser conization Removal of a portion of the cervix of the uterus, utilizing a laser knife. *See* conization.

laser iridectomy A removal of a

Larynx

portion of the iris using the laser. *See* laser.

laser therapy Treatment utilizing the laser beam.

laser vaporization The destruction of tissue utilizing the effects of the laser ray.

lasing The utilization of a laser to evaporate, cut, or excise tissues.

Lasix A powerful diuretic, causing rapid loss of large amounts of body fluid.

l. asparaginase A chemical used in the treatment of some malignant diseases, especially those involving blood cells and lymph glands.

Lassar's paste An ointment used in the treatment of certain skin diseases, particularly eczema. It contains zinc oxide, starch and petroleum jelly.

lassitude Weariness; tiredness; weakness.

latent Not obvious; present but not active. Often used in reference to a tendency, as in latent homosexuality.

latent period The time it takes for a reaction to take effect after a stimulus.

lateral Out to the side, rather than toward the midline.

　　sinus thrombosis Clot in the large vein of the lateral sinus on the inner side of the skull near the mastoid bone. It is sometimes seen secondary to the extension of a mastoid infection.

latex The juice from rubber trees; the basic substance from which rubber is made.

latissimus dorsi muscle A large flat muscle originating from the spine and attaching to the bone of the upper arm (humerus). It helps to raise the body in climbing.

laudable pus An old term referring to the discharge of large quantities of pus from an abscess. This was formerly thought to be a good sign.

laudanum A tincture of opium, sometimes given to relieve colic or diarrhea.

laughing gas Nitrous oxide, an anesthetic agent.

lavage Washing out of the stomach or other hollow organ.

law A dictum; a principle governing various phenomena.

　　all or nothing The principle that describes a type of response to a stimulus; muscles and nerves either respond completely or not at all when stimulated.

　　Courvoisier's In jaundice caused by a stone blocking the common bile duct, the gall bladder is usually not dilated and cannot be felt on examination. In jaundice caused by a tumor blocking the common bile duct, the gall bladder is usually dilated and can be felt.

　　Mendelian The law of heredity that certain characteristics are distributed in offspring on the basis of the dominance or recessiveness of the characteristics.

　　refraction A light ray entering a denser medium is turned *toward* a right angle to the surface and when it enters a rare medium it is turned *away* from that right angle (perpendicular).

　　Wolff's Change in the use of a bone will eventually lead to a change in its structure and appearance.

laxative A purge; a medication given to relieve constipation.

layman A nonmember of a profession or one of its allied fields. *See* laity.

"lazy eye" One that has lost its vision because of strabismus (crossed eyes).

LD Abbreviation for lethal dose.

L-dopa A medication used in the treatment of Parkinson's disease.

LE *See* lupus erythematosus.

lead poisoning A disease acquired by painters who, over long periods, have contact with paints containing lead. Formerly, it occurred in children who chewed on toys containing lead in their paint. It is characterized by severe abdominal cramps, weakness, anemia, black dots in the red blood cells and sometimes by paralysis and collapse. It is rare today.

learning disabilities Any of a number of learning difficulties experienced by children of average, or greater than average, intelligence. *See* dyslexia.

leather bottle stomach A thick-walled, leathery-appearing stomach in which there is an extensive cancer.

Leboyer method of childbirth A method of natural childbirth stressing the infant's welfare. Birth takes place in a quiet, dimly lit atmosphere, and the child is permitted to be born without pulling and shoving.

lecithin A group of compounds containing phosphorus and a fatlike substance, and found throughout the body. It is acted upon by various enzymes so that the fat can be utilized as a source of energy.

lectulum The nail bed, or tissue just beneath the nail.

leech A blood-sucking worm, formerly used to lower blood volume. Leeches used to be applied to the skin of the chest over the heart. The practice is no longer done.

Leeuwenhoek, Anton van (1632–1723) A Dutch scientist, one of the first people to use a microscope. He is credited with having discovered the existence of bacteria and one-celled organisms such as amebae and protozoa.

Lee-White test A test on the time it takes blood to coagulate (clot).

Le Fort's operation A surgical procedure for a "fallen womb" (prolapse of the uterus). The anterior and posterior walls of the vagina are stitched to one another, leaving just a small opening on either side.

left-handed Someone who naturally uses the left hand more than the right. This is an inherited characteristic following the Mendelian laws.

leg

    bandy Bowleg.

    bowleg Outward curvature of a leg.

    milk A swollen leg secondary to phlebitis (vein inflammation) occurring during or after pregnancy. Also called phlegmasia alba dolens.

legal blindness The condition of a person whose vision is less than 20/200 in both eyes.

Legionnaires' disease A serious form of pneumonia caused by a recently discovered bacteria. (The disease received its name because a local epidemic occurred among members of the American Legion who were attending a convention in Philadelphia.)

leiomyoma Fibroids of the uterus, a noncancerous condition.

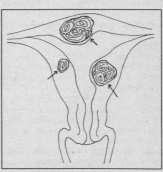

Leiomyoma of uterus

leiomyosarcoma A malignant tumor of the muscle of the uterus.

leishmaniasis A disease caused by a parasite and transmitted by the bites of certain flies. Seen in Oriental countries and in the Mediterranean area.

lens The portion of the eye lying behind the pupil. The lens bends the entering light rays so that they focus upon the retina in the back of the eyeball.

lens implant The insertion of a plastic lens to replace the natural lens that has developed a cataract and thus has lost its transparency.

lentigo A small, brownish pigmented area on the skin. Not a freckle.

leper One who is afflicted with leprosy.

lepothrix A skin condition caused by a fungus infection, which attacks those who perspire greatly. The most common sites are the armpit and the pubic region.

leprology The study of leprosy.

leprosy A chronic infection occurring in tropical countries. Symptoms include loss of sensation and subsequent loss of parts of the body. It is *not* very contagious.

lepto- Small; fine; thin.

leptocephalus One with an exceptionally small head.

leptomeninges The two main coverings of the brain and spinal cord.

leptomeningitis Inflammation of the two inner covering membranes of the brain.

Leptospira A species of spirochetes which cause such diseases as marsh fever, spirochetal jaundice, pretibial fever, etc.

lesbian A female homosexual.

lesion A change in tissue structure due to injury or disease. Ulcers, tumors, abscesses, etc., may all be referred to as lesions.

lesser circulation Pulmonary circulation; the blood flow from the heart to the lungs and from the lungs back to the heart, as opposed to the systemic circulation, which carries blood to all parts of the body.

lethal Deadly, as a *lethal* dose of a poison.

lethal gene One that prevents reproduction of a normal offspring.

lethargic encephalitis Sleeping sickness secondary to an infection of the brain; also called Economo's disease.

lethargy Inactivity; drowsiness; forgetfulness.

leucine A protein breakdown product (amino-acid) essential to human growth and development.

leukemia A group of malignant, fatally terminating diseases of the white blood cells and blood-forming organs. There are many forms of this disease, the specific type being diagnosed microscopically.

    acute A form lasting but a few weeks and terminating fatally. It is associated with rapid onset, marked anemia, hemorrhage and severe infections.

    aleukemic A form in which the white blood cells are not increased in number.

    chronic Leukemia which lasts for many years. People have been known to live for twenty or more years with chronic leukemia.

    granulocytic (myeloid, myelocytic, myelogenous) These include the most frequently encountered leukemias and are associated with increases in the number of white blood cells known as the leukocytes.

    lymphocytic A form of leukemia in which the increase in white blood cells occurs among the lymphocytes.

    monocytic A form of leukemia in which the predominating cell is the monocyte.

leukemoid A condition resembling leukemia.

leukemoid reaction The presence of blood cells usually seen in the blood in leukemia but, in actuality, due to other causes.

Leukeran (chlorambucil) An anticancer drug helpful in the treatment of certain cases of leukemia, Hodgkin's disease, and lymphosarcoma. It is not curative.

leukocidin A chemical capable of destroying white blood cells.

leukocytes White blood cells having characteristic cell nuclei. The varying appearance of the nucleus of the leukocyte, as seen under the microscope, determines whether it is a neutrophil, an eosinophil, a basophil, a monocyte, a lymphocyte, etc.

leukocytosis An increase in the number of white blood cells circulat-

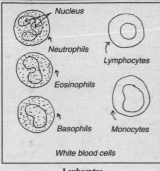

Leukocytes

ing in the blood. This occurs during most infections and toxic conditions.

leukoderma A birth deformity in which patches of the skin are devoid of pigment.

leukopenia A lower than normal number of white blood cells in the circulating blood.

leukoplakia A disease with thickening and overgrowth of mucous membrane, sometimes leading to cancer. Seen frequently in the mouth, tongue or vagina.

leukorrhea A whitish discharge from the vagina, often caused by a fungus infection (*Trichomonas vaginalis*).

levator ani muscle The muscle holding up the pelvic organs and particularly the lower end of the rectum and anus.

levitation The delusion that one is flying or floating in the air; a common hallucination occurring in dreams.

levodopa A medication helpful in the treatment of Parkinson's disease.

Levophed A patented medicine containing an adrenalinlike substance. Used to maintain blood pressure in people who are in a state of shock.

levorotatory Causing polarized light to turn toward the left, a fundamental characteristic of certain chemicals.

Levothroid The thyroid hormone,

frequently given when the gland is underactive.

levulose Fruit sugar.

lewisite A poisonous gas developed for use in chemical warfare. It causes irritation of the eyes and lungs.

libidinous Lustful; passionate.

libido Sexual desire and sex drive.

Librium A patented tranquilizing drug.

lichenification Leathery hardening of the skin due to chronic irritation.

lichen planus A common skin disease associated with reddish-purple spots on the skin, with moderate itching. It may last from a few days to several months before disappearing.

Lidocaine A useful local anesthetic agent.

lie detector A machine used to discover whether someone is telling the truth. It shows variations in pulse rate, breathing, blood pressure, etc., of a person subjected to a series of questions that may be of emotional significance.

lien The spleen.

lienitis Inflammation of the spleen.

lienorenal Referring to both the spleen and kidney.

life instinct The will to live, a much stronger instinct than the death wish in most people.

ligament of Treitz A fibrous band at the terminal point of the duodenum as it joins the jejunum, in the upper part of the abdominal cavity.

ligaments The tough connective tissue which holds bones together.

ligamentum A ligament.

    flavum The connective tissue between the vertebrae.

    pulmonis The connective tissue extending from the lungs to the covering of the heart (pericardium).

    tarsi The ligaments around the ankle joint.

    terres hepatis The connective tissue holding the liver in place.

ligation Tying off of blood vessels,

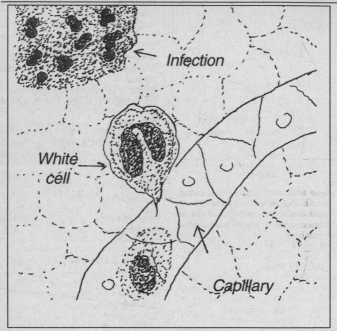

Migration of white blood cells

or other structures, during the performance of an operation.

ligature A thread for tying off a blood vessel or other structure. It may be composed of "catgut," silk, cotton, wire, Nylon, Dacron, Prolene, or other synthetic materials.

   absorbable Catgut and polyglycol ligatures that are absorbed by the body tissue.

   nonabsorbable Silk, cotton, wire, nylon, etc. Such material is surrounded by connective tissues of the body but is not absorbed.

lightening The change in sensation accompanying the descent of the unborn child into the lower part of the pelvis, which takes place during the last weeks of pregnancy and makes the abdomen look slightly smaller.

lightning pains Severe, sharp pains caused by nerve irritation. Seen in people with tabes. *See also* locomotor ataxia.

ligneous Hard or "woody" in feeling, as an organ or tumor.

limb An arm or leg.

limbus of the eye The circular area where the colored portion of the eye meets the white of the eye.

liminal Threshold; the lowest limit of perception or sensation.

Lincocin A powerful antibiotic drug.

lincomycin An antibacterial medication, effective against Grampositive bacteria. *See* Gram's stain.

linctus A syrup medicine used as a cough remedy.

linea alba The line running down the middle of the abdomen.

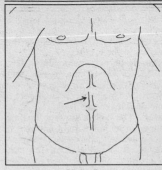

Linea alba

linae albicantes   Whitish streaks in the skin of people who have lost a great deal of weight and on the abdomen of women who have recently given birth.

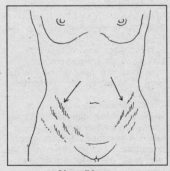

Linae albicantes

linear   In a straight line, as a linear incision.

linear accelerator   A high-powered machine for delivery of X-ray radiation, used in radiation therapy for treatment of malignancies and other conditions.

lingual   Referring to the tongue.

liniment   A liquid medicine to be rubbed into the skin for relief of underlying muscle strains; of doubtful medical benefit.

linitis plastica   A form of extensive cancer of the stomach.

linkage   The association of genes located in the same chromosome. (*See* gene and chromosome.)

linseed oil   A basic ingredient of liniments. Some laxatives contain linseed.

lipase   An enzyme manufactured in the pancreas, which aids in the digestion of fats.

lipectomy   The surgical removal of excess fat.

lipemia   An excessive amount of fat in the blood. Also called hyperlipemia.

lipid   Fats and fatlike substances normally present in the body.

lipiodol   An iodine-containing oily substance which is opaque to X rays. It is therefore used widely in X-ray examination to visualize the insides of various structures, such as the bronchial tubes.

lipodystrophy   A condition in which fat disappears from beneath the skin in patches. It is caused by a disturbance in fat metabolism.

lipoid diseases   A group of diseases in which fatlike deposits occur in the spleen, liver, etc. Gaucher's disease, Niemann-Pick disease, and others fall into this category.

lipoid pneumonia   A type of pneumonia caused by the repeated inhaling of fatty or oily substances.

lipoma   A nonmalignant fatty tumor, usually occurring beneath the skin. In all probability, the most common tumor encountered.

lipometabolism   The absorption and utilization of fat.

lipophilia   A liking and affinity for fats.

lipoprotein   Compound made up of both protein and fatlike substances.

liposarcoma   A malignant tumor originating from fat tissue.

liposuctioning   An operation in which excess fat beneath the skin is suctioned out; a cosmetic procedure.

lipping   Bony overgrowths near

joint margins, seen in older people as part of the bone-aging process.

lippitudo Inflammation of the eyelids.

lip reading Ability to understand the spoken word merely by looking at the movements of the lips. A technique developed by deaf people.

lipuria Fat in the urine.

liquefaction Degeneration of a solid structure into a fluid or semifluid mass, often as a result of infection or loss of blood supply.

liquor A liquid. A term often used in reference to certain fluid medicines.

Lister, Joseph (1827–1912) A Scottish surgeon, the founder of antiseptic surgery. He subscribed to the germ theory, and inaugurated scrubbing of the hands and cleanliness of the wound during surgery.

liter A liquid measure representing 1000 cubic centimeters or 1.056 quarts.

lithectasy Removal of a stone through the urethra. (*See* urethra.)

lithiasis The formation of stones within the body, as gallstones or kidney stones.

lithium A drug found helpful in the treatment of mental disorders, including manic-depressive states.

litholapaxy A procedure whereby a stone in the urinary bladder is crushed and washed out of the bladder. This is performed through a cystoscope.

lithotomy An operation for removal of a stone, such as one for removal of a gallstone or kidney stone.

lithotomy position On the back with the legs bent, as for a vaginal or rectal examination.

lithotripsy The breaking up or crushing of stones, especially those in the kidney, ureter, or bladder.

litmus paper 1. Blue litmus: a paper which turns red on contact with an acid solution. 2. Red litmus: a paper which turns blue on contact with an alkaline solution.

litter A stretcher.

Little's disease Cerebral palsy in infants.

Littré's glands Tiny mucus-secreting glands in the urethra.

"live-flesh" A nonmedical term often applied to muscle twitchings due to tiredness or excessive use. Such twitchings occur frequently in the muscles of the eyelids.

liver The body's largest gland, occupying the upper right and part of the upper left side of the abdominal cavity. It has dozens of functions concerned with the chemistry and metabolism of the body and is essential to life.

liver profile Chemical tests performed upon the blood in order to determine the state of liver function.

liver transplant Total removal of the entire liver with replacement of a healthy liver from a cadaver (one that has died within an hour or two of removal).

livid A grayish-blue hue to the skin.

L.M.P. Last menstrual period.

L.O.A. Left occiput anterior. The most common position of the unborn child within the uterus; head down.

lobar pneumonia One that involves an entire lobe, caused by the pneumococcus germ.

lobe A rounded segment or portion of an organ or tissue, as in the lobe of the ear; a lobe of a lung.

lobectomy An operation for the removal of a diseased lobe (one portion) of a lung.

lobotomy An operation performed upon the front portion of the brain in an attempt to relieve certain mental conditions.

lobular neoplasia A precancerous breast condition unassociated with the presence of an isolated lump; found usually on microscopic examination of biopsy material.

lobule A small portion or small lobe.

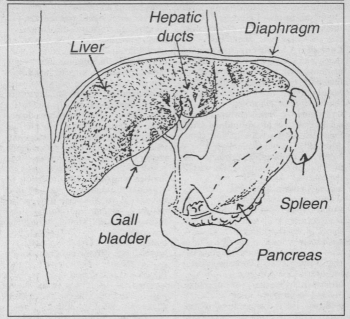

Liver and its attachments

local Not widespread; confined to one area, as a *local* infection.

localized Limited, not generalized; such as a *localized* abscess.

lochia The discharge from the vagina occurring after the birth of a child. It may last a few weeks.

lockjaw Tetanus. A severe infection due to the tetanus germ. It is associated with convulsions and severe muscle spasms preventing opening of the jaws. Untreated cases end fatally.

locomotion The ability to move from place to place.

locomotor ataxia Tabes dorsalis. Syphilis of the spinal cord resulting in loss of sense of position of the legs and a characteristic gait.

loculation The development of compartments in a structure, such as

loculation in an abscess cavity. A multiloculated abscess has many compartments, a unilocular abscess has but one cavity or compartment.

locum tenens A doctor who temporarily takes over the practice of another physician. (A British term)

locus A spot; an anatomical point or localized area.

Loestrin An oral contraceptive medication, administered for 21 days of each 28-day menstrual cycle.

logaphasia A brain disorder, often caused by a brain hemorrhage (stroke), and manifested by an inability to speak.

logasthenia Disturbance in the understanding of the spoken word.

logomania A mental illness characterized by incessant talking.

logorrhea Excessive talking, usually of an irrational kind.

loin The flank; the area just below the ribs in the back of the body.

Lomotil A highly effective drug to quiet overactive peristalsis of the intestines; used in diarrheal diseases.

longevity The length of life.

longitudinal Along the long axis of the body; lengthwise.

sinus A long vein and blood cavity traveling in the midline from the front to the back of the skull. Also called the *sagittal sinus.*

L.O.P. Left occiput posterior. A position of an unborn child within the uterus.

lop ears Ears bent over on themselves, correctable surgically.

Lopid A medication said to lower triglycerides and reduce the incidence of heart attacks.

Lopressor Trade name for a drug used in acute coronary thrombosis. It also is used as a hypotensive drug to lower blood pressure.

lorazepam A drug to reduce anxiety and to promote sleep.

lordosis Excessive arching of the back, resulting in an appearance in which the abdomen is particularly prominent.

lotion A medicated solution to be applied to the skin.

loupe A lens used to magnify or direct light upon an object.

Lovastatin An effective cholesterol-lowering drug.

LSD Abbreviation for *lysergic acid diethylamide,* a dangerous hallucinatory compound. (Used for the attainment of "thrills" and weird psychic experiences. Permanent brain damage can result from its uncontrolled use.)

L.S.P. Left sacro posterior. The breech position of an unborn child within the uterus.

lucidity Clearness of mind, as opposed to confusion or disorientation.

Ludwig's angina An infection of the floor of the mouth extending down along the neck to the region of the larynx and trachea. If unchecked it can cause suffocation.

lues Syphilis.

lumbago Lower back pain; a general term referring to almost any muscular condition causing backache.

lumbarization A birth deformity of the spinal column in which the first sacral vertebra in the lower back, instead of being fused to the other four sacral vertebrae, is unfused. (In some people, this is associated with chronic lower back pain.)

lumbar puncture The insertion of a needle through the back and into the spinal canal, permitting withdrawal of spinal fluid. Spinal anesthesia is given through a *lumbar puncture.*

lumbar region The lower back.

lumbodorsal Referring to the lower part of the back of the chest and to the lower back region.

lumbosacral Referring to the lower part of the back and the sacral area at the bottom of the spine.

fusion An operation in which the fifth lumbar vertebra is fused with the first sacral vertebra in order to remove excess motion in the joint and to obtain more stability of the spinal column.

lumbrical muscles Small muscles in the hands and feet which bend the proximal joints (those furthest from the finger or toe tips).

lumen The passageway inside a hollow organ or structure, such as the *lumen* of the bowel or the *lumen* of an artery.

Luminal A trademark for a widely used barbiturate, phenobarbital. It acts as a sedative, calming the nerves and inducing sleep.

luminous Emitting light.

lump Used to refer to a tumor or swelling.

lumpectomy The local removal of a tumor or mass, such as the excision of a lump in the breast.

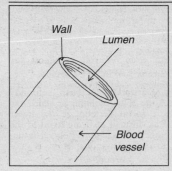

Wall

Lumen

Blood
vessel

Lumen

lumpy jaw　Actinomycosis.

lunacy　Insanity.

lunate　Crescent-shaped.

lunatic　An outmoded term for one who is mentally ill.

lungs　The organs of breathing.

lupinosis　Chickpea poisoning; an often serious disease.

Lupron　A drug used to treat cancer of the prostate that often delays the disease's progress for several years. Lupron may be given by injection every month or once every 3 months.

lupus erythematosus　An acute or chronic disease of the skin, evident mainly on the face and hands. The face rash is red, scaly, blotchy and often extends across the nose to the cheeks in a "butterfly" formation. Its cause is unknown. Certain cases are associated with disease of internal organs, and death can result.

　　vulgaris　Tuberculosis of the skin.

Luride　A lozenge containing fluorides, thought to be beneficial in preventing cavities in teeth.

Luride drops　Drops given to small children who live in an area where the drinking water contains insufficient fluoride.

luteal　Pertaining to the corpus luteum, the site within the ovary from which an egg was recently discharged.

luteinization　The changes that take place in that part of an ovary which has just discharged a mature egg. Ovarian cells in the area become enlarged and turn yellow in color.

luxation　Dislocation, as *luxation* of a vertebra.

lycine　An essential amino acid.

lycopodium　A fine powder used as an absorbent.

Lyme disease　A condition thought to be transmitted through the bite of a tick, characterized by a ring-shaped rash surrounding the bite area and attacks of recurring arthritis.

lymph　The fluid which is derived from connective tissue and tissue between organs. *Lymph* travels through lymph channels and lymph nodes (glands).

lymphadenectomy　Surgical removal of one or more lymph nodes (glands).

lymphadenitis　Inflammation of a lymph node (gland). It can be diagnosed by feeling the enlargement of the glands in the neck or groin.

lymphadenoma　Enlargement of a lymph node due either to benign or malignant tumor involvement.

lymphadenopathy　Any disease of lymph glands.

lymphangioendethelioma　A tumor originating from the tissues making up the lymph channels; a rare condition.

lymphangiogram　An X ray which shows the outlines of lymph channels, carried out by injecting an opaque dye into the lymph vessels.

lymphangioma　A benign tumor of the lymph tissue.

lymphangitis　Inflammation of a lymph vessel, a common mode of spread from a localized infection.

lymphatics　The vessels or channels which carry lymph.

lymphedema　Swelling, usually of the lower limbs, due to blockage of the lymph channels.

lymphoblastoma A malignant tumor of a lymph gland.

lymphocyte A type of white blood cell having a single, rounded nucleus (cell center).

lymphocytosis Increase in the number of lymphocytes in the circulating blood, seen in certain chronic infections; in infectious mononucleosis; in tuberculosis, etc.

lymphoepithelioma A malignant tumor often located in the back of the nose and in the throat.

lymphogenous Lymph producing.

lymphogranuloma inguinale A virus infection involving the anus and associated with enlarged lymph nodes in the groin. It tends to be subacute or chronic. A positive skin test known as the Frei test is used in making the diagnosis. It is thought by some to be venereal in origin.

lymphogranuloma venereum *See* lymphogranuloma inguinale.

lymphography X rays of lymph channels and lymph nodes following the injection of a radiopaque material.

lymphoid tissue That resembling lymphatic tissue.

lymphokine cells Powerful antitumor cells produced by incubating lymphocytes.

lymphoma A tumor composed of lymph node tissue.

lymphomatosis *See* Hodgkin's disease.

lymphopathia venereum Same as *lymphogranuloma inguinale* or *venereum*.

lymphosarcoma A malignant tumor of the lymph nodes or lymph tissue.

lyophilic A substance that goes into solution (dissolves) readily.

lyophilization The rapid-freeze and storing process used for serums, plasma, and other substances.

lysergic acid diethylamide *See* LSD.

lysin An antibody that has the ability to destroy living cells.

lysis 1. The receding of the symptoms of a disease. 2. Decline of a fever. 3. The cutting of adhesions during an operation. 4. Decomposition or dissolution.

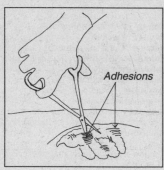

Lysis of adhesions

Lysol A patented disinfectant used principally in cleansing large areas.

lysolecithin A chemical compound with power to destroy red blood cells.

lyssa Hydrophobia; rabies.

M

McBurney's incision An oblique surgical incision in the right lower part of the abdomen, used in removing the appendix.

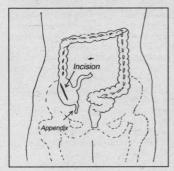

McBurney's incision

Maalox An excellent antacid medication, frequently prescribed for patients with peptic ulcer.

macerated Softened as a result of being soaked. When skin is soaked too long, the superficial layers may become macerated.

macro- Combining form meaning large; able to be seen with the naked eye.

macrobiotics The study of prolonging the life span.

macrochilia Excessively large lips.

macrocyte An exceptionally large red blood cell.

macrodactyly Marked enlargement of one or more fingers or toes; a birth deformity.

macrodontia Exceptional size of the teeth.

macroglossia Enlargement of the tongue.

macromastia Enlarged breasts.

macromolecule Exceptionally large molecules.

macrophage A large white blood cell, active in destroying and devouring bacteria or foreign matter that has entered the body.

macroscopic Of sufficient size to be seen by the naked eye.

macrostoma A birth deformity in which there is an abnormally large mouth.

macula retina The central area of the retina where the optic nerve supplies th entire retina.

macule A discolored spot on the skin, usually not raised.

Mad cow disease An infection seen in cattle and other animals such as deer, squirrels, rodents, etc. It is characterized by brain disorder and derangement. The disease can be transmitted by infected animals to humans.

Magace A medication composed of the hormone progestin. It is sometimes used in the management of patients with advanced cancer of the uterus. Its results are not curative.

magenstrasse The long channel on the inner aspect of the stomach leading from the entrance to the exit at the pylorus. Water and food travel along this groove.

maggot treatment The application of maggots (larvae of insects) to an infected wound (often a bone infection), so that dead tissue would be eaten away. This practice was more common before the days of antibiotics.

magnesium (Mg) In certain compounds this element acts as a mild laxative and as an antacid medication. (Milk of magnesia, magnesium oxide, etc.)

magnetic resonance imagining (MRI) A technique for viewing internal organs; an apparatus creating many of the images formerly revealed only by X rays. MRI uses no radioactive rays.

magnification Enlargement, as of something seen through a microscope.

maidenhead The covering tissue of the entrance to the vagina; the hymen.

maimed Crippled.

mainstreaming The taking of disabled people from institutions and attempting to place them within more normal environments.

maintenance drug therapy That which maintains a dosage sufficient to prevent recurrence of symptoms.

malabsorption syndrome Any condition characterized by inadequate, disordered absorption of nutrients from the gastrointestinal tract.

malacia Softening of an organ or part of an organ as a result of degeneration of its tissues, as softening of bone, osteo*malacia.*

maladjusted Unable to fit into the environment in which one lives.

malady An illness.

malaise A feeling of being ill or unwell.

malalignment Displacement of structures that should be lined up properly, such as teeth.

malar bone The cheekbone; the zygoma.

malaria A chronic parasitic disease transmitted by the bite of infected mosquitoes. The parasite lodges in the bloodstream, spleen, and other organs. It is accompanied by severe chills and fever at regular intervals.

mal de mer Seasickness.

male climacteric Change of life in the male. (There is considerable doubt among physicians as to the actual existence of a "male menopause.")

malemission Failure of ejaculation during intercourse.

malformation A deformity, usually present at birth.

malidone A drug used to prevent epileptic seizures.

malignancy Virulence; deadliness; a cancer.

malignant Dangerous to life; cancerous.

malignant hypertension A dangerous form of high blood pressure, often not controllable by use of the antihypertensive drugs.

malignant malaria A type associated with many fatalities. Cures have recently been obtained by giving antibiotics along with the antimalarial drugs.

malingerer One who makes believe he is sick.

malleable Soft; easily molded.

malleolus Rounded projections of the ankle.

    lateral The lower end of the fibula at the ankle; the bony point protruding on the outer side.

    medial The lower end of the tibia at the ankle; the bony point protruding on the inner side.

malleus One of the three small bones of the ear which transmit sound waves.

malnutrition State of being undernourished or poorly nourished.

malocclusion A state which exists when the upper and lower teeth do not meet properly.

malposition Abnormal position; a term applied when the embryo is lying in an abnormal position within the uterus.

malpractice Improper or negligent treatment.

malrotation A congenital deformity in which a segment of the intestinal tract fails to rotate, during embryonic development, into its normal position. (In some such

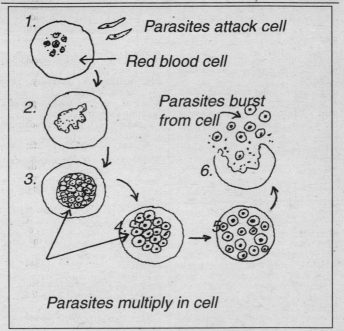

1. Parasites attack cell

Red blood cell

2. Parasites burst from cell

3.

6.

Parasites multiply in cell

Malaria; parasites in red blood cells

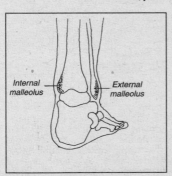

Internal malleolus   External malleolus

Malleolus

cases, the appendix and right side of the large bowel may be located on the left side of the abdomen.)

Malta fever A chronic infection caused by a germ often found in goat's milk. Seen often on the island of Malta, in the Mediterranean, where large quantities of goat's milk are drunk. (Brucellosis)

maltose An intermediate product in the breakdown of certain starches into simple sugar.

malunion Poor healing or uniting of the fragments of broken bones.

mammalgia Pain in a breast.

mammaplasty Plastic surgery upon a breast.

mammary duct curettage A procedure wherein a small curette is inserted through the duct of the nipple in order to scrape out cells from deep within the breast. The procedure is done in order to note the presence of any abnormal or pre-cancerous cells within the duct.

mammary duct fistula An abnormal duct (canal) leading from the mammary duct out onto the skin near the nipple. It is caused by an infection within the breast.

mammary glands The breasts.

mammilla Nipple of the breast.

mammography X rays of the breast, carried out by special techniques to note the presence or absence of a tumor.

mammoplasty Same as mammaplasty.

Managed Care A medical system whereby a third party, such as an insurance company, a governmental agency, a corporation, or a partnership, regulates the conditions under which doctors practice.

Mandelamine An antibacterial medication, especially effective in urinary tract infections.

mandelic acid A substance sometimes used as an antiseptic in infections of the kidney and bladder.

mandible The lower jawbone.

Mandol An antibiotic whose effectiveness, upon injection, includes destruction of many gram-positive and gram-negative bacteria.

maneuver A manual procedure or manipulation.

mange A skin condition in dogs or other animals caused by small parasites, *mange mites,* which burrow into the skin.

mania A form of insanity in which there is wild behavior; excessive desire for something; uncontrollable and violent passion.

manic-depressive A form of psychosis (insanity) associated with alternating periods of great elation and great depression.

manipulation Curing or improving a condition by use of one's hands, such as the bringing of fractured bones into line by manipulation of the fragments.

mannitol A chemical, derived from a form of alcohol, helpful in in-creasing the flow of urine. (Sometimes used after a particularly extensive and shocking surgical procedure)

manometer An apparatus used to measure the pressure of liquids, such as is used to measure the pressure of spinal fluid.

manometric block An obstruction in the flow of cerebrospinal fluid in the spinal canal, usually caused by a spinal cord tumor and determined by spinal puncture and the use of a manometer.

Mantoux test A skin test for sensitivity to tuberculosis.

manubrium The upper part of the breastbone located just below the neck.

manus The hand.

maple sugar urine disease *See* diseases. An inherited disease, often terminating fatally, in which the infant's urine has the aroma of maple sugar.

marasmus Extreme undernourishment with marked loss of weight.

marble bones A condition in which the bones become much harder than normal; osteopetrosis.

Marfan's disease *See* diseases.

Marfan's syndrome *See syndromes.*

margination The collecting of white blood cells at the edge of blood vessels, before emerging into the tissues to combat inflammation or infection.

Marie's disease An arthritis of the spine associated with curvature and deformity; also called Marie-Strümpell disease.

marijuana A plant, *Cannabis sativa* smoked like tobacco. It is habit-forming and has many effects similar to opium, causing hallucinations, loss of time sense, inhibitions, etc.

Marlex mesh A plastic material used surgically to cover over defects in large hernias that do not lend themselves to tissue-to-tissue repair.

Marplan In some patients it works as an antidepressant.

marrow The soft tissue inside long

bones. Blood cells are formed in the marrow.

marrow transplant The transplantation of bone marrow from a donor to a recipient suffering from a blood disease.

Marshall-Marchetti operation A procedure to relieve urinary stress which occurs in some women.

marsupialization An operation in which the walls of a hollow cyst are stitched to the skin. This procedure is carried out when complete removal of the cyst is not feasible.

masculinization The development of male characteristics such as hair on the face and a deep voice, occurring in females who have certain types of tumors in the ovary or adrenal gland.

masculinizing tumor of the ovary A tumor of the ovary which produces male characteristics in a female, such as hair on the face and a deepening of the voice and enlargement of the clitoris. (Such tumors are composed of cells which secrete male sex hormone.)

masking of symptoms Concealment of a condition, which may result when a narcotic or other medication is given to a patient.

masochism An abnormal mental state in which one derives pleasure from being treated cruelly.

mass A tumor; a lump.

massage Rubbing and kneading, usually carried out to relax muscles.

    cardiac An emergency measure carried out when the heart suddenly stops during anesthesia or surgery. The chest is compressed manually about 60 times per minute, thus causing the heart to pump blood and to restore the beat.

masseter muscle The main muscle of chewing, located at the sides of the face.

masseur One who gives massages (male).

masseuse One who gives massages (female).

mastalgia Pain in the breast.

mastectomy An operation for removal of a breast.

    simple The removal of only the breast, not including its underlying muscles.

    modified radical The removal of the breast and the glands in the armpit, but not including the underlying muscles.

masticate To chew.

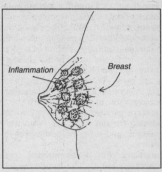

Mastitis

mastitis Inflammation of a breast.

mastodynia Pain in the breasts seen mostly before the onset of menstrual periods and associated with lumps in the breasts. It occurs mostly in young women.

mastoid bone The bone back of the ear. It is filled with air cells which can become infected following a severe ear infection.

mastoidectomy An operation for the removal of infected mastoid bone cells.

mastoiditis Inflammation of the mastoid bone cells.

mastopathy Any disease of the breast.

mastoplasty Plastic surgery of the breasts, usually carried out to reduce their size or to elevate hanging (pendulous) breasts.

masturbation Obtaining a sexual climax by self-stimulation and manipulation.

materia medica A branch of medicine concerned with the preparation and prescribing of medications and drugs.

maternal Referring to the mother.

maternity Motherhood.

matrexone An active antinarcotic agent.

matrix The basic tissue of an organ; the mold by which anything is formed.

maturate To ripen, as when bringing a boil to a head.

maturation 1. The process of developing fully. 2. The changes which take place in the maturing of a germ cell, with the cell body dividing twice but the chromosomes dividing only once. Thus, the mature germ cell has but half its original number of chromosomes.

mature cataract One that has become moderately or severely opaque, and is ready for surgical removal.

maturity Full development.

maxillary bone The upper jaw.

maxillary sinus The antrum. The sinus located in the cheekbone.

maxillofacial surgeons Surgeons who treat surgical conditions of the head and neck, exclusive of brain surgery. (Maxillofacial surgeons frequently perform plastic surgery.)

maximum The greatest possible quantity.

mayhem Committing physical, bodily harm.

Mayo, Charles Horace (1865–1939) Co-founder of the Mayo Clinic, and an outstanding American surgeon.

Mayo, William James (1861–1939) Co-founder of the Mayo Clinic, and an outstanding American surgeon.

mazopathy A diseased condition of the placenta.

Mazzini test A reliable test for syphilis.

McBurney's point The place on the abdomen where the greatest pain is usually felt in cases of acute appendicitis.

M.D. Doctor of medicine.

mean An average. An arithmetic mean is obtained by adding a set of numbers and then dividing their sum by the number of items added.

measles An effective vaccine is available. See Vaccination Tables.

measles, mumps, and German measles (rubella) A combination vaccine is effective and available.

meatitis Inflammation of the opening of the urethra, seen most often at the tip of the penis.

meatotomy Cutting and enlarging a meatus (opening), usually having reference to incising the opening in the tip of the penis.

meatus An opening.

Mebendazole A medication to rid the body of parasites such as hookworms, roundworms, and pinworms.

mechlorethamine hydrochloride (nitrogen mustard; mustargen) An anticancer drug, particularly effective in destroying malignant blood and lymph cells. (Used in the treatment of certain forms of leukemia and Hodgkin's disease)

mecism A deformity in which a part of the body is exceptionally long.

Meckel's diverticulum An outpouching of part of the wall of the small intestine (ileum), which occasionally becomes inflamed, requiring surgical removal.

mecometer An apparatus to measure the length of a newborn child.

meconium The contents of the intestinal tract of unborn and newborn infants.

meconium ileus A serious disease of the newborn infant in which there is paralysis of the small intestine associated with sticky, obstructing intestinal contents (meconium).

media The middle layer of the wall of an artery or vein.

medial Toward the midline of the body; the opposite of lateral.

median *See* mean.

median bar Enlargement of that part of the prostate gland adjacent to the outlet of the bladder. An enlarged median bar causes urinary obstruction and frequently requires surgical correction.

mediastinitis Inflammation of the tissues in the mediastinum.

mediastinotomy The creation of an opening into the mediastinum. This is usually performed by splitting the breastbone (sternum).

mediastinum The space beneath the breastbone containing the heart, aorta, vena cava, trachea, and other vessels and nerves.

medical Pertaining to medicine.

medical ethics The code and principles governing the conduct of physicians.

medical examiner A physician appointed by the local government to determine cause of death and to determine facts surrounding deaths of obscure cause.

medical group A number of physicians of various specialties who band together to treat patients. Most medical groups represent partnership practice and engage in the pooling of income.

medicament A medication or drug.

medicamentosus A rash caused by the giving of a medication or drug. Also called *dermatitis medicamentosa.*

Medicaid A federally and state financed medical insurance program for the indigent.

Medicare A popular term for national social security legislation governing hospital and health insurance for those over 65 years of age.

medicated Containing a medicine.

medication The giving of a drug or medicine in the treatment of a disease.

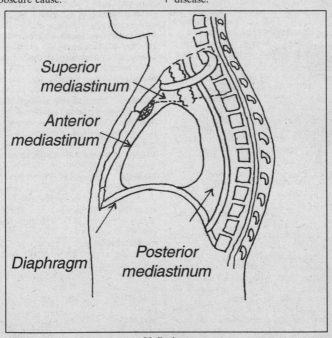

Superior mediastinum

Anterior mediastinum

Diaphragm

Posterior mediastinum

Mediastinum

medicinal Having curative or remedial properties; pertaining to a medicine.

medicine The art or science of healing.

    aviation That branch which deals with the special problems caused by traveling at great heights and at great speeds; aeromedicine.

    clinical Bedside medicine; the treatment of the sick patient.

    forensic Legal medicine.

    group The partnership practice of medicine carried out by several physicians.

    holistic A branch which emphasizes disorders that relate to the total being, both the physical, and the mental.

    internal That branch dealing with the nonsurgical treatment of diseases of the internal organs.

    legal That branch dealing with legal implications or complications.

    patent A drug or medication which is owned privately and patented so that it can be sold solely upon permission of the owner.

    physical The application of physical means to rehabilitate and restore sick or injured people. This large branch of medicine includes the use of heat, light, water, and electricity as aids to restore health. It also includes occupational therapy and the proper application of artificial limbs, etc.

    preventive That branch which concentrates upon preventing disease, preventing the spread of existing disease, and the prolongation of health and life.

    proprietary A trademarked medicine owned privately.

    psychosomatic That branch dealing with conditions whose origin is emotional, with special emphasis on the need to treat the mind in cases of physical illness.

    social That branch which concentrates upon the social implications of illness and attempts to render treatment with full consider-

ation given to environmental factors surrounding the illness.

    socialized Government-controlled medicine; medical practice in which the physician is paid by the government and the cost of medical care is assumed by the government.

    space That branch which deals with the medical aspects of travel in "outer space."

    state Another term for socialized medicine.

    tropical That branch dealing with diseases found in tropical countries.

medicolegal Referring to the legal aspects of medical problems or to the medical aspects of legal problems.

Medicone Rectal Suppositories Suppositories that help to relieve painful hemorrhoids. Relief is usually temporary.

Medihaler An aerosol device containing medications to overcome bronchial spasm, especially helpful in asthmatic attacks.

Mediterranean fever. *See* Malta fever; *also* brucellosis.

medium The substance in which bacteria are grown in a laboratory.

Medline A linkage, by computers, to rapid acquisition of medical bibliographies.

Medrol A steroid antiinflammatory medication.

medulla oblongata The lowermost portion of the brain just above the beginning of the spinal cord.

medullated Referring to nerves which are covered by a sheath (myelin sheath).

medulloblastoma A cancer of the brain, seen most often in the cerebellar region of children.

Mefoxin A trade name for cefoxitin. *See* cefoxitin sodium.

megacardia Enlargement of the heart.

megacolon Hirschsprung's disease. Huge dilatation of the large bowel, seen in infants and children, second-

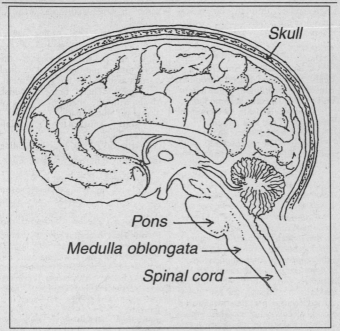

Medulla oblongata

ary to constriction at the junction of the sigmoid colon and rectum.

megakaryocyte A very large, primitive cell found in the bone marrow. It eventually forms blood platelets.

megalo- A form denoting excessive enlargement of a part or organ.

megaloblast A large primitive cell with a characteristic nuclear pattern found in certain types of anemia.

megalocyte A very large primitive red blood cell, derived from megaloblasts.

megalomania A mental illness in which the patient has delusions that he is someone of great importance.

megavolt One million volts.

Meibomian glands Small glands in the eyelids. The exit of these glands

sometimes becomes blocked off, causing a cyst to form. Such cysts are called chalazions.

meiosis A process of cell division in which each portion of the divided cell (gamete) contains only half the number of chromosomes contained in somatic (body) cells. (As an example, each male sperm and each female egg contain but 23 chromosomes, instead of the 46 present in other body cells.)

melalgia Pain in the arms or legs.

melancholia A mental depression.

melanin Dark brown pigment that occurs in the skin, in hair and in other organs such as the eye, etc.

melanoblastoma A malignant tumor of the skin originating from primitive pigment cells. Such tumors often spread through the blood-stream to other parts of the body.

melanocarcinoma Same as malignant melanoma. A highly dangerous growth usually first noted in the skin.

melanocyte A pigment cell containing melanin.

melanoma A cancer-derived from cells containing pigment. A mole which has become malignant is termed a *melanoma.*

melanosis The development of pigment in the skin, as following sunburn or the deposit of pigment in pregnant women about the nipples or on the abdomen.

melanuria A brackish, dark-colored urine caused by the presence of pigment (melanin).

melatonin The hormone secreted by the pineal gland in the brain. It inhibits function of the endocrine glands and may lead to underdevelopment of the sex glands or to diabetes.

melena 1. Black, tarry stools caused by the presence of altered blood, often occurring from bleeding from the stomach or small intestine. 2. Black vomit.

melitis Inflammation of the cheek.

Mellaril A tranquilizing drug, especially effective in treating mentally or emotionally disturbed patients.

mellitum A preparation containing honey.

melotia A birth deformity in which the ear is displaced onto the cheek.

membrana tympani The eardrum.

membrane A thin layer of tissue.

   elastic One that is capable of stretching or contracting.

   fetal Those surrounding the embryo within the uterus. They are called chorion, amnion and allantois.

   mucous Those which secrete mucus. They are the linings for the nose, throat, lungs, intestinal tract, urinary and genital tracts.

   permeable One which allows water or other substances to seep through it.

   placental That which separates the blood circulation of the mother and the child within the uterus.

   serous A thin layer of cells lining body cavities such as the abdominal and chest cavities.

   synovial The thin layers of tissue lining joints.

   tympanic The eardrum.

memory The ability to remember; also, something remembered.

menarche The beginning of menstruation; this varies anywhere from ten to sixteen years of age.

Mendel, Gregor J. (1822–1884) An Austrian botanist, the discoverer of the laws of heredity, the so-called *Mendelian Laws.*

Mendelian inheritance *See* law, Mendelian.

Menieàre's disease A disease caused by upset in sodium metabolism, characterized by intense dizziness and vertigo. Removal of salt from the diet sometimes relieves the symptoms.

meningeal Referring to the membranes covering the brain and spinal cord.

meninges The thin membranes covering the brain and spinal cord. (They are called the pia, arachnoid and dura mater.)

meningioma A tumor composed of the tissues which cover the brain or spinal cord. It is essentially nonmalignant and may be cured surgically.

meningismus Inflammation of the coverings of the brain and spinal cord, usually secondary to some disease such as measles, whooping cough, pneumonia, etc.

meningitis Inflammation of the membranes covering the brain and spinal cord. This serious disease may be caused by any of many germs, such as the meningococcus, pneumococcus, streptococcus, tuberculosis, etc.

meningocele A birth deformity in which there is a hernia of the coverings of the brain or spinal cord through a bony defect in the skull or vertebral column.

meningococcus A germ causing inflammation of the coverings of the brain or spinal cord; a cause of meningitis.

meningoencephalitis Inflammation or infection of the brain, the spinal cord and their covering membranes.

meniscectomy Surgical removal of a torn cartilage (the meniscus or semilunar cartilage) in the knee joint.

meniscus The crescent-shaped cartilage lying on the tibial bone within the knee joint, frequently torn in athletic injuries.

menopause Change of life. The climacteric. That time of life when a woman's menstrual periods cease.

menorrhagia Excessive bleeding during menstruation.

menorrhea Excessive menstruation.

menses Menstruation.

menstrual cycle The rhythmic preparation of the uterus to receive a fertilized egg and the discharge of the uterine lining (menstruation), usually at monthly intervals when no fertilized egg enters the uterus.

menstruation The discharge, at more or less regular intervals (once a lunar month), of a bloody fluid from the vagina. This continues, except for periods of pregnancy, from puberty to change of life.

    anovular Periodic vaginal bleeding without the passage of an egg from the ovary.

menstruum A solvent.

mensual Monthly.

mentality Intellect; mental ability.

mental retardation Arrested mental development. Feeblemindedness.

mentation Mental activity.

menthol An alcohol derived from the oil of peppermint, used externally as a counterirritant or as a local pain reliever.

meperidine (Demerol) A widely used narcotic medication, given to relieve severe pain.

mephitic Poisonous; foul.

Mephyton A vitamin K preparation; given by injection in cases where there is a bleeding tendency secondary to vitamin K deficiency.

meprobamate A tranquilizer, such as Miltown, Equanil, etc.

meralgia paresthetica Numbness and lack of sensation on the outer aspect of the thigh caused by failure of function of the nerve (lateral cutaneous) to that area.

meralluride (mercuhydrin) A mercury drug, highly effective in ridding the body of excess fluids. A diuretic agent, given by injection.

Mercelline mesh *See* Marlex mesh.

Mercuhydrin A medication, containing mercury, which causes an extraordinary output of urine. Used in heart cases to get rid of excess fluids in the tissues.

mercurials Preparations of mercury, formerly used in the treatment of syphilis. Now used to promote urinary output.

mercury (Hg) A chemical element useful as a medication when in combination with other substances.

    ammoniated An ointment used to treat various skin conditions, including impetigo.

    bichloride A solution used to kill germs. Formerly used to scrub operating rooms and as a dip for the surgeon's hands before operating.

meropia Partial blindness.

merosmia Partial loss of smell.

mescaline A hallucinogenic drug having similar action to LSD.

mesencephalon The middle portion of the brain.

mesenchyme The primitive tissue of the embryo which eventually forms all connective tissue, blood, blood vessels, the heart, etc.

mesenchymoma A tumor composed of cells which originated from mesenchyme. Some of these tumors are malignant; others are benign.

mesenteric arteries Two large blood vessels, the superior and inferior mesenteric arteries, which originate from the abdominal aorta and supply blood to the intestinal tract.

mesentery The tissue which connects the intestine with the posterior wall of the abdominal cavity. Through the mesentery run the blood and lymph vessels to the intestines.

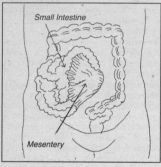

Small Intestine

Mesentery

Mesentery

mesial Toward the middle of the body; medial.

mesiodistal Referring to the inner aspect of a tooth.

Mesmer, Franz A. (1734–1815) An Austrian physician, the discoverer of hypnotism, sometimes called *mesmerism*.

mesoappendix The mesentery of the appendix, or the fatty tissue attached to the appendix through which the blood vessels travel.

mesocaval shunt An operation in which a graft (Dacron, Teflon or other substance) is inserted between the superior mesenteric vein and the vena cava. The procedure is done to relieve the portal obstruction encountered in cirrhosis of the liver.

mesocolon The mesentery of the large intestine, or the fatty tissue attached to the large intestine and the posterior abdominal wall through which the blood vessels travel.

mesoderm The primitive tissue of the embryo which goes to form the connective tissue, muscles, the kidneys, ureters, bladder, etc.

mesomorph A body type characterized by great strength and large muscles.

mesonephroma A tumor arising from the primitive embryonic tissue from which the kidneys are formed.

mesosalpinx The connective tissue which surrounds the fallopian tube.

mesosigmoid The mesentery of the sigmoid portion of the large intestine. It is a sheet of tissue through which the blood vessels of the sigmoid travel.

mesothelioma A tumor, often cancerous, derived from the cells which line the abdominal cavity, the chest cavity and the heart cavity (pericardium).

mesothelium A component of the thin tissue lining the sac around the heart, the chest, abdominal and scrotal cavities.

metabiosis A condition in which one form of life is dependent upon another for its existence.

metabolism The process by which foods are transformed into basic elements which can be utilized by the body for energy or growth.

    basal The lowest level of metabolism.

    electrolyte The changes affecting various essential minerals, such as chloride, sodium, potassium, calcium, etc.

    respiratory The exchange of gases within the lungs, specifically, the intake of oxygen and the exhalation of carbon dioxide and water.

metacarpal bones The bones of the hand to which the bones of the fingers are attached.

metachronous Occurring at a different time from something else; the opposite of synchronous.

metamorphosis A transformation; a change in appearance or structure of a part, an organ or an entire person.

Metamucil A patented preparation used as a bulk former for stool. Made from psyllium seed, it acts as a laxative in cases of constipation.

Metandren A patented preparation containing the male sex hormone, testosterone.

metaplasia A change in the structure of a tissue into that of another tissue. As one ages, cartilage sometimes changes into bone.

metaraminol bitartrate (aramine) A drug used in shock to elevate and maintain blood pressure at a satisfactory level.

metastasis The traveling of a disease process from one part of the body to another. (The spread of cancer from its original site is called a *metastasis*.)

metatarsal bones The long bones of the foot to which the bones of the toes are attached.

metatarsalgia Pain in the sole of the foot in the region of the metatarsal arch. Also called *Morton's syndrome*.

metatarsophalangeal joints The joints where the toes join the foot.

meteorism Distention of the abdomen with gas.

meter A unit of measure in the metric system, equivalent to 39.37 inches.

meth An abbreviation for methamphetamine.

methadone A drug used as a substitute for morphine, heroin, or other types of addiction. (Experiences prove this drug to be effective in overcoming narcotic addiction.)

methamphetamine An extremely dangerous hallucinatory drug, which can often lead to addiction or may cause death.

methaqualone *See* Quaalude.

methemoglobin A form of hemoglobin which is incapable of combining with oxygen and therefore is useless. It is found after poisoning with certain chemicals such as cyanide.

methemoglobinemia The presence of this form of hemoglobin in the blood, marked by shortness of breath, bluish color to the lips, dizziness, anemia, etc. If present in very large quantities, death may ensue.

methemoglobinuria The presence of methemoglobin in the urine as the result of poisoning with cyanide or other chemicals.

methenamine Also called *urotropin*. A urinary disinfectant of moderate value.

Methicillin An antibiotic particularly effective in combating staphylococcal infections.

methionine An amino acid (a break-down product of protein metabolism) essential for normal growth.

Methocarbamol A muscle relaxant. *See* Robaxisal.

Methotrexate A highly active anti-cancer drug. It acts by interfering with the multiplication and growth of cancer cells. (Has been helpful in certain types of uterine cancer, some leukemias, and some tumors of the head and neck.)

Methyldopa An effective drug against high blood pressure.

metroplasty Plastic surgery performed upon the uterus, sometimes done to correct a congenital deformity of the organ.

methyl alcohol CH_3OH. Wood alcohol. It is poisonous to drink and may cause blindness or death.

methylcellulose 1. A cellulose product used to make the stool bulky. 2. Because it swells in the stomach, it is thought to fill this organ, thus cutting down on the desire to eat.

methylene blue An aniline dye injected intravenously to counteract the effects of carbon monoxide or cyanide poisoning.

methylglucamine diatrizoate (cardiografin; gastrografin) A radiopaque iodine compound; used in outlining the blood vessels, heart, or intestinal tract.

methylsalicylate Oil of wintergreen; rubbed into the skin, it acts as a counterirritant so as to relieve muscle strain.

methyltestosterone An oral medication containing male sex hormone.

methyltheobromine Caffeine, a stimulant.

methylthiouracil An antithyroid drug, effective in treating patients with overactive thyroids (hyperthyroidism).

Meticorten A cortisone product; the same as *prednisone.*

metoclopromide A new drug, not yet·in general use, said to be effective in combating the nausea caused by chemotherapy medications.

metopic Relating to the forehead.

metrapectic disease One transmitted by a mother to a child but one which the mother herself does not have, as in *hemophilia.*

Metrazol A patented drug which, when injected intravenously, causes a convulsion; used in the same manner as electric shock in the treatment of mental depression.

metria Any infection of the uterus or inflammatory condition occurring during the period of confinement following childbirth.

metric system The French system of weights and measures; now used throughout the world. The standard unit of weight is the gram and the standard unit of measure is the meter.

metritis Inflammation of the lining and wall of the uterus.

metro- A combining form relating to the uterus.

Metrodin A fertility drug which, when taken under the guidance of expert medical specialists, may lead to multiple pregnancies or births.

metrodynia Pain in the uterus.

metronidazole A drug effective in the treatment of parasitic infestations, including amebic dysentery and whipworm.

metropathia hemorrhagica Also called *essential uterine bleeding.* It is associated with bleeding from the uterus, thickening of the lining

membrane of the uterus and cysts within the ovaries.

metroptosis A fallen womb. A "dropped" position or prolapse of the uterus.

metrorrhagia Bleeding between periods.

Meulengracht diet A diet sometimes prescribed for people suffering from a bleeding ulcer.

mev Abbreviation for 1 million electron volts.

Mg Chemical symbol for magnesium.

mgh An abbreviation for milligram-hour, or the application of one milligram of radium for one hour.

MI Abbreviation for *myocardial infarction,* a condition usually following coronary artery thrombosis.

micrencephalon An abnormally small brain.

micro- 1. Combining form indicating smallness. 2. Prefix indicating one-millionth.

micro-aerophilic A term applying to germs which thrive on but small amounts of oxygen.

microanalysis Chemical analysis performed upon extremely small samples.

microanastomosis The stitching together of very small structures, performed under magnification; a procedure often carried out in microsurgery.

microbes Bacteria; germs.

microbiology The study of bacteria, viruses, germs, etc. The science dealing with microorganisms.

microbiotic 1. Microbic. 2. Referring to an organism having a very short life span.

microcalcifations Tiny specks of white seen on a mammogram; when seen, they often denote a cancer of the breast.

microcephaly An abnormally small head resulting from premature hardening of the skull and closure of the openings (fontanels).

microchemistry That branch dealing with minute particles and the chemistry of cells rather than of a whole organ or body.

microcinematography Motion picture taken with magnifying lenses so as to visualize microscopic objects.

microcirculation The circulation in the capillaries and smallest blood vessels.

micrococcus A type of bacteria. The germs causing gonorrhea, pneumonia and meningitis fall into this category.

microcyte An exceptionally small red blood cell.

microdactylia A birth deformity in which the fingers or toes are abnormally small.

microdissection The dissection of tissues that are placed under a microscope; carried out with sharp, thin needles.

micrograph An apparatus enabling the recording and drawing of tissue seen under the microscope.

micrographia Exceptionally small writing.

micromania A form of mental illness in which a patient judges himself to be an inferior individual or to be reduced in size.

micromastia Abnormally small breasts.

micromelia *See* achondroplasia.

micrometastases Minute spreading of cells from a malignancy of such small size that they cannot be detected.

micrometer 1. One-millionth of a meter. 2. A device used in measuring the size of objects seen through the microscope.

micromethods Laboratory procedures carried out upon minute quantities of a substance.

micron (μ) One-millionth of a meter.

microorganisms Bacteria and viruses.

microphage A small cell (phagocyte), active in combating and digesting germs which may be in the tissues.

microphotograph A photograph of

cells or tissues seen through a microscope.

microscope An instrument which uses lenses to allow one to visualize objects that are so small they cannot be seen by the naked eye.

microscopic So small that it can only be seen under the magnification of a microscope.

microsurgery Operations carried out under the magnification afforded by a surgical microscope.

microtome A cutting apparatus which slices extremely thin pieces of tissue which are to be prepared for microscopic examination.

micturition Urination.

mid In the middle (an anatomical term).

midget A dwarf whose bodily parts are in normal proportion to each other.

midlife crisis A reevaluation of one's life, its goals, its accomplishments, and its satisfactions and dissatisfactions, often associated with dissatisfaction with one's sexual and social life.

midriff The upper abdomen; the waistline.

midwife A woman trained to deliver babies.

migraine Severe headache often associated with spots before the eyes, nausea and vomiting. The attacks tend to come on suddenly and are recurrent. Cause unknown.

migration A term usually referring to the traveling of an egg which has burst forth from an ovary. It migrates to the fallopian tube and down through the tube to the uterus.

Mikulicz's disease Overgrowth of a salivary gland in the neck.

Mikulicz's operation A three-staged operation for cancer of the large bowel. First, the segment of bowel containing the cancer is exteriorized on the abdominal wall. A few days later the tumor-bearing section is removed. Third, several weeks later the bowel segments above and below the tumor are

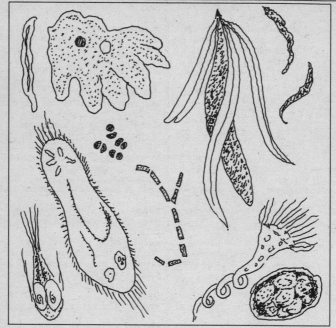

Microorganisms (many different types)

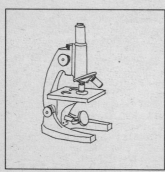

Microscope

stitched together and the bowel is replaced in the abdominal cavity.
milaria Prickly heat; heat rash. It oc-

curs mainly in hot, wet climates and is characterized by tiny blisters and itching. Occurs most often in skin folds.

Miles' operation Removal of a portion of the large intestine and all of the rectum; a surgical procedure done for cancer of the rectum.

miliaria An eruption in the sweat glands.

miliary The size of a millet seed; less than a millimeter in size.

tuberculosis Tuberculosis which has spread throughout the lungs and is characterized by thousands of small, *miliary* (millet-seed-sized) tubercles (tuberculous lesions).

milium A rounded, pearl-colored elevation on the face or genitals.

milk, acidophilus Milk containing

special cultures of a beneficial bacteria, the *Lactobacillus acidophilus*. It is helpful in certain intestinal disorders.

albumin Milk containing large amounts of protein and fat but small quantities of sugar and salt. Helpful in certain children's disorders.

butter Milk with large quantities of fat removed; the milk which remains after churning butter.

casein Same as *albumin milk.*

certified Extra pure, rich milk, certified by authorities as meeting certain standards.

condensed Milk from which a certain proportion of water has been evaporated and sugar has been added. (It is often canned and will last for long periods of time.)

crusts Scabs on the scalps of babies with eczema. So named because the eczema may be due to allergy to milk.

dialyzed Milk with the sugar removed.

evaporated Canned milk with approximately half its water removed.

fever An old term for fever occurring following childbirth. It used to be thought to be caused by excessive milk in the breasts. It is now known to be caused by infection in the uterus following childbirth.

fortified Milk to which vitamins, cream, albumin, etc., have been added.

homogenized Milk treated so that the cream (fat) is broken down into tiny particles and therefore does not separate.

leg A swollen leg secondary to phlebitis (inflammation of the veins), seen in women who have recently been pregnant. (Also called *phlegmasia alba dolens.*)

modified Milk altered so that its ingredients are in similar proportion to that of mother's milk.

mother's Breast milk.

pasteurized Milk which has

gone through the process of pasteurization, that is, heating for 40 minutes at 60 to 70° C.

protein Milk high in protein content and low in sugar and fat.

skimmed Milk from which the cream has been skimmed off.

sour Milk which has been acted upon by the bacteria (lactic acid bacteria) normally present within the milk.

treatment The treatment of an ulcer of the stomach or duodenum by the giving of milk as the sole diet.

"witch's" Milk from the breast of a newborn child.

millet seed Grass seed. Each seed is about one millimeter in size.

milli- Combining form meaning either one thousand or one thousandth.

millicurie (mc.) A measure of a radioactive substance undergoing disintegration.

milliequivalent (mEq.) The weight of a substance contained in 1 cc. (fifteen drops) of a normal solution.

milligram One one-thousandth of a gram.

milliliter One one-thousandth of a liter; 1 cc.; 15 drops.

millimeter (mm.) One one-thousandth of a meter. (A meter is 39.37 inches.)

Milontin An effective anticonvulsive medication used in the treatment of epilepsy; phensuximide.

Miltown A popular patented tranquilizer drug (meprobamate).

mimetic Pertaining to a condition which mimics, by its symptoms, another illness.

min. A drop of water.

mind The brain.

mineral Any chemical compound not containing carbon found in nature.

oil An inert oil, liquid petrolatum, used as an intestinal lubricant to promote normal bowel movements.

water Water derived from mineral springs, which contain relatively large amounts of minerals and are supposed to have medicinal qualities.

miner's lung *See* anthrocosis.

minilaparotomy A small incision into the abdominal cavity.

minim (min.) One drop of water; a fluid measure.

minimally invasive surgery Operations performed through an endoscope or laparoscope, utilizing the smallest incisions, some no more than approximately two-thirds of an inch in diameter.

Minocycline A powerful antibiotic that affects a wide range of bacteria.

Minot, George R. (1885–1950) An American physician, the codiscoverer of the liver diet treatment of pernicious anemia.

minoxidil *See* Rogaine.

miosis 1. Contraction of the pupil of the eye. 2. A special type of cell division, characteristic of maturing sex cells. 3. The phase of a disease in which the intensity of the symptoms decrease.

"miracle drugs" The antibiotics and certain chemotherapeutic drugs. (Penicillin and other antibiotics, the sulfonamides, etc.)

misanthropy Dislike of mankind; antisocial attitudes.

miscarriage Expulsion of a dead embryo or child.

misce (M.) The direction placed in front of prescriptions meaning "mix."

miscegenation Marriage or sexual intercourse between persons of different races.

miscible Able to go into solution, as, salt is *miscible* with water.

misogamist One who has an abnormal dislike of marriage.

misogyny An abnormal dislike of females.

misoneism Hatred of anything new or strange, such as new ideas.

mites Ticks; they often burrow

into the skin of animals or man. Some can cause serious disease.

mithramycin An antitumor drug used in the treatment of cancer of the testicle. Also called *Mithracin*.

mithridatism The development of immunity to a poison, obtained by taking small doses of it over a long period of time.

Mitomycin A powerful anticancer drug.

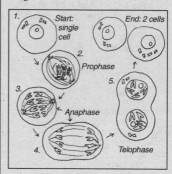

Mitosis of cells

mitosis The division of living cells.

mitral commissurotomy An operation in which the constricted mitral valve is stretched or cut. Performed to relieve mitral stenosis.

mitral stenosis Deformity of the mitral valve of the heart, usually secondary to a rheumatic fever infection.

mitral valve The valve on the left side of the heart between the two chambers, the auricle (atrium) and the ventricle.

mittelschmerz Pain in the lower abdomen occurring in between menstrual periods. It is thought to be due to escape of blood into the abdominal cavity caused by the breaking out of the egg from the ovary.

mixed infection A combination of bacteria, as in many cases of peritonitis.

mixed tumor of salivary gland The most frequently encountered growth within a salivary gland such as the

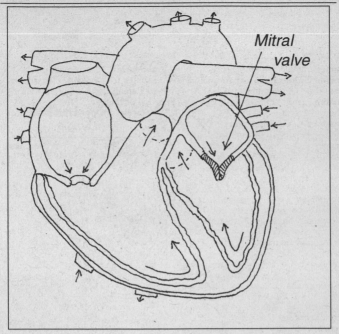

Mitral stenosis

parotid gland in the cheek or the submaxillary gland below the jawbone in the neck. A mixed tumor is usually benign and is composed of gland tissue and cartilagelike tissue; thus the name *"mixed" tumor.*

mixture The combination of two or more ingredients, each of which retains its individual characteristics, as a cough mixture.

ml Milliliter; 1/1000 of a liter; 1 c.c.; fifteen drops.

M.L.D. Abbreviation for *minimal lethal dose.*

mm. An abbreviation for millimeter.

MMR Abbreviation for mumps, measles, and German measles vaccine.

mnemonics The memorizing of material by means of a system.

mobilization 1. To free an organ

from its attachments. 2. To loosen a joint which is stiff or immovable.

modality 1. A sensation, such as taste, sight, smell, hearing. 2. A form of treatment.

modified radical mastectomy Removal of the breast and its lymph glands, but without removing the muscles beneath the breast.

Mohs operation A procedure whereby microscopically controlled tumors of the skin can be removed.

moiety 1. An indefinite portion. 2. One half of something.

molar One of the large back teeth used for chewing.

molarity The concentration of a solution, as stated in moles per 1000 cc.'s.

molding The overlapping of the

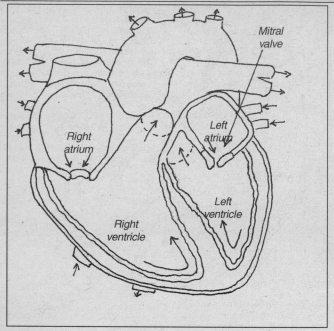

Mitral valve, normal

bones of the fetus's skull as it passes down the pelvic outlet in childbirth. This shaping allows the child to conform to the bony walls of the pelvis and thus pass through.

mole 1. A tumor of the skin, often pigmented brown or bluish black. 2. A mass formed by a dead embryo and its membranes within the uterus.

molecule The smallest particle of a substance that exhibits all its properties.

molluscum contagiosum A chronic skin condition in which there are isolated raised, rounded, pea-sized lumps of yellowish-pink hue. Microscopic examination shows characteristic "molluscum bodies."

momism Excessive attachment to a mother.

monarticular Relating to a single joint, as monarticular arthritis.

mongolian spot A bluish discoloration of the skin found in the lower back at birth. Usually it decreases in size or disappears early in life.

mongolism An obsolete term for a chromosomal abnormality associated with mental deficiency. Those affected have facial features resembling the Mongols of Asia. The condition is now known as *Down's syndrome.*

moniliasis A specific fungus infection, seen often in the vagina or on the skin or mucous membranes.

Monistat A vaginal suppository effective in treating fungal infections such as moniliasis and candidiasis.

monitor, cardiac An electrical ap-

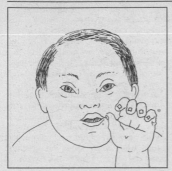

Mongolism (Down's Syndrome)

paratus which, when attached to a patient, flashes electrocardiographic tracings onto a fluorescent screen.

monitoring Measuring the performance of a service or of a project. Such as the progress of an illness or recovery process.

mono- A prefix meaning "one," "single."

monoclonal antibodies Antibodies all derived from a single clone of cells; all containing similar molecules. Recently used to increase resistance to the growth of cancers.

monocyte A type of white blood cell having one round-shaped nucleus (central portion). Monocytes are increased in number during certain infections, such as glandular fever.

monocytosis An increased number of monocytes (a type of white blood cell), as in infectious mononucleosis.

monogamy Being married to one person only.

monomania A form of insanity in which the patient's ideas concentrate on one subject.

mononucleosis See infectious mononucleosis.

monooctanoin A substance that, when injected into the common bile duct, dissolves cholesterol stones that may have been left behind inad-

vertently after surgery. The trade name is Moctanin.

monoplegia Paralysis of but one extremity (limb).

monorchidism Having but one testicle in the scrotal sac. (The other might be undescended or absent.)

monosomy See syndrome, Turner's.

monozygotic Developed from one egg.

monster A markedly deformed newborn, incapable of sustaining life.

mons veneris The prominence just above the pubic bones in females.

MOPP Abbreviation for a combination of anti-cancer drugs used in the treatment of Hodgkin's disease.

morbid Unhealthy, pertaining to disease.

morbidity rate 1. The ratio of the number of sick people to the number in the total population. 2. The number of cases of a disease occurring during the course of a year.

morbilli Measles.

morcellate To break into fragments; done to tumors which cannot be removed in one piece.

morgue The laboratory where dead people are kept until they are ready for the undertaker. Autopsies are performed in morgues.

moribund Dying; unconscious or semiconscious.

morning sickness Nausea and vomiting which occur during the second, third and part of the fourth month of pregnancy in some women. It usually takes place on getting up in the morning.

moron A mentally deficient person with an I.Q. between 50 and 75; an adult whose intellectual level is in the range of seven to twelve-year-old children.

morphine A chemical compound derived from opium. Used to relieve pain and induce sleep. Habit forming when taken regularly over a period of several weeks.

morphinism Addiction to morphine.

morphology The science of anatomy; the study of the structure of tissues.

morrhuate, sodium A solution which, when injected into a varicose vein, will cause the blood within it to clot; a sclerosing agent.

mors Death.

mortality The death rate.

motility The ability to move.

motion, active Spontaneous, voluntary movements. The opposite of *passive motion.*

passive Movement of a bodily part through the efforts of someone else, such as a physical therapist in exercising a paralyzed limb.

sickness Nausea and vomiting due to excessive motion such as one feels in an airplane or aboard ship.

Motrin A proprietary anti-inflammatory drug, helpful in treating various types of arthritis.

mountain sickness Air sickness.

mouth, trench Vincent's infection. Ulceration of the gums and mucous membranes of the throat caused by a specific germ, *Fusobacterium.* Highly contagious.

mouth-to-mouth breathing The newest suggested method of artificial respiration, carried out by the first aider who places his mouth against the mouth of the patient and forcefully blows air. This is done rhythmically about twenty times per minute until the patient resumes breathing on his own. *See also* Manual, First Aid, Artificial Respiration

movement, bowel Evacuation of the stool.

MRI Abbreviation for *magnetic resonance imaging.*

mucin Material secreted by cells lining the intestinal tract and by other glandular cells.

mucocele 1. A cavity filled with mucous secretion. 2. A tumor composed of mucous tissue. 3. Enlargement of the tear gland of the eye.

mucocutaneous junction The area where skin meets mucous membrane, as at the junction of the lips

and mucous membrane of the mouth, or at the margin of the anus and the skin of the buttocks.

mucoepidermoid tumor A malignant, but slow-growing tumor of the parotid gland at the angle of the jaw. Complete surgical removal usually results in cure.

Mucomyst A medication used to thin out mucous secretions in the bronchial tubes and lungs, thus allowing the secretions to be more readily brought up and expectorated; used as a spray in certain cases of bronchitis, emphysema, croup and asthma.

mucopolysaccharidosis A group of diseases, mostly inherited, caused by an upset in the metabolism of polysaccharides. *See* polysaccharide.

mucopurulent A discharge containing pus and mucus.

mucosa Mucous membrane.

mucosectomy An operative procedure in which the mucous membrane is removed while leaving the submucosal tissues and muscle wall of the structure intact. This is sometimes done in an attempt to retain the rectum rather than to remove it entirely. Occasionally, it is done in the pylorus of the stomach to lower the capability of the organ to secrete hydrochloric acid.

mucous Relating to mucus.

membrane A surface membrane composed of cells which secrete various forms of mucus, as in the lining of the respiratory tract and the gastrointestinal tract, etc.

patches The eruptions seen within the mouth and about the lips during the second stage of syphilis. Contact with these patches will cause syphilis.

mucoviscidosis (mucoviscoidosis) Cystic fibrosis; viscoidosis. (Old terminology: Fibrocystic disease of the pancreas)

mucus A thick liquid secreted by mucous glands, such as those lining the nasal passages, the stomach and intestines, the vagina, etc.

multi- Prefix meaning "many," "much."

multilocular abscess One containing many compartments.

multilocular cyst A sac containing many compartments.

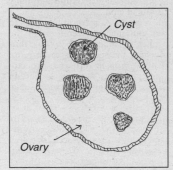

Multilocular cyst

multipara A woman who has given birth to one or more children.

multiple myeloma A widespread disease of the bone marrow. Also called *Kahler's disease.*

multiple organ failure Failure of function of more than one vital organ, such as heart, lung, liver, or kidney failure. Seen often as a terminal condition.

multiple sclerosis (disseminated sclerosis) A chronic disease of the nervous system leading to partial paralysis, changes in speech, inability to walk, etc. (This disease may last for many years.)

multivitamin preparations Capsules or fluid medications containing most of the essential vitamins, present in sufficient quantities to supply necessary requirements.

mummification A process in which a part of the body, often a toe or foot, undergoes dry gangrene, dries up and appears like the tissue of a mummy. It is caused by lack of blood supply.

mumps (epidemic parotitis) A highly contagious virus disease causing swelling of the parotid glands at the angles of the jaw. It sometimes also affects other glands, the testicles or ovaries, pancreas, etc.

Munchausen's syndrome See syndrome, Munchausen.

mural In the wall of an organ, as the wall of the heart or the wall of the uterus.

muriatic acid Hydrochloric acid.

murmur An abnormal heart sound heard when listening over the chest with an ear or stethoscope. Some murmurs are merely *functional* and do not indicate the presence of heart disease. Others are *organic* and represent disease of the heart valves.

Muscle See Manual for Important Muscles.

muscle Tissue composed of fibers which have the ability to elongate and shorten, thus causing bones and joints to move. Most voluntary muscle can contract or relax only when the nerves which supply it are normal. Failure of such nerves to transmit impulses results in a paralyzed muscle. Involuntary muscle, as in the heart, blood vessels, intestinal walls, etc., can contract and relax on their own, without the need for outside nerve stimulation. See Manual for list of Important Muscles.

muscle relaxants A group of drugs that allay muscle spasm and thus tend to relieve the pain accompanying strains and sprains.

muscular dystrophy A disease characterized by slowly progressive malfunction and wasting of muscles. Onset of this disease is usually in childhood.

musculocutaneous flap A graft of tissue composed of skin, subcutaneous tissue, and muscle.

musculoskeletal system The bones, muscles, ligaments, tendons and joints.

mustard, nitrogen An anticancer drug, highly toxic.

mutagenesis A process by which a change (mutation) in a gene is induced.

Mutamycin (Mitomycin) An anti-cancer drug, most helpful when used in conjunction with other chemotherapy agents. It is not a substitute for surgery and is not curative.

mutant gene A gene in which a change has taken place. (It is hoped that in the future harmful genes will be changed, through genetic engineering, into harmless genes.)

mutation A change in the characteristics of an animal or other organism as a result of changes in genes or other hereditary factors. A hybrid; a "sport."

mutilate To maim or do bodily harm.

mutism Speechlessness. Dumbness.

myalgia Pain in muscles, as in lumbago, rheumatism, etc.

Myambutol A powerful antituberculosis drug.

myasthenia Muscle weakness.

myasthenia gravis A serious chronic debilitating disease associated with wasting of muscles, especially those which enable a patient to swallow.

myatonia Lack of muscle tone or strength.

mycobacteria Rod-shaped bacteria. In this category one finds the germs which can cause leprosy, tuberculosis, etc. They have a characteristic "acid fast" staining quality.

Mycobacterium tuberculosis The germ that causes tuberculosis.

mycoid Resembling a fungus.

mycology The study of fungi.

mycomyringitis A fungus infection of the eardrum.

mycoplasma A type of bacteria which possesses no true cell wall.

mycosis Any infection caused by a fungus.

Mycostatin (Nystatin) An antibiotic containing anti-fungal action, used in fungal infections such as monilia.

mydriasis Dilatation of the pupil of the eye.

Mydriatic A drop that causes dilatation of the pupil of the eye.

myectomy Surgical removal of a muscle or part of a muscle.

myelemia A form of leukemia in which there are many myelocytes (primitive white blood cells).

myelin The sheath surrounding certain nerves, composed of a fatlike substance. Disease may ensue when these sheaths are damaged or destroyed.

myelitis Inflammation of the spinal cord, often associated with paralysis of the body below the level of the spinal cord inflammation.

myelo- A combining form referring to the bone marrow or spinal cord.

myeloblast The primitive cell in the bone marrow which eventually emerges as a white blood cell.

myelocele A hernia of the spinal cord through a defect in the development of the bones of the vertebral column. *See also* spina bifida.

myelocyte A primitive cell which eventually develops into a mature white blood cell.

myclocytic leukemia A very malignant form of leukemia; also called *granulocytic leukemia*.

myelography X ray of the spinal canal, carried out after the injection of a dye which will show on the X-ray film.

myeloma A malignant tumor of the bone marrow. *See also* multiple myeloma.

myelomalacia Degeneration and softening of the spinal cord leading to paralysis.

myeloradiculitis Inflammation of the spinal cord and the roots of the spinal nerves.

myelosclerosis A disease in which there is slow hardening and loss of function (as a blood-forming organ) of the bone marrow.

myenteric Referring to the muscles in the wall of the intestines.

myesthesia Awareness of one's own muscle functioning, as in realization that a muscle has contracted. This property is lost in cases of muscle paralysis and in certain other diseases.

myiasis Infestation of the body with the larvae of flies.

Mylanta An antacid medication, supplied in both liquid and tablet form.

Mylicon A patented medication used to relieve the symptoms caused by excess gas in the intestinal tract.

myo- A prefix referring to *muscle*.

myoblastoma A tumor, usually located in the arms or legs, originating from primitive muscle cells. Most such tumors are benign.

myocardial infarction Damage of heart muscle secondary to the loss of its blood supply, as in coronary thrombosis.

myocardial ischemia Lack of sufficient blood supply to the heart muscle.

myocarditis Inflammation of the heart muscle, a common complication of any severe debilitating disease; also seen in cases of rheumatic fever.

myocardium Heart muscle.

myoclonus Abnormal muscle twitchings.

myocutaneous flap A pedicle graft containing skin, subcutaneous fat, muscle, blood vessels, and nerves, used to cover large defects or to reconstruct tissues, such as a breast. *See also* graft, pedicle.

myoepithelioma A sweat-gland tumor found in the skin. They form firm, little, round, hard masses about half the size of a pea.

myofascitis Inflammation of muscle and the fibrous coverings of muscle and surrounding ligaments. Seen as one of the common causes of chronic lower back pain.

myofibroma A benign tumor composed of muscle and fibrous tissue, e.g., fibroids of the uterus.

myofibrosis Replacement of muscle tissue by fibrous tissue, often the result of long-standing inflammation of a muscle.

myogelosis A hardened area within the substance of a muscle.

myogram A tracing of muscular activity, recorded on paper, after application of an electromyographic apparatus.

myography The recording of muscle movements.

myokymia Small twitchings of parts of a muscle.

myolipoma A tumor composed of muscle tissue, fat tissue, fibrous tissue, etc. Also called *mesenchyme tumors.*

myoma Benign tumor of muscle.

myomalacia Degeneration of muscle.

myomectomy Operative removal of a fibroid tumor of the uterus. (The uterus is not removed by this procedure.)

myometrial hyperplasia Overgrowth of the muscle tissue of the uterus.

myometrium The muscle of the wall of the uterus.

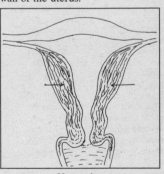

Myometrium

myoneural junction The point at which nerves enter muscles.

myopathy Disease of muscle.

myopia Nearsightedness.

myosarcoma A malignant tumor of muscle.

myositis Inflammation of muscle.

   ossificans Inflammation of muscle of long standing resulting in the formation of bone tissue (localized to a relatively small area) within the substance of the muscle. It may also occur after muscle injury.

myotomy A surgical incision of muscle.

myotonia Spasm of muscle.

myringectomy Surgical removal of the eardrum.

myringitis Inflammation of the eardrum.

myringoplasty A plastic operation to repair a damaged eardrum.

myringotomy Surgical incision of the eardrum, frequently performed to remove pus from the middle ear.

myrrh A gum resin used as a mouthwash, particularly in cases of mouth infection.

Mysteclin A patented medication, said to combat fungal growth (Can-dida and others) secondary to the use of oral antibiotic medications.

myxedema A metabolic disorder due to insufficient function of the thyroid gland (hypothyroidism). It is characterized by a puffy appearance of tissues, dryness of the skin, weight gain, etc.

myxo- A combining form meaning mucous gland, mucus, or mucous tissue.

myxochondroma A tumor of cartilage, not malignant.

myxoma A tumor of connective tissue in which there is a large amount of mucous tissue. Some of these tumors are benign, others malignant.

myxosarcoma A malignant tumor of connective tissue containing mucous tissue.

N

N Symbol for nitrogen.
Na Symbol for sodium.
nabothian cyst Small cysts containing mucus, sometimes present in the cervix of the uterus.
Naegele's pelvis Oblique distortion of the bony pelvis. In women, it may cause difficulty during labor.
nail The flat, horny growths of tissue which protrude from the finger and toe tips.
    bed The soft tissue beneath the nail.
    ingrown A painful condition in which the sharp edge of the nail, usually of the big toe, grows into the flesh alongside the nail.
    root That part of the nail beneath the cuticle and skin which covers the first portion of the nail.
nailing An operative procedure in which the parts of a broken bone are held together by placing nails through them.
naked Without clothes or covering.
nalorphine A medication used to diagnose morphine addiction.
nanism Marked smallness; dwarfism.
nape The back of the neck.
naphthalene A compound used as an antiseptic on the skin, especially in cases of itching and scabies.
Naprosyn A drug helpful in the treatment of rheumatoid arthritis; a pain-relieving medication and one which lowers elevated temperature.
Naproxen Same as Naprosyn.
narcissism Love of oneself, or libido fixation upon one's own body.
narcoanalysis Psychiatric treatment carried out while the patient is under the influence of sleep producing or narcotic drugs.
narcohypnosis The making of suggestions while the patient is under the influence of a hypnotic drug.
narcolepsy A period of deep sleep, usually not lasting very long, brought on by an epileptic attack or by an inflammation of the brain.
narcosis A state of deep stupor or unconsciousness produced by a drug.
narcotic A drug that produces sleep or stupor, simultaneously relieving pain, such as opium, morphine, etc. Many are habit-forming.
narcotism 1. Unconsciousness as the result of the taking or administration of a narcotic drug or medication. 2. Narcotic addiction.
narcotize To produce an unconscious state by administering a narcotic drug.
nares The nostrils.
nasal Pertaining to the nose.
nasal septum The tissue that separates the two cavities of the nose.
nascent Referring to a gas which has just been released from a non-gaseous chemical compound.
nasociliary nerve The nerve which supplies the eyeball and the nose.
nasogastric tube A tube placed through the nose down into the stomach, often used to drain gas and fluids from the stomach and small intestines; a Levin tube.
nasolabial Pertaining to the nose and lip.
nasolacrimal Referring to the nose and tear glands and ducts.
nasopalatine Referring to the nose and the palate.

nasopharyngitis Inflammation of the nose and throat.

nasopharynx The nose and throat.

Natalins tablets A vitamin and mineral supplement often prescribed during pregnancy or the period following childbirth.

natality Birth rate.

natant Referring to something which floats on top of a liquid.

National Formulary (N.F.) A publication compiled by members of the American Pharmaceutical Association containing lists of standard drugs and medications.

natremia A condition in which there is too much sodium in the blood. (Same as hypernatremia)

natural childbirth A method of childbirth in which as few artifical procedures as possible are carried out. Courses of instruction are given throughout the pregnancy to ready women for this type of delivery.

natural selection theory Darwin's theory of the struggle for survival; that is, that the most fit tend to mate with the most fit. Thus, the species is constantly being improved and the less fit tend to die out.

naturopath A nonmedical practitioner who claims to be able to cure illness by giving "natural" remedies derived from such things as foods, herbs, light, water, etc.

nausea The feeling that one may vomit.

navel The depression in the mid-abdomen representing the site of the umbilical cord which attached the unborn child to its mother. (The umbilicus)

navicular bone A boat-shaped bone of the wrist or ankle.

nearsightedness A condition in which the eyeball is too long and the image falls short of the retina. Nearsighted people see close objects better than distant objects (myopia).

nebulize To convert a medication or other substance into a spray.

neck That portion of the anatomy between the head and the chest.

necrobiosis The natural death of certain types of bodily cells or tissue, with preservation of some characteristics of the living state.

necrology The study of mortality statistics.

necromania An abnormal interest in dead bodies.

necrophilism 1. Morbid attraction to corpses. 2. Sexual intercourse with a dead person. 3. The death wish; a desire to die.

necrophobia Morbid fear of dying.

necropsy Autopsy.

necrosis Death of tissue, as that caused by bacterial infection.

necrospermia Dead sperm in the semen.

necrotizing enterocolitis A serious, sometimes fatal, disease of newborns, particularly premature or undernourished infants. It is thought to be caused by inadequate development of the intestinal tract, thus allowing bacteria to invade the intestinal walls and to cause gangrene or perforation.

needle biopsy Removal of a small piece of tissue from a tumor with a specially devised needle. Such tissue is then examined under a microscope.

needle holder An instrument to hold and to manipulate a curved surgical needle.

needle localization The insertion of a needle into a site in a breast that is suspected, on mammography, of being cancerous. This aids the surgeon in locating a minute tumor that cannot be felt on manual examination.

needling of lens Insertion of a needle into the lens of the eye in cases of cataract, done in the hope that the cataract will be absorbed.

negative result A method of indicating that a medical test is normal. (A *negative* Wassermann reaction means the patient does not have active syphilis.)

"negative serology" A term implying that blood tests do not show the presence of syphilis.

negativism Repeated rejection of requests to do what one is asked to do; seen at one time or another in most infants and young children.

negligence case An expression referring to the case of a patient injured under circumstances in which there has been negligence, as when someone trips over a break in the sidewalk.

Neisserian infection Gonorrhea.

Nelaton's line An anatomical landmark, helpful in diagnosing a dislocated hip.

nematodes Roundworms.

Nembutal A patented medication containing a long acting sleep inducing barbiturate.

neoarsphenamine A drug, containing arsenic, formerly used in the treatment of syphilis.

Neo-Cortef A cortisone and antibiotic (neomycin) combination used as a lotion, cream or ointment in the treatment of certain skin conditions.

Neodecadron Ophthalmic Solution An eye medication containing both an antibiotic and a cortisonelike substance; helpful in treating disorders of the covering (conjunctiva) and the anterior portion of the eye.

Neomycin A powerful antibiotic drug, especially useful against bacteria which live in the intestines.

neonatology That branch of medicine dealing with the newborn.

neonatal Newborn.

mortality The death rate among newborns and infants during their first month of life.

neoplasm Any tumor; a growth.

Neosporin A medication containing several antibiotics, namely, polymyxin B, bacitracin and neomycin.

Neostigmine A drug used to increase muscle tone; helpful in treating various conditions associated with muscle function disturbance,

such as paralysis of the bladder or intestines.

Neosynephrine (phenylephrine) A drug which constricts blood vessels; often used to relieve nasal congestion.

nephrectomy Surgical removal of a kidney.

nephritis Inflammation of the kidneys. There are many forms of this condition. The diagnosis can often be made by chemical examination of the blood and urine.

nephrolithiasis Stones in the kidney, or the condition which leads to kidney stone formation.

nephrolithotomy The surgical removal of a stone, or stones, from a kidney.

nephrology That branch of medicine dealing with disorders and diseases of the kidneys.

nephroma A malignant tumor of the kidney.

nephron That part of the kidney which secretes urine.

nephropexy An operation to replace a kidney into its normal position, carried out when a kidney has dropped out of position.

nephroptosis A "dropped" kidney.

nephrosclerosis A diseased condition of the kidney associated with high blood pressure, hardening of the arteries and impaired kidney function.

nephrosis Degeneration of the kidney; a serious metabolic disease seen in young children.

nephrostomy A surgical procedure in which a permanent opening leading to the pelvis of the kidney is constructed so as to drain the urine.

nephrotoxin Something which is poisonous to the kidney, such as mercury or some other substance.

nerve The structure which transmits impulses and stimuli to and from the brain and spinal cord. *See* Manual for list of Important Nerves.

afferent A nerve which transmits impulses from the tissues *to* the brain and spinal cord.

autonomic A nerve of the involuntary nervous system which supplies the internal organs and other structures.

block The injection of an anesthetic agent into or around a nerve in order to blot out impulses which travel through it and to produce loss of sensation to the area supplied by the nerve.

cerebrospinal A nerve having its origin in the brain or spinal cord.

cranial A nerve which originates from the brain and exits through one of the openings in the skull.

efferent A nerve which transmits impulses *from* the brain and spinal cord to the organs and tissues of the body.

ending The point at which a nerve enters the structure it supplies and transmits or receives its impulse.

motor A nerve which supplies muscles and causes them to contract.

parasympathetic A nerve of the involuntary nervous system such as those supplying the lungs, heart, intestines, etc.

sensory A nerve which travels toward the spinal cord or brain and transmits sensations such as touch, pain, heat, cold, etc.

spinal A nerve having its origin in the spinal cord.

splanchnic A nerve supplying the organs of the chest and abdomen.

sympathetic A nerve of the sympathetic nervous system which, among other things, causes blood vessels to constrict and blood pressure to rise.

tract The course a nerve takes from its point of origin to its termination.

nervousness The condition of being overly sensitive or excitable.

network A grouping of blood vessels or nerves.

neural Pertaining to nerves.

neuralgia Pain along the route of a nerve.

neuraminic acid *See* sialic acids.

neuraminidase (sialidase) An enzyme that acts upon and destroys excess sialic acid. Its deficiency causes severe congenital diseases.

neurasthenia Lack of energy, listlessness, fatigue, often associated with a neurotic state.

neurectomy, presacral An operative procedure in which the nerves supplying the uterus are severed in order to relieve severe pain on menstruation. (Surgery is carried out through an abdominal incision. Function of the uterus is not disturbed by the operation.)

neurilemma The covering or sheath of a nerve fiber.

neurilemmoma A tumor, usually benign, of the sheath of a nerve.

neuritis An inflammatory or degenerative condition of a nerve.

neuroblastoma A malignant tumor composed of primitive nerve tissue, most often located in the chest or behind the abdomen. Affects infants and children most frequently.

neurocirculatory asthenia A weakened, tired state associated with low blood pressure, dizziness, shortness of breath, rapid heart beat and poor nerve function. It is thought to be a neurotic condition.

neurodermatitis A skin disease accompanied by an itching rash seen mainly on the neck and in the folds of the elbows and knees, encountered mostly in nervous women.

neurofibroma A nonmalignant tumor composed of nerve and fibrous tissues.

neurofibromatosis An inherited condition in which there are many (from a few to thousands) tumors in the nerves to the skin and the tissues beneath the skin. The tumors are not malignant. Also called *von Recklinghausen's disease.*

neurogenic Arising from a nerve; of nervous origin.

neurogenic bladder A urinary

bladder that fails to function normally because of damage to its nerve supply.

neurolemmoma A tumor of a nerve sheath.

neuroleptanesthesia A general anesthesia combining the use of intravenous drugs to produce sleep, along with a light inhalation general anesthetic agent such as nitrous oxide.

Neurologist A physician who specializes in diseases of the nervous system.

neuroma A nerve tumor.

neuromuscular junction The point at which a nerve ends in a muscle, at which the impulse is transmitted by the nerve to the muscle.

neuron(e) A nerve, including the cell and the long fiber originating from the cell.

neuronyxis The insertion of an acupuncture needle into a nerve.

neuropathy Any disease of nerve tissue.

neurophysiology The study of nerve function.

Neuropsychiatrist A physician who specializes in both psychiatric and neurologic conditions.

neuroretinitis Inflammation of the nerve to the eye (the optic nerve) and the retina. Severe cases may end in blindness.

neurosis An emotional or psychological disorder. Not insanity.

    anxiety Emotional disturbance accompanied by inordinate worry and fears of inadequacy.

    cardiac Emotional disturbance associated with fear of a heart attack, or accompanied by pain in the heart area.

    compensation Emotional disturbance with development of painful symptoms following an accident in which there is the possibility of monetary reward or settlement.

    conversion hysteria Anxieties converted to physical symptoms.

    compulsive Disturbed behavior in which one attempts to overcome anxiety by being a perfectionist.

    sexual Emotional disturbance in which the symptoms manifest themselves through changes in sexual function, as nymphomania, impotence, etc.

    war Battle fatigue; emotionally disturbed behavior in those who are exposed to the dangers of war.

Neurosurgeon A surgeon who specializes in conditions affecting nervous system.

neurosurgery Surgery of the brain, spinal cord and nerves.

neurosyphilis Syphilis of any part of the brain or spinal cord.

neurotic One who is emotionally disturbed or unstable.

neurotoxin A poison (toxin) which affects a nerve or nerve tissue. (The virus of infantile paralysis contains a powerful neurotoxin.)

neurotripsy The surgical crushing of a nerve.

neutral Referring to a solution which is neither acid nor alkaline.

neutron An electrically neutral atomic particle, found in all elements except a variant of hydrogen; used in certain types of irradiation treatment.

Neutropen A preparation containing the enzyme *penicillinase,* used to destroy penicillin. The drug is supposedly effective in overcoming allergic reactions to penicillin.

neutropenia Decrease in the number of white blood cells in the blood.

neutrophil A white blood cell.

nevus A mole.

    junction A flat mole containing some cells that are potentially malignant or are in the early stages of malignant change. (These are small tumors that should be excised widely.)

newborn An infant up to the first three to five days of life.

new growth A tumor; a neoplasm.

N.F. *See* National Formulary.

niacin Nicotinic acid, part of the vitamin B complex.

niche An alcove or indentation in the contour of an organ, such as a niche seen on X ray of the stomach in a case of ulcer.

nicotine poisoning Weak, rapid pulse, sense of exhaustion, poor appetite, etc., associated with excessive smoking.

nicotinic acid The vitamin which prevents the disease known as pellagra. Also called niacin and *P.P. factor.*

nictation Winking of the eyelids.

nidus 1. A focus of infection; thus, an infected tooth may be the *nidus* for a generalized infection of the body. 2. A depression of one of the brain surfaces.

Niemann-Pick disease A fatal disease affecting young children in which there is enlargement of the spleen and liver, anemia and mental deterioration.

nightmare A horrible dream accompanied by fright and agitation.

night sweats Excessive perspiration during sleep. Usually thought to be associated with tuberculosis of the lungs.

night vision The ability to see in the dark.

NIH Abbreviation for National Institutes of Health.

nihilism A term used in psychiatry to describe the pessimistic thoughts of patients suffering deep depressions; the attitude that "nothing is worthwhile."

nipple The point of outlet of the milk ducts of the breasts.

Nissen operation *See* fundal plication.

Nitranitol A patented medication used to relax blood vessels and to lower blood pressure.

nitrazine paper A paper impregnated with a dye which changes color according to the acidity or alkalinity of the fluid in which it is immersed. (Used to test the acidity of urine)

nitremia An excess of nitrogen in the blood, as in uremia.

nitric acid HNO_3, an acid which is very strong and can burn tissues. Dilute solutions are sometimes used to burn warts or ulcers on the skin surface.

nitrites A group of chemicals which cause dilatation of blood vessels and lowering of blood pressure.

Nitro-Bid A pill taken twice daily to prevent attacks of angina pectoris, effective in some patients.

Nitro-Dur A medicated pad applied to the skin and left in place for periods of 24 hours. The pad contains nitroglycerin, which is absorbed through the skin and helps prevent angina pectoris.

nitrogen (N) An element making up about 77 percent of the air we breathe. It is present in all plant and animal tissue.

nitrogen, nonprotein (N.P.N.) An important element of blood. Elevation of this element may signify kidney disease.

nitrogen mustard Any of a group of chemical substances helpful in slowing the growth of certain malignant tumors, especially conditions such as leukemia, Hodgkin's disease, etc. (These chemicals were used as poisonous gases for chemical warfare.)

nitroglycerin A medication which causes dilatation of blood vessels and lowering of blood pressure. (Used under the tongue to relieve the heart pain in attacks of angina pectoris.)

Nitrol A patented medication for relief of arterial spasm; same as nitroglycerin.

Nitropatch *See* Nitro-Dur.

Nitrostat *See* nitroglycerin.

nitrous oxide An anesthetic gas; also called "laughing gas."

NMR An abbreviation for the obsolete term, *nuclear magnetic resonance.* The new name is *magnetic resonance imaging.*

NNR Abbreviation for *New and Nonofficial Remedies,* a booklet published periodically by the American Medical Association to inform the medical profession of new and approved drugs and medications.

Nobel, Alfred B. (1833–1896) A Swedish industrialist, the donator of the fund of money out of which the Nobel prizes for contributions in the fields of medicine, physics, chemistry, literature and world peace are given.

noctambulation Sleepwalking.

nocturia Getting up at night to urinate.

nocturnal Occurring during the night.

node A small, round structure, such as a lymph node.

nodules A small node, or group of cells, as a lymph nodule.

noesis The faculty of perceiving; cognition.

Nolvadex An anti-estrogen medication having an inhibitory effect upon the spread of breast cancer in some women, especially those past menopause. Nolvadex is also called *tamoxifen.*

noma A severe, sometimes fatal, ulcerating condition of the mouth.

nomenclature The terms used in a science. (Attempts have been made to standardize medical nomenclature throughout the world.)

nonallergenic A term applied to a substance which will not cause an allergy, such as a *nonallergenic* cosmetic preparation.

non compos mentis Not mentally responsible or capable of managing one's affairs.

nonconductor A substance which will not transmit an electrical impulse.

noninfectious A disorder that is not able to spread.

noninvasive procedure A procedure which enters the body through puncture wounds rather than through large surgical incisions.

noniparous A woman who has had nine childbirths.

nonmalignant Not cancerous. Benign.

nonmotile Incapable of motion. Someone who is unable to impregnate a woman may have nonmotile sperm.

nonprotein nitrogen An important element of the blood. Elevation of blood levels of nonprotein nitrogen may signify kidney disease.

nonpyogenic A term applied to certain bacteria that do not produce pus.

nonrotation of intestines A development defect in which the intestines fail to rotate into their normal position.

nonspecific General; a term applied to certain forms of treatment.

nonsuppurative Not pus forming.

nonsurgical A disease or condition not requiring surgery.

nonunion of fracture Failure of the broken fragments to fuse and form callus, (new bone tissue).

nonviable Not able to live, as an embryo or fetus which has not yet reached six to seven months in development.

Norepinephrine A drug which tends to maintain blood pressure during states of shock. (Used extensively in surgical procedures when blood pressure drops too markedly.)

Norgesic forte A pain-relieving drug, especially in muscle pain.

Norinyl An oral contraceptive medication.

Norlestrin An oral contraceptive medication.

norm The normal; the average.

normal Conforming to a standard.

normoblast An immature red blood cell.

Normodyne An anti-hypertension drug given intravenously to patients suffering from extremely high blood pressure.

normotensive Having normal blood pressure.

normovolemia Normal blood volume, as opposed to hypovolemia.

Norvasc A medication to lower blood pressure and to relieve heart pain (angina pectoris).

nose The organ of smell.

nosocomial Referring to a hospital, such as *nosocomial infection*, which has been acquired while a patient is in a hospital.

nosology The science or study of the classification of diseases.

nostalgia Homesickness.

nostril One of the orifices of the nose.

nostrum A quack, or secret medicine.

notch An indentation; a niche.

nosophobia Extreme fear of disease.

Notifiable disease Same as reportable disease.

notochord The structure in the embryo from which the spinal column (vertebrae) is formed.

Novahistine A liquid medicine to reduce cough and to combat any allergic condition of the upper respiratory tract.

Novaldex *See* tamoxifen.

novobiocin An antibiotic particularly effective against staphylococcal infections.

Novocain A patented medication containing the most widely used local anesthetic agent; procaine.

Novulin A form of insulin, also known as NPH insulin.

noxious Poisonous; harmful.

NPH An abbreviation for a brand of insulin having a long lasting effect.

N.P.N. Abbreviation for nonprotein nitrogen.

nuchal Referring to the back of the neck.

Nuck's canal A continuation of the lining membrane of the abdomen (peritoneum) through the inguinal ring in the groin, seen occasionally in women.

nuclear Referring to the nucleus or the center of a cell.

nuclear fission The splitting of certain nuclei and release of neutrons and large amounts of energy.

nuclear medicine The branch that utilizes various radioactive sub-

stances in the diagnosis or treatment of disease.

nucleic acid The substance found in the nucleus of cells. It is related to DNA and is thought to be the carrier of inherited traits.

nucleolus A small, rounded spot within the nucleus of a cell.

nucleus The central living portion of a cell; that part containing the chromosomes.

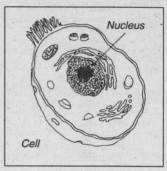

Nucleus of a cell

nucleus pulposus herniation A "slipped disk." A protrusion of the cartilage which lies in between the vertebrae.

nudist One who believes in the benefits from going about without clothes.

nulliparous A female who has never borne a child.

numbness Diminished sensation.

nummular Having the shape of a coin.

Nupercainal ointment A soothing ointment containing a local anesthetic for temporary relief of pain and itching.

nurse A person who tends the sick, wounded or infirm.

   dry One who takes care of an infant but does not suckle him. The opposite of a wet nurse.

   general duty A floor nurse assigned to the care of many patients.

   graduate A nurse holding a

diploma from an approved school of nursing.

   head   One who is in charge of a hospital or division of a hospital.

   practical   One who is trained to care for patients but has not received a diploma from a school of nursing.

   private duty   One who devotes her time on duty to the care of one patient who employs her exclusively.

   probationer   A nurse during the first few months of her training. Nicknamed "probies."

   public health   One who works for a public health agency. Most of her time is spent in prevention of disease.

   registered   (R.N.) A graduate of a school of nursing.

   scrub   An operating room nurse.

   student   One enrolled in a school of nursing.

   supervisor   One in charge of a floor or a department in a hospital.

   trained   A graduate nurse.

   visiting   One who goes to the patient's home.

   wet   Someone who suckles or breast feeds an infant not her own.

nursling   A nursing infant.

nutrient   1. Nourishing. 2. A food.

nutriment   Nourishment.

nutrition   The process of digestion and utilization of food substances.

nutritional edema   Swelling of the tissue because of inadequate protein intake.

nux vomica   A stimulant drug containing strychnine in small amounts.

nyctalgia   Pain occurring chiefly at night.

nyctalopia   Night blindness.

nyctophobia   Fear of the dark.

Nydrazid   A patented anti-tuberculosis medication. (Same as *isoniazid*)

nympha   The small vaginal lip.

nymphomania   Excessive sexual desire in a woman.

nystagmus   A rapid, rhythmic, side-to-side movement of the eyeball, seen in diseases of the brain.

Nystatin   Mycostatin; an antibiotic medication particularly effective in combating fungus infections, such as moniliasis.

nyxis   Puncturing with a needle, or tapping to draw off excess fluid.

O

O Symbol for oxygen.

oat cell cancer A type of lung cancer that spreads rapidly through lymphatic channels and is often not amenable to surgery.

obduction An autopsy; postmortem; examination of a body after death.

Ober operations Several operations in which muscles and tendons are transplanted in cases of paralysis; more particularly, operations for transplantations of tendons in the thigh or leg.

obesity Overweight.

obfuscation The process of becoming disoriented or mentally confused.

objective 1. The lens of a microscope nearest to the object being viewed. 2. Perceivable through use of the senses.

objective signs Those conditions in an illness which can be seen or felt by the examining physician, as opposed to subjective symptoms, which only the patient experiences.

obliterate Surgically, to remove a part or close it off completely.

obsession A thought which continues in one's consciousness despite all attempts to forget it.

obsessive-compulsive neurosis Emotional instability characterized by unwanted urges and thoughts.

obsolescence Something that is not useful; the loss of its usefulness.

Obstetrician A physican who specializes in delivering babies and the diseases of pregnant women.

obstetrics The branch of medicine dealing with childbirth.

obstipation Absolute inability to move the bowels; complete constipation.

obstruction, intestinal A condition in which the passage of the intestinal contents is obstructed, caused by a growth within the intestines or by something closing the passageway through pressure from outside the bowel wall.

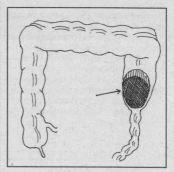

Intestinal obstruction

    pyloric Obstruction of the outlet of the stomach. In newborns this is caused by an overgrowth of the muscles in the region. In adults it may be caused either by a tumor of the stomach or by scar tissue resulting from an old ulcer.

    ureteral Obstruction of the passage of urine along the ureter, the tube from the kidney to the bladder. A stone is the most frequent cause of this type of obstruction.

    urinary Inability to expel urine from the bladder. The most

common cause of this condition in men is an enlarged prostate gland.

obtund   To lessen or do away with, as to *obtund* sensations through anesthesia.

obturator   The opening in the pelvis located between the pubic and ischial bones. It is covered by a membrane which is pierced by the *obturator nerve* and blood vessels.

obtuse   Dull.

occipital region   The lower portion of the back of the head.

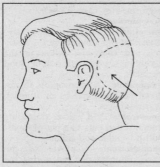

Occipital region

occipitotemporal   Referring to the back (occiput) and side (temporal) of the head.

occiput   The back of the head.

occlusion   1. A shutting off, as of the blood flow in a clotted blood vessel. Coronary *occlusion* is the clotting of blood within the coronary artery of the heart. 2. The meeting of the grinding surfaces of the upper and lower jaws.

occult   Not evident; concealed, as occult blood in the stool.

occupational disease   A disease associated with the type of work or employment of a patient, such as lung inflammation and fibrosis in miners or lead poisoning among painters.

occupational therapy   Education for an occupation to invalid or handicapped patients.

ochrometer   An instrument to determine blood pressure in the capillaries.

ochronosis   A disturbance of metabolism in which the skin of the face, the whites of the eyes, and other tissues such as muscle and cartilage become discolored brown. (It is seen in those who have a condition known as alkaptonuria. In these people, the urine is also a dark, brownish color.)

ocular   Pertaining to the eye.

oculist   An ophthalmologist; an eye doctor.

oculomotor   Referring to the movements of the eye.

Oculist   An eye specialist (physician who specializes in ophthalmology).

OD   Abbreviation for overdose.

odditis   Inflammation of the duodenum (the first portion of the small intestine) at the site where the bile duct enters.

odontectomy   Removal of teeth.

odontology   Dentistry.

odontoma   A tumor originating from a tooth.

odoriferous   Odorous.

odorimetry   Determination of the acuteness of the sense of smell.

oecology   *See* ecology.

oedema   *See* edema.

oedipal   Referring to the Oedipus complex. The psychoanalytical theory that in the development of the male child, there is a period in which love for his mother and an accompanying unconscious envy of his father are extremely important.

oestrone   An estrogenic steroid.

oestrus   Estrus. The mating period in animals.

ointment   A salve; an unguent.

olecranon   The end of the ulna bone.

   bursitis   Inflammation of the bursa of the elbow. (A bursa is a pad of fat lying upon the bone.) Olecranon bursitis is often accompanied by marked swelling, fluid or pus collection in the elbow region.

   process   The elbow tip.

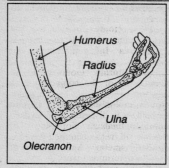

Olecranon region

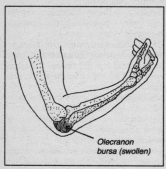

Olecranon
bursa (swollen)

Olecranon bursitis

olfactory sense The sense of smell.
oligemia Decreased blood volume; hypovolemia. Shock may ensue if blood volume is diminished too greatly.
oligo- A combining form meaning *scant, little,* etc.
oligodendroglioma A slow-growing brain tumor. Also called oligodendrocytoma.
oligomenorrhea Infrequent menstruation; menstruation once every few months.
oligospermia A condition in which the number of sperm in the ejaculate is abnormally small.
oliguria The passage of only a scant amount of urine.
olive oil The oil of olives. It has

various medical uses including that as a laxative and as an ingredient of liniments, ointments, etc.
-ology A suffix meaning *the science of.*
-oma A suffix meaning *tumor,* or *swelling.*
omentectomy Surgical removal of the great omentum.
omentopexy An abdominal operation in which the great omentum is stitched to the abdominal wall in order to short-circuit blood supply around the liver. (The operation, performed in cases of cirrhosis, is now obsolete.)
omentum A fatty, apronlike membrane hanging down from the stomach and transverse colon in the abdominal cavity. It is rich in blood vessels.
omeprazole A medication to cut down on the secretion of stomach (gastric) juices.
omnivorous An animal (including humans) that eats all types of foods, both vegetable and animal.
omphalectomy Removal of the navel, often carried out during the repair of a hernia of the navel.
omphalitis Inflammation of the navel (umbilicus).
omphalocele A birth deformity in which the umbilicus (navel) has failed to close and to have skin grow over it. Thus, a large hernia of the navel exists and abdominal organs protrude through the opening.
omphalotomy The cutting of the umbilical cord.
onanism 1. Incomplete intercourse (coitus interruptus). 2. Masturbation.
onco- Prefix indicating relationship to a tumor.
oncogene A gene possessing the ability to promote the growth of malignant tumor.
oncogenic A substance that stimulates tumor formation, such as cigarette smoking and cancer of the lung; same as *carcinogenic.*
oncology The science of tumors.

ontogeny The whole of the development of a single organism.

onychia Inflammation of the nail bed of a finger or toe.

onychomalacia Softening of the fingernails or toenails.

onychomycosis A fungus infection of the finger or toenails.

onychophagist One who has the habit of biting his fingernails.

onychotomy A surgical operation upon a fingernail or toenail.

oocyte An egg cell before it is fertilized.

oogenesis The development of an egg within the ovary, prior to its expulsion from the ovary.

oophorectomy Surgical removal of an ovary.

oophoritis Inflammation of an ovary.

oophoron The ovary.

oophorosalpingitis Inflammation of a fallopian tube (salpinx) and an ovary, often resulting from a gonorrheal infection.

opacity The quality of not being transparent; of not allowing light to pass through; a cataract within a lens exhibits opacity.

opaque Not allowing light rays to pass through; not transparent.

open heart surgery Procedures performed on an exposed heart, usually with the use of a heart-lung bypass machine.

open reduction Setting a fracture by making an incision through the skin, exposing the broken bone ends, and bringing them into proper alignment.

operable A condition for which surgery will prove beneficial or curative; opposed to "inoperable."

operation 1. A surgical procedure. 2. The mode of action of a process.

operative risk The determination of how well or how poorly a patient will withstand surgery. A patient who may succumb to contemplated surgery is termed a bad operative risk.

operator The surgeon.

ophidism Poisoning due to snakebite.

ophthalmectomy Surgical removal (enucleation) of an eye.

ophthalmia Inflammation of the eye.

neonatorum Gonorrheal inflammation of the conjuctiva in a newborn.

Ophthalmologist A physician who specializes in diseases of the eye.

ophthalmomalacia Softening of the eyeball, with decreased tension.

ophthalmometer An instrument used to determine errors in vision.

ophthalmomyotomy An operation in which one or more of the muscles that control the eyeball are severed. (This procedure is performed to straighten crossed eyes.)

ophthalmoscope An instrument used to examine the interior of the eye, particularly the retina, the back inner lining of the eye on which images are registered.

ophthalmotomy A surgical incision into the eye. (This may be carried out for any number of conditions such as cataracts, glaucoma, etc.)

opiate A medicine containing opium or an opium derivative. Given to bring about sleep and relief of pain. (Morphine, codeine, heroin, Demerol are all opium derivatives.)

opisthotonos A spasm of the muscles of the back causing such arching that only the head and the feet touch the bed. (A condition seen in tetanus during a convulsion.)

opium An extract of poppy juice. As a medication, it is used to relieve pain and to produce sleep. Its great danger is its habit-forming quality.

opponens muscles Those that bring one part of the body opposite another, such as the *opponens muscle* of the thumb which brings the thumb opposite the other fingers.

opportunistic infection One not usually caused by bacteria or viruses, but becomes a serious infection in patients with a deficient immune system, such as those with AIDS.

opsomania An extraordinary desire to eat sweets, or other special foods.

opsonin A substance in blood which acts upon bacteria making them susceptible to destruction by white blood cells (phagocytes). Immunization increases the amount of opsonin in the blood.

opsonization The process by which bacteria are rendered susceptible to destruction.

optical Pertaining to the sense of sight or to the eyes.

Optician One who makes eyeglasses or lenses.

optic nerve The main nerve to the eye, arising in the brain. Injury or disease of this nerve may cause blindness.

neuritis Inflammation and possible degeneration of the main nerve supplying the eye. (Severe cases result in blindness.)

optimum The best condition in which body functions take place.

optometer An apparatus for determining errors in vision.

Optometrist One who measures or refracts eyes to note the need for eyeglasses.

O.R. Abbreviation for Operating Room.

oral Referring to the mouth (the oral cavity is the mouth).

hypoglycemic drugs Drugs taken by mouth to lower blood sugar levels, now being prescribed in the treatment of certain cases of diabetes.

type A term used in psychoanalysis to characterize certain people who show little sense of responsibility but who depend upon a mother or mother substitute to face their problems for them.

oral contraceptive A birth control pill.

orbicular muscles Circular muscles, such as the orbicular muscles surrounding the eyes and mouth.

orbit The bony socket in the skull in which the eye is set.

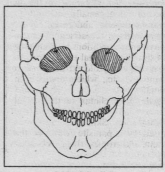

Orbit of the skull

orchidopexy An operation for undescended testicles in which the testicle is brought down into the scrotal sac and stitched in place.

orchiectomy Surgical removal of a testicle.

orchitis Inflammation of a testicle (mumps is a common cause of orchitis).

Orderly A male attendant in a hospital whose duties include helping nurses in the care of male patients.

Oreton A patented medication containing the male sex hormone, testosterone.

organ A specialized body structure which performs a specific function (the ear is the organ of hearing, the intestine is the organ of digestion, etc. *See* Manual for list of Important Organs.)

organic disease One associated with changes in the structure of an organ, as opposed to functional.

organism Anything that lives, either animal or plant.

organization 1. The process of repair of damaged or destroyed tissue. Specifically, organization means the growing into the damaged areas of new capillaries, blood vessels and connective tissue cells. 2. The characteristic relations of the elements of an organic structure.

organomegaly Enlargement of an internal organ, usually referring to organs within the abdominal cavity.

organotherapy Treatment of human diseases and conditions by the giving of extracts of animal tissue; such as the giving of thyroid extract, ovarian hormones, etc., which come from animals.

orgasm The climax of the sexual act.

oriental sore Skin ulcers and sores caused by a parasite found in the Orient and tropics, the *Leishmania tropica*.

oriented Aware of one's surroundings, as opposed to *disoriented*.

orifice An opening to a body cavity or tube, such as the mouth, the nostrils, the vagina, etc.

Ornithodoros Ticks. Some may carry germs that will affect humans. (Typhus fever, relapsing fever, etc., are thought to be caused through bites from this type of tick.)

ornithosis Psittacosis. A pneumonialike disease transmitted by an infected parrot, parakeet, etc. It is most serious and is accompanied by extremely high fever.

oropharynx The mouth and throat.

ortho- A term denoting something straight, normal, correct, etc.

Ortho Diaphragm A vaginal contraceptive diaphragm, in varying sizes to fit snugly.

orthodontia The branch of dentistry concerned with the straightening of teeth.

Orthodontist A dentist who specializes in straightening teeth and correcting improper bites.

Ortho-Gynol jelly A patented contraceptive jelly to be inserted into the vagina prior to intercourse.

orthokinetics The science of retraining muscles to perform new and different functions; advocated in some cases of advanced arthritis.

Orthomyxoviridae The group of

viruses that cause the various types of influenza.

Ortho Novum A birth control pill.

orthopedics The branch of medicine concerned with diseases and conditions involving muscles, tendons, joints, ligaments, cartilage and bones.

Orthopedist A physician who specializes in diseases of the bones, joints, muscles, tendons, etc.

orthopnea The need to sit up in order to breathe comfortably, usually associated with inadequate heart function.

orthopsychiatry The branch of psychiatry which deals mainly with mental and emotional development; it deals with prevention in that it points the way toward avoiding serious mental disorders.

orthoptics Exercises to improve the function of the eye muscles; often advocated for people with crossed eyes (strabismus) or those who have been operated upon for crossed eyes.

orthostatic Standing upright.

albuminuria Albumin in the urine in people who stand in one position for long periods of time (not a disease or abnormal condition).

os 1. A mouth. 2. A bone. *See* Manual for list of bones.

os calcis The heel bone.

oscillation Vibration.

osculate To kiss.

Osgood-Schlatter disease An inflammation of the bone of the leg (tibia) near the knee joint, seen mostly in teenagers.

Osler, Sir William (1849–1919) One of the greatest physicians of the turn of the century. He described several diseases of the blood and heart. Born in Canada, he spent much of his medical career as Professor of Medicine in various medical schools in the United States.

Osler-Vaquez disease Polycythemia, a disease characterized by the overproduction of red blood cells. It tends to be chronic and in later life may lead to the formation of clots within the blood vessels.

osmesis The act of smelling.

osmidrosis Body odor.

osmolarity The osmotic concentration of a solution. (*See* osmosis.)

osmology 1. The study of the sense of smell. 2. The branch of physics dealing with the phenomena of osmosis.

osmosis The passage of a substance through a membrane from a dilute to a concentrated solution.

osseous tissue Bony tissue.

ossicles The three small bones in the middle ear (the malleus, incus and the stapes). These bones vibrate when sound waves strike the eardrum.

ossiculectomy Surgical removal of one or more of the small bones of the ear. (Stapedectomy is frequently carried out to relieve deafness.)

ossification The transformation of nonbony tissue into bony tissue. (As people age, cartilage often turns into bone.)

osteal Pertaining to bone.

osteitis Inflammation of bone.

   deformans Inflammation of the bones, affecting mostly men in their fifties or sixties, often accompanied by marked deformity and thickening. Its cause is not known. Also called *Paget's disease* of bone.

   fibrosa cystica Inflammation and cyst formation in bones secondary to excessive parathyroid hormone activity or secondary to a tumor of the parathyroid glands in the neck.

osteo- Combining form denoting relationship to bone.

osteoarthritis A form of arthritis associated with bone and cartilage degeneration; seen most often in aging people.

osteoarthropathy Disease of the end of the bones at a joint; disease of the joint surface of the bone.

osteoarthrotomy Surgical incision into the bone surface of a joint.

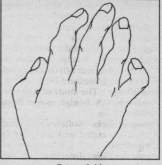
Osteoarthritis

osteochondritis Inflammation of a bone and its cartilage.

osteochondrodystrophy A type of dwarfism accompanied by an extremely short neck and body.

osteochondroma A nonmalignant tumor of bone and cartilage.

osteochondrosis Degeneration of bone growth centers in the bones of rapidly growing children. There is slow repair of the damage over a period of time but the bones may be permanently deformed.

osteoclasis A surgical procedure in which a bone is rebroken in order that it may be reset in better alignment.

osteodynia Pain in a bone.

osteodystrophy Imperfect bone formation resulting from disease, such as deformities which occur in cases of rickets.

osteofibrosis The degeneration of the bone marrow from a blood-producing structure to fibrous, nonfunctioning tissue. (Seen particularly in older people.)

osteogenesis Bone formation.

osteogenesis imperfecta A birth deformity of unknown cause in which there is imperfect bone formation, brittleness of bones and many fractures. Seen in newborns, infants and older children.

osteogenic sarcoma A highly malignant bone tumor, most often affecting the long bones in the arms or legs. It occurs mainly among teenagers or young adults.

osteoid osteoma A tumor occurring in the middle, softer portion of a bone. It is benign, causes a great deal of pain and affects mainly children and adolescents.

osteology The study of bones.

osteoma A benign, nonmalignant bone tumor.

osteomalacia Softening of bones, often associated with a lack of vitamin D.

osteomyelitis Infection of bone. This condition occurs much less frequently since the advent of antibiotic drugs.

Osteopathic physician One who uses the ordinary medical diagnostic and treatment measures, plus manipulative procedures which emphasize diseases of the bones.

osteopetrosis Hardening of the bones with increased density and destruction of the bone marrow. It is a rare, inherited disease. Also called *marble bones, ivory bones,* etc. Advanced cases may lead to severe anemia, blindness, bone fractures, etc.

osteoplasty Bone grafting.

osteoporosis A loss in bony substances producing brittleness and softness of bones; often seen in people of very advanced age or debility.

osteosarcoma A bone malignancy. These tumors tend to affect the long bones of the arms or legs, and are most common in children and adolescents.

osteosclerosis Abnormal hardening of the bones.

osteotome A surgical chisel used to cut bone.

osteotomy A surgical incision into bone.

ostium An opening or entrance to an organ or structure.

O.T. An abbreviation signifying old, outmoded terminology. Also occupational therapist.

otalgia Earache.

OTC Abbreviation for over the counter, signifying a drug that can be purchased without a doctor's prescription.

otic Relating to the ear.

otitis media Inflammation of the middle ear, seen most often in children following a cold, sore throat or some contagious disease such as measles.

otocleisis 1. Obstruction of the Eustachian tube which extends from the throat to the ear. (This condition can be caused by inflammation or by sudden change in atmospheric pressure as when descending in a plane.) 2. Obstruction of the external ear canal, as from a collection of wax.

otolaryngology The study of the ear, nose and throat, by the combination of the specialties of otology and laryngology.

otology The branch of medicine dealing with diseases of the ear.

-otomy A suffix meaning a surgical incision into an organ as cyst-*otomy* (cutting into the bladder).

otoplasty Plastic surgery on the ears, usually carried out for "lop ears" or "cauliflower ears."

otorrhea A discharge from the ear.

otosclerosis A common form of progressive deafness seen among people who are approaching middle or old age. (It is characterized by the overgrowth of bone in the area of the organ of hearing.)

otoscope A lighted instrument for examining the ear canal and eardrum.

ounce One-sixteenth of a pound.

outpatient *See* clinic.

ovarian Pertaining to the ovaries.

    follicle A sac or cavity within an ovary containing an egg. (Each month one of these follicles bursts, thus releasing an egg.)

ovariectomy Removal of an ovary (oophorectomy).

ovary The female reproductive gland, one on each side of the uterus. They are whitish-gray, oval in shape, and measure approximately 2×1 inches in diameter.

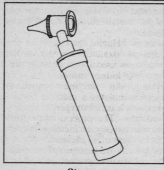

Otoscope

overbite A condition in which the teeth of the upper jaw overlap markedly the teeth of the lower jaw.

overextension Straightening of a point beyond normal limits.

overlay, emotional An upset in emotional equilibrium brought on by some physical condition.

overreaction An emotional response that is out of proportion to the stimulating factor.

overriding The sliding up of one part of a fractured bone on to the other. (Overriding must be overcome in order to properly reduce (set) the fracture.)

over the counter drug One that can be bought in a pharmacy without a doctor's prescription.

oviduct The fallopian or uterine tube; the salpinx. This hollow tube transports the egg from the region of the ovary to the uterus.

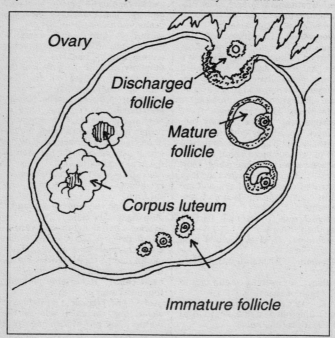

Ovary (cross-section structure)

oviparous Referring to an animal that lays eggs rather than gives birth to a live offspring.

ovotestis A sex gland in which both male and female tissues are present. (An infant born with ovotestis will suffer from hermaphroditism.)

ovoviviparous Bringing forth young after the hatching of an egg inside the body.

ovular Relating to an egg (ovum).

ovulation The process during which an egg is released from the ovary. In normal adult females this occurs once a month.

ovule The egg before it leaves the ovary.

Ovulen An anovulatory, birth control pill.

ovum An egg.

oxacillin An effective antibiotic against certain staphylococcal infections.

oxaluria Having an excess of the chemical oxalates in the urine, sometimes associated with the formation of kidney stones.

oxidase An enzyme (chemical) which stimulates a reaction involving the release of oxygen.

oxidation The process of combining with oxygen; an increase in positive valence of an element.

Oxycel A tradename for a gauze-like absorbable product used in surgery to stop bleeding and oozing from operative surfaces. (It is a cellulose material.)

oxycephaly A cone-shaped head.

oxygen An odorless gas necessary for life. The air we breathe is 20 per-

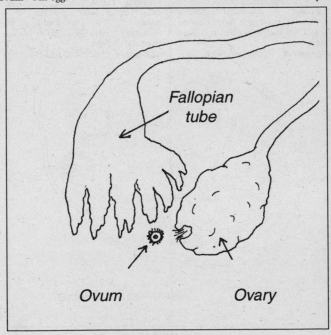

Ovulation

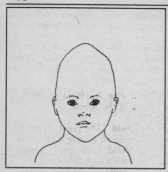

Oxycephaly

cent oxygen; the water we drink about 90 percent oxygen. The oxygen we breathe is carried to all tissues by the red blood cells.

oxygenase A chemical enzyme which extracts oxygen from inhaled air and makes it usable by body tissues.

oxygenation Perfusion with oxygen, as when a red blood cell takes on oxygen during the process of breathing.

oxyhemoglobin The combination of oxygen and the hemoglobin in the red blood cells. (This is the form in which oxygen is transported throughout the body.)

oxytetracycline (Terramycin) A powerful broad-spectrum antibiotic medication.

oxytocic A medication that accelerates childbirth.

oxytocin A hormone useful in promoting contractions of the uterus at the time of delivery; also stimulates milk production during lactation.

oxyuriasis An infestation of the intestines with pinworms, resulting in mild inflammation of the bowels and rectum.

Oxyuris Pinworms.

oz. Abbreviation for ounce.

ozone (O_3) A form of oxygen; the molecule containing three rather than two atoms.

ozostomia Halitosis; bad breath.

P

P Symbol for phosphorus.

P.A. Abbreviation for physician's assistant.

pacemaker, electrical An apparatus which stimulates the natural pacemaker mechanism in the heart, thus stimulating normal heart contractions.

pachy- Combining form meaning thickened, as in pachyderm, denoting a thick-skinned animal.

pachyderma 1. Elephantiasis. 2. Abnormal thickening of the skin.

pachydermoperiostosis An inherited condition showing swelling of the tips of the fingers, thickening of the bones, coarsening of the features of the face, and enlargement of the skin pores.

pachymeningitis Inflammation and thickening of the dura, the outer membrane covering the brain.

pacifier A rubber nipple or ring given to infants to suck upon when they cry or are teething.

pack A moist or wet application to a part of the body. It may be hot or cold, according to the specific condition it is meant to relieve.

Packed cell transfusion One in which the red and white blood cells are transfused, but not the serum.

pad A gauze dressing, usually applied to an irritated or wound area. (Foot pads are usually made of felt.)

Paget's disease 1. Paget's disease of bone is a disturbance in its metabolism associated with loss of calcium and eventually replacement in an irregular manner, causing considerable thickening and bone deformity. 2. Paget's disease of the nipple is accompanied by thickening of the skin and scaling. It is due to underlying cancer of the breast.

pain Hurt.

pain threshold The point at which one feels pain. A person with a low pain threshold feels pain sooner than one with a high threshold.

painter's colic Lead poisoning. The name refers to the severe abdominal cramps which sometimes accompany lead poisoning. (Painters used to be particularly susceptible to lead poisoning because of the high lead content of some paints.)

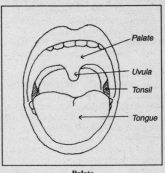

Palate

palate The roof of the mouth.

    cleft A birth deformity in which two sides of the palate have failed to meet in the midline; thus there is a direct opening between the nose cavity and the mouth cavity.

    hard That portion of the roof of the mouth which is covered by bone (the maxillary bones).

    soft That portion of the palate

behind the hard palate. It is composed only of soft tissues.

palatoplasty Surgical repair of a cleft palate, usually carried out within the first two or three years of life.

paleontology The study of fossils. (This science has given us much valuable information on animal life which existed millions of years ago.)

paliopsia Seeing something after the actual object has disappeared; afterimage.

pallesthesia The sense of vibration; unusual sensitivity to vibration.

palliation Relief of a condition but not necessarily cure of it.

palliative A medication given to relieve, not to cure; or a form of treatment directed toward relief rather than cure, as in some cases of extensive cancer.

pallidectomy Surgical destruction of ganglion cells in the thalamus of the brain, carried out to relieve the palsy of Parkinson's disease.

pallidum A portion of the brain which harbors important nerve centers.

pallor Paleness.

palm The inner surface of the hand.

palmature Webbed fingers.

palpable Able to be touched or felt, such as a palpable tumor.

palpation The act of feeling some organ or part of the body in order to make a diagnosis.

palpebral Referring to the eyelids.

palpebrate To wink.

palpitation Feeling one's own heart beat, usually associated with excessively forceful, "pounding" heart action. Seen during fright, excitement, etc.

palsy 1. Nerve paralysis or degeneration. 2. Commonly used to describe shaking of the hands. This is caused by degeneration of certain nerves at the base of the skull. 3. A tremor.

    Bell's A paralysis of one side of the face resulting in drooping of

the eyelid, inability to close the eyelid completely, and a twisting and drooping of the corner of the mouth. It is a rather common condition thought to be caused by a virus infection. It usually clears up spontaneously within several weeks but often leaves some slight permanent paralysis.

    birth Paralysis, usually of the shoulder or upper arm, brought on by injury during childbirth.

    bulbar A fatal disease in which there is degeneration of vital nerves in the brain.

    cerebral Paralysis caused by a defect within the brain. This is often a condition with which one is born.

    Erb's Paralysis of the muscles of the upper, outer arm, often resulting from a birth injury.

    shaking Parkinson's disease.

pampiniform plexus A group of veins in the male leading from the testicles and epididymis, not infrequently the site of varicose veins.

panacea A universal remedy.

panarthritis Inflammation of many joints, as opposed to one or two joints.

pancarditis Inflammation of all the structural components of the heart (often seen in severe rheumatic fever).

Pancoast tumor A malignant lung tumor located in the uppermost portion of the lung near the base of the neck.

pancreas A large gland—six to eight inches long—lying crosswise in the upper posterior portion of the abdomen. It secretes enzymes (chemicals) into the intestines for the digestion of foods and it manufactures insulin which it secretes into the bloodstream. (Insulin is essential for the proper utilization of sugar.)

pancreatectomy Surgical removal of the pancreas, occasionally performed when the gland is involved in cancer.

pancreatic cystic fibrosis An inherited disease of newborns, somewhat

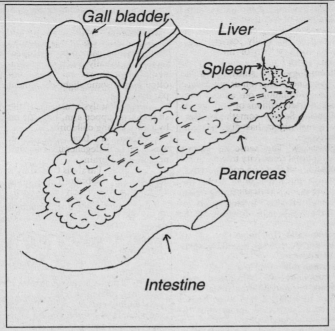

Gall bladder

Liver

Spleen

Pancreas

Intestine

Pancreas

similar to celiac disease. It is accompanied by undernourishment, large foul-smelling stools containing undigested fat, and the loss of large quantities of salt from the body. These children are very susceptible to lung infections and must be guarded against excessive heat.

pancreatic duct The tube which carries the secretions of the pancreas into the small intestine (duodenum). Also called the duct of Wirsung.

pancreatic transplant The transplantation of pancreas or pancreatic tissue. The procedure is in its experimental stage.

pancreatin An extract of hog's pancreas used as a medication for people with various intestinal disorders.

pancreatitis Inflammation of the pancreas. There are several types: 1. Acute hemorrhagic pancreatitis, sometimes associated with hemorrhage, shock and death. 2. Chronic interstitial pancreatitis associated with indigestion, inability to properly digest foods, foul-smelling stools, etc.

pancreatoduodenectomy Removal of both the pancreas and duodenum (first portion of the small intestine), performed for cancer of the pancreas.

pancreatolithiasis Stones in the duct of the pancreas.

pancytopenia Diminished amounts of red and white blood cells and blood platelets.

pandemic disease A disease occurring in epidemic proportions covering a whole state or an entire country.

panhysterectomy Complete removal of the uterus, cervix, tubes and ovaries.

panmetritis Inflammation of all the component structures of the uterus along with the tissues (broad ligaments) adjoining it.

panniculitis Inflammation of the fat beneath the skin on the abdomen, seen most often in stout people.

panniculus A layer of fat beneath the skin.

pannus The growth of tiny blood vessels and other tissue in the cornea of the eye, thus obscuring vision.

panophthalmitis Inflammation of all the component structures of the eye.

pansinusitis Inflammation of all the sinuses (frontal, maxillary, sphenoid, ethmoid).

pantaphobia Fearless.

Pantopaque A radiopaque substance injected into the spinal canal prior to taking X rays. It is used in cases of suspected spinal cord tumors or slipped disks.

pantothenic acid An important part of the vitamin B complex.

pantropic viruses Those which affect many organs.

panus An inflamed, swollen lymph gland.

Panwarfin A medication to prevent blood clotting. Its actions are similar to coumarin.

Papanicolaou test Examination of a vaginal smear for cancer cells. The vagina and cervix of the uterus are swabbed with cotton and the cells so obtained are placed under the microscope. Also called *Pap smear.*

papaverine A drug derived from opium which has the effect of relaxing muscles. It is therefore given to relieve many conditions in which spasm is a prominent feature.

papilla A small nipple-shaped prominence of tissue, such as the papilla of Vater in the duodenum at

the site where the bile duct enters the intestine.

papilledema Swelling of the optic nerve in the back of the eye. When seen through an ophthalmoscope, it may indicate increased pressure within the skull.

papillitis Inflammation of the optic nerve supplying the eye.

papilloma Any benign growth of surface lining cells, such as mucous membranes. Papillomas often grow on a stalk. Some of them may undergo cancerous changes.

papillomatosis The presence of many papillomas.

papillotomy An incision into the papilla of Vater at the terminal end of the common bile duct, sometimes done to relieve a stricture of the duct.

papule A pimple, or a pimple-like formation such as occurs in chickenpox or other diseases with skin eruptions.

para- A prefix meaning next to, resembling, related to, etc.

para-aminobenzoic acid Part of the vitamin B complex, used in the treatment of many conditions.

para-aminosalicylic acid (PAS) A valuable drug in the treatment of tuberculosis.

paracentesis Tapping a body cavity, such as the abdominal cavity, with a needle in order to draw off accumulated fluids.

Paradione An anti-epilepsy drug.

paraffinoma A tumor caused by the injection of paraffin beneath the skin. (This procedure has been carried out for cosmetic purposes to smooth out wrinkled skin.)

paraganglioma *See* pheochromocytoma.

paraglossia Swelling and enlargement of the tongue.

paragraphia Distorted writing secondary to a brain disease.

paraldehyde A medication given to produce sleep and calm the nerves. It gives an exceedingly un-

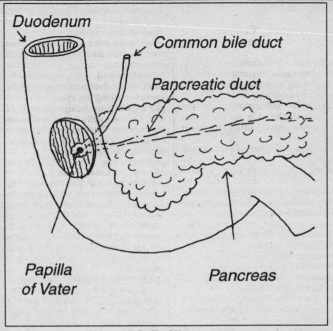

Duodenum

Common bile duct

Pancreatic duct

Papilla
of Vater

Pancreas

Papilla of Vater

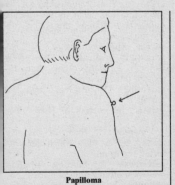

Papilloma

pleasant odor to the breath. (Used often to calm acute alcoholics.)

parallax The apparent change in the position of an object caused by a change in the position of the observer.

paralogia Inability to think logically.

paralysis Inability to use muscles because of disease or injury of the nerves which supply them.

paralysis agitans Parkinson's disease.

paralytic One who is paralyzed.

paramecium A form of one-celled organisms; protozoan.

paramedian Located alongside the midline, as the *paramedian* incision in the abdomen.

paramedical personnel Nurses, social service workers, technicians, dietitians, medical secretaries, etc., all of whom are part of the "medical team."

parameter A mathematical term.

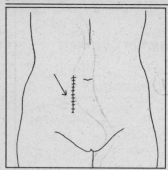

Paramedian incision, abdominal

A quantity whose value varies with the circumstances of its application.

parametritis Inflammation of the tissues surrounding the uterus, occasionally seen as a complication of childbirth.

parametrium The loose connective tissues which surround the uterus.

paranasal sinuses Those located surrounding the nose.

paranoid state One in which a person is affected by delusions of persecution.

paraphimosis Inflammation of the foreskin with constriction below the head of the penis.

paraplegic A person with both lower limbs paralyzed.

parapsychology The study of extrasensory perception, mental telepathy, etc.

pararectal abscess One located alongside the rectum.

parasexuality Any sex perversion.

parasitic disease One caused by an invading parasite, such as malaria, amebic dysentery, hookworm disease, etc.

parasitology The study of parasitic organisms, particularly those which invade animals and humans.

parasympathetic nerves The involuntary or autonomic nervous system which supplies nerves to the eyes, glands, heart, lungs, abdominal organs, genitals, etc.

parasympatholytic Referring to the blockage of the actions of the parasympathetic nerves.

parasympathomimetic drugs Those which stimulate the parasympathetic nerves.

parathormone The hormone secret- ed by the parathyroid glands.

parathyroid glands Four small endocrine glands located in the neck behind the thyroid gland. They secrete the hormone which controls calcium and phosphorus metabolism.

parathyroidectomy Surgical removal of one or more parathyroid glands; performed when the gland or glands are the site of a tumor.

paratrichosis Hair which grows abnormally or which grows in places where it is not ordinarily seen.

paratyphoid fever A disease resembling typhoid fever but caused by a different germ, the *Salmonella*. It is usually not as serious as typhoid fever.

paravertebral region The area located alongside the spinal column.

paregoric A medication used to stop diarrhea and severe colic. (Camphorated tincture of opium)

parenchymal tissue That part of an organ which is responsible for its main function, such as the glands lining the intestines, the air cells in the lungs, etc.

parent Mother or father.

parenteral medication One given through a route other than by mouth; thus, an injection.

parenting The art of being a parent.

paresis Incomplete or partial paralysis.

  general A form of insanity caused by syphilis which has affected the brain.

paresthesia A burning, tingling sensation often felt in neuritis.

pareunia Sexual intercourse.

parietal Referring to the wall of a cavity such as the parietal peritoneum which lines the abdominal cavity.

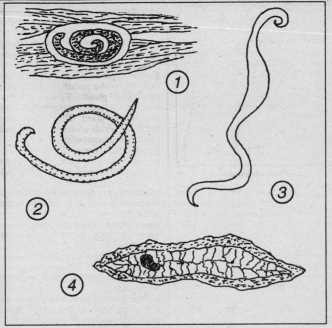

Parasites (assorted drawings of common ones)
1. Whipworm—life size
2. Hook worm
3a. Trichinosis larva in muscle
3b. Trichinosis adult
4. Liver fluke—life size

parietal bones Major bones of the skull lying behind the frontal bones. They make up the top of the head.

parietal cell vagotomy The cutting of those branches of the vagus nerve that supply the acid-secreting cells of the stomach. Frequently used in the treatment of duodenal ulcer.

parietes A wall, such as the chest or abdominal wall.

Paris green A valuable insecticide, extremely poisonous if eaten by man.

parkinsonism (Parkinson's disease) A nervous disease involving a rhythmic tremor, mask-like appearance to the face, rigidity of muscle action and slowing of all body motion. Also called *paralysis agitans* or *shaking palsy.*

parodontitis Inflammation around a tooth.

paronychia An inflammation around the fingernail or toenail. If pus develops, it must be opened surgically.

parosmia Distorted sense of smell, sometimes encountered in certain brain tumors or in mental illness.

parotidectomy Surgical removal of the parotid gland.

parotid gland The salivary gland

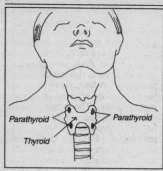

Parathyroid glands

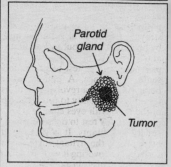

Parotid tumor

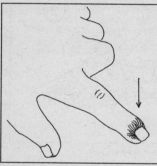

Paronychia

located at the angle of the jaw in front of and below the ear. Inflammation of this gland by a contagious virus is known as "mumps." The parotid secretes saliva into the mouth.

parotitis Inflammation of the parotid gland.

parous Referring to a woman who has had at least one child.

parovarian Located by the ovary, such as a *parovarian* cyst.

paroxysm A convulsion; a sudden, unexpected attack; a severe spasm.

paroxysmal fibrillation Episodes of irregular rapid heart action, usually abrupt in onset and termination.

paroxysmal tachycardia Episodes of rapid heartbeat, usually abrupt in onset and termination. The rate may fluctuate from 100 to 250 beats per minute.

parrot fever *See* psittacosis.

pars A part of an organ or structure.

parthenogenesis Reproduction without the necessity of fertilization, occurring only in some lower forms of animal life.

partial ileal bypass An operation excluding part of the small intestines; a procedure found effective in lowering cholesterol levels.

partial mastectomy An operation for removal of part of the breast, occasionally performed for a localized malignant tumor.

parturition Childbirth.

parumbilical pain Pain near the navel, encountered in cases of intestinal disorder or inflammation.

PAS Abbreviation for para-aminosalicylic acid.

passage A channel through an organ or structure.

passive Caused without active effort, such as *passive motion* of a limb carried out by someone else in the patient's behalf.

Pasteur, Louis (1822–1895) A French bacteriologist, generally regarded as the father of bacteriology. Among many contributions, he discovered the cause of pneumonia, rabies, anthrax, etc. Also, he was the first to use vaccine as protection against disease.

pasteurization The process of destroying the harmful germs in milk by heating it for about forty minutes at 60° C to 70° C.

past-pointing A test to note one's sense of balance. A patient, after being rotated in a revolving chair, is tested for the ability to touch the tip of the nose with eyes closed.

patch test A test to determine sensitivity to irritants. It is performed by applying the irritant to the skin surface and covering it with an adhesive patch. This is inspected a day or two later for characteristic reactions.

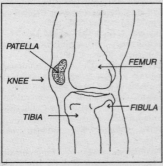

Patella

patella The kneecap.

patent Wide open, as the passageway through a blood vessel or the opening of the cervix during labor.

patent ductus arteriosus Failure of closure of the blood vessel connecting the pulmonary artery to the aorta in the fetus; such closure should take place at birth. Failure may require surgical ligation or cutting of the vessel.

patented medicine One that has a brand name or is owned by a pharmaceutical company or individuals. (Many do not require prescriptions.)

paternity test A test to determine if a man is the father of a child. If the blood type of the mother and

suspected father do not combine to create the blood type of the child, the man is not the father. However, the fact that the woman's and man's blood types are compatible with that of the child does not necessarily prove that he is the father.

pathogen A bacteria or virus capable of causing infection or disease.

pathogenesis The origin of a disease and the course leading up to its full development.

pathogenic Relating to the ability to cause disease (*Pathogenic* bacteria are those able to cause disease.)

pathognomic Referring to special signs and symptoms which distinguish a particular disease from all others.

pathological fracture One that takes place without injury or with minimal injury. This happens most often when a bone is involved in a disease process, such as a cyst or a tumor.

Pathologist A physician who specializes in the study of the exact nature of disease by examination of tissues grossly and microscopically.

pathology The science dealing with the nature of disease on the basis of examination of diseased tissues.

pathway A group of nerve fibers that transmit impulses from the nerve cell of origin, along a specified route, to other nerve cells and other nerve fibers.

patient One who is under the care of a physician.

patulous Open, as a *patulous* cervix.

pavex A machine used to increase circulation to the lower limbs in conditions in which there is disease of the blood vessels.

Paxil A drug for the treatment of mental depression.

Pb Symbol for lead.

PBI Abbreviation for *protein-bound iodine,* a test to determine thyroid function.

pCO₂ Symbol for the tension of carbon dioxide. When elevated, it indicates presence of acidosis; a *blood gas* determination.

PCP An abbreviation for *pneumocystis carinii pneumonia.*

peau d'orange The appearance of the skin of a patient who has an advanced breast cancer, looking like the skin of an orange. (French)

pectinase An enzyme which digests pectin, a sugar found in the rinds of citrus fruits and in apples.

pectinate Arranged like the teeth in a comb.

pectineal Referring to the region of the pubic bone.

pectoral muscles The chest muscles located in the upper chest region. They bring the arm close to the body and they move the shoulders forward.

pectus A general term denoting the chest or breast.

pederasty Anal intercourse with a boy.

Pediatrician A physician who specializes in diseases of children.

pedicle graft A skin graft transferred from one part of the body to another by use of a stalk or "pedicle."

pedicular Infested with lice.

pediculosis A skin condition caused by lice.

    capitis Head lice.

    corporis Body lice.

    palpebrarum Lice in the eyebrows.

    pubis Pubic-hair lice; "crabs" is the slang.

pedology Pediatrics; pediatry.

pedometer 1. A scale to measure a newborn child. 2. An apparatus attached to the leg to measure the distance one walks.

pedophilia Love of children. (A term sometimes used to describe an abnormal sexual love by adults for children.)

pedunculated Attached by a narrow stalk, as a *pedunculated* tumor which hangs down from the surface of the skin.

peeling Used to describe skin that is losing its outermost layer or layers.

PEEP Letters standing for "positive end-expiratory pressure," a method of mechanical ventilation of the lungs so as to retain more gas in the lungs after exhaling.

Pel-Ebstein's disease A disease resembling leukemia but not actually a true leukemia. Also called *pseudoleukemia.*

pelage The hairy part of the body.

pellagra A vitamin deficiency disease characterized by a rash on exposed body surfaces, diarrhea, ulcerations in the mouth and mental disorientation. It is due to a lack of nicotinic acid (P.P. factor) in the diet and may be seen among alcoholics who drink rather than eat.

pellicle The cuticle of the skin.

pelotherapy Treatment by the use of various muds or earth.

pelvic cavity The space occupied by the uterus, tubes, ovaries, and portions of the large bowel.

pelvic exenteration An operation which removes the organs and surrounding tissues from the pelvis.

pelvic inflammatory disease *See* PID.

pelvimetry, x-ray X rays taken prior to childbirth in order to determine the size of the walls of the pelvis and the child's head.

pelvis 1. The bony ring formed by

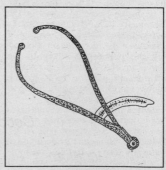

Pelvimeter

all the bones in the hip region, namely, the sacrum, coccyx, ilium, ischium and pubic bones. 2. Any basinlike structure, as the pelvis of the kidney.

contracted One in which the bones are smaller than normal and may interfere with normal childbirth.

flat One in which the diameter from front to back is shorter than normal.

frozen One that is involved in metastatic (spreading) cancer in organs such as the uterus, ovaries, or large bowel.

funnel One in which the outer measurements are normal but the outlet is so small that it may interfere with normal childbirth.

masculine A term applied to a female pelvis which is shaped like that of a male.

Naegele A pelvis deformed in an oblique diameter.

renal That portion of the kidney where the ureter commences. It is large and surrounds the section of the kidney which excretes the urine.

pelvisection Surgical cutting of one of the pelvic bones.

pemphigus A most serious skin disease with formation of large blisters, areas of skin slough, etc. (Before the advent of cortisone and the antibiotic drugs, most of these cases terminated fatally.)

pendulous Hanging down, as *pendulous* breasts.

penetrating An ulcer or wound

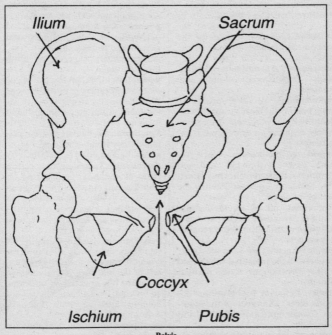

Ilium

Sacrum

Coccyx

Ischium

Pubis

Pelvis

which is eating through the wall of an organ or is piercing a body cavity.

penetration The entrance of the penis into the vagina.

penicillin An antibiotic (antibacterial) derived from the fungus, *Penicillium notatum*. It is the first truly antibiotic drug and is still among the most useful.

penicillinase A substance present in bacteria which combats the effect of penicillin.

penile prosthesis A silicone tube-like structure implanted into the penis in impotent men in order to permit them to have an erection.

penis The male sex organ.

penis envy A term used in psychoanalysis to denote the envy of the female child for the organ which she lacks.

Penrose drain A "cigarette drain." A soft rubber tube with gauze in its center which is inserted into the depths of a surgical wound for the purpose of drainage of pus, blood, etc.

pentaquine An antimalarial drug, often administered along with quinine.

pentobarbital A sleep-producing drug; one of the barbiturate group.

Pentothal A patented drug used widely as an intravenous general anesthetic.

Pepcid A medication which reduces gastric (stomach) acid and secretions, thereby relieving heartburn and indigestion, and aiding the healing of ulcers.

peppermint, oil of A medication used to stop nausea, to decrease gaseous distention and to overcome intestinal colic.

pepsin An enzyme (chemical) secreted from the intestinal tract to aid in the digestion of food, particularly protein.

peptic Referring to digestion.

peptic ulcer An ulcer of the stomach, duodenum or lower end of the esophagus.

peptones Basic proteins which are

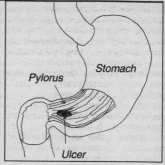

Peptic ulcer

changed, through metabolism, into amino acids which are absorbed through the intestinal wall into the blood stream.

Perandren A patented medication containing the male sex hormone.

percent Per hundred.

percentile A figure denoting what percentage of those taking a test a person equals, exceeds, or scores less well than.

perception The ability to recognize and interpret external stimuli.

Percodan A narcotic, pain-relieving medication; may become habit-forming.

Percorten A patented drug containing cortisone, a secretion of the adrenal gland.

percussion Tapping of various parts of the body and noting the sound which ensues. (This is an aid to diagnosis; *percussion* of the chest may indicate congestion of a lung.)

percutaneous Through the skin, as a *percutaneous* injection.

percutaneous cholangiography X-raying the bile ducts after inserting a needle through the chest wall into one of the bile ducts within the liver. After the bile duct has been located, an opaque dye is injected in order to demonstrate the bile ducts on X-ray film.

percutaneous transluminal coronary angioplasty X-ray demonstration of the coronary arteries of the heart after needling a blood vessel in the skin and passing a catheter (a polyester tube) into the heart. An opaque dye is then injected so as to outline the coronary arteries.

perennial Lasting throughout the year or for several years.

perforated Pierced, ruptured; having a hole through it.

perforated ulcer One which has broken through the structure, as in the stomach, that harbors it. Ruptured ulcer. In most instances, surgical repair is required.

perfusion The pouring or injecting of a fluid into or through an organ or structure of the body, in order to thoroughly permeate it.

peri- A prefix meaning *around; near; surrounding.*

perianal Located near the anus (the outlet of the rectum).

periappendicitis Inflammation of the outer coat and tissue surrounding the appendix.

periarteritis nodosa A disease, often fatal, involving inflammation along the course of arteries.

periarthritis Inflammation of the tissues surrounding a joint, sometimes leading to great restriction of joint motion.

pericardiectomy Removal of a portion of the pericardium, the sheath surrounding the heart; a procedure performed to relieve constriction of the heart by a pericardium which is thickened and tight.

pericardiocentesis Tapping the pericardial sac which surrounds the heart; carried out to remove collections of fluid, pus, or blood.

pericardiotomy A surgical incision into the pericardium, often performed to release adhesions of the pericardium to the heart muscle or to empty a collection of fluid or pus surrounding the heart.

pericarditis Inflammation of the sheath surrounding the heart. It may be acute or chronic; it may be accompanied by an outpouring of fluid

or a collection of pus in the pericardial sac.

pericardium The sheath of tissue encasing the heart. See illust. p. 266.

pericholecystitis Inflammation surrounding the gall bladder, in most instances secondary to an inflammation of the gall bladder.

perichondritis Inflammation around the cartilage of a joint.

periduodenitis Inflammation and adhesions about the duodenum.

perimetritis Inflammation of the tissues surrounding the uterus.

perimetry The limits of a visual field.

perimysium The sheath enclosing muscle fibers.

perinatal Referring to the time just preceding, during, or after birth.

perinatology That branch of medicine dealing with the fetus before it is born and the infant immediately after its birth.

perineoplasty Surgical repair of the tissue between the vagina and rectum. (This area is often torn during difficult childbirth.)

perineorrhaphy Same as perineoplasty.

perinephric abscess An abscess located around the kidney, often originating from the kidney.

perineum The tissue between the anus and scrotum in the male, or that between the anus and the vaginal opening in the female.

perineuritis Inflammation of the sheath surrounding a nerve (perineurium).

period, childbearing That from the onset of menstruation until the change of life (menopause), in which ova are extruded and are capable of being fertilized.

    gestation The period of pregnancy, or approximately 280 days.

    incubation The time from exposure to the germs until the development of the disease.

    monthly The menstrual period.

    "safe" Those times of the month when pregnancy cannot take

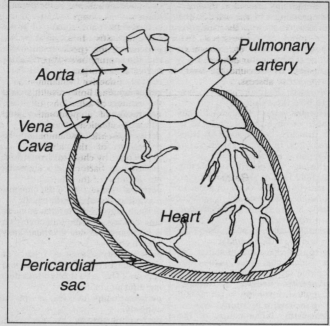

Pericardial sac

place. This varies markedly in different females.

periodicity The tendency for a thing to recur at regular intervals.

periodontia The dental specialty which concerns itself with the tissues, including the gums, immediately surrounding the teeth.

Periodontist A dentist who specializes in conditions which surround the teeth.

perioperative The period immediately preceding, during, and after a surgical procedure.

periosteum The thin tissue encasing bones.

periostitis An inflammation or infection of the tissue covering bones (the periosteum).

peripheral Near the surface; dis-

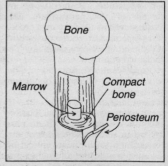

Periosteum

tant. (The opposite of proximal) Peripheral nerves are those supplying the arms and legs, etc.

peripheral vascular disease Abnormalities of the arteries or veins located outside of the chest. (Arteriosclerosis of the vessels in the legs, varicose veins, etc., constitute peripheral vascular diseases.)

perirectal Around the anus, as a *perirectal* abscess.

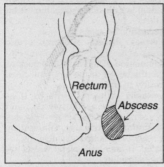

Perirectal absecess

perirenal Around the kidney, as a perirenal abscess.

perisplenitis Inflammation of the covering of the spleen.

perispondylitis Inflammation in the vicinity of the vertebrae.

peristalsis Contractions of the intestines, occurring in waves, which propel the intestinal contents onward.

peritendinitis Inflammation of the sheath covering a tendon.

perithelium Tissue surrounding small blood vessels and capillaries.

peritoneal cavity *See* abdominal cavity.

peritoneal dialysis Removal of fluid from the abdominal cavity.

peritoneoscope An instrument which is inserted through a small incision in the abdominal wall for the purpose of diagnosing disease within the abdominal cavity. It is a long metal tube through which the examining physician inspects the various organs. A type of laparoscope.

peritoneum The lining membrane of the abdominal (peritoneal) cavity. It is composed of a thin layer of cells.

peritonitis Infection of the abdominal lining (peritoneum) following the rupture of an appendix or other intestinal organ.

   adhesive Inflammation of the abdominal lining resulting in the formation of adhesions; often the end result of a peritonitis associated with infection.

   aseptic Inflammation of the lining of the abdominal cavity caused by chemical irritation rather than by bacteria, as after rupture of an ulcer of the stomach.

   diffuse An inflammation of the entire abdominal lining.

   localized Inflammation of one area of the abdominal lining, such as that associated with an appendix which has just ruptured.

   pelvic Inflammation of the abdominal lining associated with the disease in the ovaries and fallopian tubes.

   puerperal That type found following childbirth.

   purulent That type associated with pus formation, as after the rupture of an infected appendix.

   septic That associated with pus and a severe, generalized toxic reaction.

   tuberculous Inflammation of the abdominal lining caused by tuberculosis.

peritonsillar abscess Quinsy sore throat. An abscess of the tonsil which has spread to the tissues in the throat surrounding the tonsillar region.

peritonsillitis *See* quinsy sore throat.

Peritrate A medication to dilate blood vessels that have a tendency to go into spasm. Recommended for patients who suffer from angina pectoris.

perityphlitis Inflammation in the region of the bowel in the right lower portion of the abdomen (a term used frequently before appendicitis was known and recognized).

perivascular Located around a blood vessel.

PERLA Abbreviation used in describing physical examinations, meaning *Pupils equal, react to light and accommodation.*

perle A container (capsule) in which medications are placed so that they can be swallowed easily.

perlèche Cracking of the skin in the corners of the mouth, thought to be due to a vitamin B (riboflavin) deficiency or a fungus infection.

permeability of capillaries The characteristic of small blood vessels (capillaries) which permit certain molecules to pass through their walls.

permeable Allowing solutions and fine particles to pass through, as a *permeable* membrane.

permeate To pass through, as blood cells when they *permeate* the capillary membrane and thus gain access to the tissue spaces surrounding cells.

pernicious anemia Addison's anemia. Primary anemia. A specific type of anemia associated with lack of acid in the stomach, inflammation of the tip of the tongue and nervous disorders. It responds well to treatment with liver and stomach extracts, folic acid, vitamin B_{12}, etc.

pernicious (falciform) malaria A severe form of malaria, including symptoms relating to the brain, intestinal tract, and kidneys.

pernio Chilblains.

perodactylus One with absent or only partially developed fingers or toes.

peroneal region The region on the outer side of the leg.

peroral Through the mouth, as passing a stomach tube perorally.

per os By mouth, as the giving of a medicine *per os*, or food by mouth.

peroxide (H_2O_2) A common name for hydrogen peroxide, a mild anti-septic which releases oxygen and forms water.

per rectum Through the rectum, as giving a medication per rectum.

perseveration Continued repetition of words or actions. Excessive persistence.

personality The behavior, attitudes and total makeup of an individual which distinguish him from others.

perspire To sweat.

Perthes' disease A characteristic disease of the bone involving inflammation of the head and neck of the thighbone at the hip joint. Seen mostly in children.

pertussis Whooping cough. It is caused by *Hemophilus pertussis* and is accompanied by severe episodes of strenuous coughing, followed by a whooping sound when air is inhaled. It may last several weeks before subsiding.

perversion A deviation from the usual; a term often referring to abnormal sexual practices.

pes Foot.

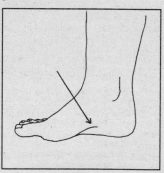

Arch of the foot

pes cavus Flatfoot.

pessary An appliance inserted into the vagina, usually as an aid toward maintaining the normal positions of the uterus and bladder.

pesticide A chemical used to kill lice, insects, etc.

petechiae Small, dot-sized hemorrhages into the skin or mucous membranes, encountered in patients who have a disease, often a fever, involving the whole body.

petit mal A minor epileptic attack associated with momentary loss of awareness but not accompanied by major convulsive episodes.

pétrissage Deep massage with kneading of muscles.

petrolatum A petroleum base used in the preparation of ointments. Also called petroleum jelly.

petrositis Infection of the petrous bone in the skull. This occurs as an extension of a mastoid bone infection.

petrous bone Part of the temporal bone on the side of the skull. It is close to the mastoid bone behind the ear and sometimes becomes infected in severe cases of mastoid infection.

Peyer's patches Patches of lymph-like tissue on the mucous membrane of the intestines.

Peyronie's disease A fibrous inflammation of the shaft of the penis resulting in a deformity (a bend) of the organ.

pH A symbol denoting acidity or alkalinity. A solution of pH 7 is neutral; below 7 is acid, above 7 is alkaline.

phacitis Inflammation of the lens of the eye.

phacocele A condition in which the lens of the eye is out of place.

phacolysis Surgical procedure for removal of the lens.

phacoscotasmus A condition of the lens of the eye in which clouding occurs and vision is impaired.

phacocystectomy An operation that removes part of the capsule of the lens of an eye.

phagocyte A body cell which can eat or destroy foreign matter or bacteria.

phagocytosis A process in which phagocytes destroy circulating bacteria, viruses or foreign bodies.

phagomania An uncontrollable desire for food.

phalanges The bones of the fingers or toes.

phalanx A bone of the fingers or toes.

phallic Pertaining to the penis.

phallus The penis.

phantasy Fantasy. A mental impression based upon imagination or unconscious wishes, not reality.

phantom limb A pain or sensation that a person imagines he has in a limb which has been amputated.

pharmaceutical Referring to pharmacy.

Pharmacist Druggist. Apothecary.

pharmacology The science dealing with the nature and action of drugs and medicines.

pharmacopeia (P) The standard book for drugs and drug formulas. The United States Pharmacopeia is the authoritative work in the field.

pharyngitis Sore throat. Inflammation of the mucous membrane of the pharynx.

pharyngoglossal Pertaining to the tongue and throat.

pharyngolaryngitis Inflammation of the pharynx (throat) and larynx (voice box).

pharyngorhinitis Inflammation of the nose and throat.

pharynx The area in the back of the nose and mouth. The throat.

Phazyme A medication given to reduce the amount of gas in the stomach and lower intestinal tract.

phenacaine A local anesthesia, frequently used to anesthetize the surface of the eye.

phenacetin A most useful drug for relieving headache and muscular pain, having much the same uses and effectiveness as aspirin. Acetophenetidin.

Phenaphen A drug to relieve pain and lower elevated temperature. (The medication does not contain salicylate.)

Phenergan A medication to relieve coughing, especially that related to allergic conditions.

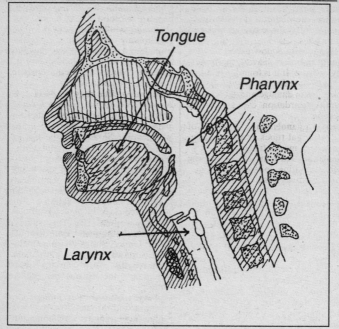

Pharynx

phenglutarimide Aturban, an anti-histamine drug used to combat sea-sickness or to control the symptoms of Ménière's disease.

phenmetrazine (Preludin) An appetite depressant; used to help obese patients curb their appetites.

phenobarbital One of the barbiturates, useful in calming the nerves and inducing sleep.

phenol Carbolic acid. In varying dilutions, it is used as an antiseptic and disinfectant.

phenolphthalein A basic ingredient of many laxatives; also used in chemical reactions.

phenomenon A sign or manifestation of a disease. Certain phenomena occur only in one particular disease and thus enable the physician to make a specific diagnosis.

phenotype A term used in genetics to denote an individual's particular inherited characteristics, especially those characteristics which display variations in inheritance.

phenylalanine An essential amino acid.

phenylbutazone Butazolidin, a drug used in the treatment of bursitis, sacroiliac sprain, arthritis, etc.

phenylhydrazine hydrochloride A drug used to reduce the number of red blood cells in cases of polycythemia, a disease characterized by an excess of red cells.

phenylketonuria (PKU disease) A congenital disease of newborns due to inability to metabolize the substance phenylalanine. As a consequence, the children develop brain damage, often have convulsions and skin rashes.

Every child is now tested for this condition before leaving the maternity division. If it is found, a diet low in phenylalanine is given. By so doing, brain damage and subsequent mental retardation can usually be prevented.

phenylpropanolamine A dilator of the bronchial tubes and a nasal decongestant medication.

phenytoin An anti-convulsion drug used in treating epilepsy.

pheochromocytoma A tumor of the adrenal gland often associated with markedly increased blood pressure. Surgical removal of the growth is followed by clearing of symptoms.

pheresis A technique in which blood is taken from a donor and is separated from some of its constituents, and the rest is given back to the donor.

phenotype A person distinguished by his visual appearance rather than by his hereditary characteristics.

Ph.G. Graduate pharmacist.

philiater A medical student or a person interested in medical science.

phimosis A condition in which the foreskin cannot be withdrawn over the head of the penis. In such cases, circumcision should be performed.

pHisoHex An antibacterial soap, used widely in surgical scrubs.

phlebectomy Excision of a vein; in eradicating varicose veins, the procedure is known as *stripping*.

phlebitis Inflammation of a vein; as evidenced by pain, swelling and tenderness in the area. If a superficial vein is involved, the *phlebitis* can be felt as a cordlike thickening along the vein.

phlebolith A calcified deposit in a vein, seen on X ray.

phleboplasty An operation to repair veins.

phlebothrombosis The development of a blood clot in a vein; not uncommon following surgery.

phlebotomy Bloodletting; occasionally carried out to reduce congestion in the lungs or high blood pressure.

phlegm Mucus secreted from the lungs or bronchial tubes.

phlegmasia alba dolens Milk leg, an infection of the veins following childbirth. (It sometimes leads to a permanently swollen limb.)

phlegmatic Slow; sluggish; lacking in alertness.

phlegmon An infection of soft, connective tissues usually extending over a wide area.

phobia An excessive fear; morbid dread.

phocomelia A birth deformity of the arms or legs.

photochemotherapy The use of chemotherapy drugs that have been or are exposed to ultraviolet light, thus enhancing their effectiveness in the treatment of certain malignancies.

phonate To vocalize; to speak.

phonetics That branch of medicine which deals with pronunciation and speech.

phonophobia Excessive fear of sound or of the spoken word.

phoresis The process of transmitting ions into the tissues by means of an electrical current.

phosphatase, acid A laboratory test for the presence of acid phosphatase. When present in excess amounts it sometimes indicates the spread of cancer of the prostate gland.

alkaline A laboratory blood test for alkaline phosphatase. When present in excess quantities it sometimes indicates the presence of obstruction to the outflow of bile from the liver to the intestinal tract.

phosphaturia Excessive excretion of phosphates in the urine.

phosphorus (P) A normal constituent in human blood.

phosphorus-32 Radioactive phosphorus, useful in the treatment of certain bone and bone marrow (blood-producing) diseases.

phossy jaw Slang term for destruction of the jawbone occurring in people who fail to take proper precautions when working with phosphorus.

photism A sensation of light or color resulting from stimulation of another sense, such as that of taste, smell, or hearing.

photo- Combining form meaning light.

photocoagulator A device which generates an intense light beam, of sufficient strength to destroy tissues. *See* laser.

photodermatitis A skin rash on areas exposed to light but stimulated originally by sensitivity to some drug.

photofluorography Photography of the images seen on a fluoroscopic screen.

photomania An abnormal desire for light.

photometer An instrument used to measure the intensity of light.

photomicrograph A photograph taken through a microscope to demonstrate the material on the microscopic slide.

photophobia Inability to withstand light; fear of light.

photopsia Seeing flashes of light, usually due to disease within the eye or in the nerve to the eye (optic nerve).

photoreceptor cells Those located in the retina; known as rod and cone cells.

photoretinopathy Diminished vision caused by overexposure to intense light.

photosensitization Excessive sensitization to sunlight after taking certain drugs or foods.

photosynthesis The process by which plants manufacture carbohydrates (sugars) from carbon dioxide and water. This process must be carried out in the presence of light.

phototherapy Treatment of disease with light, especially beneficial in certain cases of jaundice of the newborn.

phrenetic Frantic.

phrenic 1. Pertaining to the diaphragm. 2. Pertaining to the mind.

phrenicectomy Surgical cutting of the nerve to the diaphragm (phrenic nerve) in order to put a diseased lung to rest; an operation formerly performed in some cases of tuberculosis.

phrenic nerves The nerves supplying the diaphragm. They originate in the neck and travel through the chest to the diaphragm.

phrenocardia A neurotic condition associated with pain in the region of the heart and shortness of breath.

phrenology A bogus theory that one can tell fortunes by feeling and noting the shape of the skull.

phthisis An obsolete term for tuberculosis.

phylogeny The complete development of the species, from their simplest to their most complex form.

physiatrics Physical medicine, including physical therapy and rehabilitation techniques.

physic A laxative.

physical examination The inspection and examination of the body by a physician, including investigation with such instruments as the stethoscope, blood pressure apparatus, fluoroscope, laboratory testing equipment, etc.

physical medicine Rehabilitation medicine to aid people with physical disabilities.

physical therapy Treatments with manipulation, exercises, massage, diathermy, heat, cold, water bottles, electrical devices, etc.

Physician One licensed to practice medicine.

physician's assistant. *See* P.A.

physiochemical Referring to matters in which chemistry and physics are both involved.

physics The science which deals with matter and the laws of nature.

physiognomy Physical appearance, especially of the face.

physiology The science dealing with the study of the function of tissues or organs.

physiotherapy Treatment which utilizes physical agents such as heat, light, rays, water, etc.

physostigmine salicylate A drug which stimulates involuntary muscles such as those in the walls of the intestines. Useful in treating intestinal paralysis and certain muscular diseases such as myasthenia gravis.

phytobezoar A ball of foreign body such as hair, vegetable matter, etc., found in the stomachs of people (usually mentally unbalanced people) who have eaten large quantities of such material.

phytosis A disease caused by a vegetable parasite, such as athlete's foot.

phytotoxin A poison produced by a plant, often causing the body to react by forming an antitoxin.

pia arachnoid Two of the membranes covering the brain and spinal cord, composed of the pia mater and arachnoid.

pia mater The membrane covering the brain and spinal cord which contains the blood vessels.

pica The craving for odd foods sometimes encountered during pregnancy.

Pick's disease *See* Alzheimer's disease.

picrotoxin A drug used to combat the effects of barbiturate poisoning.

PID Abbreviation for *pelvic inflammatory disease,* a not uncommon condition associated with disease of the ovaries and fallopian tubes.

piebald skin Skin with patchy areas lacking in pigment; vitiligo.

pigeon-breast A deformity of the breastbone causing it to resemble the breast of a pigeon.

pigeon-toe A foot deformity characterized by walking with the toes and forefoot turned in.

pigmentation Discoloration by pigment, as on skin surfaces, etc.

pigmented Colored.

pilary Referring to hair.

pile A lay term for hemorrhoid.

sentinel A thickening of the membrane of the anus at the lower end of a fissure.

piliform Hairlike.

pill A tablet containing medicine.

Pill, the A slang expression for any one of the many birth control medications.

pilleus The caul; the membranes occasionally found covering the head of a newborn.

pilo- Combining form meaning hair.

pilocarpine A drug which stimulates the involuntary nerves and thus has the opposite effect of atropine. It is used to induce constriction of the pupil of the eye, urination and perspiration.

piloerection Hair standing on end.

pilonidal cyst A cyst located at the base of the spine, usually containing an accumulation of hairs. When irritated, infected or draining, such a cyst should be removed surgically.

pilosis Excessive growth of hair.

pimelorrhea Diarrhea with fat in the stool.

pimeluria Fat in the urine.

pimple A small abscess; a pustule.

pinch graft Skin grafting in which many pea-sized "pinches" of skin are placed in the raw area.

pinealectomy Surgical removal of the pineal gland, necessitated when it undergoes tumor formation.

pineal gland A small gland in the brain whose function is not clearly known. Tumors of the structure occasionally occur in children and are accompanied by precocious development of all sex characteristics.

pinealoma A tumor of the pineal gland.

piniform Cone-shaped.

pink-eye An inflammation of the

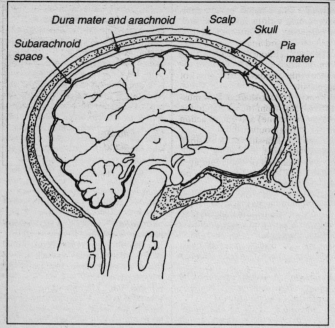

Dura mater and arachnoid   Scalp   Skull

Subarachnoid space   Pia mater

Pia mater

lining membrane of the eye; also known as Koch-Weeks conjunctivitis.

pinna The outer ear; the projecting portion of the ear.

pint Half a quart; sixteen fluid ounces.

pinta A tropical skin disease characterized by patchy changes in skin color and skin texture.

pinworm A parasite which sometimes invades the intestinal tract and rectum, causing inflammation of the bowel wall and rectal itching.

piperazine A chemical used to rid the body of certain worm infestations, such as round worms and pinworms.

pipe smoker's cancer One that develops on the lips.

pipette A glass tube used to suck up and transfer measured quantities of liquids. Used extensively in laboratories.

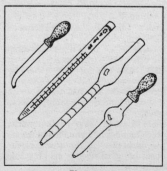

Pipettes

Pipracil Trade name for an antibiotic used in serious infections, such as peritonitis. It is effective against both aerobic and anaerobic bacteria. To be used cautiously because of adverse reactions.

piptonychia Spontaneous loss of fingernails.

piriform 1. Pear-shaped. 2. A muscle extending from the sacrum to the femur (thighbone) and whose action turns the thigh outward.

pisiform 1. Pea-shaped. 2. A small bone in the wrist.

pit An indented or depressed area of the body such as the armpit, pit of the stomach, etc.

pitchblende An ore containing both uranium and radium.

pithiatism Treating disease by suggestion, as in the treatment of hysterical paralysis.

Pitocin A patented medication causing powerful contractions of the uterus; employed sometimes during labor.

Pitressin A patented medication used to induce contraction of involuntary muscles, such as those of blood vessels, the uterus, etc.

pitting Making small indentations, such as the pitting of chickenpox.

pituitary gland An important endocrine gland located at the base of the brain. Its hormones regulate growth and seem to control the secretions of other endocrine glands, such as the thyroid and adrenals.

Pituitrin An extract of the posterior portion of the pituitary gland.

pityriasis rosea An acute skin disease sometimes accompanied by fever for a few weeks and characterized by pale red patches over the body; the patient gets well spontaneously.

PKU disease *See* phenylketonuria.

placebo A medicine having no active ingredient, given for the purpose of pleasing or calming the patient.

placenta The structure by which

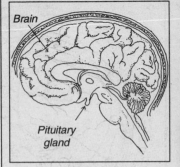

Pituitary gland

the embryo is attached to the wall of the uterus; the afterbirth.

    abruptio Separation of the placenta prematurely.

    previa A condition in which serious hemorrhage occurs during the latter part of pregnancy, caused by the placenta being located too low in the uterus.

    retained One not passed after childbirth. It usually has to be expressed or removed manually by the obstetrician.

placentography X-ray examination after injection of a radiopaque dye that lights up the placenta and permits diagnosis of its contours.

Placidyl A sleep-inducing medication. Advisable not to be used for more than a week or two at a time.

plagiocephaly An asymmetrical, deformed skull. Also called *wryhead*.

plague A highly contagious, often fatal, epidemic disease with high fever, enlargement of lymph glands, hemorrhage and mental confusion. It is transmitted to man by the bite of infected fleas from rats.

plane A natural dividing line between tissues, as the plane between muscles.

planing, skin A cosmetic surgical procedure in which the skin is planed with a rotating wire brush in

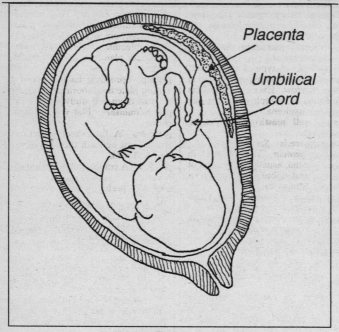

Placenta

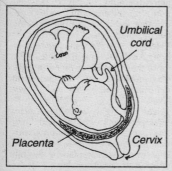

Placenta previa

order to smooth out its surface. Used in treating acne scars.

planotopokinesia Loss of sensation and appreciation of space.

plantar warts Painful warts on the sole of the feet.

plaque A circumscribed patch on a mucous membrane, the skin, or within an artery involved in aterios-clerosis. Also a deposit found on teeth.

plasma The fluid portion of blood, minus the red and white blood cells.

 antihemophilic A specially prepared plasma, obtained from a whole group of donors, containing large quantities of antihemophilic globulin. Used to stop bleeding in someone with hemophilia.

 dried Plasma from which the fluid has been removed. It can be stored for long periods of time, to be hydrated when required for use.

 plasma expander A substitute for plasma; often used in states of shock as an emergency procedure until blood or plasma can be obtained. *Dextran.*

plasma substitute Same as plasma expander.

plasma cell A type of white blood cell akin to the lymphocyte, found in bone marrow. Excessive numbers are found in multiple myeloma. *See* multiple myeloma.

plasma cell mastitis *See* ectasia, mammary.

plasmapheresis *See* pheresis.

plasma protein That found in blood plasma, usually in the form of albumin and globulin. *See* section on Blood Chemistries.

Plasmochin A medication effective in the treatment of malaria.

Plasmodium The parasite (protozoan) that causes malaria.

plasmolysis Shrinkage of a cell brought on by water loss.

plaster cast A hard appliance made of plaster of Paris encasing a limb which has been injured or fractured.

plastic surgery Surgery devoted to altering the shape of parts of the body or to the restoration of lost tissues.

plastron The breastbone and the rib cartilages attached to it.

platelets, blood Thrombocytes, the small colorless disks in circulating blood which aid in blood clotting.

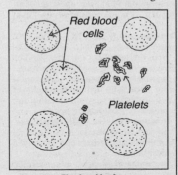

Platelets, blood

platelet transfusion The intravenous administration of blood platelets, usually employed when patients have a bleeding tendency due to inadequate platelets in the bloodstream.

plating Spreading bacteria onto a culture plate in a laboratory in order to grow them and study them.

platyhelminthes Flat worms; tapeworms.

platysma A thin sheet of muscle located just beneath the skin of the chin and neck.

pledget A cotton ball or cotton applicator.

pleo- A prefix denoting the word "more."

pleomorphic Referring to malignant cells which have a common origin but which have widely different appearances upon microscopic examination.

pleoptics Special exercises for those with impaired vision who have no demonstrable, organic (physical) disease of the eye.

plethoric Having an excess of blood in the body and therefore looking reddish.

pleura The membrane lining the chest cavity and covering the lungs. It is made up of a thin sheet of cells.

pleurectomy Surgical removal of the pleura.

pleurisy Inflammation of the lining of the chest cavity. It is associated with pain, aggravated on deep breathing or coughing.

pleuritis Pleurisy. Inflammation of the pleura.

pleurodynia A condition in which there is onset of sudden, severe pain in the side of the chest and down along the ribs. It lasts a few days and disappears spontaneously.

pleuropneumonia The coexistence of pleurisy and pneumonia.

plexus A network of nerves or blood vessels, as the celiac *plexus* in the upper abdomen.

plica A fold of tissue.

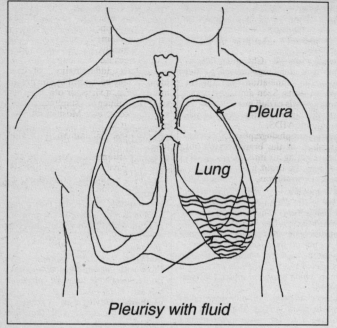

Pleura

Lung

Pleurisy with fluid

Pleurisy

plicate To fold tissue so as to form a double layer; carried out in surgery in the repair of certain hernias and muscle weaknesses.

plombage Injection of paraffin inside the chest cavity but outside of the lung in order to collapse a tuberculous lung. This procedure is no longer used since the advent of the new antituberculous drugs.

plug, cervical The plug of mucus normally found at the entrance to the uterus.

mucous Secretions obstructing the bronchial tubes in certain cases of lung collapse following surgical procedures.

plumbism Lead poisoning.

plutonium An element capable of undergoing nuclear fission.

pneum-; pneuma-; pneumo- Combining form meaning air.

pneumarthrography X-ray examination of a joint after injection of air or an opaque substance to "light up" the joint.

pneumatology 1. The science of gases, especially with reference to their therapeutic capacities. 2. The science of respiration or breathing.

pneumatosis cystoides intestinalis Gas formation within the walls of the intestine, a rare condition caused by gas-forming bacteria.

pneumaturia Gas in the urine, usually due to a fistula (an abnormal communication) between the bowel and bladder.

pneumobacillus Klebsiella, a form of bacteria causing infection of the lungs.

pneumococcemia Blood poisoning (septicemia) caused by the presence of the pneumococcus in the blood.

pneumococcus A germ causing pneumonia.

pneumoconiosis Chronic inflammation of the lungs caused by the prolonged inhalation of certain types of dusts. Seen among miners.

pneumocystis carinii pneumonia A viral pneumonia often seen in patients with AIDS.

pneumoencephalography X-ray examination of the brain carried out after injecting air into the space surrounding the brain.

pneumohemothorax Air and blood in the chest cavity surrounding the lungs, sometimes the result of a stab or bullet wound of the chest.

pneumolysis The cutting of adhesions between the lung and the chest wall. Such adhesions are found in old cases of tuberculous infection.

pneumonectomy Removal of a lung surgically, most often performed because of a lung tumor.

pneumonia Inflammation of the lungs. It may be caused by the pneumonia germ, a virus, or other germs such as influenza, staphylococcus, streptococcus, etc. Most cases can now be cured.

pneumonitis Inflammation of the lung.

pneumoperitoneum Air in the abdominal cavity. This condition is sometimes created artificially in order to obtain by X ray an outline of the various abdominal organs.

pneumothorax Air in the pleural (chest) cavity surrounding the lung.

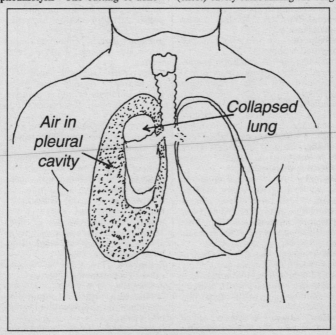

Air in pleural cavity

Collapsed lung

Pneumothorax

Often, this condition is the result of the rupture of a bleb (blister) on the lung surface.

Pneumovax An effective vaccine that protects against pneumonia caused by the pneumococcus bacteria.

pO₂ Symbol for tension of oxygen. When lower than normal, it indicates presence of acidosis; a *blood gas* determination.

pock mark The scar left from a small pimple associated with an erupted fever, such as from smallpox or chickenpox.

podalic Referring to the feet.

podalic version Changing the position of the baby within the mother's uterus so that it will be delivered feet first.

Podiatrist A specialist in conditions affecting the feet.

podophyllum A laxative. Also called *mandrake.*

poikilocyte An irregularly shaped large red blood cell.

poikilocytosis A condition characterized by the presence of deformed red blood cells, as in certain types of anemia.

poikilothermic Cold-blooded, unable to regulate body temperature to counter the environment; referring to a variable body temperature.

pointing Said of an abscess which is "coming to a head," or approaching the surface.

poisoning A toxic condition caused by bacteria, drugs, medications, spoiled foods, bites, contact with certain plants, etc. Almost any substance can cause poisoning if the particular person reacts unfavorably to it.

poison ivy A vine, *Rhus toxicodendron,* which on contact can cause a skin inflammation and dermatitis.

poison oak A plant which causes a dermatitis similar to that from poison ivy.

poison sumac A shrub which causes a skin condition similar to that from poison ivy.

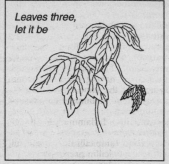

Leaves three, let it be

Poison ivy

poker-back A stiff spine caused by arthritis of the vertebrae of long duration.

polarity The quality of having two opposite poles, as in a magnet.

polio An abbreviation for poliomyelitis (infantile paralysis).

polioencephalitis Inflammation of the brain, especially of the gray matter.

poliomyelitis Infantile paralysis.

    abortive A mild form of infantile paralysis in which paralysis does not develop. It subsides within a few days.

    bulbar A severe, often fatal, form of infantile paralysis involving the base of the brain.

    nonparalytic Poliomyelitis without paralysis.

poliosis Early graying of the hair.

Politzer's bag An apparatus, used by nose and throat specialists, to inflate the middle ear.

pollen The microspores of flowering plants which are carried by the air. They may act as irritants to allergic people.

pollenosis Hay fever or asthma caused by sensitivity to pollen.

pollex The thumb.

pollicization An operation in which one of the fingers is converted into a thumb. (The procedure is performed when a thumb has been lost in an accident or when none has developed because of a birth deformity.)

pollinosis Hay fever.

pollution Unclean.

poly- Combining form meaning "many"; "excessive."

polyandry The socially sanctioned practice of having more than one husband at the same time.

polyarteritis Inflammation of several arteries.

polyarthritis Inflammation of several joints.

Polycillin (ampicillin) A powerful synthetic penicillin preparation.

polycystic kidneys A condition in which the kidneys have innumerable cysts. This condition usually is present from birth and eventually results in inadequate kidney function.

polycythemia A disease characterized by too many red blood cells. It is associated with an enlarged spleen, hemorrhages from the nose, mouth, intestinal tract, etc.

polydactyly Having more than five fingers or toes on each hand or foot, respectively.

polydipsia Excessive thirst.

polyethylene A plastic material which can be molded into the shape of a tube. Such tubes are used as a stomach tube, as a tube inserted into the veins for intravenous feedings, etc.

polygamous Referring to a society in which a man or woman can have more than one spouse at the same time.

polygraph A lie detector.

polymer Something with a high molecular weight. (Starch is a polymer of sugar.)

polymorphic Occurring in several forms.

polymorphonuclear leukocyte A white blood cell in which the nucleus has several parts.

polymyositis Inflammation of several groups of muscles.

polymyxin B An antibiotic drug particularly effective in treating infections of the urinary tract and in meningitis. It is the drug of choice against the Pseudomonas bacteria. (Also known as Aerosporin.)

polyneuritis Inflammation of many nerves; a condition sometimes encountered in diabetes, chronic alcoholism, etc.

polyp A growth, usually nonmalignant, of mucous membranes. Such tumors usually arise from stalks or pedicles.

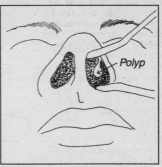

Polyp of the Nose

polypectomy Removal of a polyp.

polyphagia Excessive eating.

polypoid Polyp-shaped.

polyposis Having many polyps. A congenital (birth) condition of the large bowel in which there are many thousands of polyp growths. Such polyps usually become cancerous.

polysaccharides Starches; carbohydrates.

polyserositis *See* Pick's disease.

polysomy One or more extra chromosomes in the cells, often found in newborns with birth defects.

polythiazide (Renese) A drug used to reduce blood pressure and to increase the output of excess body fluids.

polyuria The passage of large quantities of urine.

polyvalent serum An antiserum containing several immunizing substances, such as influenza vaccine.

pompholyx A skin disease charac-

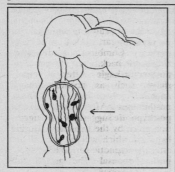

Polyposis of the large intestine

terized by blisters and peeling of the skin, particularly of the palms of the hands and the soles of feet.

pons 1. Part of base of the brain. 2. A slip of tissue connecting two parts of an organ.

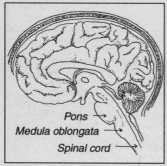

Pons
Medula oblongata
Spinal cord

Pons

Pontocaine A local anesthetic agent, used as a spinal anesthetic.

Popliteal bypass An operation in which a vein graft, or one composed of Dacron or Teflon, is hooked into the circulation in the thigh and leg, thus bypassing a blocked artery in the knee (popliteal) region.

popliteal region The back of the knee.

popliteus muscle A muscle located in the back of the knee.

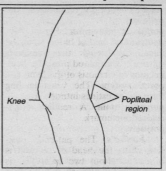

Knee
Popliteal region

Popliteal region

porcine Referring to pigs.

pore A tiny opening, such as the opening of a sweat gland on the surface of the skin.

porencephaly The presence of abnormal cavities in the cerebral portion of the brain.

pornography Obscene writings, paintings, etc.

porosis A condition in which the solidity of bone is impaired and calcium is replaced by cysts and soft tissue.

porphyria An upset in metabolism resulting in inadequate utilization of chemicals known as *porphyrins*. In certain people this condition leads to abdominal colic, paralysis, mental disturbance, skin eruptions and a brackish colored urine.

porrigo Skin disease of the scalp, such as dandruff, ringworm, dermatitis, etc.

Porro section Cesarean section operation for delivery of a child followed, during the same operation, by removal of the uterus (hysterectomy).

portacaval shunt An operation performed to relieve cirrhosis of the liver. The portal vein is stitched to the inferior vena cava, thus permitting blood from the intestines to bypass the obstructed cirrhotic liver.

porta hepatis That part of the liver which receives the important blood vessels (the portal vein and the hepatic artery).

portal hypertension Partial obstruction of flow of blood from the intestines through the liver, resulting in high blood pressure. Seen in cases of cirrhosis of the liver.

portal system The veins leading from the intestines into the liver.

portwine stain A reddish, wine-colored birthmark.

position

    Fowler's The patient's position when the head of his bed is raised up about two feet. This is used in cases of peritonitis so that the pus drains down to the pelvic region where its effects are somewhat less toxic.

    knee-chest A bent posture with the knees and chest touching the examining table. This position is sometimes used for examination of the rectum. It is also recommended to women who have recently given birth, in order to get the uterus to fall forward into its normal position.

    lithotomy The patient lies on her back with knees spread apart and bent. This position is used in order to perform a pelvic (vaginal) examination.

    recumbent Lying down or reclining.

    Sims' The patient lies on the left side with the right knee and thigh drawn up. This position permits a satisfactory rectal examination.

    Trendelenburg's The bed or operating table is tilted so that the patient's head is a foot or two below the level of the knees. This position is used in order to get more blood to the head and thus prevent shock. Also called *shock position.*

"positive serology" A loose term implying that the blood test shows the presence of syphilis.

post- A prefix meaning "after."

postconcussion neurosis Symptoms of an emotional nature that persist

long after a trauma, usually minor, to the head.

posterior Located in the back, or toward the rear.

postero- Combining form referring to the back.

posthemorrhagic After a hemorrhage, such as posthemorrhagic anemia.

posthumous After death.

posthypnotic suggestion A suggestion given by the hypnotizer during hypnosis which will be carried out after the hypnotic period has ended.

postmenopausal The period following menopause.

postmortem Autopsy. Necropsy. After death.

postnasal drip A discharge of mucus or pus which goes down the back of the nose into the throat.

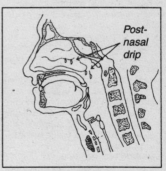

Postnasal drip

postnatal The period ensuing immediately after birth.

postoperative After surgery.

postpartum Following childbirth.

postpartum depression A depressed state of mind occasionally seen after childbirth. It may last several weeks or months, and usually clears up spontaneously.

postpartum hemorrhage That which originates during or after childbirth.

postprandial After eating.

post-traumatic After an injury, as

a *post-traumatic* neurosis following a head injury.

potable Fit to drink.

potassemia Excess potassium in the blood.

potassium (K) An element normally found in the blood.

potassium chloride The salt of potassium. Tablets are taken by people with potassium deficiency or for those who have low levels because of taking diuretic medications.

potassium permanganate An antiseptic solution, usually administered as a local application.

potency 1. Power, as the ability of the male to have sexual intercourse. 2. The power of a medication.

potentiation Improvement of the effects of one medication by addition of another medication.

potion A liquid medicine.

Pott's disease Tuberculosis of the spine.

Pott's fracture The most commonly encountered fracture above the ankle. It involves both the tibia and the fibula.

pouch Any anatomical area which forms the shape of a pocket or sac.

poultice A semisolid application of the skin for the purpose of bringing heat and added blood supply to the area, such as the old-fashioned mustard plaster.

pound (lb.) Sixteen ounces.

Poupart's ligament The ligament in the groin extending from the pubic bone to the crest of the hipbone. It marks the division between abdomen and thigh.

powder A mixture of medications pounded into fine powder for easy swallowing.

   Dover's A powder containing ipecac; used to promote perspiration.

   dusting A powder applied to the skin to decrease irritation.

   Sippy An antacid powder used in treating patients with peptic ulcer.

pox A small pus-pimple, as seen in chickenpox, smallpox, etc.

P.P. factor The factor in the vitamin B complex which prevents pellagra.

pragmatism A philosophy that teaches that things are only worthwhile if they are useful.

prandial Pertaining to a meal.

Pranone A patented medication composed of one of the ovarian hormones (progesterone).

prazepam A tranquilizer.

PRBC An abbreviation for packed red blood cells.

pre- A prefix meaning "before," "in front of," etc.

preagonal Just before death.

preanesthetic medication Medication given to quiet the patient prior to giving anesthesia.

preauricular In front of the ear.

precancerous mastopathy Diseases of the breast which show, on microscopic study, a tendency toward future cancer development.

precancerous Tumor tissue which is presently benign but which may develop into cancer.

precipitation A process by which a substance in solution is brought out of solution. This can be done by evaporation, freezing, adding chemicals, etc.

preclinical stage 1. The phase of a disease before the signs and symptoms have become apparent. 2. The end of the incubation period.

precocious Developing earlier than normal.

precognition Foretelling.

preconscious Thoughts that are not quite conscious, but can be recalled and brought to consciousness.

precordial pain Pain in the heart region.

precordium The region overlying the heart.

precursor A substance that goes to form another substance, as an inactive compound that is converted to an active one.

predigested Treated for easier digestion, as *predigested* food.

predisposition The state of being particularly susceptible to a certain condition or disease.

prednisone Cortisone tablets, administered in many conditions where steroid therapy appears to be indicated.

Prednisolone A patented cortisone preparation, often used in treating arthritis.

preeclampsia A toxic condition of pregnancy in which there is increased blood pressure, kidney damage, edema, but no convulsions.

prefrontal lobotomy A brain operation sometimes used in treating certain types of mental illness, such as melancholia.

pregnancy The condition of having a developing baby inside the body; "being with child." The normal human pregnancy lasts about 280 days.

   abdominal Pregnancy in which the embryo is developing within the abdominal cavity rather than in the uterus.

   ectopic Pregnancy developing outside the uterus, usually in the fallopian tube.

   false Phantom pregnancy; pseudocyesis. A hysterical condition in which the woman develops many of the signs of being pregnant, including enlargement of the abdomen, but is actually not pregnant.

   ovarian Pregnancy which takes place within the ovary; an extremely rare occurrence.

   phantom *See* pregnancy, false.

   tubal One developing in the fallopian tube; ectopic pregnancy.

pregnancy kits Devices for detection of pregnancy which are available for home use. (Most pharmacies sell them.)

prehension The act of grasping, as a newborn child will close its fingers around an object placed in its hand.

premalignant *See* precancerous.

premalignant dysplasia Microscopic findings suggestive of a benign tumor changing into a malignant one.

Premarin A patented medication containing estrogen, the female sex hormone.

premature Taking place before the proper time.

   ejaculation Discharge or expulsion of semen prior to insertion, or just after insertion, of the male organ into the vagina.

premature ventricular contractions *See* PVC.

prematurity Usually referring to delivery before forty weeks of pregnancy have elapsed.

premedication Giving quieting drugs prior to surgery.

premenstrual Before menstruation, as a premenstrual swelling of the breasts, or premenstrual tension.

premenstrual syndrome *See* premenstrual tension.

premenstrual tension A period of tension, irritability, headache, nervousness, swelling and pain in the breasts, seen in some women for the few days prior to menstruation.

premonition Foreknowledge; foreboding.

prenatal care Care of the mother during pregnancy, before childbirth.

   influence The theory that an unborn child can be influenced, either physically or psychically, by events which occur to its mother. "The child is nervous because his mother was frightened by a burglar while she was carrying him." Very few physicians place credence in this theory!

   period The period from the time of conception until the onset of labor.

prenatal screening Detection of an abnormality or disease prior to birth.

preoperative procedures Measures carried out to prepare a patient for surgery.

prepatellar In front of the kneecap.

prepuce   The foreskin of the penis.

prepyloric   The region of the stomach just before the pylorus.

presacral neurectomy   The cutting of a nerve located in front of the sacrum, sometimes carried out to abolish severe menstrual pains.

presbyopia   Farsightedness due to old age.

prescription   Written instructions concerning medications or drugs to be administered.

presentation   The position of the baby within the uterus, particularly the position of the part which can be expected to emerge first from the cervix of the uterus.

    breech   The baby's buttocks and feet first.

    brow   The brow of the child's head first (a difficult position for delivery).

    cephalic   The baby's head first.

    face   The baby's face, usually the chin, first.

    footling   The baby's foot, or feet, first.

    transverse   The child lies crossways in the uterus. It cannot be delivered unless this position is changed.

    vertex   The back of the baby's head first. This is by far the most common and normal position.

pressor   A drug which causes a rise in blood pressure.

pressure   Stress, pull, tension.

    abdominal   Changes brought on by attempting to move the bowels, urinate, coughing, etc.

    arterial   The tension of the wall of the blood vessel.

    atmospheric   The pressure of the atmosphere. At sea level it is fifteen pounds to the square inch. It decreases as one moves upward.

    blood   The pressure exerted against the heart muscle by the blood within the heart. Measured with a blood pressure machine (a sphygmomanometer).

    intracranial   The pressure of the brain and its blood supply upon the bones of the skull

    intraocular   The tension within the eyeball.

    osmotic   The pressure existing between two solutions of differing strengths when they are separated by a permeable membrane.

    pulse   The difference in blood pressure when the heart is contracting and when it is relaxing.

    venous   The tension of blood in the veins.

presystolic   The interval just preceding heart contraction.

pretibial   Referring to the front of the leg; the shinbone area.

preventive medicine   The branch of medicine which concerns itself with the prevention of disease, whether communicable or not.

prevesical   Located in front of the urinary bladder.

priapism   An abnormally persistent erection of the male organ.

prickly heat   A skin rash, seen particularly in children, brought on by excessive heat and perspiration.

Prilosec   A medication found to be highly effective for the treatment of stomach ulcers.

primal scene   The first instance of a child observing his or her parents having intercourse.

primary cancer   The original site of the cancer.

primary medical care   The type in which the physician makes the initial contact with the patient.

primary union   Healing quickly and without infection.

Primaxin   Trade name for an antibiotic with effectiveness against an extremely wide range of bacteria.

primidone   Mysoline, an anticovulsant drug used in the treatment of epilepsy.

primipara   A woman who is having her first child.

primordial   Simple; undeveloped; primitive.

primrose dermatitis   A skin rash

brought on by sensitivity to a primrose plant.

Priscoline A patented medicine used in cases of arterial and venous disease of the legs. It acts by dilating small blood vessels.

privileged communication Confidential information given by a patient to his physician. A physician should not give out this information without the patient's consent.

Privine A nasal decongestant, usually used in drops or through spraying.

p.r.n. A prescription abbreviation signifying *pro re nata,* "whenever necessary."

proband The member of a family who calls attention to the need to study the family genetically.

Pro-Banthine A medication given to ulcer patients to decrease the amount of acid secreted in the stomach.

probe Any slender metal instrument used to explore wounds or orifices.

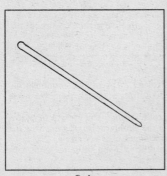

Probe

Probenecid A pain-relieving medication, especially beneficial in relieving the pain of acute gout.

proboscis The nose.

procainamide A drug that decreases irritability of heart muscle and is helpful in regulating an irregular heart, often used in conjunction with digitalis.

procaine A local anesthetic agent. Novocain is a patented form of procaine.

procarbazine A chemical agent used to treat certain malignant conditions, including Hodgkin's disease.

Procardia (mifedipine) A medication to prevent arterial constriction and spasm, thus lowering the incidence of attacks of angina pectoris.

procedure Any form of treatment, such as an operation or a regime for treating a medical condition.

process 1. A prominence; a bony outgrowth. 2. A set of circumstances or a group of occurrences leading to a given result.

    xiphoid The bony projection of the breastbone which extends downward.

procidentia A falling down, especially a "falling womb."

procreate To reproduce; to produce young ones.

proctalgia Pain in the anus or rectum.

proctectomy Surgical removal of the anus and rectum.

proctitis Inflammation of the anus and rectum.

proctocolitis Inflammation of the anus, rectum and large bowel.

Proctologist One who specializes in conditions of the anus and rectum.

proctoplasty Surgical repair of the anus and rectum.

proctoscope A hollow, metal tube inserted into the anus and rectum for the purpose of examination.

proctotomy, posterior An operation in which the rectum is opened through an incision made below the sacrum and coccyx in the lowermost portion of the back. Performed to remove a tumor of the rectum.

prodromal symptoms Early manifestations of a disease before it has developed.

professional Referring to a person thoroughly trained and certified in his occupation, or to the methods, manners, etc., of such a person.

professorial ranks Promotion differences between the teachers of a college. From lowest to highest: Assistant Professor, Associate Professor, Professor, Professor Emeritus (retired).

profundoplasty An operation to produce widening of an obstructed or narrowed deep femoral artery in the thigh.

progenitor A parent or ancestor.

progeny Offspring.

progeria Premature aging, a rare disease seen in children or adolescents. All the appearances of aging may be present. The cause is unknown.

progsterone The corpus luteum hormone secreted by the ovaries.

progesterone receptor test One to discover the influence of the ovarian hormone, progesteron, upon the growth of a breast cancer cell. (Positive receptors in postmenopausal women indicate the giving of a substance called *tamoxifen*.).

prognathism Having a jaw which juts forward.

prognosis Prediction as to the duration, course and outcome of a disease.

prognosticate To tell what outcome will eventuate.

progessive Referring to a disease that is advancing, usually unfavorably.

progressive muscular atrophy A disease of the spinal cord characterized by slow degeneration of some of the nerve cells within the cord. This process leads to wasting of certain muscles.

Progynon A patented medication containing the female sex hormone, estrogen.

projection In psychiatry, the process whereby someone displaces his own unconscious feelings onto someone else.

prolactin An anterior pituitary gland hormone that stimulates milk production.

prolactin adenoma A tumor of the pituitary gland in the base of the skull, often leading to cessation of menstruation and the secretion of milk from the breasts.

prolamine sulfate A medication that, when injected, tends to counteract some bleeding tendencies, especially when caused by an overdose of heparin. *See* heparin.

prolan The hormone secreted by the anterior portion of the pituitary gland.

prolapse The falling down (out of position) of an organ.

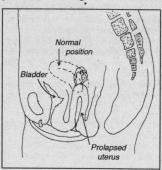

Prolapse of the uterus

Prolene A synthetic, nonabsorbable suture material, used by some surgeons as a substitute for silk.

proliferation The growth of tissue, as the proliferation of skin over the raw edges of a wound.

prolific Giving birth to many offspring.

Prolixin A drug used to treat certain types of psychosis, including schizophrenia. It is administered by injection.

Prolosec *See* omeprazole.

promazine A compound that helps to control the itching encountered in various skin diseases.

promethazine Phenergan. A drug with many clinical uses, including the prevention of motion sickness, the relief of allergic symptoms, the relief of cough, the control of nausea and vomiting associated with early pregnancy, etc.

promontory A projection; an anatomical term.

pronate To turn into a face down (*prone*) position. To *pronate* the arm means to turn the palm downward.

prone Lying face down; turned downward.

Pronestyl A medication to relieve heart irregularities, especially those due to irritability of the ventricles. (It reduces heart muscle excitability.)

propagate To reproduce; to have children.

Propecia A medication that is said to cause hair to grow on bald scalps of men and to diminish hair loss. It is estimated to be effective in approximately 80 percent of men. Propecia must be taken once a day for the remainder of one's life. Not to be used by women.

prophylactic Preventive.

prophylaxis Measures carried out to prevent disease.

propranolol An agent that tends to block the action of the autonomic nervous system, thus tending to lower blood pressure and to help patients with certain types of heart disease.

proprietary 1. A patented drug. 2. A privately owned hospital.

proprioceptive Referring to impulses from joints, tendons, muscles, etc. This sense is essential to proper position, balance, walking, etc.

proptosis Falling out of position of an organ, such as bulging of the eyes seen in some cases of overactivity of the thyroid gland; prolapse.

propylthiouracil A drug to slow down thyroid activity; used in cases of hyperthyroidism and toxic goiter.

Proscar A drug used in the treatment of enlargement of the prostate gland.

prostaglandin Fatty acids, found naturally in all people, that affect many body activities. They tend to lower blood pressure, regulate body temperature, stimulate contractions of the uterus and other involuntary muscles, and regulate acid secretion of the stomach.

Prostaphlin A synthetic penicillin preparation, reportedly effective in combating staphylococcal infections.

prostate The male gland behind the outlet of the urinary bladder.

prostatectomy Surgical removal of the prostate gland. It may be carried out in a number of different ways. The need for this procedure is occasioned by the overgrowth of the gland in older men.

Prostate Specific Antigen (PSA) Elevated amounts may indicate possibility of a cancer of the prostate gland.

prostatic calcium A calcium stone in the prostate gland.

prostatic massage Massage of the prostate done by inserting the finger into the rectum, to relieve congestion of the gland.

prostatism Noncancerous enlargement of the prostate gland, a frequent condition in men during their later years.

prostatitis Inflammation of the prostate gland. This condition may give pain in the bladder region, frequency of urination, blood in the urine, etc.

Prostep A medicated patch attached to the skin to help people stop smoking.

prosthesis An artificial part, such as an artificial limb, denture or eye.

Prostygmine Neostygmine, a useful drug for encouraging normal intestinal function and urination. Also used in certain muscle diseases, such as myasthenia gravis.

prostitution Sexual relations for money.

prostrated Exhausted; extremely weak.

protamine insulin A long-acting

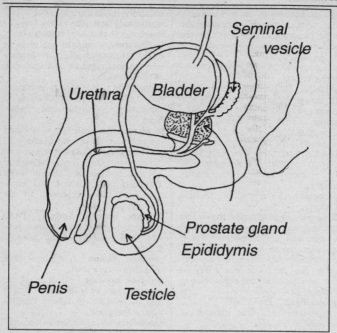

Prostate gland

insulin preparation absorbed slowly by the body, thus necessitating fewer injections each day.

protean Having many appearnaces and forms. A *protean* disease is one which has many characteristics, differing symptoms, and affects many different parts of the body.

protease An enzyme (chemical) which digests proteins.

protease inhibitors One of several drugs that act as anti-viral agents, especially against the HIV virus. These medications are most effective when used in combination with other drugs such as the widely used AZT.

protein-bound iodine test (PBI) A test for thyroid activity.

proteinosis A group of diseases as-

sociated with excess production of protein materials. When such materials collect in the lungs they can impair pulmonary function markedly.

   pulmonary alveolar A chronic lung disease, seen in adults, accompanied by collection of protein materials in the air sacs.

proteins A basic food substance containing nitrogen, characteristic of all living matter. Found in meats, vegetables, etc.

proteinuria Albuminuria. The appearance of any protein in the urine, frequently an indication of kidney disease.

proteolytic Referring to the destruction of proteins.

Proteus A genus of bacteria. Certain ones cause severe infections, particularly of the urinary tract and intestinal tract, very difficult to cure be cause of their great resistance to antibiotic drugs.

prothrombin A body protein which goes to form thrombin, an essential substance in blood clotting. Lack of adequate amounts of *prothrombin* may lead to excessive bleeding.

prothrombin time The time it takes blood to clot after adding calcium and thromboplastin. An increased clotting time may indicate presence of a blood abnormality, as in hemophilia.

protocol The clinical notes and records of a patient's case

proton The positively charged portion of an atom, constituting the nucleus. It is surrounded by negatively charged electrons.

protopathic Referring to a generalized, not highly defined sensation.

protoplasm The essential materials making up living cells.

Protostat A medication effective in combating trichomonas infections.

prototype An original model.

protozoa One-celled organisms; the lowest form of animal life. Some protozoa act as parasites and can cause serious disease in humans.

Protropin A growth hormone,

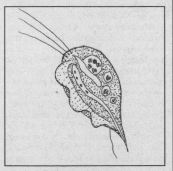
Trichomonas protozoan

sometimes given to children who are dwarfed or markedly undersized.

protrusion The projection outward of an organ or part of the body, as the *protrusion* of intestines through a hernia.

protuberance A localized swelling, something that sticks out from a flat surface.

proud flesh Overgrown tissue in a wound which has not yet healed. It is composed of many tiny blood vessels and connective tissue but still is not covered with skin (epithelium). Also called *granulation tissue*.

Proventil A medication to relieve spasm of the bronchial tubes.

Provera A patented medication composed of chemicals similar to the progesterone produced by the ovaries. It is given to women who fail to have abnormal uterine bleeding. It should not be given to women during the first few months of pregnancy.

Provest An effective birth control medication.

proximal Near the center of the body, as opposed to peripheral or distal. The elbow is proximal to the wrist.

proximal vagotomy Same as *parietal cell vagotomy.*

Prozac An anti-depressant medication, to be used only under medical supervision.

PRSO Abbreviation for Professional Standards Review Organization. This organization checks on the quality of care being rendered people through Medicare, Medicaid and other government supported programs.

prurigo Chronic inflammation of the skin with severe itching and little pink, irritated spots. The condition may continue on and off for many years.

pruritus Itching.

    ani Itching of the anus, a chronic condition usually of unknown origin. The scratching tends to bring on a dermatitis of the anal area which often proves difficult to cure.

    senilis Itching due to the aging process in the skin.

    vulvae Itching of the vulva and surrounding parts.

PSA An abbreviation for prostate specific antigen. When the results of this test are elevated, it may indicate the presence of a prostate gland cancer.

psammoma A tumor of the coverings (membranes) of the brain. When operated upon early, this type of tumor is curable.

pseudo- Combining form meaning false; or resembling but not actually a certain thing or condition.

pseudoacanthosis nigricans See acanthosis.

pseudoangina An emotional condition accompanied by pain in the heart region but with no concrete evidences of true heart disease.

pseudoarthrosis A false joint, usually the result of long-standing failure of fractured bone ends to unite.

pseudocyesis See pregnancy, false.

pseudocyst A false cyst; a collection of fluid in a sac that has no true cyst lining, as a *pseudocyst* of the pancreas.

pseudogout See chondral calcinosis.

pseudohermaphrodites An individual born with internal genitals of one sex but whose external characteristics resemble the opposite sex. Their sex organs and sex glands are usually incompletely formed.

pseudomembrane A false membrane.

pseudomembranous colitis A serious inflammation of the large bowel produced by the administration of large doses of antibiotics.

Pseudomonas A group of bacteria, some causing serious infections in humans.

pseudomucinous cystic tumors Tumors, often originating in the ovaries, which produce a mucouslike

secretion. They tend to grow and spread rapidly.

pseudopod A projection of the cell wall of an ameba enabling it to move about and to surround matter which it intends to eat.

pseudopolyposis Warty growths of the lining of the intestines seen in some cases of long-standing colitis; to be distinguished from true polyposis of the bowel, a birth deformity in which there are thousands of true polyp growths.

pseudopregnancy False pregnancy. A hysterical state in which a female to all outward appearances is pregnant, including the cessation of menstruation and the progressive enlargement of the abdomen, but no pregnancy exists.

psittacosis Parrot fever; a severe form of lung disease in humans, sometimes fatal, caused by a virus affecting parrots and other tropical birds. It is characterized by very high temperature reactions.

psoas muscles Muscles arising from the abdominal aspects of the vertebrae and running down along the posterior part of the abdomen to the pubic and thigh bones.

psoriasis A noncontagious, chronic skin disease with reddish silvery patches located on the chest, knees, and elbows. It may come and go throughout the patient's entire life.

psyche The mind.

psychedelic drugs Drugs that may produce hallucinations and/or distorted mental functioning.

psychiatric Referring to psychiatry.

Psychiatrist A physician who specializes in disorders of the mind.

psychoanalysis 1. A method of treating some mental disorders through analysis of the character, personality and mind. It is more applicable in treatment of neuroses than psychoses. 2. The theory that mental disorder results form repression from consciousness of unacceptable desires.

psychogenic disorder Any illness or imbalance of mental origin.

Psychologist A specialist, not necessarily a physician, who studies the function of the mind.

psychology The study of the mind and its functions.

psychomotor Concerned with voluntary, conscious movements.

psychomotor epilepsy A condition in which there may be only partial loss of consciousness. Such attacks may be brought on by fits of extreme anger or temper tantrums. Loss of memory of the attack sometimes occurs.

psychoneuroses Mental and emotional imbalance associated with anxiety states but not associated with loss of insight or loss of reality perception.

psychopathic Pertaining to severely disturbed behavior.

psychophysiology The study of the relationship between psychological and physiological processes.

psychosexual Pertaining to the emotional aspects of sex and sexual activity.

psychosis An extreme mental disorder, usually involving the functioning of the mind rather than organic disease; mental illness; insanity.

psychosomatic Pertaining to the mind and body.

psychosurgery Surgery upon the brain to relieve some forms of mental disorders. *See* lobotomy.

psychotherapy Treatment of mental disturbances.

psychotic Associated with psychosis; insane; mentally ill.

psyllium seeds A mild laxative, derived from the seeds of the psyllium plant.

pterygium A growth of mucous membrane extending over the inner portion of the conjunctiva of the eye.

pterygoid Wing-shaped.

ptilosis Loss of eyelashes.

ptomaine poisoning Food poison-

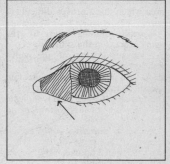

Pterygium

ing. A popular, nonmedical term for gastroenteritis caused by eating spoiled food.

ptosis 1. The dropping or falling out of position of an organ, as *ptosis* of the stomach; 2. a drooping eyelid.

PTH Abbreviation for *parathyroid hormone*.

ptyalin The chemical in saliva which starts the process of digestion of starches.

ptyalism Secretion of more saliva than necessary.

ptyalolithotomy Incision into a duct of a salivary gland in order to remove a stone.

ptysis Spitting.

ptysma Saliva.

puberty The period of life when the sex organs begin to mature; pubescence. Usually between twelve and eighteen years among residents of the United States.

pubescent Adolescent; during puberty; between the ages of twelve and eighteen years.

pubic hair Hair located on the skin of the lower abdomen around the pubis.

pubis The bones forming the front of the pelvis located at the bottom of the abdomen.

pudendum The external genitals, especially of the female.

puerile Childish.

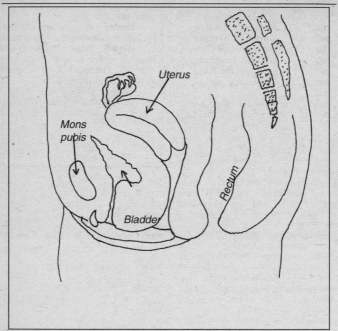

Mons pubis

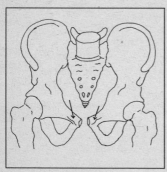

Pubic bones

puerperal Referring to or caused by childbirth, as *puerperal fever*.
   fever An infection following childbirth; "childbed fever." Before the days of antisepsis this was a common occurrence and caused many maternal deaths. Today, this condition is rare and when it does happen, the antibiotic drugs bring about a cure.

puerperium Childbirth; labor.

Pulex A type of flea. The Indian rat flea carries the germ causing plague.

pulmonary Pertaining to the lungs.
   edema The filling up of the lungs with fluid, as seen in certain types of heart failure. It can frequently be relieved by aiding heart function.

pulmonary embolism A blood clot to the lungs, often causing sudden death.

pulmonologist A physician specializing in diseases of the lungs.

pulmotor A machine to resuscitate those who have been asphyxiated. It establishes artificial respiration by pumping oxygen into the lungs.

pulsation A beating, as of the pulse.

pulse The wave felt when a finger is placed over an artery. The intermittent beat or wave is caused by heart contractions and in people with normal heart action, every heartbeat will create a pulse beat. A pulse can be felt over any sizable artery in the neck, head or limbs.

deficit The difference between the number of heart beats per minute and the number of pulses per minute. In normally beating hearts there should be no pulse deficit.

pulse generator A pacemaker that electrically sets heart rate.

pulsus alternans A pulse in which there are stronger and weaker beats, occurring at more or less regular intervals.

pulvule A capsule containing a powdered medicine.

pump

breast An apparatus to remove milk from a nursing breast.

cardiac Any one of many machines used in heart surgery to circulate blood while the surgeon works upon the heart.

stomach An apparatus to empty the stomach; used especially in cases of poisoning.

pump-oxygenator A heart-lung machine that substitutes for the patient's heart and lungs during open-heart surgery.

punch drunk A state of acquired feeblemindedness seen in prize fighters after many years of head blows which have caused small hemorrhages within the brain.

punctate Mark with many tiny dots; *punctate hemorrhages* are many, tiny, pinpoint areas of hemorrhage.

puncture

lumbar A spinal tap; placing a syringe needle into the spinal canal.

sternal Puncturing the breastbone in order to get a sample of marrow. Carried out to diagnose various blood diseases.

wound One made with a pointed object; particularly dangerous if germs are thus carried into the deep tissues.

PUO *See* FUO.

pupil The place in the center of the eye through which light is admitted. It contracts in bright light and dilates in the dark.

pupillary Pertaining to the pupil.

purgative Laxative; cathartic.

Purinethol Brand name for a chemical agent used in the treatment of acute lymphocytic leukemia; mercaptopurine.

purpura Hemorrhage into the skin, characterized by a bluish appearance of the skin. There are several causes of this condition, one of the most frequent being an inadequate number of platelets in the blood.

purse-string operation A surgical procedure in which the cervix of a pregnant woman is closed tightly with a purse-string in order to prevent a subsequent miscarriage. Also called *Shirodkar's procedure*.

purulent Containing pus.

pus The end product of many infections; fluid containing dead cells, dead tissue, and white blood cells.

pustule A small abscess, filled with pus.

putrefaction Decomposition of tissue as a result of the action of bacteria, as seen in gangrene.

putrified Rotten; decayed.

PVC Abbreviation for *premature ventricular contractions,* an extrasystole, or "skipped heartbeat."

PVD Abbreviation for *peripheral vascular disease.*

pyelitis Infection of the pelvis (outlet) of the kidney.

pyelograms X-ray plates, taken

after specific dyes have been given to outline the pelvis (outlet) of the kidneys.

pyelonephritis Inflammation, due to the action of bacteria, involving the kidney and its outlet, the pelvis of the kidney.

pyelotomy An incision into the pelvis of the kidney, usually performed to remove kidney stones.

pyemia A generalized condition associated with bacteria in the blood and the development of abscesses where the bacteria finally lodge.

pyknic Having a thick and stocky body build.

pyknolepsy An inherited form of minor epilepsy, occurring in females.

pylephlebitis Inflammation of the portal vein, the vein bringing blood from the intestines to the liver. (It is usually caused by infection somewhere in the intestines which spreads up to the portal vein.)

pylorectomy Surgical removal of the pyloric portion of the stomach; a form of partial stomach removal.

pyloric stenosis Constriction of the outlet of the stomach. The congenial type is seen during the first few weeks of life and is characterized by overgrowth of the muscles surrounding the outlet of the stomach.

pyloric ulcer An ulcer of the stomach near its outlet. *See* helicobacter pylori.

pyloroplasty A surgical operation to broaden the passageway from the stomach into the duodenum. Sometimes carried out in cases where an ulcer has caused a constriction of the pylorus.

pylorospasm Severe spasm of the sphincter muscle of the pylorus causing severe pain in the upper abdomen.

pylorus The far end of the stomach just before the duodenum.

pyo- A prefix referring to the word "pus".

pyoderma A pustular (pus-formed) condition of the skin. The pus lesions may be in the form of small pimples, abscesses or carbuncles.

pyogenic Pus-forming, as *pyogenic* bacteria.

pyometritis An inflammation of the lining of the uterus, accompanied by the discharge of pus from the vagina.

pyonephritis Inflammation of the kidney with the discharge of pus.

pyopneumothorax A condition in which there is pus and air in the pleural cavity surrounding the lung; a type of empyema.

pyorrhea 1. A discharge composed of us. 2. An inflammation of the gums about the teeth with pus formation.

pyosalpinx Pus in the fallopian tube. Often the result of an infection caused by gonorrhea.

pyrazinamide An antituberculosis drug.

pyretic condition One associated with fever (elevated temperature).

pyrexia Fever.

Pyribenzamine A patented medication containing antihistamines. Used to relieve the symptoms caused by certain allergies such as hay fever, hives, etc.

Pyridium A patented medication given to relieve urinary symptoms such as frequency, burning and pain on urination.

pyro- Combining form meaning heat or fire.

pyrogallol A medication applied locally in the treatment of psoriasis and other skin conditions.

pyrogen A substance, usually composed of protein, which will cause fever when injected. (Pyrogens often cling to tubing or are found in sterile solutions and when an intravenous injection is given, the patient develops chills and high fever which may last for several hours.)

pyrogenic Causing fever.

pyromania An irrational desire to set fires.

pyrosis Heartburn.

pyuria Pus in the urine, denoting an inflammation within the urinary tract.

PZI Initials for protamine zinc insulin, a common form of the medication.

Q

Q fever An infection caused by one of the rickettsia, the bacterialike parasites which are carried by ticks and lice. The bite of such an infected tick or louse causes the symptoms of Q fever: high fever, inflammation of the lungs, nausea and vomiting. Recovery in a few days is the rule.

q.h. A prescription symbol meaning *quaque hora,* every hour. *q 2 h* is every two hours, *q 3 h* is every three hours, etc.

q.i.d. A prescription symbol meaning *quater in die,* four times daily.

QRS complex A phase in heart action, noted on an electrocardiogram.

q.s. A prescription symbol meaning *quantum satis,* as much as is sufficient.

qt. Abbreviation for quart.

quack A fake doctor; an untrained person posing as a physician.

quadrant A quarter of, such as the right upper quadrant of the abdomen.

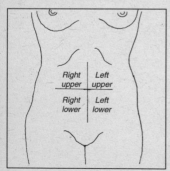

Quadrants of the abdomen

quadriceps The large muscles in the front of the thigh. They straighten the knee joint.

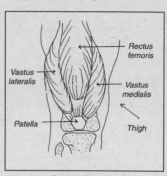

Quadriceps muscles

quadriplegia Paralysis of all four limbs, as in certain spinal cord injuries.

quadruplet Any one of four children born at one birth.

qualitative Referring to quality.

quantitative Referring to quantity.

quantum A certain amount.

quarantine The detaining and isolating of people who have been exposed to contagious diseases. When the incubation period (the time during which they might develop the disease) has elapsed without their manifesting the disease, they are allowed to go their way.

quartan Occurring every fourth day, as in certain fevers wherein there is a marked temperature rise and chill every fourth day.

Queckenstedt's test *See* tests.

querulous Complaining; argumentative.

Quibron An effective medication for relieving spasm of the bronchial tubes.

quick 1. Alive; pregnant with a moving baby; 2. the fingernail bed.

quickening The first sensations the mother has of the movements of her unborn child. This usually comes on during the fourth or fifth month of pregnancy.

Quick test A blood test to determine adequacy of liver function. Also, a test used to determine the ability of the blood to clot.

Quinacrine *See* Atabrine.

Quinamm A quinine preparation helpful in preventing muscle cramps.

quinidine A medication used to stop irregularities of the heart beat, such as flutter.

quinine A drug extracted from cinchona bark, specific in the treatment of malaria. Also used to relieve symptoms of grippe.

quinsy sore throat A severe infection of the tonsil associated with the formation of an abscess alongside the tonsil. This condition may require surgical incision of the abscess.

quintuplet Any one of five children born at one birth.

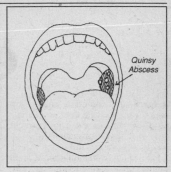

Quinsy
Abscess

Quinsy sore throat

quotane A local anesthetic agent, effective by surface application to the skin.

quotidian Occurring every day, as the quotidian chills and fever in certain forms of malaria, etc.

quotient, intelligence *See* intelligence quotient.

respiratory The ratio of the amount of carbon dioxide created to the amount of oxygen consumed in the lungs and other tissues. It is an index of the efficiency of lung function.

q.v. An abbreviation meaning *quantum vis,* as much as is desired.

R

Ra Chemical symbol for radium.

rabbit fever An infectious disease with high fever, swollen glands and weakness, due to a germ which gets into the body from handling infected rabbits.

rabid Having rabies (hydrophobia).

rabies A specific fatal infectious disease of animals such as dogs, cats, rabbits, squirrels, wolves, etc. It can be transmitted to man by the bite of one of these infected animals. Vaccination can prevent the onset in man if carried out soon after a bite.

rachiotomy *See* laminectomy.

rachis The spinal column.

rachitic Having rickets, a vitamin D deficiency disease.

rachitis Rickets.

radar kymography An instrument that permits the visualization of the heart's action on a video screen.

radial 1. Leading out from the center. *A radial incision* of the breast is one which extends out from the nipple. 2. Referring to the radius bone in the forearm.

radial keratotomy A procedure for the relief of nearsightedness, done by making several incisions in the cornea.

radiation The passage of energy through space. The energy may be transmitted by ultraviolet rays, X rays, gamma rays, cosmic rays, etc.

  sickness Nausea, vomiting and weakness as a reaction to large doses of X rays or other radiations from radioactive substances.

  therapy Treatment with X rays, or radium, cobalt and other radioactive materials.

radiation burn Burn that is caused by excess exposure to X rays, radium, nuclear products, sun, etc.

radiation cataract Cataracts formed in eyes that have been overexposed to X rays, radium, or other radioactive rays.

radiation dermatitis Inflammation of the skin caused by exposure to X-ray radiation.

radical hysterectomy Removal of the uterus, tubes, ovaries, upper vagina, and surrounding connective tissue, performed for a cancerous condition.

radical mastectomy Breast removal including the pectoral muscles and the lymph glands in the armpit. (The procedure was considered to be "radical" 75 or more years ago; today it is an operation fraught with little risk or danger as recovery from the surgery itself takes place in almost 100% of cases.)

radical treatment Extensive treatment. When applied to surgery, it implies an "all-out" attempt to eradicate a disease.

radicular Referring to the nerves originating in the spine.

radiculitis Inflammation of the root of a nerve, particularly of a nerve going to the spinal cord. It is accompanied by excruciating pain along the course of the nerve.

radiculopathy Disease of the spinal nerves.

radioactive Referring to any substance which emits radiant energy, such as radium.

radioactivity The emission of radioactive particles, such as alpha, beta or gamma particles.

radiocinematology A motion picture showing the movements of organs on X-ray examination.

tb**radiodermatitis** Skin condition (dermatitis) caused unavoidably by administration of X rays in a course of radiation treatment. (Taking an X-ray picture does *not* cause dermatitis.)

radiography The making of X rays.

radiohumeral Pertaining to a bone (the humerus) of the upper arm and one of the bones (the radius) of the forearm.

radioimmunoassay A method of determining, through immunological techniques, minute quantities of antibodies or antigens. *See* antibody; *see* antigen.

radioiodine Radioactive iodine, especially I^{131}, used as a medication in treating patients with certain forms of overactive thyroid disease and certain thyroid cancers.

radioisotope A stable, nonradioactive element which is bombarded in a nuclear reactor with neutrons, protons, or other particles so as to make it radioactive. Examples are radioactive iodine, cobalt, gold, and phosphorus.

Radiologist A physician who specializes in the use of X rays and radioactive substances, both for diagnostic and for treatment purposes.

radiology The branch of medicine dealing with radioactive substances and their use in diagnosing and treating disease.

radiolucent Permitting the passage of X rays through certain structures while not permitting them to pass through others, thus creating variable shadows on an X-ray film.

radionecrosis Destruction of tissue as a result of its having been exposed to radiation.

radiopaque Not transparent to X rays, such as barium. Thus, when barium is swallowed, it casts a shadow which outlines the various intestinal tract organs.

radioresistant Resisting the effects of radiation and therefore not destroyed, as a *radioresistant tumor*.

radiosensitive Changeable or destroyable by radiation.

radiosurgery The use of radium in surgical treatment.

radiotoxemia Radiation sickness caused by exposure to X-ray treatments. (It is accompanied by feelings of nausea, headache, and weakness.)

radiotherapy Radiation therapy.

radio-ulnar Pertaining to the bones of the forearm.

radium A radioactive metal from pitchblende used in the treatment of certain malignant diseases. It has the property, through its radiation, of destroying malignant cells.

    implantation Placing metal needles containing radium into tissues, allowing them to remain in place for a specified period of hours, and then removing them.

radius The outer bone of the forearm.

radon The radioactive element given off by radium when it disintegrates; radium emanation.

    implantation The placement of small metal "seeds" containing radon into tissues harboring cancer.

    seed A metal container for radon. These "seeds" are placed into tumor tissue and give out radioactivity, thus destroying the tumor.

rag-sorters' disease *See* anthrax.

ragweed The weed, genus *Ambrosia,* found throughout the United States, whose pollen causes a type of hay fever.

rale Clicking sounds heard through a stethoscope placed over the chest of someone suffering from a lung condition, such as pneumonia, bronchitis, tuberculosis, etc. It is evidence of excess mucus in the lungs.

raloxifene A new composition of estrogen (the female sex hormone) which is said to strengthen the bones against osteoporosis and decrease the chances of heart attacks. At the

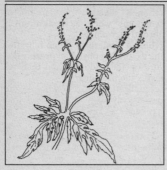
Ragweed

same time, it does not increase the risks for breast or uterus cancer. Investigators believe raloxifene reduces the risks, and may prevent some cases of cancer.

ramification A branch, usually referring to a nerve or blood vessel.

Ramstedt operation A surgical procedure in which the overgrown muscle tissue surrounding the outlet of the stomach is cut. It is performed on newborns who have a condition known as pyloric stenosis.

ramus A branch, usually of a nerve or blood vessel.

random sampling A selection by chance.

Ransahoff's operation Cutting the adhesions of the pleura (lining of the chest cavity) in cases of old empyema (abscess in chest cavity).

ranula A cyst of the salivary gland beneath the tongue. It appears as a thin-walled, fluid-containing, ball-shaped cyst under the tongue.

rape 1. Forceful sexual intercourse against the will. 2. Statutory rape is sexual intercourse with a minor, even when consent has been given.

raphe A seam; a ridge indicating the fusion of two sides, such as the ridge down the center of the tongue or the roof of the mouth.

rarefaction of bone Loss of calcium in bone. This process makes a bone more brittle and subject to fracture.

rat bite fever A disease brought on by the bite of an infected rat. It may cause joint pain and swelling along with patches of redness on the skin. Also, a chronic ulcer may form at the site of the bite.

Rathke's pouch A projection or pouch found in the embryo in the roof of the mouth. It extends upward toward the brain and helps to form the pituitary gland.

rationalization A mental attempt to justify an unacceptable situation or attitude; an explanation invented for something one wishes to do or believe.

rauwolfia A tropical herb which, when refined, has been found of great use in reducing high blood pressure and calming nerves; Reserpine.

ray Radiant energy, occurring in many forms such as actinic rays, alpha rays, beta rays, cosmic rays, gamma rays, infrared rays, ultraviolet rays, X rays, etc.

Raynaud's disease A disease, affecting women more than men, in which there is chronic constriction and spasm of the blood vessels in the fingers, toes, tip of the nose, etc. It occasionally leads to gangrene of the affected part.

RBC Abbreviation for red blood cells.

reaction 1. Any response to stimulation. 2. Chemical process.

   anaphylactic An allergic reaction resulting from contact with a substance to which a person is sensitive. Some anaphylactic reactions can be severe enough to cause death.

   coordinated Normal muscle responses.

   delayed A reaction which takes place some time after exposure to the stimulus. The length of time may be seconds, hours, or days.

   false negative A reaction to a

test that appears to be negative but is in reality positive.

false positive A reaction to a test that appears to be positive but is in reality negative, such as a falsely positive Wassermann reaction in someone not afflicted with syphilis.

immune A reaction to a test which shows that an individual is not susceptible to a certain disease.

infusion Chills and temperature which occasionally follow an intravenous injection.

irreversible One that cannot be changed or reversed.

local A reaction that occurs in the area where the stimulus has been applied, as the vaccination reaction following smallpox inoculation.

manic-depressive The periods of great elation alternating with periods of marked depression which characterize a type of mental disorder.

paranoid A feeling of being persecuted which characterizes a type of mental disorder.

schizophrenic A term used to describe a form of schizophrenia.

time The period which elapses between the stimulation and the response to it.

transfusion The results in the recipient of a transfusion of incompatible blood.

tuberculin Redness and swelling of the site of injection of tuberculin. Such a "positive" reaction indicates that the patient has had contact with the germs causing tuberculosis but it does not necessarily mean an active infection is present.

reactive To make something active again.

reagent Any substance used in a chemical reaction.

reattachment procedure A maneuver whereby the eyeball is treated with electrical diathermy in order to induce a detached retina to reattach itself to the other coats of the eyeball.

rebound reaction A flare-up of symptoms when a medication is abruptly terminated.

rebound tenderness Pain felt after the examining physician exerts pressure on the abdomen and then releases the pressure.

recanalization Restoration of the passageway of a blood vessel that has been blocked by a blood clot, as following phlebitis.

receptor An organ, or part of an organ, that receives an impulse or antigen.

recessive characteristics Those characteristics which have a tendency not to be visible or active when inherited.

recidivation Relapse of an illness.

recombinant DNA DNA that contains a new combination of genes, thus altering, to an extent, inherited characteristics. *See* DNA.

recovery room A part of a modern surgical suite where patients are taken to be observed and treated during the first few hours, or even days, after surgery.

recrudescence A relapse in the course of a disease which had seemed to be subsiding.

rectal pull-through operation A surgical procedure wherein the anal (rectal) sphincter is preserved by stitching the small intestine to the anal outlet, thus doing away with the need for a colostomy. *See* colostomy.

rectalgia Pain in the rectal area.

rectocele A protrusion of the rectum into the vagina, sometimes encountered in women who have been torn during childbirth.

rectocolitis Inflammation of the large bowel and rectum.

rectosigmoid The last few feet (in the adult) of the large intestine.

rectosigmoidectomy Surgical removal of the sigmoid and rectal portions of the large intestine.

rectovaginal Referring to the vagina and the rectum.

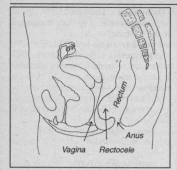

Rectocele

rectovesical Referring to the urinary bladder and the rectum.

rectum The lower or terminal eight to ten inches (in the adult) of the large intestine. The anus is the termination of the rectum.

rectus abdominis The long straight muscles of the abdominal wall extending from the ribs down to the pubic region.

recumbent position Lying down; reclining.

recuperation Convalescence; the period during which one recovers from an illness.

recurrent disease One which has a tendency to come back after having apparently subsided.

reduction When applied to a fracture, it means setting the fracture and bringing the broken fragments into alignment.

reduplication Doubling, such as a birth deformity in which certain parts of the intestinal tract may occur twice.

Reed-Sternberg cells Cells whose presence indicate Hodgkin's disease.

referred pain Pain which is felt some distance from the site of its origin.

reflex An uncontrollable (involuntary) response to a particular stimulation.

    Achilles An ankle jerk obtained by striking the large tendon above the heel.

    Babinski Elevation, rather than bending, of the big toe when the sole of the foot is scratched. It often indicates disease within the brain or spinal cord.

    chain A series of coordinated reflexes.

    ciliary Changes in the size of the pupil of the eye caused by contraction or dilatation of the iris muscles in response to variations in light intensity.

    conditioned An acquired reflex in which one responds automatically because of constant repetition (repeated association with the stimulus).

    conjunctival Blinking of the eyelids when the surface of the eyeball is touched. This can determine whether someone is conscious or unconscious.

    corneal *See* reflex, conjunctival.

    cough Coughing when the back of the throat or larynx is irritated or stimulated.

    instinctive A natural reflex; an inherited reflex. Many of these take the form of *protective reflexes,* such as ducking when something is thrown at one's head.

    laughter Laughing as a result of being tickled.

    light Contraction of the pupil of the eye when a bright light is shined at it.

    nasal Sneezing as a result of stimulating the inside of the nose.

    patellar Knee jerk.

    protective An automatic reflex against anything which threatens bodily harm.

    skin "Gooseflesh" and other skin reactions from irritating or stimulating the skin.

    sucking An instinctive reflex of a newborn when anything comes into contact with its lips.

    tendon A muscle contraction resulting from striking a tendon, as a knee jerk or ankle jerk. Failure to respond sometimes indicates a disturbance in nerve function.

    vasomotor Contraction or dilatation of blood vessels in response to stimulation.

    vomiting Throwing up the contents of the stomach as a result of irritation of the back of the mouth or throat.

reflux Flowing in a backward direction, as the flowing of intestinal contents back to the stomach.

reflux esophagitis Inflammation of the lower portion of the esophagus caused by the repeated backing up (regurgitation) of the acid stomach contents into the esophagus.

refraction Testing the eyes for glasses.

refractory A term referring to an illness which does not respond to treatment.

refrigeration 1. Cooling the body, or a part of the body, prior to performing surgery. 2. Cooling the body after surgery when the temperature is too high. Also referred to as hypothermia.

regeneration The healing of tissues; the formation of new tissues after the old ones have been destroyed by disease or injury.

regimen A planned course of treatment.

region A part of the body, as the lumbosacral *region*, referring to the lower back.

    axillary The armpit.

    cubital The crook of the elbow.

    deltoid The outside of the upper arm near the shoulder joint.

    epigastric The upper abdomen, just below the chest.

    femoral Below the groin and on to the thigh.

    gluteal The buttocks.

    iliac The crest of the hip bones.

    inframammary Below the breasts.

    infrascapular The area below the scapulae (wing bones) on the back, alongside the vertebral column.

    inguinal The groin.

    ischiorectal Out of the sides of the rectum.

    lumbar The lower back.

    perineal 1. In the female, between the vagina and the rectum. 2. In the male, between the bottom of the scrotal sac and the rectum.

    precordial Over the heart.

    sternal The area covered by the breastbone.

    submental Beneath the chin.

    supraclavicular Above the collarbones.

    umbilical Around the navel.

regional ileitis An inflammatory disease involving the lower portion of the small intestine. It tends to be chronic and to be characterized by quiescent periods and flare-ups.

registry A place where data is accumulated and organized.

regression 1. A relapse. 2. The subsiding of symptoms.

regurgitation A backward flow.

rehabilitation Treatment directed toward the restoration of people who have had a severe, prolonged, debilitating illness.

rehydration The restoration of water, as after dehydration. (Rehydration can be effected either by taking fluids by mouth or by giving them intravenously.)

Reidel's struma A disease in which fibrous tissue invades the thyroid gland.

reimplantation *See* replantation.

reinfection Another infection with the same germ, an occurrence sometimes caused by inadequate precautions in handling the primary infection.

rejection reaction The body's destruction of a foreign body, including a structure or organ that has been transplanted from another person, or animal. (Successful grafts must overcome the *rejection reaction*.)

relapse The return of a condition after apparent recovery from it.

relapsing fever A louse or tick-borne fever characterized by recurring bouts of fever, each lasting a few days and then subsiding for a few days.

relaxant A drug that relaxes muscles, often used during anesthesia to relax the abdominal muscles. Also used to relax muscles that are sprained or strained.

remedial Referring to something which attempts to cure.

remineralization The restoration to the body of minerals that have been excreted during dehydration or have been lost through illness. (Calcium, sodium, chloride, and potassium are most frequently in need of replenishment.)

remission A clearing up of a disease or its symptoms.

renal Pertaining to the kidneys.

renal colic Excruciating, sudden pain in the kidney region and down along the course of the ureter, caused by a kidney stone which has moved from the kidney region down toward the bladder.

rennin A substance, found in the stomach juice, which curdles milk.

reoperative surgery Surgery necessitated by failure or complications resulting from an initial operation; corrective surgery.

replacement therapy Treatment that supplies the patient's deficiencies, such as vitamins or hormones, in instances where they are insufficient.

replantation Stitching a severed part of the body back into place.

replication The repetition of an experiment to prove its validity.

reposition To put back a misplaced organ or part into its normal position.

repression A psychological term used to describe a mental mechanism whereby an individual pushes out of his conscious mind those ideas which are incompatible with his routine existence. Such ideas are held in the unconscious mind.

reproduction The process of producing one's kind, a basic drive of all animal life.

repulsion An aversion; a marked dislike.

RES Reticuloendothelial system.

resectable Referring to a tumor or other tissue which lends itself to surgical removal.

resection Surgical removal or excision.

resectoscope The instrument used in carrying out transurethral (through the penis) resection of the prostate gland.

Reserpine A medication which lowers high blood pressure. Rauwolfia.

reserve An ability or capacity for use on special occasions.

    alkaline Chemicals in the blood which are able to neutralize acids. Sodium bicarbonate, phosphates, etc.

    cardiac The power of the heart to pump more blood than is ordinarily necessary.

    diminished The inability of an organ to respond when extraordinary demands are made upon it.

Resident physician A physician in hospital training, learning a specialty of medicine or surgery. Resident training begins after completion of internship.

residual urine The urine remaining in the bladder after voiding. Normally, the bladder should contain practically no residual urine.

resistance The opposing force.

resolution The clearing up of an infection, such as pneumonia subsiding.

resolve To return to a normal state.

resonance The vibrations which are heard over the chest when the lungs are normally clear and filled with air.

resorb To absorb again.

Resorcinol A medication used effectively in certain skin diseases.

respiration Breathing.

respirator An iron lung; a machine

which performs artificial respiration, such as the Drinker respirator used in certain cases of infantile paralysis.

respiratory acidosis A condition encountered when the lungs are unable to expel sufficient carbon dioxide.

respiratory alkalosis A condition encountered when an excessive amount of carbon dioxide is exhaled by the lungs, as when there is a severe decrease in the oxygen-carrying capacity of the blood.

respiratory arrest Cessation of breathing.

respiratory capacity *See* vital capacity.

respiratory center The part of the brain that controls breathing.

respiratory distress syndrome Inability of the heart and lungs to maintain a normal exchange of oxygen and carbon dioxide. Also *see* ARDS.

respiratory failure Inability of the lungs to carry out an adequate exchange of gases, particularly oxygen and carbon dioxide. *See* ARDS.

respiratory rate The number of breaths per minute. The normal adult inhales approximately twenty times per minute.

respiratory system The nose, throat, larynx, trachea, bronchial tubes and the lungs.

restraint Inhibition; the condition of being held in check.

resuscitation The revival of a patient who appears to be dead, or almost dead.

resuture To stitch a wound again. A procedure sometimes required if the first suturing fails to hold.

retardation Slow or below normal development.

retching Attempting to vomit.

rete A network; a term applied mainly to a network of blood vessels.

retention 1. The condition of being held in, as the *retention* of urine. 2. *Retention* sutures are specially placed stitches to give additional support to a weak surgical wound.

reticular Forming a structure resembling a net or network.

reticulocyte A young (immature) red blood cell.

reticuloendothelial system (RES) All the phagocyte cells of the body. It includes cells located in the lymphatic channels, bone marrow, connective tissues, lungs, liver, adrenal glands, etc.

reticuloendotheliosis Marked overgrowth of primitive blood cells which takes place at first within the spleen, bone marrow, and liver. In the late stages, this condition may turn out to be a malignant form of leukemia (monocytic leukemia).

Reticulogen A potent liver extract and vitamin preparation, given intramuscularly in cases of pernicious anemia and other types of severe anemia.

reticulum cell sarcoma A sarcoma (malignant tumor) derived from cells of the reticuloendothelial system (phagocytes).

retina The innermost layer of the eye, the sensitive organ upon which light rays are focused.

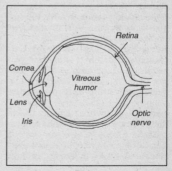

Retina

retinaculum A structure that holds an organ in place.

retinal artery The artery supplying

the retina of the eye. A clot in this vessel results in blindness.

retinal detachment *See* detachment of the retina.

retinal schisis A splitting of the retina, as distinguished from a tear. Treated either by cryotherapy (freezing) or by use of a laser beam.

retinitis Inflammation of the retina of the eye.

retinoblastoma A malignant tumor of the retina of the eye.

retinochoroiditis An inflammation of two layers of the eye, the retina and choroid.

retinology A branch of ophthalmology specializing in diseases and disorders of the retina.

retinopathy Disease of the retina.

retinopexy A procedure to repair a torn retina.

retinoscope An instrument for determining errors in vision; skiascope.

retinoscopy A procedure in which, by use of an instrument known as a retinoscope, the retina of the eye can be viewed and inspected for abnormalities or disease.

retort A glass container used in distilling and other chemical processes. It has a long neck and an oval base.

retract A surgical term meaning to hold back the tissues so that the surgeon can perform work more easily on deeper structures.

retraction 1. The pulling back or causing a structure to indent, such as *retraction* of the nipple. 2. The pulling aside of a structure during surgery to afford the surgeon a better view.

retractor Any one of many instruments devised for drawing back superficial tissues to give the surgeon a better view of deeper structures.

retro- A prefix meaning "in back of," "behind."

retrobulbar Located behind the eyeball.

    neuritis Inflammation of the optic nerve supplying the eye. Severe, prolonged retrobulbar neuritis

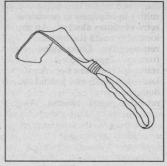

Retractor

may result in loss of vision in the involved eye.

retrocecal Located behind the cecum, such as *retrocecal* appendicitis.

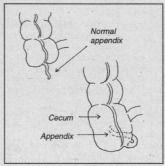

Normal appendix

Cecum

Appendix

Retrocecal appendix

retrocession A relapse.

retrocolic Behind the large intestine.

retroflexed Bent backwards. This term is often applied to a poorly positioned uterus.

retrograde Going in the opposite direction from the normal, as *retrograde* flow of blood in a vein which has incompetent valves.

retrogression A deterioration of a tissue or structure; degeneration.

retrolental fibroplasia Embryonic

tissue behind the lens of the eye, resulting in blindness in newborns.

retromammary abscess An abscess located beneath the breast.

retrospective Conclusions drawn from past experience.

retroperitoneal abscess An abscess located beneath and behind the abdominal cavity.

retropharyngeal abscess An abscess located behind the membrane of the back of the throat.

retroplasia Degeneration of an organ or a tissue structure.

retroposition A term applied to a uterus which is displaced in a backward position.

retrosternal Behind the breastbone.

retroverted Tilted or tipped backwards, as a *retroverted* uterus.

Retrovir Trade name for AZT. *See* AZT.

retrovirus A virus that frequently attacks T-lymphocyte white blood cells. Thought to be involved in causing AIDS and certain forms of leukemia.

retrusion Backward movement of the lower jaw.

Retuxan A medication said to be helpful in the treatment of lymphomas of the non-Hodgkin's type.

revascularization The operative procedure in which grafts are inserted in order to reestablish blood supply to a part or organ.

reversion A biologic term applied to a "throwback," or someone who has inherited some characteristic from a remote ancestor.

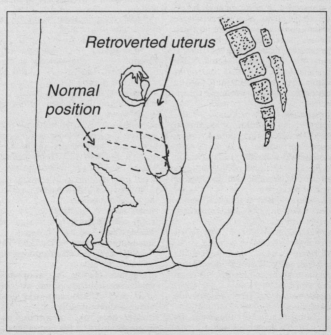

Retroverted uterus

revive To bring back to life.

revulsion A lessening of a disorder.

Reye's syndrome *See* syndrome, Reye's.

rhabdomyoma A tumor of muscles.

rhabdomyosarcoma A malignant tumor of muscles.

Rh blood groups *See* Rh factor.

Rh D Immune Globulin An injection given to an Rh(D) negative mother within 72 hours after the birth of an Rh(D) positive infant in order to prevent Rh disease in a subsequent child.

rheography A noninvasive light reflection technique to determine the circulation of the small veins and capillaries in the legs.

rheumatic fever An inflammatory disease, seen most often in children, associated with bouts of high fever, painful swelling of joints, and inflammation of the valves and muscles of the heart.

rheumatic heart disease Inflammation of the heart muscle and distortion of the valves of the heart (especially the mitral and aortic valves) due to a rheumatic fever infection.

rheumatism A word used to describe many conditions associated with diseases of the joints, tendons, muscles or bones.

rheumatoid arthritis Inflammation of joints associated with symptoms resembling rheumatism (a specific type of arthritis).

Rheumatologist A specialist in diseases involving the joints, particularly arthritic conditions.

rhexis Rupture of a vessel or organ.

Rh factor A blood component. Its presence may be involved with destruction of the red blood cells of an unborn or newborn infant (erythroblastosis). Also, it may be involved in the causation of blood transfusion reactions. A serious situation exists when an Rh negative mother is carrying an Rh positive baby in her uterus. This, in some instances, leads to the loss of the infant.

    negative A term referring to people whose blood does not contain the Rh substance. Fifteen per cent of people fall into this category.

    positive A term referring to people whose blood contains the Rh substance. Eighty-five per cent of all people are Rh positive.

    sensitization The process of becoming sensitized to Rh substances.

    testing Examining the blood to determine whether one is Rh positive or negative. This is an important test to perform upon all expectant mothers.

Rh factor diseases Erythroblastosis.

rhinencephalon That part of the brain which controls the sense of smell.

rhinitis Inflammation of the lining membrane of the nose.

    allergic Hay fever.

    vasomotor An allergic inflammation of the mucous membranes of the nose, due to vasomotor neurosis.

rhinodynia Pain in the nose.

rhinopharyngitis Inflammation of the nose and throat.

rhinophyma Enlargement and redness of the entire nose with large pores and blood vessels in the skin of the nose. Also called toper's nose, whisky nose, although its occurrence is not limited to heavy drinkers.

rhinoplasty Plastic surgery upon the nose; nasoplasty.

rhinorrhea A "running" nose. Nasal mucous discharge.

rhizonychia The root of a nail.

rhizotomy Surgery to cut the roots of spinal nerves, carried out to relieve incurable pain.

Rhogam This is a substance which, when injected into an Rh negative woman who has just borne an Rh positive baby, will prevent her from developing immunization to the Rh factor. Thus, her next child will be protected against Rh factor disease (erythroblastosis). Rhogam should be given within 72 hours after the birth of the Rh positive baby.

rhomboid muscle A large rectangular muscle in the upper part of the back.

rhonchus A loud, wheezing sound heard when listening to the chest with a stethoscope. A *rhonchus* is caused by mucus in the larger bronchial tubes or in the trachea.

Rhus The generic name of the shrub which causes poison ivy.

Rhus Tox Antigen An injectable substance to build up immunity against poison ivy.

rhythm Regularity. Occurring according to a regular pattern, as the *rhythm* of the heart beat.

    cardiac The even, regular heartbeat of sixty to eighty per minute.

    ectopic Extra heartbeats originating from other than the normal area in the heart muscle.

    gallop A heartbeat having three, rather than two, components, thus sounding somewhat like the galloping gait of a horse.

    method A system of preventing pregnancy by avoiding sexual intercourse during the time when ovulation (the egg bursting forth from the ovary) occurs.

    regular sinus The normal heartbeat.

rhytidectomy A plastic operation to remove wrinkles in the skin.

rib The bones forming the chest cage. There are twelve ribs on each side.

    cervical An extra short rib in the neck. It sometimes presses upon the nerves going to the arms, thus producing pain.

    floating The bottom two ribs which are not attached, by cartilage, and thus appear to "float."

riboflavin Vitamin B_2. Lack of this vitamin causes skin cracking and dryness, inflammation of the eyes and tongue, etc.

ribonucleic acid (RNA) This material and deoxyribonucleic acid (DNA) are present in all living cells. They are responsible for the characteristics of a species and for the transmission of inherited traits.

rickets A disease of infancy caused by lack of vitamin D, evidenced in marked cases by bone deformities such as bow legs, funnel chest, beading of the ribs, etc.

Rickettsial diseases A group of diseases caused by bacterialike organisms, which are parasites. These parasites are carried by ticks, lice, etc. which, in turn, transmit the diseases to man. Examples are: typhus fever, Q fever, psittacosis (parrot fever), etc.

Riedel's lobe A tongue-shaped projection of liver in a downward direction. It has no significance and is found only infrequently.

rigidity Hardness and stiffness of muscles. In cases of peritonitis, appendicitis, or other abdominal infections, the muscles of the abdominal wall show *rigidity* when pressed upon by the physician.

rigor mortis Stiffness of the muscles which sets in after death.

rima A cleft (an anatomical term).

ring, inguinal The circle of tissue in the groin through which the structures going to the testicle pass. Ruptures usually take place through the *inguinal ring.*

ringworm A contagious disease caused by a fungus. Its typical eruption often is in the shape of a ring.

Riopan Antacid medication to be used for excess acid, dyspepsia, heartburn, etc.

risorius A facial muscle which manipulates the corners of the mouth and thereby helps to control facial expressions.

Ritalin A central nervous system stimulant, administered in certain cases of attention disorders.

R.N. Registered Nurse, a licensed

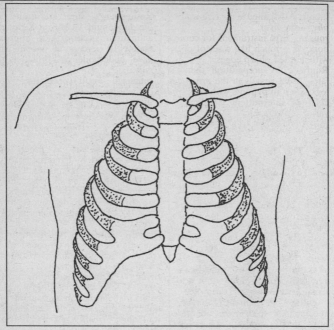

Rib cage

graduate of an approved nurses' training school.

RNA *See* ribonucleic acid.

R.O.A. Right occiput anterior, a normal position of the baby within the uterus at the time of delivery.

Robaxisal A muscle relaxant drug, sometimes efficacious in relieving pain from muscle sprains.

Robitussin An effective cough mixture, helpful in bringing up phlegm.

Rocky Mountain spotted fever A dangerous disease caused by the bite of an infected tick. It occurs in the Rocky Mountains and other areas in the United States. Vaccination against this disease has recently proven most effective.

rodent ulcer A common form of

skin cancer, seen most often on the face. Also called *basal cell epithelioma*. It is curable when treated early.

roentgenography Photography utilizing X rays.

roentgenology The branch of medicine dealing with the use of X rays, both in diagnosing and in treating disease.

roentgen therapy X-ray therapy; treatment with *roentgen* rays (X rays).

Rogaine A liquid supposed to be helpful in stimulating the growth of hair in balding men. It is not uniformly successful.

Rokitansky's disease A severe poisoning of the liver with rapid destruction of liver tissue. It often ends fatally. Also called *acute yellow atrophy* of the liver.

rongeur An instrument for cutting bone. It is much like a set of pliers with cupped, sharp edges.

Roniacol A preparation that dilates blood vessels in the arms and legs, given to patients with poor circulation, intermittent claudication, varicose ulcers, etc.

root The origin of a part or of an organ.

R.O.P. Right occiput posterior, one of the normal positions of the baby prior to delivery.

Rorschach, Hermann (1884–1922) A Swiss psychiatrist who developed a test of personality, particularly effective in determining the extent of neurotic tendencies.

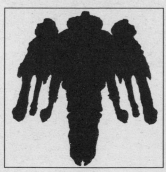
Rorschach test

rosacea Whisky nose. *See* rhinophyma.

rose fever An allergy, much like hay fever, caused by sensitivity to the pollen of roses.

roseola infantum A contagious disease of childhood in which there is fever for a few days followed by a light rose-colored rash and then a sudden drop in fever. Also called *exanthem subitum*.

rose water ointment Cold cream.

rotavirus A virus that causes diarrhea in children, especially among infants.

Rothenberg's sign Deformity of the duodenum, visible on X-ray examination, occurring in approximately 10 percent of people who have undergone gall bladder removal.

roughage Food containing material which will not be absorbed from the intestinal tract, such as cellulose. Celery, lettuce, fruit skins, etc. contain much *roughage*.

round ligament; of the liver A fibrous band of tissue extending from the underside of the navel to the liver. It represents the course of the large umbilical vein in the embryo. Also called *ligamentum teres*.

of the uterus A fibrous, round band of tissue extending from either side of the uterus into the inguinal canal in the groin and attaching to the lips of the vagina. It helps to keep the uterus in its proper position.

round shouldered Someone with poor posture who hunches his shoulders forward and drops his head.

roundworm A worm which sometimes inhabits the intestinal tract; a nematode.

Roux-en-Y anastomosis A cutting across and restitching of small intestine so as to create a diversion of the flow of feces away from one limb of the intestine.

Roxanol A tablet containing morphine. It can be habit-forming.

R.Q. Abbreviation for respiratory quotient.

R.T. A licensed, registered X-ray technician.

rubefacient A substance causing redness and increased blood supply when rubbed into the skin. Most liniments are rubefacients.

rubella German measles. It can be diagnosed by its light pink rash and by swollen glands in the back of the neck.

rubeola Measles.

rubescent Reddish, flushed.

rubor Redness caused by inflammation.

ructus Belching.

rudimentary Only partially formed; undeveloped. The coccyx bone at the bottom of the spine is supposed to represent a *rudimentary* tail.

RU-486 A French pill capable of causing abortions.

rugae Folds or ridges of tissue, as seen in the lining of the stomach and in the vagina.

rumination Psychologically, the pondering and hashing over and over again of a thought or idea.

rump The buttocks.

run-around An infection surrounding a finger or toenail. A paronychial infection.

rupture A hernia; tearing of a part, as a ruptured muscle, ruptured bowel, etc.

   of bag of waters Same as rupture of the membranes.

   of membranes A tear in the membranes surrounding the unborn child. This is followed by leakage of the fluids out through the vagina.

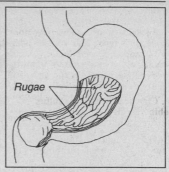

Rugae of stomach

   artificial A procedure carried out by the obstetrician in order to bring on labor.

rutin A chemical given to decrease the fragility of red blood cells, thus preventing them from rupturing easily.

Rythmol A drug useful for overcoming irregular heart rhythms.

S

S Chemical symbol for sulfur.

Sabin vaccine An oral vaccine for the prevention of infantile paralysis.

sac An anatomical term denoting a pouch or covering of a body cavity, as the *peritoneal sac,* which contains the abdominal organs.

saccharin A chemical possessing the sweetening powers of sugar but containing few calories.

saccharose Cane sugar; sucrose.

saccular Pouch-shaped.

saccule A small sac.

sacralization A spinal deformity in which the fifth lumbar vertebra in the lower back is fused to the first sacral vertebra.

sacrococcygeal region The area at the very bottom of the spine, just above the anal region.

sacroiliac Referring to the area where the sacrum and the iliac bones form a joint. These areas are on either side of the spine in the lower back region. The muscles and ligaments in the region are exceptionally prone to injury, thus causing the condition known as *sacroiliac strain.*

sacrolumbar Referring to the region of the lower back and the loins; a region particularly subject to muscle sprains.

sacrospinalis The long, large muscles extending up along either side of the vertebral column from the sacrum to the ribs. These muscles are often strained by strenuous work.

sacrouterine ligaments The ligaments extending from the uterus to the sacrum. They help to maintain the normal position of the uterus (womb).

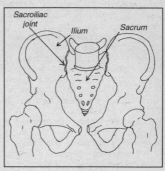

Sacroiliac joint

sacrum One bone, shield-shaped, composed of five fused vertebrae. It is located toward the base of the vertebral column and forms the back wall of the pelvis.

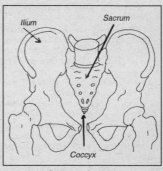

Sacrum and coccyx

sadism Pleasure derived from hurting people.

sadist One who takes pleasure in hurting others.

sadomasochism Love of cruelty and pain, either active (sadistic) or passive (masochistic).

"safe" period That time during the menstrual cycle when a woman supposedly is unable to become pregnant; thought by some to be the week before and the week after the menstrual period.

safe sex Any practice which diminishes the risks of transmitting a contagious disease to a sex partner.

sagittal plane An anatomical term applied to the "front to back" plane of the body, as the *sagittal suture* of the skull running from the front to the back of the head.

St. Anthony's fire Erysipelas; a streptococcal infection of the skin.

St. Martin's disease Alcoholism.

St. Vitus Dance Chorea, a disease of the nerves characterized by irregular and involuntary movements of the muscles of the limbs and face. Sometimes associated with rheumatic fever.

salicylate drugs Medications particularly useful in relieving pains in muscles, joints, and in rheumatic fever. Also helpful in relieving headaches of a transient nature. Aspirin is a salicylate.

salicylic acid The active ingredient of many medications such as aspirin, and in ointments, lotions, and powders used in treating various skin diseases.

saline solution Salt solution; sodium chloride in water.

saliva The secretion of the salivary glands into the mouth. It moistens food and aids in swallowing. It also contains an enzyme (chemical) called ptyalin which helps to digest starches.

salivary calcium A stone usually lodged in the duct leading from the salivary glands into the mouth.

salivary glands Those glands which produce and secrete saliva. They are connected to the mouth through ducts (tubes). The three salivary glands are: the parotids, the submaxillaries, and the sublinguals.

salivation Excess secretion of saliva from the various salivary glands (the parotid, submaxillary, and sublingual glands).

Salk, Jonas (1914–1995) An American physician, the discoverer of poliomyelitis (infantile paralysis) vaccine.

Salk vaccine Polio vaccine. A full course of four injections will protect about 80 to 85 percent of people from infantile paralysis.

salmonella infection Paratyphoid fever, a disease similar but milder than typhoid fever, caused by the *Salmonella* bacteria. Its main symptoms are fever, nausea, vomiting, and diarrhea.

salpingectomy Surgical removal of a fallopian (uterine) tube, performed when infected or when a pregnancy takes place within the tube (ectopic pregnancy).

salpingitis Inflammation of the fallopian (uterine) tubes which extend out from both sides of the uterus.

salpingography X-ray visualization of the fallopian tubes after intrauterine injection of a radiopaque substance. Performed to note whether the passageway in the tube is open.

salpingo-oophorectomy Removal of a fallopian tube and ovary.

salpingoplasty An operation which attempts to reopen the channel through a fallopian tube; performed in certain cases of sterility caused by closed tubes.

salpinx A tube. The term is applied mainly to the fallopian or uterine tube.

salt 1. Sodium chloride. 2. Any chemical resulting from the interaction of acids and bases.

salt depletion Loss of sodium and chloride from the body, frequently leading to electrolyte imbalance. Perspiration, diarrhea, or vomiting of a severe nature can cause such depletion.

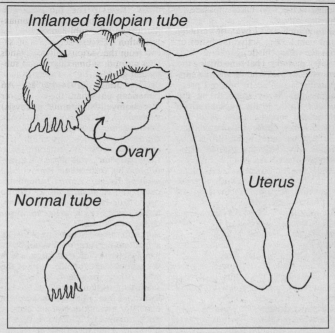

Inflamed fallopian tube

Ovary

Uterus

Normal tube

Salpingitis

salting-out A method of abortion whereby saline solution is injected into the pregnant uterus to stimulate expulsion of its fetus.

saltpeter Potassium nitrate, a chemical supposedly reducing one's sexual desires.

Salvarsan A patented preparation used extensively in the treatment of syphilis in the days prior to the antibiotic drugs. It contains arsenic.

salve Any ointment.

same-day surgery That which is performed in a hospital in the morning, with the patient going home later in the day.

sample Any specimen to be examined, such as a *sample* of urine, feces, blood, spinal fluid, sputum, etc.

sanatorium An institution specially designed and equipped to treat people suffering from long-lasting illnesses.

sandfly fever A three-day fever, accompanied by severe aches and pains in bones and muscles, caused by the bite of an infected sandfly. Seen mostly in the Mediterranean area, South America, and Africa.

sanguine 1. Bloody. 2. Optimistic.

sanguineous Containing blood, as a *sanguineous* discharge from a wound.

sanitarian A public health or preventive medicine practitioner.

sanity Mental balance; the opposite of insanity. A term used more often in legal than in medical circles.

San Joaquin Valley fever A chronic

lung infection seen among residents of San Joaquin Valley in California. Also called *coccidioidomycosis* or *valley fever.*

Sansert An anti-headache medication, especially for those who have frequent attacks; used also for migraine.

saphenous veins The large system of veins in the legs and thighs which drain the superficial tissues of the lower limbs. These veins empty into the femoral veins in the groin. The saphenous veins are prone to develop varicosities.

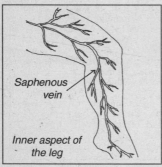

Saphenous vein

Inner aspect of the leg

Saphenous vein

saponification The transformation of a fat into a soap.

sapphism Lesbianism; female homosexuality.

saprogenic Causing rotting; putrefied.

saprophytes Germs which live by eating dead tissue rather than living matter.

Saquinavir *See* protease inhibitor.

sarcoendothelioma A malignant tumor of the covering (sheath) of a tendon.

sarcoidosis Boeck's sarcoid, a chronic disease affecting mostly young adults. It has many of the characteristics of tuberculosis but is not caused by any known bacteria. It involves lymph glands, lungs, skin, and other structures but does not

cause them to undergo degeneration. It lasts for many years, does not usually cause death but often does not subside.

sarcolemma The covering or sheath surrounding a muscle fiber.

sarcoma A malignant tumor made up of connective tissues, such as bone, muscle, fat, etc.

sarcomatous Resembling a sarcoma.

sarcoplasm The connective tissue between the individual small muscle fibers.

sartorius muscle A long muscle in the thigh which aids the act of crossing one leg over another.

satellite lesion A small tumor located in the vicinity of, and often originating from, a larger one. Also, a small cyst or skin lesion accompanying a larger one.

satiation A state of being satisfied.

saturated Having all the solids or gases dissolved in a solution which the solution can take. If more of the solid or gas is added, it does not readily dissolve.

saturated fats Animal fats, high in cholesterol content. Not advised for people with high blood pressure or high blood cholesterol levels.

saturnism Lead poisoning.

satyriasis Excessive sexual lust in males.

satyr tip A pointed ear.

saucerization of bone Cutting out a saucer-shaped portion of bone in cases of osteomyelitis (bone infection).

SBE Abbreviation for *subacute bacterial endocarditis,* a serious infection of the valves of the heart.

scabies A contagious skin condition caused by an insect which burrows under the superficial layers of the skin. It causes great itching and the diagnosis can often be made by noting extensive scratch marks.

scalene node biopsy An operation in which a lymph node is excised from the lower neck to see if a cancer of the lung has spread. (If the lymph node shows cancer, it indicates that the lung malignancy has progressed so far that further surgery will be of no avail.)

scalenotomy Cutting the scalene muscles in the neck in order to relieve pressure of these muscles on the nerves which go to the arm (the brachial plexus).

scalenus anticus syndrome Pain, weakness, pins-and-needles, numbness in an arm secondary to pressure of the scalene muscles in the neck on the brachial plexus (the group of nerves which supply the arm).

scalenus Muscles in the neck which arise near the spinal vertebrae and extend to the front portion of the first two ribs. The brachial plexus nerves which supply the shoulder and arm are located beneath these muscles.

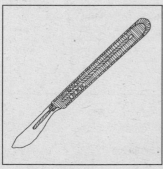

Scalpel

scalpel A surgical knife.

scanning *See* scintiscanner.

scaphoid Small bones in the wrist and ankle which are boat-shaped.

scapula The shoulder blade.

scarification The making of many small superficial incisions.

scarlatina Scarlet fever.

scarlet fever A contagious disease caused by a streptococcus. It is associated with high fever, sore throat, swollen glands, and a typical strawberry rash. During the healing period, the skin peels. A common complication is inflammation of the kidneys. Recovery takes place in two to three weeks.

scarlet red ointment A medication particularly helpful in stimulating the healing of open wounds. It promotes growth of new skin.

scatology The study of feces, as a means of diagnosing disease.

scatoma A hard lump of stool in the bowels, giving the impression of a tumor when felt by an examining hand.

scatophagy Eating feces; seen occasionally among infants and mentally ill patients.

Schick test A skin test to note if one is immune to diphtheria. Discovered by a well-known American pediatrician, Bela Schick.

Schilder's disease An inflammatory disease of the brain and nerves leading from the brain.

Schimmelbusch's disease "Lumpy breasts," "shoddy breasts." A chronic condition of the breasts in which there are many areas of cysts and overgrown gland tissue. Not malignant.

schisis A splitting of a membrane, as in *retinal schisis.*

schisto- A combining form meaning "split," "divided," "slit."

schistocyte A broken red blood cell.

schistosomiasis 1. "Swimmer's itch." A skin condition incurred by swimming in waters infested with a parasite of snails. 2. In Asian and tropical countries it is a serious disease caused by infestation with the parasite known as bilharzia.

schizo- A term meaning split, as in schizophrenia.

schizoid Resembling schizophrenia.

schizophrenia A form of mental illness in which there is a withdrawal from reality. Occurs mostly in young adults. Dementia praecox.

schizophrenic reaction A general term to describe any one of the many forms taken by schizophrenia.

Schüller-Christian disease A lipoid

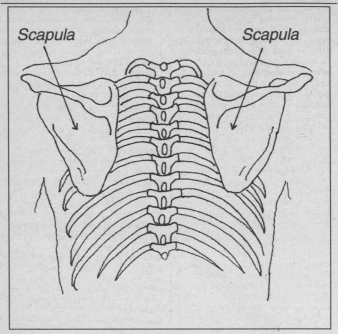

Scapula *Scapula*

Scapula

(fatlike) disease of childhood with involvement of bones, skull, and other organs.

Schultz-Charlton test A skin test to note if one is immune to scarlet fever.

schwannoma A cancerous tumor of the nerves.

sciatica A condition in which there is severe pain in the lower back and down the back of the thigh and leg along the route traveled by the sciatic nerve. It is associated with an inflammation of the sciatic nerve and may lead to numbness, tingling and wasting of the muscles supplied by the sciatic nerve.

sciatic nerve The large, long nerve originating in the spinal cord, exiting near the base of the spine, and sup-plying the muscles of the lower limbs.

scintillation Seeing flashes of light or sparks before one's eyes.

scintiscanner A device for determining the presence of radioactive substances which have been given. When placed over a body area, such as the thyroid gland, it acts in the same manner as a Geiger counter if radioactive iodine has been given and has been absorbed by the gland.

scirrhoid tissue Hard tissue.

scirrhous cancer A firm, hard tumor containing large amounts of fibrous tissue.

scission The dividing or splitting of a cell. Nuclear splitting.

sclera The white of the eye.

scleral buckling A surgical procedure in which tucks are placed in the sclera to shorten the eyeball from front to back; sometimes performed in cases of detached retina.

sclerectoiridectomy A surgical procedure in which the sclera (the white portion of the eye) and the iris (the colored portion of the eye) are incised in order to relieve glaucoma.

scleritis Inflammation of the white of the eye.

scleroderma A skin disease in which there are very hard patches with color changes. Other organs of the body may also become involved with hardening (calcification) of muscles and blood vessels.

sclerokeratitis Inflammation of both the white portion (sclera) and the colored portion (cornea) of the eye.

sclerosing tenosynovitis An inflammation and overgrowth of a tendon sheath causing intense pain, most often seen in the wrist near the base of the thumb.

sclerosis Hardening of tissues, with deposit of fibrous tissues to replace the original structure, as sclerosis of the walls of arteries.

sclerotherapy The injection of an agent or medication into a vein in order to clot it and to get fibrous tissue to form within it. Done in treating varicose veins. Also called *sclerosing treatment.*

sclerotic Hardened, such as *sclerotic* blood vessels.

sclerotomy A surgical incision into the sclera, the white portion of the eye.

scolex The head of the tapeworm. Unless this is removed, the worm will continue to grow within the intestines.

scoliokyphosis Curvature of the spine in both front to back and side to side directions.

scoliolordosis Curvature of the spine in which there is both side-to-side and front-to-back deformity.

scoliosis Abnormal curvature of the spine. This condition tends to occur during adolescence, more often in girls. When the deformity is severe, it may require a fusion operation upon the spine.

scope Any device for examining an organ or part of a patient, as a stethoscope or a cystoscope.

scopolamine "Truth serum." It is a drug, derived from an herb, with many actions, such as dilating the pupil, producing a sleepy relaxed state, and making a patient much more susceptible to suggestion. It aids and fortifies the action of morphine and other hypnotic and pain-relieving medications.

scopophilia An abnormal desire to view nude bodies; a characteristic of voyeurs (Peeping Toms).

scopophobia Abnormal fear of being seen.

scorbutic Pertaining to scurvy.

scotoma A blind spot on the retina.

scrapings Tissues scraped off surfaces for the purpose of examining them under the microscope.

screening The practice of examining large groups of supposedly healthy people to see if they have developed a disease for which they are at high risk, as mammographic screening to note the presence of a hidden breast cancer.

scrofula Tuberculosis of the lymph glands in the neck. Formerly, this occurred from drinking milk infected with tuberculosis germs; the condition occurs only rarely today.

scrofuloderma Tuberculosis of the skin.

scrotum The pouch, located beneath the penis, which contains the testicles.

scrub nurse An operating room nurse.

scrub typhus A rickettsial infection causing headache, fever, and a rash. Seen mostly in Japan and in other Pacific islands. Also called *tsutsugamushi fever.*

scrum-pox A slang expression for

impetigo, sometimes affecting soccer, football, and rugby players. It is characterized by eruptions on the face and head.

scurvy A deficiency disease caused by lack of vitamin C. Anemia, weakness, bleeding gums, and other bleeding tendencies are common symptoms.

scybala Hard, round feces, secondary to marked constipation.

seasickness Nausea, vomiting, dizziness caused by the rolling motion of a boat. Also called motion sickness.

sebaceous cysts Wens; cysts in and just beneath the skin, containing a greasy, smelly substance.

seborrheic dermatitis A skin disease due to oversecretion of the sebaceous glands. When it affects the scalp, this condition often leads to baldness.

sebum The material secreted by sebaceous glands. It is an oily, waxy substance.

Seconal An effective short-acting barbiturate, often prescribed as a "sleeping tablet."

secondary cancer Cancer that has spread from its original site.

secondary medical care The type in which the physician acts as a consultant to the primary physician.

second sight Improved vision which sometimes occurs in older people if they become somewhat nearsighted.

secreta Material which has been secreted by a gland.

secretagogue A chemical which stimulates a gland to secrete, such as a hormone.

secrete To produce a special substance and to expel it, such as the salivary glands *secrete* saliva, the pancreas *secretes* insulin, etc.

secretin A name given to a specific hormone (chemical) which is secreted by the cells of the duodenum, is absorbed through the wall of the small intestine into the bloodstream and when it reaches the pancreas,

causes that gland to secrete digestive juices which are fed into the intestines in the region of the duodenum.

secretory Relating to secretion.

section A slice of tissue.

secundines The afterbirth; the placenta, umbilical cord and membranes which follow after delivery of the child.

sedative A drug given to calm the nerves and to decrease a state of excitement, such as the barbiturates.

sediment Any material (usually a solid) settling to the bottom of a liquid.

sedimentation rate (ESR) The rate at which red blood cells settle to the bottom of a test tube. A rate above normal may indicate the presence of an infection.

segment A portion of tissue.

segmental bone resection The removal of a portion of a bone, leaving other tissues such as muscles, nerves, and blood vessels in place.

segmental mastectomy The operative removal of a portion of the breast.

segmentation Cleavage, as in the division of cells; a term applied to a fertilized egg which is growing by the process of cell *segmentation*.

Seidlitz powder A laxative and antacid powder (formerly very popular in relieving indigestion and constipation).

seizure A sudden attack of a condition, such as the abrupt, severe pain caused by a stone in the kidney or ureter, or a sudden convulsion as seen in epilepsy.

Seldane A patented anti-allergic medicine, most effective in treating allergic conditions of the nose and throat.

selection, natural See natural selection.

self-abuse An old term for masturbation.

self-hypnosis Hypnosis of oneself.

self-limited A term applied to a condition or disease which lasts but a specific length of time and then disappears.

sella turcica The depression, cup-shaped, in the base of the skull, in which the pituitary gland is lodged.

Selsun A liquid suspension that is highly effective in overcoming dandruff and dermatitis of the scalp.

Selye, Hans (1907–1984) The exponent of the theory of stress as a cause of organic disease; a Canadian physician.

semen The fluid which carries the male sperm. It is stored in the seminal vesicles and is ejaculated when orgasm is reached.

semi- A prefix meaning "half."

semicircular canals The bony canals of the inner ear. They are important in maintaining the sense of equilibrium (balance).

semicomatose A state of partial unconsciousness from which a patient can be aroused with difficulty.

semiconscious Partially conscious.

semilunar Crescentic in shape.

cartilages The cartilages lying on top of the tibial bone (the main bone of the leg) in the knee joint. These cartilages are often torn in athletic injuries; surgical removal is often necessary.

semimembranosus muscle One of the large "hamstring" muscles extending down the back of the thigh. It acts to bend the knee.

seminal vesicles Small glands near the prostate and urethra where semen is stored prior to its discharge.

semination The ejaculation of semen into the vagina.

seminoma A tumor of the testicle, sometimes malignant. Also called *dysgerminoma* or *spermatocytoma*.

seminuria Semen in the urine.

semirecumbent position Partially sitting up in bed.

semitendinosus muscle One of the large "hamstring" muscles extending down the back of the thigh. It bends the knee.

Semmelweis, Ignaz (1818–1865) The doctor who discovered that dirty hands and instruments caused infections among women who were delivered. One of the founders of antisepsis; an Austrian physician.

senescence Aging; growing old.

senile psychosis A form of mental illness seen among some elderly people who have marked arteriosclerosis of the arteries in the brain.

senility Old age.

senium The later years of life; from sixty years of age onward.

senna A mild laxative, derived from an herb.

senopsia The aging eye, with particular reference to people who lose their nearsightedness during their fifth, sixth, or seventh decades of life.

sensation A kind of feeling, as the result of a particular type of stimulation; something of which one becomes aware through the use of one's senses.

sense The appreciation and realization of a sensation. *Cold* sense would be from the knowledge that it is cold because one's skin is stimulated by a low temperature.

sense organ Special nerves equipped to receive and pass along specific stimuli. The fingers are the site for extremely sensitive nerve endings for the sense of *touch*.

sensibility The ability to feel and transmit impulses, impressions, stimuli, etc.

sensitivity The greater or lesser capacity of receiving and transmitting sensations.

sensitized Having developed a sensitivity to stimuli; a person with hay fever is *sensitized* to the pollen of ragweed.

sensorium The part of the brain which receives and interprets sensations.

sensory Pertaining to sensation.

sensualism Condition of being governed by desires, emotions and instincts.

sentient Capable of feeling.

sepsis A reaction of the body to

bacteria which circulate in the blood, characterized by chills and fever. Once fatal, now often curable through use of antibiotics.

septal defect An abnormal opening between a right and left chamber of the heart; atrial defects occur between the two auricles, ventricular ones between the two ventricles.

septectomy An operation for correction of a deviated septum of the nose.

septic Not free of bacteria; infected.

septicemia A serious condition caused by bacteria living and growing in the bloodstream.

septotomy An operation in which the nasal septum (dividing the two nasal cavities) is cut.

Septra *See* Bactrim.

septum A partition between two structures or cavities, as the *nasal septum.*

sequelae Symptoms developing as a consequence of an illness. Sequelae may come on long after the original illness has subsided.

sequestration 1. The passing out of the body of a dead piece of tissue, as the *sequestration* of bone from an area of infected bone. 2. The isolation of diseased persons for treatment or for quarantine.

serendipidity An accidental finding when one is looking for something else.

seriograph An apparatus for taking several X rays in rapid succession; used often in x-raying the vessels of the brain.

serofibrinous exudate A discharge composed of serum and fibrin; the type of material which oozes from a burned body surface and goes to form a scab.

serology The branch of clinical medicine which studies the serum of the blood.

seronegative The absence of a previous infection.

seropositive The finding of a previous infection or the finding of an existing one.

seropurulent exudate Discharge from an infected area containing serum and pus.

seroma A collection of serum, usually following a surgical incision, located beneath the skin.

serosa The membranes which cover the heart, the lungs, all the abdominal organs, as well as the various body cavities in which they are lodged.

serosanguineous A discharge containing both blood and serum. It is pink in color and much thinner than blood alone.

serositis An inflammation of a membrane lining the chest, or abdominal cavity.

serotonin A chemical found in the blood which causes blood vessels to constrict and contract. It is present in large amounts in people who have a spreading "carcinoid" tumor in the intestines.

serous fluid A discharge of material resembling the serum of the blood.

Serpasil A patented medication used to reduce high blood pressure. Reserpine; rauwolfia.

serpiginous Serpentine; shaped like a snake; a term applied to ulcers of the skin and other conditions which extend in a snakelike fashion.

serration A notched or toothlike border to a structure.

serratus muscle A large muscle extending from the back of the chest and inserting into the ribs.

serum That part of whole blood which remains after blood has clotted. It is yellowish in color.

    immune A serum containing antibodies which can fight against a specific disease. It is injected into patients to protect them from that disease.

    pooled Serum used from a number of people.

    truth One that is obtained from a patient while he or she is under the influence of a drug and/or medication.

serum sickness Illness following the injection of a serum into someone who is allergic to an ingredient in the serum. Hives, pain and swelling at the site of injection, pain in joints and, in some instances, shock and collapse may result.

sesamoid bones Small extra bones, about the hands and feet, which develop in tendons which have been subject to great use and pressure.

sesqui- A combining form meaning "one and one-half."

sessile Having a broad base, as a *sessile* polyp of the rectum. Not possessing a stalk.

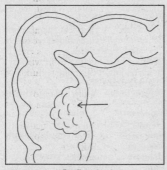

Sessile polyp

seton Threads which are placed through tissues in order to create an artificial tract (tunnel). Used in certain rectal operations.

sex cells Those produced either by the ovaries or the testicles; also known as *germ cells*.

sex chromosome The X and Y chromosomes; the chromosomes which determine the sex of the individual.

sex-linked disorder A disorder caused by an abnormality of the sex chromosomes, X or Y. Hemophilia, Klinefelter's syndrome, and Turner's syndrome are examples.

sexology The science of sex and sexual relations.

sexual deviation Departure from usual sexual practices. It includes such deviations as sexual attraction to minors, sexual sadism, sexual fetishes, etc.

S.G.O. The Surgeon General's Office. There are four Surgeon Generals; those of the Army, the Navy, the Air Force, and the Public Health Service.

SGOT Abbreviation for a laboratory test known as a *transaminase test*. It is elevated in certain cases of coronary thrombosis, in liver disease, and other conditions in which there has been tissue damage.

shaking palsy A nervous disease involving shaking, rhythmic tremor of the hands. Also called *Parkinson's disease* or paralysis agitans.

shank That portion of the leg extending from above the ankle to the knee.

sheath A tissue covering, such as those surrounding nerves, muscles, tendons, etc.

shell shock Battle fatigue. An emotional reaction to the fear of being injured or killed in battle which prevents the person from continuing his duties.

"shift to the left" An increase in number, as of young forms of white blood cells when an acute infection invades the body. This is seen on performing a blood count.

shigellosis A form of dysentery (diarrhea) caused by the bacillus *Shigella* of the *Salmonelleae* group.

shin The bony margin of the tibia on the front of the leg.

shingles Herpes zoster. A disease of the nerve endings in the skin characterized by the formation of blisters, crusts and severe pain along the course of the involved nerve. It is a virus infection and may last several weeks.

shin-splints Muscular tenderness and pain in the front portion of the leg, often caused by overexertion.

shock An upset caused by inadequate amounts of blood circulating in the bloodstream. It manifests itself by a drop in blood pressure, rapid weak pulse, pale moist clammy skin, marked thirst and a state of great anxiety. Shock can be caused by marked blood loss, overwhelming infection, severe injury to tissues, by emotional factors, etc.

anaphylactic Shock produced by injecting a medication or substance to which the patient is allergic or sensitized.

cardiogenic Shock brought on by a heart attack.

endotoxin Profound collapse secondary to the poisons of bacteria circulating in the bloodstream. This type of shock is seen with septicemia secondary to Gram-negative bacteria.

hematogenic Shock caused by great blood loss, as in a hemorrhage.

hypovolemic Shock caused by an insufficient amount of circulating blood.

insulin Shock caused by injecting too much insulin, resulting in too little sugar in the circulating blood.

irreversible Shock which has lasted so long that recovery cannot take place. Surgical shock lasting twenty-four hours or more is usually irreversible and death ensues.

neurogenic Shock caused by such dilatation of blood vessels that there is insufficient circulation to maintain proper blood pressure. This may be caused by injuring the brain, the spinal cord or by excessive nerve stimulation.

primary Shock occurring immediately after an injury.

reversible Shock that can be overcome by treatment.

secondary Shock occurring several hours after a severe injury.

treatment Electric current administered to the brain causing momentary unconsciousness and convulsions, given in the treatment of mentally disturbed people. Most helpful in treating manic-depressive states.

shock lung One that is incapaci-

tated by shock, with diminished ability to accommodate air because of fluid and collapse of its air spaces.

shortening of eye muscles Surgery performed to correct a cross-eye (strabismus).

short-term memory The ability to remember recent events. (Some elderly people have good memory of events that took place many years ago but forget many recent events.)

"shot" A common expression denoting an injection or inoculation, such as a *polio shot, typhoid shot,* etc.

shoulder The region where the arm joins the body.

show Loose expression for the blood-tinged discharge of mucus from the vagina seen just prior to the onset of labor.

shunt A bypass; an alternate route. A *shunt operation* is one in which blood is detoured so that it alters its course, performed to bypass clotted (thrombosed) vessels.

sialadenitis An inflammation of a salivary gland.

sialic acids Derivatives of neuraminic acid.

sialidase *See* neuraminidase.

sialo- Combining form meaning related to saliva or the salivary glands.

sialoadenectomy Surgical removal of a salivary gland.

sialodenitis Inflammation of a salivary gland. Also written as *sialadenitis.*

sialogogue A medication causing secretion of saliva. Also written as *sialagogue.*

sialography X-ray examination of the salivary glands after injection of a radiopaque material into their ducts.

sialolithotomy The surgical incision for removal of a stone from the duct or removal of one of the salivary glands.

sialorrhea Secretion of flow of saliva.

Siamese twins Twins whose bodies are joined together.

sibling A brother or sister.

sibling rivalry Jealousy between brothers or sisters.

sickle cell anemia A type of anemia, characterized by a sickle shape to the red blood cells. It is seen mostly in dark-skinned people.

sickle cell trait The coexistence of both normal and abnormal hemoglobin in a person without symptoms of sickle cell anemia. Such a person can, however, transmit sickle cell anemia to an offspring.

sicklemia *See* sickle cell anemia.

side-effect A result that has not been anticipated from a certain specific course of treatment. Side-effects are sometimes beneficial, at other times harmful.

sideropenia Iron deficiency in the body, primarily in the blood.

siderosis Chronic inflammation of the lungs seen among miners who work in iron mines. Also called arcwelder's disease.

sig. A prescription abbreviation meaning in Latin *signetur;* let it be labeled. This is an instruction from the physician to the pharmacist.

sigmoid colon Part of the descending colon on the left side of the abdomen; that part of the left large bowel just before the beginning of the rectum.

sigmoidectomy The surgical removal of the sigmoid portion of the large bowel.

sigmoiditis Inflammation of the sigmoid colon.

sigmoidoscope A long, hollow, lighted tube used to look into the rectum and sigmoid colon. It is inserted through the rectum and is about 10 inches long.

signa A prescription notation preceding instructions on how a medication is to be taken. Abbreviation is *sig.*

sign Objective evidence of disease, such as when a rash is a *sign* of a disease.

Argyll Robertson A specific reaction of the pupil in which it reacts to accommodation (changing the distance of one's gaze) but does not react to changes in light; seen in certain cases of advanced syphilis.

Battle's Bluish discoloration behind the ear, diagnostic of a fractured skull.

Chvostek's In tetany, tapping the muscles of the face causes them to go into spasm.

Cullen's Following the rupture of an ectopic pregnancy with marked hemorrhage into the abdominal cavity; the navel is discolored blue.

fontanel Bulging of the openings in the skulls of infants is present in meningitis and in conditions where pressure within the skull is increased.

Hegar's A softer than normal feel to the lower portion of the uterus, coming on about 7 to 8 weeks of pregnancy.

Homan's In cases of phlebitis of the deep veins of the leg, jerking the foot upward will cause pain in the calf.

Kernig's In cases of meningitis, attempts to straighten the knee completely when the thigh is flexed meet with pain and resistance.

Koplik's Spots in the mouth occurring a few days before the onset of measles.

Laseàgue's In cases of sciatica, attempts to raise the leg when the patient is lying flat on his back are accompanied by pain and resistance.

McBurney's In appendicitis, pain, tenderness, and muscle spasm are present in the right lower portion of the abdomen.

moulage Absence of the feathery appearance of the lining of the small intestine, as seen on X ray in cases of sprue.

Murphy's Pain in the right upper portion of the abdomen on finger pressure, seen in cases of

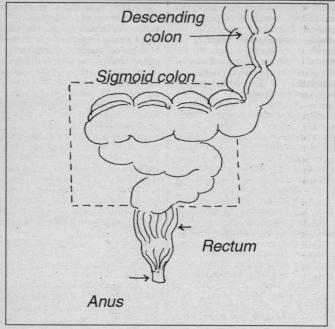

Sigmoid colon

acute inflammation of the gall bladder.

Romberg Inability to keep one's balance when standing with eyes closed; seen in cases of syphilis of the spinal cord.

Silastic bag A sac made of rubber and silicone, often filled with silicone or salt solution. It produces little or no reaction when buried in tissues and is therefore used in plastic surgery to augment the size of the breast.

sildenafil Medication, taken orally, which is said to be helpful in creating an erection in some men who are impotent.

silicone A plastic material with many uses, including the coating of glass receptacles for the collection of blood, injection into tissues to fill out defects, etc. (Silicone, because it causes so little tissue reaction, has been used in plastic surgery to obliterate wrinkles and to enlarge the appearance of the breasts.)

silicosis A chronic fibrous lung condition found among miners who have inhaled silicon dust over a period of years.

silver nitrate A chemical used to shrink inflamed mucous membranes; also used as an astringent on proud flesh.

simethicone A medication to cut down on the amount of gas in the lower intestines.

Similac Trade name for several types of infant formulas.

Simmond's disease A set of symptoms with extreme emaciation and exhaustion, caused by failure of the pituitary gland.

simple mastectomy Surgical removal of the breast without the removal of the underlying muscles or the glands in the armpit (axilla).

simulation A disease that mimics or resembles another.

sinew Tendon.

singultus Having hiccups.

sinister Left.

sinistrality The development of the right side of the brain to a dominant position over the left side, as seen in left-handed people.

sinistro- Combining form meaning left, or related to the left side.

sinoatrial block Disturbance in heart action due to interruption of normal impulses which travel between the atrium (auricle), and the sinoatrial node (the point of origin of the normal heart beat).

sinuous Twisting and turning, such as the twisting and turning of the sinus tract.

sinus 1. A hollow body cavity. 2. A channel containing blood from the veins. 3. The hollow spaces in the bones surrounding the nose, the paranasal sinuses.

    ethmoid *See* ethmoid sinus.

    frontal *See* frontal sinuses.

    maxillary *See* maxillary sinus.

    sphenoid *See* sphenoid sinus.

sinusitis Inflammation of one of the sinuses about the nose.

sinusotomy Incision into a sinus; an artificial opening drilled into a bony sinus for the purpose of allowing drainage of pus.

sinus rhythm The normal, regular heart rhythm.

Sinutab Medication for relief of symptoms of allergies and sinus disorders.

siphonage Washing out the stomach or any other cavity by applying negative pressure (siphoning).

Sippy diet One composed mainly of milk and cream, advocated for

those suffering acutely from an ulcer of the stomach or duodenum.

sister A registered nurse (British).

Sister Kenny treatment A method of treating infantile paralysis, directed toward the relief of muscle spasm seen in the early stages of the disease.

sitology The science of dietetics.

sitomania Excessive craving for food.

situs inversus A birth deformity in which the organs are on the opposite side from normal, such as a right-sided heart.

sitz bath A sitting bath, frequently used to relieve pain and congestion in the rectal or pelvic areas.

skatole A breakdown product of protein found in the feces and partially responsible for the characteristic odor of the feces.

Skelaxin A muscle-relaxing medication.

skeleton The bony support of the body.

Skene's glands The small mucous glands located on either side of the urethra (the tube leading urine from the bladder to the outside) in females.

skiagram An X-ray picture.

skin tabs Excessive "tabs" or projections of skin about the anus; seen often after the removal of hemorrhoids (piles).

skip area An area that is unaffected by a disease process that affects other parts of the same organ; seen not infrequently in ulcerative disease of the small and large intestine.

skipped generation A situation wherein someone inherits a condition or trait from a previous ancestor, but not from an immediate relative such as a parent.

skull The bony structure containing the brain.

sleeping sickness Inflammation of the brain (encephalitis). The disease is so-named because its frequent symptoms are lethargy and sleepiness.

slide A rectangular piece of glass on which material to be examined under the microscope is mounted.

sliding flap operation A plastic surgery procedure in which flaps of skin are fashioned so that they cover a raw surface. Such flaps are obtained from the sides of the raw area.

sling A bandage placed around a bodily part in order to support it, such as an arm *sling* placed around the neck.

slipped disk *See* disk.

slipped epiphysis An epiphysis that is out of place, seen occasionally in children. *See* epiphysis.

slough Dead tissue which separates from a wound, abscess, burned area, etc.

SMA Iron-Fortified Infant Formula A ready-to-feed infant formula.

smallpox A highly contagious, sometimes fatal disease tending to occur in epidemic form. It is accompanied by high fever and a characteristic skin eruption. It can be prevented by periodic vaccination.

smear Cells which have been smeared or spread onto a glass slide and stained for examination under a microscope.

smegma The material secreted by the sebaceous glands of the foreskin and the labia minora. This material is thought by some to irritate the cervix of the uterus and possibly cause it to undergo tumor formation.

smooth muscle Muscle that contracts and relaxes involuntarily, such as the muscles in the blood vessels, intestines, and bladder. (To be distinguished from voluntary muscles, such as those in the limbs, etc.)

SMO steel A steel alloy used in bone surgery. It causes little or no tissue reaction and is therefore well tolerated by the body.

Snellen test A test of vision; a normal reading on this test is 20/20.

social medicine That branch of medicine which concerns itself with environmental and community factors as they relate to health and disease. Not to be confused with socialized medicine.

socialized medicine Government medicine, usually accompanied by compulsory health insurance for all citizens. Medical costs are paid out of taxes; physicians are paid by a governmental agency.

sociology The study of the origin and evolution of human society, its people, their organizations and institutions, various group functions and interrelationships.

sociomedical Referring to the welfare of the patient as it relates to the society in which he lives.

sodium (Na) A metallic element found in large amounts in many combined forms in body fluids and cells.

    bicarbonate A mild alkali used extensively to neutralize excess stomach acid. It is ordinary baking soda.

    bromide A chemical which, when taken internally, tends to calm the nerves.

    chloride Salt.

    solution, isotonic Such a salt solution approximates the strength which exists in the body tissues. It contains 0.9 grams of salt in every 100 cc. of water.

    citrate solution A solution added to transfusion blood to prevent it from clotting.

    perborate A chemical used as a mouthwash, particularly effective in trench mouth infections.

    salicylate A drug with the same pain-relieving effects as aspirin.

    sodium-24 Radioactive sodium, sometimes used in the treatment of malignancies of the bladder.

    succinate A drug used to arouse patients after anesthesia with barbiturates.

    sodium sulamyd As an ointment or eyedrop, this medication is effective in overcoming many forms of conjunctivitis due to bacteria.

sodomy 1. Unnatural methods of intercourse, such as anal intercourse, between humans. 2. Intercourse between a human and an animal.

softening A decrease in the normal firmness and consistency of an organ or tissue. ("Softening" of the brain is associated with senile changes.)

solar plexus A nerve center in the upper abdomen containing nerves which supply the stomach, liver, gall bladder, pancreas, etc.

soleus muscle One of the two large muscles making up the calf of the leg.

solipsism 1. The belief that the self can only know itself and its environment. 2. The belief that the universe consists only of the self and its experiences.

soluble Capable of dissolving, as salt is *soluble* in water.

solution The mixture of a solid, liquid or gas with another liquid. The dissolved substance is called the solute; the liquid is called the solvent. The solvent is usually in excess of the solute.

    isotonic A solution corresponding in strength to a dissolved substance encountered in body tissues, as an *isotonic salt solution* is of the same concentration as the salt solution within the bloodstream.

    Ringer's An artificially made solution containing many of the minerals found in body fluids, including sodium chloride, potassium chloride, and calcium chloride.

    saturated One containing all the solids it can hold in a dissolved state.

Solu-Cortef A cortisone solution used for intravenous injection. It will bring about a reaction within a short period of time. *See* cortisone. Used in cases of shock or severe allergic reactions.

Solu-Medrol An antiinflammatory steroid drug given by injection. Its actions are similar to prednisone, a cortisonelike medication.

solvent A liquid which can dissolve a substance.

Soma compound A medication to relieve muscle spasm and pain. Certain of its ingredients also act to lower elevated temperature.

somatic 1. Pertaining to the body. 2. Pertaining to the "framework" of the body, as differentiated from the organs of the body. 3. In psychology, pertaining to the body as distinguished from the central nervous system.

somatization A psychological term referring to the conversion of anxiety symptoms into physical ones.

somato- Combining form referring to the word *body*.

somatoplasm Body cells, as contrasted to cells found in the ovaries of testicles.

somatotype A body type, such as endomorph, ectomorph, mesomorph.

somnambulism Sleepwalking.

somnambulist One who walks in his sleep.

somnifacient 1. Causing sleep. 2. A sleep-producing drug.

somniloquy Talking in one's sleep.

somnolence Sleepiness.

sonography Sonography is a diagnostic method based upon the reflection of ultrasonic sound waves that occur at the boundaries between different tissues within the body. These reflections are recorded photographically and show the clear outlines of various organs and tissues. The reflections of the various sound waves are translated via a computer into actual images. The variations in images often make the diagnosis when viewed on a viewing screen or photograph.

sophomania A delusion in which one believes he is tremendously gifted mentally.

soporific 1. Causing deep sleep. 2. A sleep-producing drug.

sorbefacient An agent that aids

absorption, such as a medication that has been applied to the skin.

sorbitol A diuretic agent.

sordes The matter, often brownish-black in color, which collects on the lips and teeth of chronically ill people who are extremely weak and who are unable to clean it away.

S.O.S. A symbol written by physicians after an order for a drug, meaning *si opus sit, if necessary.*

sotalol A beta-blocking medication helpful in eliminating irregular heart rhythms, such as fibrillation, etc.

Sotradecol A patented preparation injected into varicose veins in order to produce a blood clot and thus obliterate the varicosity.

sound A long metal instrument used for insertion along a body channel in order to determine if the passageway is open; a *urethral sound* is passed through the penis into the bladder to discover if the urethral channel is open.

sp. *See* specific gravity.

spa A resort with mineral water springs, supposedly helpful in the treatment of certain conditions. A health resort.

space An anatomical region.

dead The vacant space left behind after the surgical removal of an organ or structure.

distal closed The tissue space of the finger tip, an area particularly prone to infection.

epidural The area just outside the spinal canal. Anesthetic drugs are sometimes injected into this space in order to anesthetize body areas in the vicinity.

fascial Areas in between bundles of ligaments, muscles, tendons, etc.

intercostal The space between ribs.

mediastinal The area in which the heart and great blood vessels are located in the chest.

palmar Compartments in the anterior portion of the hand.

peritoneal Areas in between the intestines and other abdominal organs.

perivascular Those areas surrounding blood vessels.

popliteal The back of the knee.

prevesical The area above and in front of the urinary bladder.

retroperitoneal The area behind the abdomen in which the kidneys, adrenal glands, aorta, vena cava, etc., are located.

retropharyngeal The area behind the throat.

subarachnoid A space, surrounding the brain and spinal cord, and beneath the arachnoid (a membrane), which contains cerebrospinal fluid.

subdural A space containing blood vessels, surrounding the brain, but beneath the dura mater (a membrane). A severe head injury may cause hemorrhage into this space, called a *subdural hematoma.*

subphrenic The area beneath the diaphragm.

space medicine That branch of medicine which is concerned with the biological effects on the individual of flying to extremely high altitudes at extremely high speeds.

spallation Bombarding elements with protons, alpha particles, etc., in order to cause changes in the structure of such elements.

Spanish fly *See* cantharides.

spasm An abrupt and forceful contraction of a muscle, usually maintained for several minutes or hours and frequently associated with marked pain.

carpopedal A simultaneous forceful contraction (spasm) of the hands and feet, as seen in tetany, which is caused by calcium deficiency.

clonic Muscle contractions and relaxations occurring intermittently; a series of "convulsions."

tonic Muscle contractions which

continue steadily without periods of relaxation.

spasmodic Pertaining to or characterized by spasms.

spastic Characterized by spasms.

spasticity Prolonged and continued contraction of a muscle.

spatula A flat wooden or metal instrument, used to spread an ointment.

Specialist A physician who limits his practice to the study and treatment of one class of diseases or who confines his interest to specific organs or systems within the body.

specific Pertaining to a particular organ or disease. A *specific* drug is one which affects a particular disease.

specific gravity The weight of a volume of a substance compared with the weight of an equal volume of another substance used as a standard. Water is usually the standard for solids and liquids.

specimen radiography Removal of tissue and submission of the tissue for X-ray examination; a procedure sometimes practiced after excision of a lump in a breast.

spectography An apparatus to photograph the spectrum; used in detecting and noting the characteristics of certain isotopes.

spectrochemistry The identification and study of substances through spectroscopy.

spectroscopy A method of measuring various light rays in a spectrum. (Different chemicals emit different rays and can therefore be identified by using a spectroscope.)

speculum Any instrument inserted into a body opening so that the examiner may view inside it better, such as a *vaginal speculum, nasal speculum,* etc.

speech center The part of the brain that controls the power of speech. In right-handers it is on the left side of the brain; in left-handers on the right side.

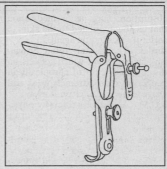

Speculum (vaginal) bi-valve

"speed" Slang for the drug methamphetamine.

sperm The male germ cell, manufactured in the testicle; a spermatozoon.

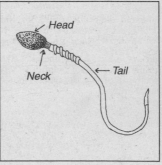

Sperm

spermatic cord The tubular structure leading from the testicle to the seminal vesicle and conveying semen.

spermatocele A cyst of the testicle or epididymis which connects with the testicle. Such growths contain sperm manufactured by the testicle.

spermatocyte The forerunner of the mature sperm (germ cell).

spermatogenesis The process by which male germ cells (sperm) are formed.

spermatorrhea The flow of semen and sperm from the male organ without sexual stimulation; an abnormal condition not under the control of the individual afflicted with it.

spermaturia The passage of semen in the urine.

sperm count An estimate of the number of sperm in an ejaculation, usually several hundred million. Low sperm counts may indicate lack of male fertility.

sperm donor A male who contributes his sperm toward the impregnation of a female. Sperm donors are used in cases where the husband is sterile.

spermicide A contraceptive which kills sperm on contact with it.

sphenoiditis Inflammation of the sphenoid sinus, associated with fever, headache, pain in the eyes, and a discharge down the back of the nose.

sphenoid sinus A cavity in the skull behind and above the nose. It has an outlet which drains into the nasal cavity.

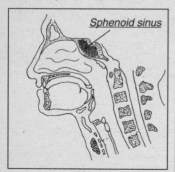

Sphenoid sinus

sphenopalatine ganglion An important nerve center in the face, the nerves of which supply the nose and the palate in the mouth.

spherocytes Red blood cells which are round all over instead of having two concave sides. They are particularly fragile and are easily ruptured and destroyed.

spherocytosis A disease in which the red blood cells are spherocytes and rupture easily. It is an inherited disease associated with anemia, jaundice, and an enlarged spleen. Also called *chronic familial jaundice* or *hemolytic anemia.*

sphincter A ringlike muscle which controls opening and closing of a bodily opening. In the intestinal tract there are the *pyloric sphincter*, the *ileocolic sphincter*, the *anal sphincter*, etc.

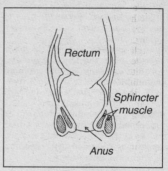

Sphincter anal muscle

    anal The one surrounding the anus (the termination of the rectum).

    cardiac The one surrounding the lower end of the esophagus (food pipe) at the entrance to the stomach. (This has no relation to the heart.)

    of Oddi The one surrounding the termination of the bile duct and pancreatic duct at the entrance to the duodenum (small intestine).

    pyloric The one surrounding the outlet of the stomach at the entrance of the duodenum.

    urethral The one surrounding the urethra (the tubular structure leading from the bladder to the outside). The action of this sphincter is under voluntary control.

vaginal The muscles surrounding the entrance to the vagina.

sphincterismus A muscle spasm, usually painful, involving the sphincter surrounding the anus.

sphincterotomy The surgical cutting of a sphincter, as the anal sphincter, in cases of painful fissure.

sphygmomanometer Device for measuring the blood pressure.

sphygmus The pulse.

spica A figure-of-eight bandage applied to an extremity, such as a thumb, arm, or thigh, usually because of a fracture.

spicule A small, sharp piece of something hard, such as bone.

spider, black widow A jet-black spider, the female having a red hourglass-shaped marking on its underside. Only the female bites and her bite can cause severe reactions including intense abdominal pain and rigidity of the muscles. Occasional fatalities, especially among children, result from the bite.

spider bursts Small reddish-blue marks in the skin of the legs caused by many small-sized varicose veins. These marks are often in the shape of a spider.

spike 1. A sharp rise in the tracing made during electroencephalography (the recording of brain waves). 2. A sudden, abrupt rise in temperature with a return to normal or near-normal within a few hours.

spina bifida A severe birth defect in which there has been incomplete formation and fusion of the spinal canal. A hernia (rupture) occurs in which the spinal cord and nerves protrude through the back and appear beneath the skin.

occulta A birth deformity in which there is incomplete formation of the spinal canal but no hernia or protrusion takes place.

spinal accessory nerve The eleventh cranial nerve, exiting from the skull and supplying muscles in the throat and neck.

spinal canal The area, filled with

spinal fluid, immediately surrounding the spinal cord. It is tapped when performing a lumbar puncture.

spinal cord That part of the central nervous system contained within the vertebral (spinal) column.

spinal fusion An operation for fusing and making the spinal column rigid. Often carried out for marked curvature of the spine (scoliosis).

spinalis muscles Muscles along the vertebra which help to straighten the head and spine.

spine The backbone or spinal column.

cervical That portion of the spine which is in the neck; the first seven vertebrae.

dorsal That portion of the spine which is in the chest. Also called thoracic spine. There are twelve dorsal vertebrae.

lumbar That portion of the spine which is in the lower back. There are five lumbar vertebrae.

sacrococcygeal That portion of the spine which forms the posterior wall of the pelvis. There are five fused sacral vertebrae and four fused coccygeal vertebrae in the sacrococcygeal spine.

spirochete A type of bacterium. The germ causing syphilis is of the *spirochete* type. So called because of its spiral shape.

spirometer An apparatus for measuring the amount of air breathed in and out.

splanchnicectomy An operation cutting the splanchnic nerves in the abdomen. It is sometimes performed in an attempt to reduce chronic hypertension (high blood pressure).

splanchnic nerves Those supplying the abdominal organs such as the intestines, stomach, liver, spleen, pancreas, etc.

spleen An abdominal organ located in the left upper portion of the abdomen. It is a lymph organ which, during the life of the embryo, manu-

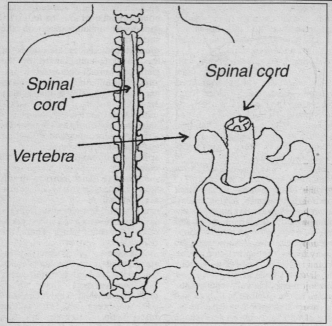

Spinal cord

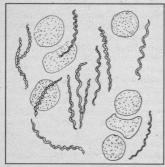

Spirochetes

factures blood cells. After birth, one of its functions is related to disposal of old, worn-out red blood cells. Other functions are not yet completely determined.

accessory Small additional spleens sometimes found in the vicinity of the main spleen.

splenectomy Surgical removal of the spleen, advocated for certain blood diseases and for certain types of overactivity of the spleen (hypersplenism).

splenic artery The blood vessel supplying the spleen.

splenic infarct A clot of a vessel of the spleen leading to a segment of the organ. As a result, that portion becomes functionless. *See also* infarct.

splenic puncture The insertion of a needle into the spleen and the withdrawal of cells for microscopic examination; a form of biopsy.

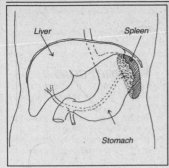

Liver   Spleen

Stomach

Spleen

splenitis Inflammation of the spleen.

splenohepatomegaly Enlargement of both the spleen and liver.

splenomegaly Enlargement of the spleen.

splenoportography Visualization on X-ray films of the circulation of the spleen and portal vein which goes to the liver. (This is accomplished by the injection of a radiopaque substance into the spleen.)

splenorenal shunt Surgical connection of the large vein of the spleen (splenic vein) to the large vein of the left kidney (renal vein) in an attempt to have the blood bypass the liver. This is sometimes performed in cases of cirrhosis of the liver, in which blood cannot pass through the liver.

splenorrhaphy An operation to repair an injured spleen.

splint A support for an injured extremity or other part of the body. It may be constructed out of wood, metal, plastic, etc. Its object is to stop movement of the injured part.

    airplane One designed to keep the arm up and out from the side of the body, usually at right angles.

    banjo A wire and rubber hand splint to put traction (pull) on a broken finger, so called because it is shaped like a banjo.

    T One applied to the upper

back in cases of fractured collarbone. It is shaped like the letter T.

spondylitis Inflammation of the vertebrae.

spondylolisthesis A deformity of the spinal column caused by the gliding forward of one vertebra, usually the fifth lumbar vertebra, on to the sacrum. At times, this is very painful.

spondylosis Fusion of the vertebrae with one another. This process tends to occur in elderly people or those afflicted with certain types of arthritis of the spine.

sponge A piece of gauze or a gauze pad, used in surgery to absorb blood, pus, or other fluid collections.

spongioblastoma A tumor originating from the supporting connective tissue of brain or other nerve cells. They often form within the skull.

spongiocyte 1. A cell which is present in the coverings of certain nerves; 2. Certain cells in the cortex of the suprarenal gland.

spontaneous abortion A miscarriage that occurs naturally, without any attempts to induce it.

spontaneous fracture One that is not caused by an injury, such as a fracture of a bone due to a cancer.

spontaneous pneumothorax Air in the chest (pleural) cavity; an abnormal condition of unknown cause.

sporadic Occurring once in a while.

spore The reproductive cell of certain lower organisms, such as the tetanus germ. It is covered by a thick shell and survives great heat and great cold, thus making it difficult to destroy.

sporicide Anything which destroys the spores of germs.

sporotrichosis A chronic fungus infection found especially among farmers. It is due to a fungus found in dirt. The skin is most often affected but other organs may also be involved.

sport A form of animal or plant

life which has many characteristics differing markedly from those of its parents; a mutation.

spotting A nontechnical term meaning a slight bloody discharge from the vagina not coming at the time of the expected menstrual period. It may signify some abnormality of the female organs.

sprain A tear, rupture or marked stretching of a muscle, ligament or a joint.

spray A medicine which is applied by vaporizing it and *spraying* with a specially designed container.

spring catarrh An allergic inflammation of the conjunctiva (membrane of the eyeball), usually coming on in the spring, lasting a few weeks or months and disappearing spontaneously; vernal conjunctivitis.

sprue A nutritional deficiency disease, chronic in nature. Its cause is unknown. The symptoms are: anemia, sore red tongue, large frothy stools, loss of weight and weakness.

spur A pointed growth on a bone, often seen in the heel bone (calcaneus). It is not malignant.

sputum Mucous material spit out of the mouth. It may rise from the nose, throat, windpipe or lungs.

squamous Resembling in shape the scales of a fish. *Squamous* cells line certain body surfaces.

squill A medication having many of the same effects as digitalis. Occasionally used to support the action of heart muscle.

squint A condition in which the eyes are crossed; strabismus.

ss. A prescription symbol meaning *semis,* one-half.

stab Puncture.

stable 1. Referring to an individual who makes it a practice to exercise emotional control. 2. Referring to a chemical or compound which resists destruction and maintains its normal composition.

stabilization procedure An operation to create stability in an unstable joint, usually done by fusing some of the bones of the joint.

staff, attending The active group of physicians who are in charge of the ward patients in a public or voluntary hospital.

   consultant Experienced older physicians whose positions in the hospital are mainly those of an advisory nature.

   house The interns and residents who live in a hospital.

   visiting The physicians who come to a hospital to see ward or private patients.

stage A period during the course of a condition or disease.

   eruptive The period when a rash appears during the course of a contagious disease.

   of labor There are three stages. First: When the baby's head is in the pelvic canal and the cervix of the uterus is dilating; Second: When the baby emerges; Third: When the afterbirth (placenta) is expelled.

   pre-eruptive The period before a rash comes out.

staggers A common word, used by tunnel workers and divers, for the symptoms of caisson's disease. The symptoms include dizziness, vertigo, weakness, and mental confusion.

stagnation A term usually applied to blood which is not flowing as fast as is normal; the blood in large varicose veins *stagnates.*

stain A dye. Tissues to be examined under the microscope are first *stained* with various pigments, resulting in certain parts of the tissues appearing red, blue, green, yellow, etc., according to the manner in which they absorb the dye in which they are immersed. There are hundreds of tissue stains producing characteristic color effects which aid in diagnosis.

stalk An elongated portion of tissue, as the *stalk* of a polyp.

stamina Strength, ability to undergo physical strain.

stammer To speak haltingly.

standard deviation (SD) The degree of deviation from the average.

standstill, cardiac Sudden stoppage of the heart; cardiac arrest. A condition occurring rarely during surgery and requiring immediate massage of the heart to start it beating again.

stapedectomy An operation in which the stapes bone of the middle ear is removed as part of a procedure to restore lost hearing.

stapes One of the three small bones of the ear (the incus, malleus, and *stapes*).

    mobilization operation An operation to relieve deafness in which the small bones of hearing, such as the stapes bone, are freed of adhesions and manipulated so that they vibrate normally.

Staphcillin A penicillin preparation particularly useful in overcoming staphylococcus infections.

staphylectomy Surgical removal of the uvula, the pointed projection of tissue into the mouth from the palate.

staphylococcemia Blood poisoning (septicemia) due to the presence of staphylococcus germs in the circulating blood.

staphylococcus A type of germ (bacteria). It appears round under a microscope. Probably the most prevalent type of germ in existence. It may cause simple pimples, boils, etc., or more important infections in organs of the body.

    antitoxin Antibodies obtained from the serum of horses who have been injected with staphylococcus toxin. This material is injected into humans to combat a staphylococcus infection.

    toxoid The poisons of the germ which have been altered sufficiently so that they do not create the effects of a staphylococcal infection but can, nevertheless, stimulate the formation of antibodies which will combat a staphylococcus infection.

staphylorrhaphy Surgical repair of a cleft palate.

stapler A mechanical device used to clip tissues together; a procedure sometimes performed instead of the usual stitching with ordinary suture material.

stasis Stagnation. Sluggishness of function.

Stat. An abbreviation for *statim,* immediately. Used as an instruction when prescribing for a patient.

static In balance; quiescent.

statistical significance The probabilities that a study or investigation will or will not be reliable or important.

status A condition.

    anginosus Repeated, uncontrollable attacks of pain in the heart area (angina pectoris).

    asthmaticus Continuous, unrelieved asthmatic attacks, sometimes ending fatally.

    epilepticus Repeated attacks of epilepsy occurring one after another.

    lymphaticus A state of suffocation and sudden death, supposedly caused by enlargement of the thymus gland beneath the breastbone. Death of children under anesthesia was often attributed to *status lymphaticus.* This entire theory is now being challenged by most physicians.

statuvolence Self-induced trance; self-hypnotism.

STD Abbreviation for sexually transmitted disease.

steady state Constancy; a state which does not change.

steapsin An enzyme (chemical) originating in the pancreas, which digests fats secreted into the intestines.

steatitis Inflammation of fat tissue.

steatolysis Emulsification of fats prior to their absorption from the intestines.

steatoma A sebaceous cyst; a wen.

steatorrhea 1. Increased discharge

from sebaceous glands. 2. Fatty feces.

Steinmann pin A metal nail, driven through the ends of bones such as the femur (thighbone) or tibia (leg bone), in order to obtain traction in cases of fracture.

Stelazine A drug sometimes helpful in treating psychotic disorders (mental illness).

stellate Star-shaped.

stenocephaly An exceptionally narrow skull.

stenose Narrowed, such as a *stenosed* blood vessel or heart valve.

stenosis Constriction or narrowing of a passageway or opening, such as *pyloric stenosis* in which the exit of the stomach is constricted.

    aortic Narrowing of the value of the aorta (which is near the heart).

    mitral Narrowing of the mitral valve of the heart. This condition can now be treated surgically, by mitral commissurotomy.

    pyloric Narrowing of the outlet of the stomach.

    tricuspid Narrowing of the tricuspid valve of the heart (which is on the right side).

Stenson's duct The duct (tube) leading from the parotid gland at the angle of the jaw to the inside of the cheek. It transports saliva to the mouth.

stent A mold, used to shape tissues which have been operated upon and stitched into new positions. It helps tissues to retain their new shapes.

stercolith A very hard piece of stool.

stercus Stool; feces.

stereo- A prefix referring to something that is three-dimensional.

stereoanesthesia Inability to recognize objects merely by handling them.

stereochemistry The branch of chemistry dealing with atoms and the space they occupy in compounds.

stereognosis The ability to recognize objects merely by handling them.

stereogram An X-ray picture giving the impression of being three-dimensional; a stereoscopic X ray.

stereopsis Three dimensional vision.

stereoradiography Three dimensional X-ray pictures.

stereotaxis Three-dimensional.

sterile 1. Unable to have children. 2. Germ free.

sterile abscess One that contains no bacteria or other organisms.

sterility 1. Incapable of bearing children. Unable to reproduce. 2. Creating an area in which no bacteria can live; such as a *sterile* field for surgery to be performed.

sterilization 1. Destruction of germs. 2. An operative procedure performed to make an individual sterile, such as by tying off the uterine tubes in females or the vas deferens in males.

sterilizer An apparatus for making instruments, drapes, or other materials free from germs (bacteria).

sternal puncture Inserting a specially devised needle into the marrow of the breastbone (sternum). This is done to obtain bone marrow cells which are then submitted to microscopic examination. Sternal puncture is frequently advocated in cases of suspected blood disease.

sternoclavicular region Referring to both the collarbone and breastbone.

sternocleidomastoid muscles The large muscles on either side of the neck extending from behind the ears down to the junction of the breastbone and collarbones.

sternodynia Pain in the breastbone (sternum).

sternomastoid muscle Same as sternocleidomastoid.

sternothyroid A small neck muscle extending from the sternum (breastbone) to the thyroid cartilage (the voice box). Its action is to pull the larynx in a downward direction.

sternotomy Cutting the sternum, an operation performed in order to

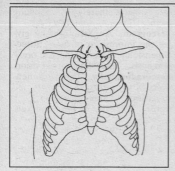

Sternoclavicular joint

gain surgical access to the mediastinum (the space in which the heart and great vessels are located).

sternum The breastbone in the front of the chest.

steroids Drugs of hormone origin, especially those from the pituitary and adrenal glands. These are often used in the treatment of various disease states. Examples are: cortisone, ACTH, etc.

stertorous breathing Loud, harsh sounds heard in certain types of breathing; snoring.

stethoscope An instrument used by physicians to amplify sounds heard from the body, such as heart sounds, breath sounds, etc.

Stewart-Morel syndrome A condi-

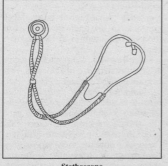

Stethoscope

tion mostly affecting women past menopause, characterized by overgrowth of the skull above the eye region, obesity, and headache.

sthenic type A vigorous, energetic person.

stigma A mark or sign signifying the existence of some special condition.

stilbestrol Diethylstilbestrol, a preparation containing the female sex hormone.

stillbirth The birth of a dead child.

stillborn A child born dead.

Still's disease A chronic infectious arthritis in childhood, in which many joints are attacked.

stimulants Any drug whose action produces stimulation (caffeine, Benzedrine, etc.).

stimulation Causing an exciting reaction in the body. The smell of cooking food *stimulates* the secretion of saliva in a hungry person.

stimulus Something which stimulates or results in a specific reaction.

   threshold The least stimulation which will produce a desired reaction.

stippling Small black dots, as seen in red blood cells in cases of lead poisoning.

stitch 1. Suture. 2. A sudden, sharp pain.

stockinet A cotton stocking applied to an arm or leg prior to the application of a plaster cast.

Stokes-Adams disease *See* Adams-Stokes disease.

stoma 1. A minute opening, a skin pore. 2. The opening in the abdominal wall formed in certain surgical procedures for the passage of intestinal contents.

stomach That part of the digestive tract located between the esophagus (food pipe) and the duodenum (the first portion of the small intestine). It is dilated and saclike in shape. Its main function is to churn food and to start the processes of digestion.

   hourglass One constricted in

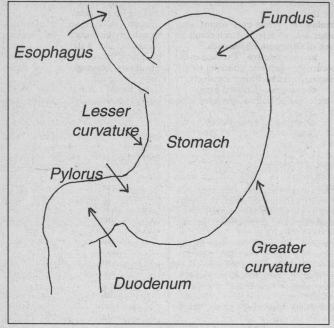

Stomach

its midportion so that it takes the shape of an hourglass.

    J shaped One shaped like the letter J.

    steerhorn One shaped like the horn of a steer.

    "upside-down" One which has protruded through a hernia (opening) in the diaphragm so that a portion of it lies within the chest cavity.

stomachic A medication to stimulate the appetite.

stomatitis Inflammation of the mucous membranes of the mouth.

stomatology The branch of medicine that concerns itself with diseases and functions of the mouth.

stomodeum The mouth of an embryo during the early stages of its development.

stone 1. 14 pounds (British terminology). 2. A calculus; a solid mineral concretion, such as a gall bladder or kidney calculus (stone).

stool Feces.

    fatty Feces containing large amounts of fat, seen in diseases of the pancreas, such as celiac disease, etc.

    lead pencil Very narrow feces, as seen in stricture of the anus, rectum or descending colon.

    mucous Feces mixed with mucus, as seen in some cases of inflammation of the bowel lining.

    tarry Jet-black stools, seen when there has been hemorrhage in the upper portion (stomach or duodenum) of the intestinal tract.

storm, thyroid Severe toxic reaction associated with over-activity of the thyroid gland.

strabismus Cross-eye, squint and other muscle defects which result in lack of alignment of the eyes.

    accommodative Crossed-eyes occurring when one attempts to accommodate his vision excessively.

    convergent Crossed-eyes in which one or both of the eyes turn in.

    divergent Crossed-eyes in which one or both of the eyes turn out.

strain Pain in a muscle due to excessive stretching or overuse.

straitjacket A cloth jacket with arms so long that they can be wrapped around the patient's body, thus restraining his movement. Used on delirious or insane patients.

stramonium A drug causing relaxation of blood vessels; the same effect as atropine, scopolamine, etc.

strangulation 1. Inability to breathe because the air passage is blocked. 2. Death of a part because the circulation is cut off, as *strangulation* of a loop of bowel caught in a hernia.

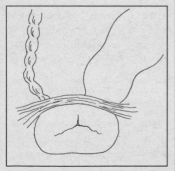

Strangulation of bowel due to adhesive band

strangury Difficult, painful urination with passage of only a small amount at a time.

stratification Occurrence of tissues

in layers, as in the case of the cells making up the skin.

stratum A layer, such as of tissues.

strawberry birthmark One looking somewhat like a strawberry, caused by dilated blood-vessels in the skin.

strawberry hemangioma *See* strawberry birthmark.

strep throat An infection of the pharynx and tonsils due to the streptococcus. It can cause high fever, chills, malaise, swelling of lymph glands, etc. It is treated with antibiotics.

streptococcemia Blood poisoning due to streptococci growing in the blood stream.

streptococcus A type of germ (bacteria). It may cause severe infections in humans. Under the microscope, these germs appear round and often occur in long chains.

streptokinase An enzyme whose action helps to dissolve blood clots and adhesions. It is used frequently following an acute coronary artery thrombosis.

streptomycin A powerful antibiotic drug useful against many bacteria, particularly the germ causing tuberculosis.

streptothricosis *See* actinomycosis.

stress incontinence Involuntary loss of urine under conditions of stress, seen most often among women in their middle or later years.

stress reactions Abnormal conditions or disorders caused by undue stress or the tensions of living.

stretch marks Lines on the abdominal skin sometimes occurring in women during the later months of pregnancy.

striae Streaks or stripes, as in the skin seen on the abdomen of a pregnant woman.

striated muscle Voluntary muscle, as in the arms and legs. It is so called because on microscopic examination it appears to have cross stripes.

stricture An abnormal narrowing,

as a *stricture* of the esophagus or rectum.

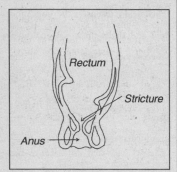

Stricture of the anus

stridor Loud, harsh breathing, caused by failure of the larynx to be open sufficiently during respiration.

stringent Binding.

stripping 1. The last of the milk to be gotten from a breast. 2. An operative procedure for varicose veins in which large sections of the veins are removed with a metal "stripper," an instrument inserted into the passageway of the veins which are to be removed.

stroke Apoplexy. The sudden rupture or clotting of a blood vessel to the brain. It may lead to unconsciousness, partial paralysis, and in some instances, death.

stroma The connective tissue of an organ. The tissue not actively concerned with the function of the organ, such as the fibrous tissue, nerves, blood vessels, etc., of a gland whose function it is to secrete.

strontium-90 A radioactive substance resulting from fallout after an atomic explosion. (Excessive amounts absorbed into the body may lodge in bones and cause harmful radiation effects.)

strophanthin A chemical used to aid the action of heart muscle. It has much the same action as digitalis.

structure 1. The arrangement of the elements that make up an organ or bodily part. 2. An organ or part of the body.

struma A goiter.

Hashimoto's A lymph tumor of the thyroid gland, an uncommon form of goiter.

Riedel's An inflammation of the thyroid gland; "woody thyroiditis."

strychnine A chemical obtained from nux vomica. It is valuable as a stimulant when given in small doses. In large doses, it acts as a dangerous poison, producing violent convulsions and death.

stunting Stopping growth. Contrary to common belief, there are no foods or medicines which cause *stunting* of growth.

stupe A poultice, often containing turpentine, for applying heat or counterirritation, as a *stupe* applied to the abdomen to promote passage of gas.

stupefaction Bewilderment; stupor; mental sluggishness.

stupor Semiconsciousness; lack of alertness to the degree that one is only partly sensible.

stye An infection of a sebaceous gland of an eyelid. Hordeolum.

stylet 1. A metal rod inserted into a rubber catheter to give it firmness for insertion into the urethra. 2. A thin metal wire inserted into a hypodermic needle so that it does not become clogged.

stylomandibular joint The joint between the lower jaw and the temporal bone of the skull, located beneath the temple.

styptic A medication causing capillaries (tiny blood vessels) to contract and thus stop superficial hemorrhage.

sub- A prefix meaning "beneath," "under."

subacromial Referring to the region just beneath the front of the shoulder joint.

subacute In between acute and chronic.

subacute bacterial endocarditis An

infection of the heart valves with *Streptococcus viridans*. Until the discovery of the sulfa drugs and the antibiotics, this disease ended fatally within several months or years. Today, most patients can be cured. This condition affects mainly those who have rheumatic valve disease.

subaqueous Under water, as a *subaqueous drainage tube* whose end is placed beneath the level of the water in a bottle.

subarachnoid hemorrhage Hemorrhage around the brain beneath the arachnoid membrane which covers the brain. A bloody spinal tap is evidence of such a hemorrhage.

subarachnoid space The area beneath the arachnoid membrane which covers the brain.

subclavian Beneath the clavicle (collarbone), as the *subclavian artery*.

subclinical disease A condition whose signs and symptoms are so mild and slight that they go unnoticed.

subconscious That portion of the unconscious mind whose contents, such as memories, can be recalled at will.

subcostal Beneath the ribs.

subcutaneous Underneath the skin.

subdeltoid Beneath the deltoid muscle on the outer surface of the shoulder joint and down on to the arm, as *subdeltoid bursitis*.

subdiaphragmatic Under the diaphragm in the uppermost reaches of the abdomen.

subdural Beneath the dura (a

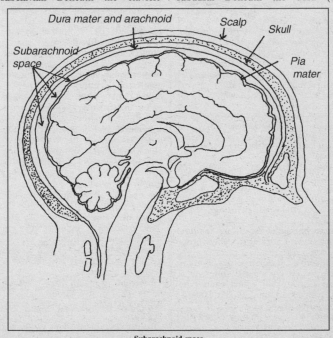

Subarachnoid space

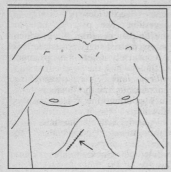

Subcostal incision

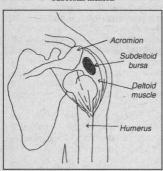

Acromion

Subdeltoid bursa

Deltoid muscle

Humerus

Bursa, subdeltoid

membrane covering the brain and spinal cord).

subdural hematoma A blood clot within the skull lying beneath the dura (the outer covering of the brain) but on top of the arachnoid and pia (the inner coverings of the brain).

subinvolution of the uterus Failure to return to normal size after pregnancy.

subjective Referring to symptoms the patient knows and states he is experiencing but which cannot be seen or ascertained by the examining physician.

sublethal Less than fatal, as the *sublethal* dose of a poison.

sublimate To convert base or

primitive instincts into socially acceptable aggressive acts.

sublimation The mental process whereby base or primitive instincts and desires are converted into socially acceptable conduct.

subliminal A term referring to stimulation which does not reach the patient's consciousness.

sublingual Located under the tongue, as the *sublingual gland.*

subluxation A slight dislocation of a bone or joint.

submandibular Underneath the lower jaw.

submaxillary Lying under the lower jaw, as the *submaxillary* gland.

submental Under the chin.

submucosa The connective tissue lying beneath a mucous membrane.

submucous resection An operation upon the nose to correct a deviated septum.

subnormal Below normal, as *subnormal* temperature.

suboccipital Under the back of the head.

subperiosteal region An area beneath the covering tissue (periosteum) of bone. Hemorrhage secondary to injury sometimes occurs in this region.

subpleural bleb A blister on the outer surface of the lung just beneath the pleura (the thin covering membrane of the lung). Should this burst through the pleura, a pneumothorax will result.

subscapular Beneath the shoulder blade (scapula).

subserous Beneath the serosa (the outer covering of organs such as the stomach and intestines).

subsidence Symptoms of a disease subside or disappear and there is a return to normal.

substernal Beneath the breastbone. The most common cause of *substernal* pain is coronary artery disease.

substitution In psychiatry, the replacement of an unacceptable emotion or thought with an acceptable one; an unconscious mental process.

substrate 1. An under layer; a term often applied to layers of liquid; 2. The substance on which an enzyme acts.

subtentorial Located beneath the cerebellum of the brain.

subtotal Less than complete. A subtotal thyroidectomy is an operation in which some of the gland is not removed.

subungual Beneath a finger or toenail, as a *subungual* infection.

Succinylcholine A powerful muscle relaxant drug, often used when giving shock therapy to protect the patient from dislocations or fractures.

succinylcholine chloride *See* Anectine.

succulent Juicy.

succus entericus The intestinal juices which contain the enzymes that digest food.

suckle To nurse from a breast.

sucralfate An aluminum-containing medication, taken to reduce stomach acid and help the healing of ulcers.

sucrose A sugar.

suction apparatus Any one of many machines to suck out secretions, discharges or fluids from the body.

suction dissector An instrument that dissects and removes tissue by suction; sometimes used in removing parts of the liver.

Sudafed A nasal decongestant.

sudamen Sweat clogging the pores.

sudation Sweating.

Sudeck's atrophy Degeneration of bone following a severe injury.

sudoresis Profuse perspiration.

sudorific A medication to bring about sweating.

suffocate To be unable to draw air into the lungs.

suffused Bloodshot.

suffusion The pouring out of body fluids into the tissues.

sugars Saccharides.

suggestion The psychic state in which a patient senses things which the psychiatrist suggests that he feel or, conversely, when he stops sensing things which the psychiatrist suggests he not feel; also, something communicated in this manner.

    hypnotic One made by a psychiatrist to a patient under hypnosis.

    posthypnotic One made to a patient under hypnosis which is to be carried out at a later time.

suicide Self-destruction; taking one's own life.

Sulamyd A sulfa drug used as an eye medication for inflammation of the conjunctiva (lining membrane of the eye).

sulcus A groove or lined depression in the surface of an organ, bone, etc.

sulfadiazine An antibacterial drug, very effective against staphylococci, streptococci and pneumococci bacteria.

sulfa drugs A group of drugs (sulfonamides) which have remarkable powers in inhibiting the growth of certain infectious bacteria. Some of the most widely prescribed ones are: sulfadiazine, sulfaguanidine, sulfanilamide, sulfasuxidine, sulfathalidine, etc.

sulfanilamide The first sulfa drug to be used.

Sulfasalazine A tablet given in conjunction with other medications in the treatment of mild cases of ulcerative colitis.

sulfhemoglobin A combination of a sulfonamide with the hemoglobin of the blood.

sulfide Any one of many sulfur compounds.

sulfobromophtalein A chemical used in testing liver function.

sulfonamides The sulfa drugs.

sulfur (S) An element which forms the base for many useful medications. It is prescribed extensively, in combined form, for various skin conditions such as acne, psoriasis, ringworm, scabies, etc.

sumach A reddish shrub (Rhus) often causing a severe skin rash and itch similar to poison ivy. Also called *poison sumac*.

sunstroke Being overcome by excessive heat and inability of the body to get rid of the excessive heat. Body temperatures may go as high as 106 to 108° F.

super- A prefix meaning "upon," "above" or "too much."

superalimentation Overfeeding.

superalkalinity The condition of being excessively alkaline.

superego A term referring to one of the three basic divisions of the personality recognized in psychoanalysis. The conscious manifestations of the *superego* are popularly termed *conscience*.

superfecundation One pregnancy taking place while another is in progress. This is extremely rare and only occurs when an egg bursts forth from an ovary after another one has been discharged and has been fertilized.

superfetation The implantation and growth of a fertilized egg in a uterus which is already pregnant. A rare condition.

superficial Near the surface, as a *superficial* infection; not serious or profound.

superinfection A second infection by a different germ, occurring as a complication of the first infection.

superior An anatomical term referring to an organ or part which is located above another organ or part of the body.

superiority complex A neurotic's manifestation of a superior attitude when, in actuality, the person has feelings of inferiority.

supernumerary Referring to an extra organ or part of the body, as a sixth finger or extra breast nipples.

supersaturated Containing more solid dissolved in solution than a solution can ordinarily hold.

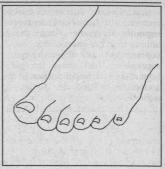

Supernumerary digit

supersonic Referring to sound waves of such high frequency that they cannot be heard.

supinate To turn the palm of the hand upward. The opposite of pronate.

supine Lying down with face upward. The opposite of prone.

supplementary vitamins Vitamins given by pill or injection to patients who lack a sufficient amount of vitamins in their bodies.

suppository, rectal A medication prepared for insertion into the rectum. Its active ingredients may treat a local rectal condition, be absorbed into the body to treat distant conditions, or may induce bowel evacuation.

    vaginal A medication prepared for insertion into the vagina.

suppression 1. The stoppage of a secretion or excretion, such as the cessation of urination. 2. In psychiatry, it means the deliberate, conscious pushing into the "background" (unconscious) of the mind those desires and thoughts which would result in socially unacceptable behavior or in great emotional conflict; cf. repression.

suppurate To form pus.

suppurative wound A wound from which pus is discharged.

supra- A prefix meaning above.

supraclavicular Just above the collarbones, the *supraclavicular region*.

supradiaphragmatic Above the diaphragm; in the chest cavity.

supraorbital Just above the eye.

suprapubic Just above the pubic bones; the lowermost portion of the abdomen covered, in adults, by pubic hair.

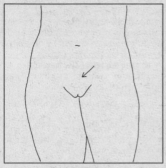

Suprapubic region

suprarenal Just above the kidneys. The adrenal glands are also called the *suprarenal glands*.

Suprarenin A patented preparation containing epinephrine (one of the chemicals secreted by the adrenal glands).

suprascapular Located above the scapula (shoulder blade).

supraspinatus muscle A muscle extending from the upper portion of the scapula (wing-bone) to the humerus (the bone of the upper arm). It helps to lift the arm away from the body.

suprasternal notch The depression just above the sternum (breastbone) at the base of the neck.

Suprax An antibiotic most helpful in combating infections of the ears, nose, and throat, and of the bronchial tubes.

suramin A preparation used in parasitic infestations, such as trypanosomiasis.

surface tension The tension on the top of a liquid. It tends to form a spherical shape and resists the outflow of liquid beneath its surface.

surfactant Any substance that acts to alter surface tensions, such as those in the lungs. A lack of *surfactants* is noted in premature infants suffering from respiratory distress.

Surgeon A physician who specializes in treating people through operative procedures (surgery).

surgery That branch of medicine dealing with operative treatment of disease.

surgical microscope One permitting the surgeon to operate upon minute structures under great magnification.

surgical pathology A branch of medicine in which tissue is removed from a patient and is examined by a pathologist in order to make a diagnosis.

Surgicel An absorbable cellulose product, used to control surgical bleeding. (It is applied to a bleeding surface as a gauze tampon, where it exercises its property of causing blood to clot.)

Surital An intravenous drug widely used in the induction of sleep prior to administration of an anesthetic gas.

surveillance An observation, usually ongoing.

survey An investigation.

susceptibility The tendency to develop a disease if exposed to it. The opposite of immunity.

susceptible Not having acquired immunity.

suspension A liquid in which tiny solid particles float. (Not a solution, since the solid particles are not dissolved.)

suspension operation An operation in which the uterus is stitched to the under surface of the anterior abdominal wall. (Occasionally done in cases of "tipped womb.")

suspensory A cloth fashioned so as to support the testicles.

Sustagen A powdered preparation

containing all essential nutrients. It is composed of milk solids, casein, maltose, dextrose, vitamins, and iron. (Administered by mouth or through a stomach tube to patients who are unable to eat solids or who cannot be fed orally. Before giving, it is diluted with water.)

suture To stitch tissue surgically; to sew a wound or laceration.

    material Thread used in sewing tissue. It may be made of various substances such as sheep's intestines (catgut), silk, cotton, wire alloys, nylon, plastic materials, etc.

Swan-Ganz catheter A catheter with a balloon at the tip, inserted through a vein in the arm and advanced in the circulation until it enters the main artery leading from the heart to the lungs. Its purpose is to measure arterial pressure.

swayback Excessive arching of the back.

sweat glands Small structures in the skin which produce sweat.

sweat test Examination of sweat for its chemical composition. Performed in infants in cases of suspected cystic fibrosis.

swelling, cloudy A microscopic finding of early degeneration of tissues, such as *cloudy swelling* of the liver in cases of liver disease.

sycosis Inflammation of the hair roots.

Sydenham's chorea Purposeless, involuntary movements of the muscles of the face, arms and legs. It is caused by disease within the nervous system.

symbiosis The living together of organisms of different species for their mutual benefit.

symbol 1. A sign. 2. An abbreviation for a chemical element.

symbolism The act of substituting an object or sign for some thing or idea. In psychiatry, a mental process in which the unconscious masks problems which face the conscious mind and presents them in a distorted form, as in dreams.

symmetry Similarity between the two sides of the body.

sympathectomy Removal of some of the sympathetic nerves; usually performed to improve circulation or to dilate blood vessels.

sympathetic nervous system The involuntary part of the nervous system, such as that which controls blood vessel contractions, sweating, etc.

sympathetic ophthalmia A severe inflammation of an eye, often leading to blindness, caused by an injury or disease of the other eye.

sympathomimetic Referring to medication which produces the same effects as stimulation of sympathetic nerves (constriction of blood vessels, etc.).

symphysis The joining together or meeting of two bones, as the *symphysis* pubis, where the two pubic bones meet one another.

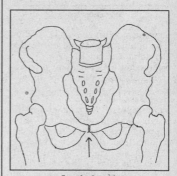

Symphysis pubis

symptom Evidence of a disease; a complaint, such as a subjective feeling occurring during a disease (pain, nausea, dizziness, etc.).

symptomatic treatment Treatment which is directed toward relieving the patient's complaints rather than toward getting at the basic cause of the illness.

symptomatology All of the symptoms which are present in a particular illness.

symptom complex All the symptoms of a disease; a syndrome.

syn- A prefix referring to something which is "joined."

Synalar A cream applied to the skin to combat inflammation; to be used for a limited period of time only.

synapse The area where one nerve ends and another begins. Impulses pass over the *synapse* from one nerve to another.

synarthrosis An immovable, or only slightly movable, joint where the bones dovetail and lock into one another. For example, the junctions of the various bones of the skull.

synchondrosis A junction of two bones in which cartilage lies in between, as the joining of the bones in the sacroiliac joint.

synchronism Things that take place at the same time; simultaneous.

synchrotron An apparatus which generates high speed protons and electrons.

syncope Fainting.

syncytium A mass of conglomerated cell substance (protoplasm) with many nuclei, produced by the merging of cells.

syndactyly Webbed fingers or toes.

syndesmology The study of ligaments and joints.

syndrome *See* also *disease* A group of symptoms and signs which, when appearing simultaneously, form a definite pattern of a specific condition, disease or abnormality.

  Acute (or adult) respiratory distress syndrome. *See* ARDS.

  Adams-Stokes Fainting, slow pulse, convulsions, usually brought on by heart block. *See* heart block.

  adaptation Reactions of the body to stress. Such reactions are divided into three stages: alarm reaction; resistance; exhaustion.

  Adie's A condition in which the pupils of the eye react incorrectly to light, and the knee and ankle jerks are not present.

  adrenogenital Various sexual changes seen as the result of excess secretion of male-type hormone from the cells of the adrenal gland. It affects males and females in different ways.

  anginal Pain in the heart region or beneath the breastbone on excitement, eating, physical exertion, cold exposure, walking, etc. Also called *angina pectoris*.

  Banti's An anemia, usually ending fatally, associated with marked enlargement of the spleen.

  Battered Child Various injuries caused by a beating from a parent.

  Bernheim's Blockage of free passage of blood through the right heart ventricle because of a certain deformity in the heart.

  Blount-Barber Bowlegs in infants (not due to rickets). It corrects itself without treatment.

  Brown-Séquard A nerve disease in which there is paralysis of movement limited to one side of the body and loss of sensation limited to the opposite side of the body.

  carcinoid A set of symptoms resulting from the release of a substance known as serotonin from a carcinoid tumor in the abdomen. It is characterized by attacks of skin flushing, diarrhea, asthmatic attacks, and heart valve involvement.

  carotid sinus Weakness, dizziness and fainting due to excess stimulation or irritability of the carotid sinus in the neck.

  carpal tunnel Numbness, tingling, loss of sensation in the middle three fingers and swelling of the hand due to pressure upon the median nerve in the wrist.

  cavernous sinus Swelling of the eyes, loss of use of several of the eye muscles, etc., due to thrombosis (clotting) of the large vein (cavernous sinus) in the brain.

  celiac Celiac disease. Underdevelopment, weakness, and anemia in infants, due to improper absorption of fats. The abdomen is swollen and stools are large and foul-smelling.

cerebellopontine angle tumor A specific brain tumor resulting in ringing in the ear, loss of hearing on the side of the tumor and paralysis of certain of the nerves to the face.

cervical disk Excruciating pain associated with marked muscle spasms and areas of numbness in the neck, caused by a herniated intervertebral disk.

cervical rib Pain, "pins and needles" sensations, with feelings of cold and numbness in an arm and hand, due to an extra rib which presses on the nerves supplying the upper extremity. (The extra rib is located in the lower neck.)

Chauffard-Minkowski An anemia, present at birth, characterized by jaundice due to destruction of red blood cells. Also called congenital hemolytic jaundice.

Chiari's Clotting of the veins leaving the liver. It is associated with marked enlargement and tenderness of the liver, and the development of large veins beneath the skin of the abdomen and lower chest.

chiasmatic Partial loss of vision, headache and dizziness caused by a tumor or lesion within the brain located at the site where the optic nerves (to the eyes) cross one another (the chiasm).

Clarke-Hadfield Slowed physical development in a child, secondary to disease of the pancreas.

Conn's Extreme muscle weakness, high blood pressure, convulsions, intense thirst, and an exceptionally large output of urine, secondary to overactivity of the cortex of the adrenal glands.

costochondral Pain at the junction of a rib and the breast bone due to inflammation or injury; often misinterpreted by the patient as being caused by heart trouble.

cough Dizziness and occasional fainting after a severe, prolonged coughing spell.

crush Failure to secrete urine because of severe crushing injury to one or more limbs. This is a toxic reaction affecting the kidneys.

Cushing's Extreme fatness, high blood pressure, bluish streaks on the skin, excess hairiness, diabetes, etc., seen in people having overactivity of the adrenal glands or a tumor in the adrenal glands or pituitary gland in the base of the skull.

Down's Mongolism; a birth defect associated with the presence of an extra chromosome in the cells.

dumping Weakness, faintness, sweating, rapid heart beat, nausea, seen in some people who have had part of their stomach removed (gastrectomy). It is thought to be caused by food entering, and being absorbed from the intestines too rapidly.

effort Shortness of breath, palpitation and pain in the heart region, weakness on physical exertion of even a mild or moderate degree in people who have no true organic heart disease. Also called neurocirculatory asthenia. It is thought to be a functional or neurotic disorder.

exhaustion Weakness, lassitude, lack of appetite, thought to be caused by inadequate function of the adrenal glands.

Fanconi An inherited type of anemia, usually coming on in childhood. It may be accompanied by dwarfism, crossed-eyes, mental defects, and other abnormalities.

Felty's Rheumatoid arthritis, associated with an enlarged spleen and deficient white blood cells in the circulation.

Friderichsen-Waterhouse Blood poisoning associated with a meningitis infection. It leads to hemorrhage in the adrenal glands, collapse and death. It is a rare condition.

Froelich's A lack of pituitary gland function in children, resulting in marked obesity and underdevelopment of the genitals.

Gardner's An inherited condition in which there are great numbers of polyps in the large bowel. Such patients may also have tumors of the skull and cysts of the skin.

Guilain-Barre Inflammation of nerves (neuritis) associated with fever.

Hedblom's An acute inflammation of the diaphragm.

hepatorenal Failure of liver and kidney function, usually terminating fatally, in people who have undergone major surgery or have suffered injury to the liver.

Horner's A depression of the eyeball, a drooping of the eyelid, contraction of the pupil of the eye and flushing of the face seen in people who have had destruction to the sympathetic nerves in the neck.

Howship-Romberg Pain in the thigh and knee region due to pressure on the obturator nerve because of a hernia in the groin (obturator hernia).

hyperventilation Dizziness, numbness and tingling in the arms and legs, convulsions and occasional loss of consciousness from overbreathing. Also called *oxygen poisoning*.

inferior vena caval Swelling of the legs and enlargement of the superficial veins in the legs and abdomen due to blockage of the large vena cava (vein) in the abdomen.

Jeghers-Peutz Innumerable small tumors (polyps) of the large bowel. An inherited condition often terminating in cancer unless the entire large bowel is removed.

Klinefelter's An inherited disease in males, associated with sterility on attaining adulthood, enlarged breasts, and an abnormal chromosome pattern in their cells.

Korsakoff's A mental disorder caused by chronic alcoholism, associated with pain in the arms and legs, hallucinations and a tendency to falsify the truth.

Leriche Marked pain and cramps in the legs on walking or exercise and impotence in men, caused by clotting (thrombosis) of the aorta in the lower part of the abdomen.

Leschke's Diabetes, brown spots on the skin, excessive fatigue. Also named *dystrophy pigmentosa*.

Libman-Sacks An inflammation and bacterial infection of the heart valves (endocarditis).

Loeffler's Inflammation of the lungs and a characteristic blood picture showing a large increase in certain types of white blood cells (eosinophils).

Lorain-Levi Dwarfism due to underactivity of the pituitary gland.

lower nephron A form of nephritis (kidney malfunction) associated with lowered uninary output or complete urinary stoppage. Seen after certain major surgical procedures.

low salt Heat exhaustion, abdominal cramps, lowered urinary output, seen when the sodium in the blood is reduced to very low levels.

malabsorption Any one of a number of conditions due to inadequate absorption of nutrients, vitamins, and minerals from the intestinal tract. Symptoms may include poor appetite, weakness, weight loss, diarrhea, anemia, bleeding tendencies, etc.

Mallory-Weiss Severe hemorrhage from the lining of the stomach, caused by alcoholism, excessive vomiting, or inflammation of the stomach lining.

Marfan's A heritable disorder of the connective tissue that affects many organ systems, including the skeleton, lungs, eyes, heart, and blood vessels.

Meigs' A special type of tumor of the ovary associated with large amounts of fluid in the abdominal cavity (ascites).

Ménière's Severe dizziness, ringing in the ears, deafness, nausea and vomiting, and twitching of the eye muscles. Thought to be an allergic reaction. (Treated by low salt diet)

middle lobe Collapse of the right middle lobe of the lung due to pressure, possibly by a tumor, upon the bronchial tube supplying this portion of the lung.

Milkman's Brittleness of the bones; small multiple fractures and loss of calcium in the bones.

Morquio's An inherited defect characterized by skeletal deformities and extremely short stature.

Morton's Severe pain and tenderness in the sole of the foot, also called *metatarsalgia*.

MSG The "Chinese restaurant" syndrome; headache, burning sensations over various parts of the body, felt after eating foods to which monosodium glutamate has been added.

Munchausen's A condition in which a patient gives a logical explanation of symptoms which would lead to a diagnosis of disease, but the patient's statements are untrue, and in reality, no organic disease is present.

Osler-Libman-Sacks *See* lupus erythematosus.

Pancoast Pain in the arm and shoulder region, plus Horner's syndrome, paralysis of a vocal cord, all due to a tumor in the top (apex) of a lung.

Parkes-Weber Enlargement of an arm or leg due to a birth deformity in which there is a tremendous increase in the number of blood vessels in the limb.

Peutz-Jeghers An inherited disease characterized by polyposis (innumerable warty growths) in the small and large intestine, with brownish pigmentation of the skin, bleeding, and anemia.

Plummer-Vinson A rare condition in which there is difficulty in swallowing due to degeneration of muscles in the esophagus (food-pipe); associated with anemia.

postcholecystectomy Continuation of symptoms of gall bladder disease after the organ has been removed.

postcommissurotomy Chest pain, fever, with fluid in the chest, appearing several weeks after a heart operation to relieve valvular disease. (The condition clears by itself within a week or two.)

postconcussion Dizziness, headache, sleeplessness, irritability in people who have sustained a recent head injury (concussion).

post-thrombotic Swelling, blueness, pain, eczema of the leg due to clotting (thrombosis) of deep veins within the leg.

post-traumatic Multiple symptoms including headache, dizziness, weakness, blurred vision, muscle aches and pains, occurring and persisting after an injury has apparently healed. (Many of the symptoms are thought to be neurotic in origin.)

Raynaud's Blanching, redness, blueness, coldness, severe pain in the toe or finger tips. Seen mostly in young women. It sometimes leads to superficial gangrene of the skin of the toes or fingers.

Reye's A set of symptoms seen in some children following a viral infection, such as chickenpox or influenza. Symptoms include mental confusion, vomiting, convulsions, occasional coma, and respiratory failure. The cause of the condition is unknown and no specific treatment exists.

scalenus anterior Pain, numbness and weakness in the arm because of pressure upon the nerves in the neck (brachial plexus) by the *scalene* muscles which are located above these nerves. Relieved by cutting the scalene muscles.

shoulder-hand Pain, stiffness and numbness leading to shrinking of the muscles; all in the shoulder, arm and hand. Thought to be brought on by lack of proper function of the nerves supplying this area of the body.

sick sinus Irregularities of heartbeat originating in the sinus of the atrium of the heart. Conditions of this kind sometimes require the insertion of a pacemaker to regulate the heartbeat.

splenic flexure Pain, bloating, flatulence, beneath the ribs on the left side, thought to be due to trapping of gas in the splenic flexure loop of large bowel. (It is sometimes misinterpreted by patients as heart pain.)

Stokes-Adams Fainting and convulsions seen in people with an extremely slow heart beat due to a special type of heart dysfunction (heart block).

Sudeck's Degeneration of one of the bones in the hand or foot following a relatively minor injury to the soft parts of the area.

sudden death Crib death; the sudden death of an apparently healthy infant.

superior mesenteric artery Constriction and obstruction of the third portion of the duodenum (the beginning of the small intestine) due to pressure from blood vessels which cross over it. Relieved surgically.

superior vena caval Blockage of the return of the blood to the heart from the head, neck and upper extremities, due to clotting (thrombosis) of the large superior vena cava vein.

Tietze's Pain and swelling of a rib cartilage. The cause is unknown. The condition usually subsides without treatment.

toxic shock High fever, shock and blood poisoning occurring in a woman who uses a vaginal tampon during menstruation. (A rare condition.)

trisomy D A set of abnormalities due to an extra (47th) chromosome of the D type appearing in the cells of a newborn. Mental defi-

ciency, malformed ears, cleft palate, hare-lip, and many other deformities occur in this condition.

trisomy E A set of abnormalities due to an extra (47th) chromosome of the E type appearing in the cells of a newborn. (*See* trisomy D for list of defects found.)

trisomy 21 Mongolism; Down's syndrome.

Turner's An inherited chromosomal condition in females, accompanied by underdeveloped sex organs, absence of menstruation, and occasionally dwarfism.

Waterhouse-Friderichsen *See* Friderichsen-Waterhouse syndrome.

Werner's A rare inherited disease displaying underdevelopment of the sex organs, cataracts, diabetes, and thickening of the skin.

withdrawal Emotional and physical upset caused by withdrawal of a drug to which a person is addicted. Also called *abstinence syndrome.*

Zollinger-Ellison Stomach and duodenal ulceration secondary to extreme hyperacidity caused by overactivity or tumor of the insulin-producing cells of the pancreas.

synechia Adhesions; fibrous bands extending from one part of an organ to another or from organ to organ.

synergetic Referring to two or more organs working in harmony.

synergism Working together, as two muscles which together produce a certain movement that neither could accomplish alone.

synergy The cooperative action of two or more chemicals, substances, organs, etc.

synesthesia The transference of sensations from that which one originally experiences, that is, smelling what one sees or tasting what one smells, etc.

Synkayvite A synthetic vitamin K preparation, given in certain cases where there is a hemorrhagic tendency. (Used in newborn infants who show bleeding tendencies and in patients who bleed because of lack of vitamin K absorption from the intestinal tract.)

synorchism Fusion of the two testicles; a rare condition.

synostosis The union of two or more bones which originally were separate.

synovectomy Surgical removal of the lining membrane of a joint. (Performed in cases of chronic infection, etc.)

synovial fluid The clear amber fluid usually present in small quantities in a joint.

synovial membrane The thin lining tissue of a joint.

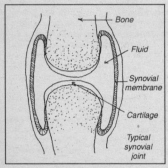

Bone

Fluid

Synovial membrane

Cartilage

Typical synovial joint

Synovial membrane

synovioma A malignant tumor originating in the membrane or covering (sheaths) of joints, tendons or bursae.

synovitis Inflammation of a joint lining membrane.

synthesis Formation of complex substances out of a combination of simple substances.

Synthroid A patented medication containing thyroxine, the thyroid hormone.

syntropy The tendency of two or more conditions to blend into one.

syphilid An eczema or skin eruption caused by syphilis.

syphilis A communicable venereal disease, characterized by a primary

sore (chancre) and subsequent involvement of all the organs of the body. It can be cured through intensive treatment.

    acquired That which is caught from another through sexual contact, as distinguished from congenital syphilis.

    cardiovascular Late effects of syphilis, years after the original infection, upon the heart and blood vessels. It may cause weakening (aneurysm) and rupture of large blood vessels.

    congenital That with which a child is born, having acquired it during development in the uterus.

    extragenital That in which the first (primary) lesion, a chancre, is located elsewhere than on the sex organs.

    latent Quiescent syphilis. Syphilis without any symptoms or manifestations. This stage of the disease may last for several weeks after the initial sore has healed or it may last many years until the disease becomes active again.

    nonvenereal Syphilis not acquired through sexual intercourse.

    primary That stage in which the initial reaction, the chancre sore, is present. It lasts several weeks and heals.

    secondary The stage in which there is a rash over the body, sores in the mouth, and swelling of lymph glands. This may come on several weeks after the chancre has disappeared.

    tertiary Late stages of the disease in which damage to the brain, spinal cord, heart, blood vessels, etc. becomes apparent. This may take place many years after the original infection.

syphilitic Having syphilis.

syphilology That branch of medicine dealing with the treatment of syphilis in all its phases.

syphilophobia Fear of contracting syphilis.

syringe The glass or metal container and plunger which, when attached to a needle, allow for the injection of a substance into the body.

syringotomy Surgical opening of a fistula.

syringomyelia A disease of the spinal cord, lasting many years, in which there are many and extensive partial paralyses of various parts of the body.

system A set of organs performing one main function, such as the *respiratory system* for breathing, the *central nervous system* for brain and nerve function, the *gastrointestinal system* for nutrition, the *genitourinary system* for elimination and reproduction, the *endocrine system* for hormone secretion, etc.

systemic Referring to a condition or disease involving the entire body; as opposed to a localized condition.

systole The phase of heart beat during which the heart contracts and expels the contained blood.

systolic blood pressure The force with which blood is pumped when the heart muscle is contracting.

T

tabacosis *See* tobacosis.

tabes Locomotor ataxia; a degeneration of a portion of the spinal cord. It results in knifelike pains in the legs, unsteady gait with loss of the sense of position of the legs, a slapping gait and characteristic changes in the reaction of the pupils. It is often caused by syphilis.

tabetic Affected with syphilis of the spinal cord. It leads to locomotor ataxia with its characteristic gait. *See also* locomotor ataxia.

Tables of Immunization and Vaccination *See* page 530.

tablet

    buccal One that dissolves slowly when held in the mouth against the cheek.

    enteric-coated One that is coated so as not to dissolve until it reaches the intestine.

    sublingual One that is placed under the tongue, where it is absorbed.

    sustained release One that is absorbed slowly over a period of hours.

tache cérébrale A French term for a sign sometimes present in meningitis. It consists of a red line seen when a fingernail is rubbed across the skin of the abdomen.

tachistoscope An apparatus for measuring time reactions.

tachography The measurement of the speed of blood flow through the arteries, an important consideration in determining competence of heart action.

tachy- A prefix meaning "rapid."

tachycardia Rapid heart beat. (More than 100 beats per minute)

    paroxysmal Extremely rapid heart beat, anywhere from 150 to 250 beats per minute, coming on suddenly and lasting several minutes to several hours. The condition is encountered often in highly emotional young people.

tachylogia Excessively rapid and voluminous talking, as seen in the manic phase of a mental illness.

tachypnea Excessively rapid breathing.

tactile Referring to the sense of touch.

taenia Tapeworms.

taenia coli The long bands of fibrous tissue extending along the outside of the large bowel. (So named because the structure has a resemblance to the long, narrow appearance of the tapeworm.)

taeniafuge A medication given to get rid of tapeworm.

tag An extra piece of skin; a skin polyp. (Skin tags often remain after removal of hemorrhoids.)

Tagamet *See* cimetidine.

tagged Referring to the addition of a radioactive isotope to an inactive chemical compound. This enables one to follow the course of a drug within the body.

taint An inherited tendency toward development of a disease or condition.

Takazyme A patented antacid medication.

talcosis A lung disease similar to silicosis; occasionally seen among workers in the talc industry.

talipes Deformity of the foot, such as clubfoot and other malformations.

talus Astragalus. The large ankle bone lying between the leg and foot.

Talwin pentazocine A drug having some of the pain-relieving features of morphine but none of its addictive qualities.

tamoxifen An anti-estrogen (female sex hormone) substance used to combat the spread of certain breast cancers in postmenopausal women.

Recent investigations suggest that tamoxifen helps to prevent many breast cancers, particularly in high-risk women, and perhaps in others, too.

Tampax A patented product for insertion into the vagina to absorb the menstrual flow.

tampon A cotton sponge, particularly one used to plug a cavity such as the nose, vagina, etc.

tamponade Stopping a discharge or flow of blood by inserting a cotton sponge.

    cardiac Compression of the heart caused by blood or pus in the sac (the pericardial cavity) surrounding the heart. This must be relieved or death may ensue.

tannic acid An acid obtained from nutgall. When applied to a raw wound or burned area, it tends to stop oozing and bleeding and forms a scar or scab.

tantalum A metal element. When stitched into tissues in the form of a mesh, it acts as a support; used as a graft in large hernias because it creates practically no irritation within the body. It becomes surrounded by fibrous tissue, thus curing the weakness in the abdominal wall.

tantrum Rage; uncontrollable temper.

TAO Abbreviation for thromboangiitis obliterans; Buerger's disease.

tapeworm Long, narrow flat worms which live in the human intestinal tract. They cause weight loss, anemia and a voracious appetite.

tapping The insertion of a needle

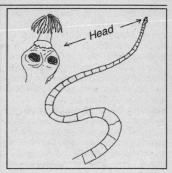

Tapeworm

into the body in order to remove fluids such as serum, blood, pus, etc.

tarantula A large spider whose bite is extremely painful. However, contrary to popular belief, its bite is not fatal to humans.

target cell A cell with a specific receptor for a hormone, antigen, or antibody.

tarsalgia Pain in the foot.

tarsometatarsal Referring to the bones of the foot.

tarsus The ankle.

tartar The brownish-black, hard deposits around the base of teeth (also called dental calculus). It is composed of calcium and iron salts.

TAT Abbreviation for tetanus antitoxin, given when a laceration or puncture wound is the result of contact with a dirty knife, nail, glass, etc.

taxol An anti-cancer drug, said to be helpful in advanced cancer of the ovaries and breast. The drug is derived from the bark of the yew tree.

taxonomy The study and classification of living organisms.

Tay-Sach's disease Amaurotic familial idiocy. A progressive, fatal disease occurring in infants and associated with blindness and brain deterioration.

TB *See* Tuberculosis.

T-cells Lymphocytes (white blood cells) that have a capacity for killing tumor cells or tissue that has been transplanted into the body from another individual.

tear duct *See* nasolacrimal duct.

teat The nipple.

technetium-99 A radioactive substance used in performing brain scans. By its use, diagnosis of a brain cyst or tumor can sometimes be made.

technique The methods used in performing surgery. Also, one refers to "good technique" or "poor technique" when speaking of the skill of the operating surgeon.

Tedral An effective medication to overcome spasm of the bronchial tubes; frequently prescribed in asthma.

Teflon A synthetic, nonabsorbable material used as a graft, especially valuable in blood vessel grafting.

tegmen A tissue covering.

Tegretol An anti-convulsion drug, used in preventing seizures.

telalgia Pain radiating to another part of the body; referred pain, such as heart pain which travels down the left arm.

telangiectasis Small, reddish areas on the skin caused by enlargement and dilatation of a group of blood capillaries.

    hereditary Enlargement of small blood vessels located in various parts of the body such as the nose, throat and intestinal tract. They sometimes bleed, causing extensive blood loss.

telangitis Inflammation of small blood vessels (capillaries).

Teldrin An antihistamine, probably effective for the relief of symptoms of hay fever and other allergic respiratory disorders.

telectrocardiogram A cardiogram taken from a patient and recorded on a machine located a distance away. Telectrocardiograms can be transmitted through telephone systems.

telediagnosis Diagnosis resulting from data received from a distant station.

telemetry Taking measurements of certain bodily functions at a distance from the patient, such measurements being transmitted by radio signals.

telencephalon The front portion of the brain.

teleology The belief that there is design and purpose in all nature. (The disbelief that things in nature "just happen")

Telepaque A radiopaque substance, an iodine compound, used to outline the gall bladder and biliary tract so that it will be noted on an X-ray film.

telepathy The theory that one can know another's thoughts without spoken communication; extrasensory perception.

TEM A substance used in the treatment of certain leukemias. Technically named triethylenemelamine.

temperature Body heat. Normal is 98.6° F.

temple The side of the head in front of and slightly above the ear.

temporal Referring to the region of the temple.

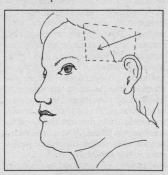

Temporal region

temporal arteries Inflammation of the temporal artery, located in the temple. Pain and headache are associated with the condition, which affects females more than males.

temporal-cortical bypass An operation in which an artery outside the brain (the temporal artery) is sutured to one on the surface of the brain, thus bringing blood to an area of the brain that has been deprived of its blood supply.

temporization Treating disease by waiting to see its course. Expectant treatment.

temporomandibular joint The junction of the lower jawbone (the mandible) and the temporal bone, located just in front of the ear.

temporoparietal Referring to the junction of the temporal and parietal bones of the skull. The area is above the ear toward the top of the skull.

tenaculum A long, thin, metal clamp with sharp tongs at its end. It is used to grab and hold a part, such as the cervix of the uterus.

tenderness Pain on touching a part, such as tenderness in the right lower part of the abdomen in someone who has appendicitis.

tendinitis Inflammation of a tendon.

tendinoplasty A plastic operation upon a tendon, often performed in cases of paralysis or when there is a tendon contracture.

tendon The fibrous portion of muscles which extends to their attachment to bones.

   of Achilles The large tendon just above the heel. When its attached muscle, the gastrocnemius in the calf, contracts, the foot is bent down.

tendonitis Same as *tendinitis.*

tendon transplant Moving a tendon to another area in order to create another function for it.

10-EDAM An experimental drug that improves survival rates in some types of lung cancer.

tenesmus Pain and spasm when attempting to pass urine or evacuate the bowels. Various inflammatory conditions can produce *tenesmus.*

tenia An anatomical term denoting a bandlike structure.

teniafuge Any medication that can rid the intestinal tract of tapeworms.

tennis elbow An inflammation of the epicondyle of the humerus (upper arm bone) at the elbow.

tenodesis Transferring a tendon's point of insertion from one site to another, done in an attempt to compensate for paralysis of muscles previously serving the area.

tenoplasty Plastic surgery or repair of a tendon.

tenorrhaphy An operation to repair torn tendons.

tenosynovitis Inflammation or infection of a tendon and the sheath which covers it.

tenotomy Cutting a tendon, an operation sometimes performed upon the tendon of Achilles in order to relieve certain foot deformities.

tenovaginitis Inflammation of the covering (sheath) of a tendon.

tension Stretched or strained. (Tissues should not be stitched to one another under *tension* as this may cause them to pull apart.)

   headache Any headache caused by or associated with stress or tension.

   intraocular The tension of the fluid within the eyeball. (When increased it may result in glaucoma.)

   premenstrual Emotional disturbance, irritability, etc., preceding the onset of menstruation, occurring in some, but not all women.

tensile strength The maximum amount of stress a material can maintain without rupturing.

tentative diagnosis A trial diagnosis, subject to change when more information is obtained about an illness.

tentorium The fibrous tissue shelf separating two main portions of the brain, the cerebrum from the cerebellum.

tenuous Thin.

TEPA An anti-cancer chemical with the same effects as TEM. *See* TEM.

tepid Lukewarm; approximately body temperature.

teratocarcinoma A cancerous tumor composed of cell elements found in embryos; teeth, hair and other organ cells can all be found in a *teratocarcinoma*.

teratogen Any substance that interferes with the normal development of a fetus.

teratoma A tumor composed of tissue which usually does not grow in the region where the tumor is located. Thus, a *teratoma* in the ovary may contain hair, teeth, stomach tissue, etc. Teratomas are formed out of embryonic tissues.

term The end of the ninth month of pregnancy when delivery is expected.

terminal The end; a term referring to a patient who is about to die.

terminology A method for naming and classifying medical terms.

terpin hydrate In liquid form, a helpful medication in cases of inflammation of the windpipe and bronchial tubes. It is an important ingredient of many cough mixtures.

Terramycin An antibiotic effective against a wide range of bacteria.

tertian Recurring every other day, as the fever in *tertian* malarial fever.

tertiary medical care That given by specialist consultants who have had patients referred to them by other physicians.

tertiary syphilis The third stage of syphilis, often affecting the brain and nervous system.

test A procedure to aid in making a diagnosis.

   acid phosphatase A blood test which sometimes indicates the presence of a cancer of the prostate gland and its spread to other parts of the body.

   after image An eye test demonstrating the degree of strabismus (crossed eyes).

   agglutination A test to demonstrate the presence of antibodies in the blood.

   albumin The presence of albumin in the urine may indicate kidney disease.

   alkaline phosphatase A blood test which, when elevated, indicates obstruction of the flow of bile into the intestine. A valuable test in cases of jaundice.

   allergy Any test used to demonstrate the presence of an allergy.

   amylase A blood test which, when elevated, may indicate an inflammation of the pancreas (pancreatitis).

   amyloid A test which, when elevated, indicates the presence of degeneration (amyloidosis) in certain of the organs such as the liver, kidney, spleen, etc.

   Apgar Performed on newborn infants to give some indication of the general state of health. Respirations, heartbeat, skin color, and muscle tone are all checked and evaluated.

   aptitude A psychological test to determine the potential ability of someone in a special field of endeavor.

   Ascheim-Zondek A test for pregnancy. It is performed by injecting a mouse with the patient's urine. If, two days later, the mouse's ovaries become swollen, it indicates that the patient is pregnant.

   association A psychological test in which the patient is given a series of words and is asked to state what other words they make him think of.

   auditory The use of the audiometer to determine the ability to hear.

   Bachman A test to determine the presence of trichinosis (an infection caused by eating diseased pork or ham).

   Bárány's A test to determine the presence of disease in the inner ear (labyrinth).

   Bence Jones protein A urine test which, when positive, indicates the presence of a tumor known as myeloma.

Benedict's A urine test for the presence of sugar.

benzidine A test for the presence of blood. It can be performed on urine, stool, sputum, etc.

benzodioxane The intravenous injection of this substance brings about a lowering of the blood pressure in people who have a tumor (pheochromocytoma) of the adrenal gland.

bilirubin A blood test for the presence of bile pigment. Increased bilirubin indicates the presence of jaundice.

bilirubin clearance The ability of the liver to remove injected bilirubin from the blood stream is a test of adequacy of liver function.

Binet-Simon I.Q. test. A psychological test of intelligence.

biopsy The surgical removal of tissue in order to determine the exact diagnosis.

bleeding time Puncturing the finger and noting how long it takes for the bleeding to stop.

blind A *blind test* is one in which both the observer and the one being tested are unaware of the end result.

bone conduction A hearing test in which a vibrating tuning fork is placed against the mastoid bone behind the ear. Failure to hear the vibrations indicates bone conduction deafness.

bone marrow One in which a small amount of marrow is obtained from the breastbone or some other bone by placing a needle into it. It enables the physician to see how well the blood is being formed and whether it contains abnormal cells

breath-holding An index of adequacy of heart and lung reserve. A normal adult can usually hold his breath for 30 seconds; decreased amounts may mean diminished heart or lung reserve.

Bromsulphalein Failure of the liver to eliminate injected Bromsulphalein is an indication of impaired liver function.

capillary resistance A test for the resistance of small blood vessels (capillaries) to stress. A tourniquet is applied to an arm; if capillaries break it shows lowered resistance.

Cattell infant A test for the intelligence of infants under two and a half years of age.

cephalin flocculation A liver function test based upon its ability to flocculate (clot) cholesterol.

cholesterol A blood test to determine the quantity of cholesterol in circulating blood.

circulation time A test to determine how rapidly blood circulates throughout the body. It is impaired in certain types of heart disease.

clearance A test of the efficiency of the kidney in clearing certain substances which come to it in the circulating blood.

coagulase A test for the virulence (strength) of staphylococcal germs. A positive coagulase test shows these germs to be more dangerous and resistant to destruction.

coccidioidin A skin sensitivity test to determine the presence of a coccidioidomycosis (fungal) infection. This infection is also called *San Joaquin Valley fever*.

coin Striking coins against one another on the chest wall while the physician listens with a stethoscope on the opposite chest wall. A clear bell tone indicates pneumothorax, or air in the space between the lung and the chest cage. (The normal sound is dull and muffled.)

cold agglutination A test for blood antibodies which are present in certain peculiar types of pneumonia (atypical pneumonia).

cold pressor People with a tendency to high blood pressure will show a marked rise in their pressure when a hand is immersed in ice cold water for one minute.

colloidal gold A test for syphilis of the brain or spinal cord.

color vision The viewing of multi-colored cards with numbers upon them; given to determine if a man is color blind.

complement-fixation A test formerly used to detect the presence of gonorrhea, especially in women.

concentration-dilution A test for adequacy of kidney function based upon its ability to concentrate and dilute urine.

Congo red A test to detect amyloid degeneration of organs or tissues.

conjunctival An allergic test in which the substance suspected of being the cause of the allergy is dropped into the eye. Inflammation and redness shows a positive reaction.

Coombs' A test upon the blood to detect the presence of Rh antibodies.

cross-matching A test to determine whether the donor's and recipient's blood will mix without clotting; performed before giving a blood transfusion.

Davidsohn differential A test to determine the presence of infectious mononucleosis; a heterophil test.

Dick A skin test to determine susceptibility or immunity to scarlet fever.

exercise tolerance A test for heart function, angina pectoris, etc. A patient steps up and down two stairs in the physician's office. It is noted how much exercise he can do before developing chest pain.

Fehling's A urine test for the presence of sugar.

ferric chloride A urine test for the presence of diacetic acid, an indication of acidosis.

finger to finger A test of brain (cerebellar) function in which the patient, from an outstretched arm position, must bring his two index fingers together. Normally, this is easy to do.

finger to nose A test of brain (cerebellar) function in which the patient, from an outstretched arm position, must bring his index finger smoothly to the tip of his nose.

Fishberg's A test for kidney function in which the concentration (specific gravity) of the urine is calculated twelve hours after not drinking. Normally, the kidneys concentrate urine without difficulty.

Folin-Wu A blood chemical test for the amount of urea. Excess amounts of urea in the blood may lead to uremic poisoning.

fragility A test to note the strength of red blood cells by putting them in salt solutions of varying strengths.

Frei A skin sensitivity test to determine whether the patient has lymphogranuloma venereum.

Friedman A pregnancy test using the woman's urine and injecting it into a female rabbit.

frog A pregnancy test using the woman's urine and injecting it into a female frog.

galactose tolerance A test for liver function to see if it can utilize galactose (milk sugar). Failure to do so indicates poor liver function.

Gesell A psychological test for the mental development of children under five years of age.

glucose tolerance A blood test to determine the presence of diabetes or a tendency toward its development. It also is used to determine the presence of hypoglycemia.

Gmelin's A test to detect the presence of bile in the urine.

Gofman A blood test to determine tendencies toward development of hardening of the arteries (arteriosclerosis).

Graham-Cole A test for gall bladder function and to see if it contains stones. A dye is swallowed or injected, following which X rays are taken.

guaiac A test for the presence of blood in the stool, urine, sputum, etc. A positive guaiac test result denotes the presence of blood.

heterophil A test to detect the presence of infectious mononucleosis.

hippuric acid A chemical test to determine adequacy of liver function.

histamine The injection of histamine normally causes secretion of hydrochloric acid in the stomach.

icterus index A test for the presence of bile pigments in the blood. It is elevated in cases of jaundice.

indigo carmine This chemical dye is injected intravenously. If the kidneys are functioning normally the dye should appear in the urine within seven minutes.

intelligence Any one of many psychological tests to determine the degree of intelligence.

iodine tolerance A test for overactivity of the thyroid gland.

Kahn A blood test for the presence of syphilis.

kidney function Any one of many tests to determine adequacy of kidney function.

Kline A blood test for syphilis. A positive test indicates the presence of the disease.

Kveim A skin test to determine the presence of sarcoidosis (Boeck's sarcoid).

latex A test done upon a patient's serum to diagnose rheumatoid arthritis.

L.E. A test for the presence of lupus erythematosus.

liver function Any one of the many tests to determine the adequacy of the numerous liver functions.

manometric A test performed upon the spinal fluid, after spinal puncture, to note the pressure of the fluid within the cerebrospinal space.

Mantoux A skin sensitivity test for tuberculosis.

Mazzini A test for syphilis. (A positive test indicates the presence of syphilis.)

medicolegal blood Tests performed upon old dried blood to determine whether it is human blood and what type it is.

methylene blue This dye is injected and should appear in the urine within thirty minutes if kidney function is adequate.

Mosenthal A kidney function test in which the various levels of concentration of the urine are determined over a twenty-four-hour period.

Naffziger's Pressing the jugular veins in the neck will cause increased pain in the back in a patient with a herniated disc.

pancreatic function Any one of several tests to determine the adequacy of pancreatic function.

Papanicolaou A cancer smear test.

parallax An eye test to detect cataracts or opaque areas in other parts of the eyeball.

patch An allergy test in which the substance suspected of causing the allergy is applied to the skin and held in place for a day or two with an adhesive patch.

paternity A test attempting to prove that a particular man *might* be the father of a child. More important, such a test (performed on the blood) might prove conclusively that a particular man is *not* the father of a child.

penicillin sensitivity A test to discover how sensitive a particular germ is to the action of penicillin.

Perthes A test performed to discover whether the deep veins in the legs are open or clotted. (This test is sometimes performed before operating for varicose veins.)

phenolsulfonphthalein (P.S.P. test) This dye is injected intravenously and its presence is noted in the urine. Failure to find it in the urine indicates kidney disease.

plasma L.E. A test for the presence of lupus erythematosus.

potassium tolerance A potassium salt is swallowed. If the patient has inadequate adrenal gland function, the potassium blood quantity is markedly increased.

pronation-supination A test of brain (cerebellum) function determined by having the patient rapidly rotate his hands up and down.

prostigmine This chemical is injected and if menstruation does not ensue, it suggests that the patient is pregnant.

prothrombin time A blood test to determine adequacy of the blood clotting mechanism. A prolonged *prothrombin time* indicates impairment of this mechanism.

Queckenstedt-Stookey Pressing the jugular veins in the neck normally causes a rise in the pressure of the cerebrospinal fluid surrounding the brain and spinal cord. Failure of this to take place indicates disease within the skull (intracranially).

radionucleotide A test to determine heart damage. It is performed by injecting a radioisotope into the patient's arm.

reduction Any test demonstrating the presence of sugar, as in the urine.

Rh A blood test for the presence of the Rh factor. It is now performed upon all pregnant women.

Rorschach A psychological test for the presence of neurotic tendencies.

rose bengal A liver function test based upon its ability to remove this dye from the circulating blood.

Rubin (tubal insufflation test) Air is injected through the cervix into the uterus. If the fallopian tubes are open the air (or oxygen) easily passes up and causes pain in the shoulder blades.

Schick A skin test to determine susceptibility or immunity to diphtheria.

Schultz-Charlton A skin test to determine the presence of scarlet fever.

scratch An allergy test in which the skin is scratched and the substance suspected of causing the allergy is applied to the scratched area.

sedimentation The time it takes blood cells placed in a glass tube to settle out and separate from the serum. (It happens more rapidly in people harboring infections.)

serologic One performed on the serum of the blood.

sickle cell A test to show whether people have a tendency toward sickle cell anemia. It is performed upon red blood cells, and the number of cells which become sickle-shaped is noted.

Shellen An eye test to denote the presence or absence of near-sightedness.

Stanford-Binet An I.Q. test, usually performed upon children rather than adults.

stress One which tests the capacity of heart function. It is carried out by having the patient "walk up-hill" on a specially constructed device.

sweat A test on perspiration to determine its sodium and chloride levels, thus enabling one to make a diagnosis of cystic fibrosis.

Test, T3 and T4 Blood chemical tests denoting the activity of the thyroid gland. (These tests have replaced the B.M.R., or basal metabolism rate, as a gauge of thyroid activity.)

Takata-Ava A liver function test.

tannic acid A test for the presence of carbon monoxide in the blood.

therapeutic Any test in which the response to treatment is used as an aid to diagnosis, such as giving iodine to a suspected case of overactivity of the thyroid gland. If the patient improves it indicates that the diagnosis was correct.

thymol turbidity A liver function test, used to determine whether the outlet of the bile duct is obstructed.

tine A tuberculin test performed upon the skin. *See* tuberculin test.

Töpfer's A test to determine the presence of hydrochloric acid in the gastric (stomach) juice.

tourniquet *See* test, capillary resistance.

transaminase A blood test which, when markedly positive, points to the presence of heart muscle damage, liver damage, or inflammation of the pancreas.

Trendelenburg's A test to note the extent of varicosities of the veins in the legs.

tuberculin A skin test to determine the presence of the germ causing tuberculosis in the system. A positive response does not necessarily indicate that an active tuberculosis infection exists, but rather that the person has at one time or another harbored the tuberculosis germ in his body.

two-step An exercise test performed to note the response of the heart to exertion. In angina pectoris, this test may bring on heart pain.

urea clearance A test of kidney function depending upon the amount of urea (a waste product) the kidneys can remove (clear) from the blood in one minute.

van der Bergh's A blood test to determine whether jaundice is caused primarily by liver disease or by obstruction of the bile ducts leading to the intestines.

VDRL A reliable test for syphilis.

vestibular Tests to determine the adequacy of function in the inner ear. Disturbance of such function may indicate the presence of a brain tumor.

vital capacity Tests to determine the adequacy of lung function.

von Pirquet A skin test for the presence of the tuberculosis germ in the body.

Wassermann A blood test for the presence of syphilis. A positive Wassermann result usually indicates the presence of syphilis.

water A test of adrenal gland function. People with diseased adrenal glands do not urinate in large quantities after drinking large quantities of water.

Weber's A tuning fork hearing test carried out by placing the vibrating tuning fork on the forehead.

Weill-Felix A test for the presence of one of the rickettsial infections.

Widal A test for the presence of typhoid fever.

testicle The male organ which produces sperm; located in the scrotum.

undescended One that has not descended into the scrotal sac but remains in the abdomen or groin. This is a birth deformity, usually correctable through hormone treatment or surgery.

testis A testicle.

test meal Food is eaten and after a certain number of minutes or hours is removed from the stomach by means of a tube. Analysis of the retrieved substance demonstrates how well the stomach is functioning.

testosterone The male sex hormone, manufactured and secreted by the testicles.

test tube baby One born as a result of fertilization taking place outside the female's body. Eggs are removed from the female by laparoscopy and are mixed with sperm and cultured. If pregnancy takes place, the egg (or eggs) is inserted into the woman's uterus.

tetanus Lockjaw. An infectious disease, often fatal, caused by the tetanus germ which enters the body through a cut or injury. It is associated with convulsions and severe muscle spasms.

tetanus antitoxin *See* TAT.

Tetanus toxoid Tetanus vaccine

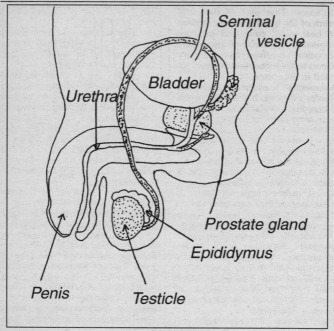

Seminal vesicle

Bladder

Urethra

Prostate gland

Epididymus

Penis

Testicle

Testicle and attachments

which stimulates active immunity against the disease. (There are no allergic reactions to toxoid, since it is not derived from animal serum.)

tetany A disease caused by insufficient calcium in the blood, sometimes associated with disease of the parathyroid glands. It is characterized by muscle spasms and convulsions. In infants, tetany may be caused by lack of vitamin D in the diet.

tetracycline The technical name for several of the antibiotic drugs such as *Achromycin, Terramycin,* etc.

tetralogy of Fallot A birth deformity of the heart involving defects in the blood vessels and walls of the heart chambers. In certain cases, this

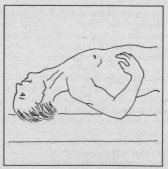

Tetany (showing typical opisthotonos and finger and hand spasm)

condition can be corrected through surgery.

thalamus That part of the cerebrum of the brain where sensations of heat, cold, pain, and pressure originate. The thalamus also relays sensations received from sensory nerves to the higher brain centers located in the cortex.

thalassemia Mediterranean anemia; Cooley's anemia. It is thought to be a hereditary disease and is characterized by onset in early childhood, enlargement of the spleen, underdevelopment of the body and a marked anemia.

thalidomide A tranquilizer drug, withdrawn from use, after it caused birth deformities when pregnant women ingested it during the early months of the embryo's life.

thallium A metal which, when converted into a radioactive isotope, is valuable as a diagnostic scanner.

thanatoid Deathlike.

thanatology The study of death.

thanatomania Death occurring in a hysterical state in people who believe they are going to die; seen sometimes in savages who think they are bewitched.

thanatophobia Morbid fear of death.

theca The covering or sheath of a tendon.

thecitis Tendon sheath inflammation.

thecoma An ovarian tumor composed of thecal cells.

thelalgia Pain in the nipple of the breast.

thelasis Suckling a breast.

theleplasty Plastic surgery upon a nipple.

thelerethism Erection of the nipple, brought on by stimulation or excitement.

thelitis Inflammation of a nipple.

thelium The nipple.

thenar region The palm of the hand, especially that region located adjacent to the base of the thumb.

theobromine A medication which stimulates the heart muscle and causes the excretion of large

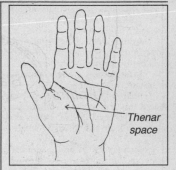

Thenar space

Thenar space

amounts of urine; used in people with heart disease or high blood pressure.

theomania A form of insanity in which the patient is a religious fanatic, sometimes believing himself to be God or some other divine being.

theophylline A chemical having the same effects as theobromine.

theory A credible scientific idea; a supposition backed up by many scientific facts.

    Cohnheim The theory or concept that cancer originates in misplaced or undeveloped cells which have been in the body since embryonic life. Due to some unknown stimulation in later life, they begin to grow and form tumors.

    germ The theory that all infections are caused by germs (bacteria or viruses).

Theragran A patented multivitamin tablet.

therapeusis The science of treatment of disease.

therapeutic malaria Malaria produced intentionally during the treatment of syphilis of the nervous system. (Not used at the present time.)

therapeutics The branch of medicine that concerns itself with the treatment of disease.

Therapist One who treats an illness, disease or condition.

therapy Treatment.

anticoagulant The giving of heparin or other substances to forestall blood clotting or thrombosis.

chemotherapy The treatment of disease with chemicals.

collapse Collapsing an infected tuberculous lung by injecting air into the chest cavity. This is designed to keep the diseased lung at rest.

electroshock Causing convulsions and unconsciousness through electrical shock. This form of treatment is sometimes used on mentally ill patients.

endocrine The treatment of disease through the giving of hormones.

fever Treatment of disease, such as syphilis of the brain, by bringing on fever. (The fever is artificially produced.)

group The psychiatric or psychological treatment of several patients at the same time. Their reaction to one another may produce a good result.

hormone Endocrine (glandular) treatment.

inhalation The use of various gases, positive pressure devices and medications to overcome breathing difficulties.

insulin shock Giving large doses of insulin to produce unconsciousness and convulsions in mentally ill patients.

malarial Giving a patient malaria, with its chills and high fever, in order to cure syphilis of the brain.

nonspecific protein Giving protein by injection in order to produce a high fever and thus benefit certain illnesses which are unrelated to the protein which is being injected.

occupational Treatment of a disease by getting the patient to keep himself busy, such as doing arts and crafts, gardening, making bandages, or any other simple occupation.

oxygen Applying an oxygen tent or feeding oxygen to the patient through a mask or rubber tube inserted into the nose.

physical Treatment of disease utilizing physical aids such as heat, light, water, electricity, etc. This field also includes rehabilitation techniques for the handicapped or chronically ill.

psychotherapy Any form of treatment for emotional or mental disorders of a non-organic (nonphysical) nature.

radiation Treatment with X rays, radium or other radioactive substances.

replacement The use of hormones to replace those which the body has stopped producing and secreting, as the giving of ovarian hormones to a woman who has had her ovaries removed.

roentgen X-ray treatments.

shock *See* electroshock therapy; *also* insulin shock therapy.

vaccine Vaccination; giving a vaccine in order to stimulate immunity.

thermal Relating to heat.

thermesthesia The sensation of heat.

thermoanesthesia The loss of the sense of heat.

thermocautery A surgical instrument which destroys tissue by burning.

thermocouple A method for measuring skin temperatures.

thermography A technique for measuring the heat given off by a particular organ or region of the body. A thermogram is extremely sensitive and records small temperature changes. Disease, including cancerous growths, show up on the thermogram as areas of greater than normal heat.

thermolabile Referring to a substance which is readily destroyed by heat.

thermometer An instrument for measuring temperature.

thermonuclear Referring to nuclear changes that take place by extremely high temperatures. Specifically, the fusion of hydrogen and helium at 100,000,000° Centigrade.

thermoplegia Sunstroke.

thermostable Referring to a substance which is not easily destroyed by heat.

thermotaxis The regulation of body heat.

thermotherapy Treatment of any condition by utilizing heat.

thesis 1. A paper written to obtain a degree or to pass a course in an institution of learning. 2. A theory.

thiamin Vitamin B_1. Found in grains and cereals.

thiamine hydrochloride Same as thiamin.

thiazides Medications that cause diuresis. *See* diuresis.

Thiersch grafts Small pieces of skin which are placed onto raw areas in the hope that they will grow in their new location.

thigh That part of the leg extending from the groin to the knee.

    amputation Leg removal above the knee joint.

thiocarbamide A medication helpful in treating leprosy.

thiopental sodium An intravenous anesthetic agent.

Thiouracil A drug used to combat overactivity of the thyroid gland; an antithyroid medication.

Thomsen's disease A lack of muscle function and coordination due to a defect present from birth. Thought to be a hereditary condition.

thoracentesis Tapping the chest cavity to withdraw and examine any fluid that might be present.

thoracic Referring to the chest.

thoracic duct The main lymph channel in the chest which collects lymph from organs in the chest and abdomen and empties into the large subclavian vein in the left side of the neck.

thoraco- A term relating to the chest (thorax).

thoraco-acromial Referring to the tip of the shoulder and the chest.

thoracolaparotomy An operation in which both the chest cavity and abdominal cavity are entered, as for operations upon the lower end of the esophagus or the upper end of the stomach.

thoracolumbar spine The parts of the spine extending from the chest down to the sacrum in the lowermost portion of the back.

thoracoplasty An operation upon the chest wall in which several ribs are removed; sometimes performed in cases of tuberculosis in order to collapse the lung and keep it at rest.

thoracoscope A hollow, lighted instrument that permits inspection of the pleural (chest) cavity.

thoracoscopy A procedure in which a hollow lighted metal tube is inserted into the chest cavity in order to diagnose an abnormal condition.

thoracotomy A surgical incision into the chest cavity, performed either for diagnostic purposes or to carry out treatment.

thorax The chest.

Thorazine A patented drug used to calm nerves; chlorpromazine.

thorium A radioactive element sometimes used instead of radium, as in certain skin conditions (thorium X).

Thorotrast A thorium preparation which, when injected, shows the outlines of blood vessels on X rays. Used as an opaque dye which will cast shadows on X-ray films.

thready pulse A very small pulse when felt by an examining finger.

threonine An essential amino acid.

threshold The level of stimulation which will produce a response.

    auditory The least sound which can be heard.

    pain The least pain which can be felt.

thrill A vibration felt by the physician's examining hand when placed upon a heart in which there is a murmur, or over a blood vessel containing an aneurysm.

throat The pharynx.

> **sore** Pharyngitis.

thrombectomy Surgical removal of a blood clot from the passageway of a blood vessel.

thrombin A chemical (enzyme) which becomes active when blood leaves its natural place within the blood vessel system. *Thrombin* induces blood clotting. Lack of it may lead to fatal hemorrhage.

thromboangiitis obliterans Buerger's disease. A chronic inflammatory disease of the arteries and veins; sometimes leading to gangrene of portions of the lower limbs.

thromboarteritis Inflammation of an artery with formation of a clot (thrombus) within the artery.

thrombocyte A blood platelet. It is essential to the normal blood clotting mechanism. Normal blood contains 250,000 to 500,000 platelets (*thrombocytes*) per cubic millimeter.

thrombocytopenia A condition in which there are an insufficient number of platelets in the blood.

thrombocytopenic purpura A generalized disease associated with hemorrhages into the skin, improper blood clotting, a deficiency of blood platelets. Most cases can be cured by surgical removal of the spleen.

thrombocytosis The condition in which the number of blood platelets is very large.

thromboembolism The clotting of a blood vessel as a result of a clot having broken away from the wall of a distant blood vessel and traveling through the circulation.

thromboendarterectomy The surgical removal of a blood clot that has formed within an artery.

thromboendarteriectomy An operation upon a sclerotic (hardened) artery in which the vessel is opened and the inner layer is reamed out.

This may lead to improved flow of blood through it.

thrombogen Prothrombin; a blood element instrumental in bringing about coagulation (clotting). Its presence in diminished quantities may lead to bleeding tendencies.

thrombokinase A chemical (enzyme) present in the blood which is essential to the formation of thrombin and thus is essential to blood clotting.

thrombolectomy Surgical removal of an embolus.

thrombolysis Dissolution of a blood clot (thrombus) within a vessel.

thrombolysis therapy Treatment to help dissolve blood clots, as after a thrombosis of a coronary artery of the heart.

thrombopenia Decrease in the number of blood platelets. This may lead to a bleeding tendency.

thrombophilia A tendency to form blood clots (thrombi).

thrombophlebitis Inflammation of a vein with blood clot formation within the vein.

thromboplastin A substance which aids in the formation of thrombin and thus promotes the normal blood clotting mechanism.

thrombose To clot.

thrombosis Formation of a blood clot.

> **coronary** Clotting of the coronary artery in the heart; coronary occlusion.

thrombus A clot of blood within the heart or a blood vessel.

> **antemortem** A clot that has formed in the circulation during life.

> **ball-valve** A clot that intermittently obstructs a heart valve.

> **mural** A blood clot attached to the wall of the heart.

> **postmortem** A clot that has formed after the death of an individual.

throwback The appearance of a type which resembles a primitive ancestor.

thrush A fungus infection (monilia) of the mouth often seen in children. It can be diagnosed by white patches on the tongue and membranes of the mouth.

thymectomy Surgical removal of the thymus gland in the chest. This is an infrequently performed operation as tumors of the thymus gland are quite rare.

thymic Referring to the thymus gland.

thymol A form of carbolic acid, used to kill germs and fungi.

thymoma A tumor of the thymus gland, seen rarely in infants.

thymus gland A lymph gland located beneath the breastbone in newborns. Its main function is carried out during development of the embryo and it undergoes degeneration during the first two years of life.

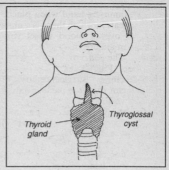

Thyroglossal cyst

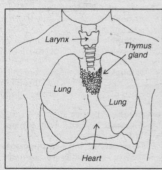

Thymus gland

thyro- Combining form denoting thyroid.

thyroarytenoid The cartilage in the neck located just above the thyroid gland.

thyroglossal cyst A cyst in the front of the neck composed of cells originating from the tongue and thyroid gland; usually occurring in children and young adults.

thyrohyoid Referring to the thyroid cartilage which makes up a portion of the voice box and the hyoid bone under the chin.

thyroid crisis Severe, life-endangering, toxic state due to extreme overactivity and excess secretion of the thyroid gland. Also called *acute thyrotoxicosis*.

thyroidectomy Surgical removal of the thyroid gland, or portions of it.

thyroid gland The endocrine gland, located in front of the neck, which regulates body metabolism. It secretes a hormone known as thyroxin.

thyroiditis Inflammation of the thyroid gland.

thyroid storm A serious condition caused by the uncontrolled release of huge quantities of thyroid hormone into the bloodstream. It causes high fever, very rapid pulse, and impairment of heart function. If untreated, it may lead to death. Antithyroid drugs often control the condition.

thyrotoxicosis Overactivity of the thyroid gland with all the consequent symptoms, such as rapid pulse and heart beat, irritability, increased metabolism, weight loss, etc.

thyroxin The hormone manufactured by the thyroid gland. It contains large quantities of iodine.

TIA Abbreviation for transient ischemia attack. The sudden loss of nerve function, usually lasting only

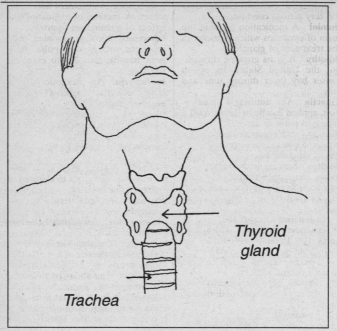

Thyroid gland

Trachea

Thyroid gland

several hours; secondary to blood loss to the brain.

tibia The larger of the two leg bones, located on the inner side of the leg and responsible for weight bearing.

tibialis muscles Two long muscles of the leg responsible for flexing and extending the foot.

tibiofibular Pertaining to the tibia and fibula; the bones of the leg.

tic Twitching; a habit spasm, often accompanied by spasmodic contraction of muscles of the face.

tic douloureux Trigeminal neuralgia. A condition in which there are severe, excruciating pains along the course of the nerve (trigeminal) which supplies the eye region, cheek and lower jaw. The pains come on in sudden attacks.

tick fever Any one of several diseases caused by a tick bite. (A tick is a blood-sucking insect.)

ticks Insects or bugs (arthropods) which live on plants or animals. Their bite often transmits serious diseases to man.

Ticlid (ticlopidine) The medication is effective in helping to prevent strokes caused by blood clots. Its activity inhibits clumping of blood platelets which might result in embolus formation.

t.i.d. An abbreviation meaning "three times daily."

tidal drainage An apparatus for automatically draining urine from a paralyzed bladder.

Timentin A powerful antibiotic given intravenously to combat a wide range of bacteria. Used mainly for very serious conditions.

timolol A medication given in the form of eyedrops which is useful in the treatment of glaucoma.

timothy A grass growing throughout the United States. Its pollen causes hay fever during June and July.

Tinactin An antifungal medication, applied locally in the form of a cream, powder or aerosol.

tincture A 10 percent alcoholic solution of a medication or drug.

tinea Ringworm.

tinnitus Ringing in the ears.

tissue An aggregation of cells which are similar in type, such as *fat tissue, brain tissue, connective tissue,* etc.

    cicatricial Scar tissue.

    connective Tissue which supports the tissues responsible for body functions (parenchyma).

    erectile Tissue which can become hard and erect.

    fibrous Dense connective tissue, such as ligaments, tendons, fascia, etc.

    granulation Healing tissue, composed largely of new blood vessels and new connective tissue.

    lymphatic That composed of lymph spaces and lymph cells.

    parenchymal The functioning tissue of an organ, as opposed to the connective tissue of an organ; the secreting cells of a gland, the air cells of the lungs, etc., are *parenchymal tissue.*

    subcutaneous The connective tissue beneath the skin.

tissue typing The matching of tissues between donor and recipient when an organ transplant is considered. Good matching will reduce the incidence of the rejection reaction.

titration Measurement of the volume or strength of a solution.

titubation Staggering, loss of balance due to disease within the brain or spinal cord.

TNM Abbreviation for tumor site, lymph node involvement and metastases. A method of evaluating the extent of a malignant tumor.

tobaccosis Nicotine poisoning. Toxic reactions, such as rapid pulse, dizziness, nausea, etc., due to excessive smoking.

tobramycin An antibiotic particularly effective against Gram-negative bacteria.

tocograph An instrument that records the force of contractions of the uterus prior to delivery.

tocopherol Vitamin E; wheat germ oil.

Tofranil A drug used to combat depression; also given to children to overcome bedwetting.

tokology An old term for *obstetrics.*

Tolbutamide An anti-diabetic tablet, given orally.

tolerance The ability or inability to endure the influence of a medication or drug.

    sugar The ability of a diabetic patient to utilize sugar.

tomogram An X ray taken to get a clear picture mainly of one plane of the body. (It is also called *section X ray.*)

tongue The muscle of speech arising from the floor of the mouth and back of the throat. It is also the organ of taste and aids in chewing.

    bifid A birth deformity in which the front portion of the tongue is split into two parts.

    coated A whitish-colored tongue, thought by some to be due to indigestion or an upset bowel function.

    furred Same as *coated tongue.*

    geographic A deformity in which there are thickened areas and deep furrows on the surface of the tongue.

    hairy A tongue which is brownish in color and contains long, wavy projections upon its surface. Usually this is harmless.

    parrot A dry, shriveled tongue,

seen in people who are markedly dehydrated.

strawberry The reddened tongue seen in scarlet fever.

-tie A tongue which has an abnormally short frenum (band) beneath it which anchors it to the floor of the mouth. This is a birth deformity, easily corrected by cutting the frenum.

tonic 1. A medication given to stimulate a person who feels "below par." 2. Referring to a continuous muscle contraction or spasm, such as a *tonic convulsion.*

tonicity The state of relaxation or contraction of a muscle or other organ.

tonometer An instrument, placed on the eyeball, to measure pressure within the eye. (It is elevated in cases of glaucoma.)

tonsil Lymph glands located in the mouth near the back of the tongue. They frequently become enlarged and infected. Their exact function is not known.

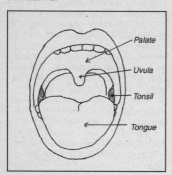

Tonsil

tonsillectomy Removal of the tonsils.

tonsillitis Inflammation or infection of the tonsils, characterized by chills, high fever, sore throat and weakness. Seen often in children.

tonus The normal degree of contraction present in most muscles.

This keeps them always ready to function when needed.

tooth, bicuspid The premolar teeth.

canine The sharp, pointed teeth next to the front four incisor teeth.

deciduous Baby teeth. There are twenty in number instead of the thirty-two adult teeth. Milk teeth.

impacted One lying obliquely or one on its side against another tooth.

incisor One of the front four teeth in the upper and lower jaws.

molar The back three teeth on both sides, upper and lower jaws. Used for chewing and grinding.

premolar The two teeth in both jaws, on both sides, lying behind the canine and in front of the molars.

wisdom The third (last) molar, located in back of the mouth. They usually do not break through the gums until early adulthood.

tophus A small, hard lump, usually about the size of a fingernail or smaller, located near a joint. It is composed of urates and usually signifies the presence of gouty arthritis. Seen often in the sacroiliac region.

topical application The application of a medication or anesthetic agent to the skin or mucous membrane.

topography The study of body surfaces.

toponeurosis An emotional disturbance concerning one topic.

torpid Sluggish as *torpid liver.*

torpor A "below par" feeling.

torsion A twisting.

of the omentum A twist in the omentum, the large apron of fatty tissue which hangs down from the transverse colon (large bowel).

of the testicle An acute condition in which the cord leading to the testicle becomes twisted. (Immediate surgery is necessary to save the testicle from becoming gangrenous.)

torso The trunk of the body.

torticollis Wry neck. A spasm or contraction of the muscles on one side of the neck, causing the head to be tilted and twisted.

tortuous Containing many turns and twists, as an enlarged varicose vein.

torulosis A yeast infection involving the brain, skin and lungs. The condition is very difficult to cure and may last for months or years. Also called *cryptococcosis*.

torus A ridge or prominence on the surface of the body.

total parenteral nutrition (TPN) *See* hyperalimentation.

tourist's disease Diarrhea, often with vomiting and fever, of tourists who visit foreign countries; also called traveler's disease.

tourniquet An apparatus for controlling hemorrhage; constriction is placed above the bleeding point.

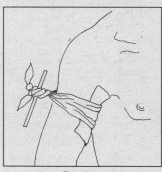

Tourniquet

toxemia A condition characterized by poisonous products (toxins) in the blood, with resultant illness of the patient.

   of pregnancy A serious disease of pregnancy caused by poisons circulating in the blood, often associated with inadequate kidney function, high blood pressure, convulsions, etc.

toxic Poisonous.

toxicity The quality of being toxic. The ability to produce toxemia, a term often applied to drugs or poisons.

toxicodendron Plants such as poison ivy, poison oak, sumac, etc.

toxicology The study of poisons and their effects. Also, the detection of poisons in a live or dead body.

toxicosis Poisoning of the entire body, whether from the toxins of bacteria or from chemical poisons.

toxic shock syndrome A condition marked by high fever, chills, diarrhea, low blood pressure and overwhelming weakness. It is encountered occasionally in females who use vaginal tampons during menstruation but is thought to occur also in other people, including males. The symptoms are thought to be caused by a toxin (poison) from the staphylococcus aureus germ.

toxin The poison manufactured by germs or other forms of animal or vegetable life. When it gains access to the body of humans, it acts as a poison and stimulates the formation of antibodies (antitoxins).

toxoid A toxin (poison) which has become inactivated but which retains its ability to stimulate the formation, within the body, of antibodies (antitoxins). Useful in building up immunity to disease.

toxoplasmosis A serious disease caused by the parasite *Toxoplasma*. In young people it may cause inflammation of the brain.

TPA An abbreviation for a substance that aids in dissolving a blood clot that has formed following a heart attack.

TPN Abbreviation for *total parenteral nutrition*, or feeding exclusively by injecting nutrients into the veins. Also known as *hyperalimentation*.

tr. A prescription abbreviation meaning *tincture*.

trabecula A band of fibrous tissue which helps to support the structure of an organ.

trabulectomy An operation to aid those who have glaucoma. The laser is often utilized in performing the operation.

tracer A radioactive particle or

group of particles which can be detected as it travels through the body. Important in noting the action and location of chemicals in the body.

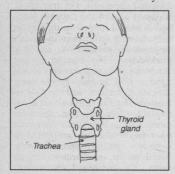

Trachea

trachea The windpipe.

tracheitis Inflammation of the trachea (windpipe).

trachelectomy Surgical removal of the cervix and neck of the uterus.

trachelitis Inflammation of the cervix of the uterus; cervicitis.

tracheloplasty Surgical repair of a torn or overgrown cervix of the uterus; trachelorrhaphy.

tracheobronchial Referring to the trachea (windpipe) and the bronchial tubes which extend from it.

tracheobronchitis Inflammation of the trachea and bronchial tubes.

tracheolaryngeal Referring to the trachea and the larynx (voice box).

tracheoesophageal fistula (TEF) A birth deformity in which there is a false communication between the trachea (windpipe) and the esophagus (foodpipe).

tracheotomy A surgical incision into the trachea (windpipe), often performed to relieve suffocation.

trachoma A virus disease of the eyelids, seen most often in North African countries. A turning of the eyelids often leads to serious scratching of the eyeball (conjunctiva).

tracing A recording, such as the *tracing* of heart action in electrocardiography or the *tracing* of brain waves in electroencephalography.

tract A pathway, as the gastrointestinal *tract*.

    afferent A nerve pathway carrying impulses toward the spinal cord and brain.

    alimentary The digestive tract.

    biliary The bile ducts leading from the liver to the intestine, including the gall bladder.

    efferent A nerve pathway carrying impulses from the brain or spinal cord outward to the organs and muscles.

    gastrointestinal Same as the alimentary tract.

    motor A nerve pathway from the brain carrying nerves which will eventually cause organs or muscles to function.

    respiratory The nose, throat, larynx, trachea, bronchial tubes and the lungs.

    sensory Nerve pathways carrying *sensations* (sensory impulses) to the brain, such as smell, sight, taste, touch, hearing, etc.

    urinary The kidneys, ureteral tubes, urinary bladder, urethra.

traction Pulling or exerting force to stretch a part.

    head Application of tension

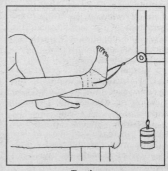

Traction

to the head, used for injuries to the spine in the neck region (cervical spine).

Trade-named drug A patented, named drug. (It is frequently much more expensive than the same drug under its generic, non-patented name.)

tragacanth A gummy base into which dyes, powders and other medications are placed so that they will adhere to body surfaces.

tragus The small cartilage pointing backwards over the opening of the external ear.

trait, dominant One that is transmitted to an offspring as a dominant characteristic, resulting from the fusion of similar dominant genes or a dominant and a recessive gene.

    recessive One that is transmitted to an offspring as a recessive characteristic, resulting from fusion of dissimilar genes or two recessive genes.

trance The hypnotic state.

tranquilizer drugs Drugs given to calm the nerves and to allay apprehension, such as Miltown, Equanil, Librium, Valium, etc.

trans- Prefix meaning "through"; "across."

transactional psychosis A type of mental illness having a great deal to do with actual relations with important people in the patient's life.

transaminase An enzyme (body chemical) which helps in the transformation of one amino acid (the basic component of proteins) into another amino acid. Useful in testing for certain diseases.

    alamine amino transferase (ALT) Increased amount of this enzyme may indicate faulty liver function or damage to the heart muscle.

    asparate amino transferase (AST) Increased amount of this enzyme may indicate faulty liver function or damage to the heart muscle.

Transderm-Nitro An adhesive patch

containing nitroglycerin, applied to the skin once daily to allay attacks of angina pectoris.

transducer The long arm of an ultrasound apparatus. The transducer is placed against the patient's body and is moved in various directions, thus showing differences in the recordings. *See* sonography.

transduction The transfer of genetic material from one cell to another. This takes place with utilization of viral infection.

transection The cutting across, as the *transection* of bone in performing an amputation.

trans fat These fats are found in large amounts in deep-fried foods, baked goods, margarines, and in some vegetable oils. Large quantities of these fats may increase the risk of heart attack, especially in women.

transferase Enzymes that cause the movement of chemical groups from one compound to another.

transference The feeling of affection and love or of hostility and hate that a patient being analyzed develops for the psychoanalyst. It is akin to the love and hate he may have had, in childhood, for his mother or father.

transfer-RNA *See* ribonucleic acid.

transfixion The piercing of a structure.

transformation The changing of one tissue into another, such as cartilage to bone.

transfusion The giving of blood from a donor into the vein of a recipient.

    arterial One in which the blood is pumped into an artery rather than a vein.

    direct The immediate transfer of blood from one individual to another through a connecting apparatus.

    exchange One in which practically 80 to 90 percent of an infant's blood is removed and is replaced by transfused blood; done in cases of Rh factor disease.

fetal Transfusion of blood to a fetus while it is in its mother's uterus.

indirect The donor's blood is collected and treated with citrate so that it does not clot. It is then, several hours or days later, given intravenously to the recipient. This is the usual method employed in most cases today.

peritoneal Injection into the abdominal cavity, from whence it is absorbed into the circulation. Performed mainly upon fetuses.

reaction One caused by giving incompatible blood. It may be mild with merely a reaction similar to hives, or may be severe enough to cause death.

transillumination The lighting up of an organ or part of the body as an aid to diagnosis, as the *transillumination* of the sinuses to see if they are infected.

transitional cell A cell that represents a phase in the transformation of one type of cell into another type.

translocation The transposition of two segments of a chromosome.

translucent Partially transparent; permitting the passage of some light.

transmigration The passage of cells from their usual habitat out into the tissues or to another location; the moving of an egg from the ovary to the fallopian tube; the moving of white blood cells out from a blood vessel into inflamed tissues.

transmissible A condition which can be given to another; a contagious disease.

transmutation The method by which one species of animal life develops into another; the evolutionary process.

transoral Through the mouth.

transparent Allowing light to pass through, as the pupil and lens of the eye.

transpiration 1. Exhaled air. 2. The

transfer of air, sweat or fluid through the skin.

transplant Tissue taken from one part of the body and implanted in another; a graft.

transplantation Grafting. *See* grafts.

transplantation immunity The rejection phenomenon; the rejection reaction; the destruction of a transplanted tissue or organ by the body's defense mechanisms. The treating of the grafted tissue as a foreign body, thus destroying it.

transposition A birth condition in which an organ or organs are located on the wrong side of the body, such as a heart on the right side or a liver on the left side.

transsex procedures Operations to alter an individual's external sex organs so that they resemble those of the opposite sex.

transsexual surgery Operations which transform the external genitals from one sex to another.

transudate Fluid which exudes from a blood vessel out into the tissues or on to a body surface; serum.

transureteral lithotomy A procedure in which stones are removed from the uterer by passing an instrument through the urethra and bladder up into the ureter.

transurethral resection An operation performed via the urethra, such as *transurethral prostatectomy* in which a portion of the prostate gland is removed through the penis.

transvaginal Through the vaginal opening.

transversalis fascia The fibrous sheath of tissue lying on top of the lining of the abdominal cavity, beneath the abdominal muscles. A tear in this fascia often leads to the development of a hernia.

transverse Across; at right angles to the longitudinal axis of the body.

colon That part of the large bowel which lies across the upper abdomen.

transvestitism A desire to wear the clothes of the opposite sex; men dressing as women or women dressing as men.

trapezius muscles Large muscles arising from the back of the head and vertebrae in the neck and chest. They extend to the collarbones and scapulae (shoulder blades). They raise and straighten the shoulder.

Trasentine A patented medication having the ability to relieve spasm of involuntary muscles, as that in the intestines, uterus, etc.

trauma Injury.

traumatic Caused by an injury or accident.

traumatology That branch of medicine dealing with the treatment of injuries and accidents.

traveler's diarrhea The type which is usually caused by traveling to a distant place and drinking or eating unfamiliar fluids or foods.

treatment, conservative That which disturbs the natural course of a disease as little as possible.

  empirical Experimental or practical treatment, usually not based upon proved scientific data.

  expectant Conservative treatment which withholds aggressive intervention until absolutely necessary.

  palliative Treatment which attempts to relieve symptoms rather than to ·eradicate the cause of the disease; applied when true cure is not possible.

  perennial That which is carried on throughout the year, as for hay fever when, in actuality the condition only is active for a few months.

  preseasonal Treatment of an allergic disease before its expected onset in order to prevent its onset.

  symptomatic The treatment of the symptoms caused by the illness rather than treatment of its underlying cause.

trematodes Flat worms or flukes. They can cause serious disease in humans.

trembling Muscle quivering, seen often during emotional excitement.

tremor A shaking of a hand, arm, leg or head due to muscle quivering. It is found in certain diseases of the nervous system, such as "shaking palsy."

  intention One which comes on when attempting to perform a muscular act, as in multiple sclerosis.

  pill rolling A continuous motion of the fingers and hands as if one is rolling a pill, seen in Parkinson's disease (paralysis agitans).

tremulous Trembling.

trench foot A disturbance of the smaller arteries and veins in the feet whereby they fail to contract and relax properly; seen in soldiers who have been exposed for long periods to wet and dampness. Such feet are cold, blue and painful.

trench mouth *See* Vincent's angina.

Trendelenburg position Lying supine with the foot of the bed elevated; the shock position sometimes used after surgery to stimulate flow of blood to the head.

trepanning An operation in which a hole is bored in the skull.

trephining An operation in which a coin-shaped hole is bored in the skull, done to relieve increased pressure within the skull or for purposes of diagnosing brain disease.

trepidation Anxiety; fear; hesitation.

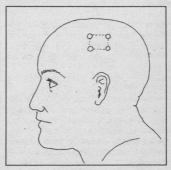

Trephining

treponema pallidum The germ, a spirochete, which causes syphilis.

triacetin A medicine applied locally to cure a fungal infection.

triad A combination of three symptoms or signs which make the diagnosis of a particular disease.

  Charcot's Eye twitching (nystagmus), tremor, and peculiar speech; seen in multiple sclerosis.

  Hutchinson's Deformed teeth, deafness and eye inflammation; seen in infants with inherited syphilis.

  Whipple Shaking and faintness, low blood sugar levels, recovery after eating sugar; seen in hyperinsulinism, a condition in which there is an excess of insulin.

triage Sorting out the wounded so that the most serious cases are treated first. Also, sorting out the wounded so that they are treated by the appropriate specialist.

triangle A triangularly shaped area or region in the body, such as the *femoral triangle* in the upper inner corner of the thigh.

triceps The muscles in the back of the upper arms. They extend the elbow.

trichesthesia The sensation one experiences when hair is touched or gently brushed.

trichiasis 1. A disease of the eyelashes which irritates and affects the eyeball. 2. An anal condition caused by irritation from hair about the anus.

trichinosis A parasitic disease affecting muscles and causing nausea, vomiting, dizziness and diarrhea. Caused by eating infected pork or ham.

tricho- Combining form referring to hair.

trichobezoar A ball of hair in the stomach or intestine; sometimes seen in mentally ill patients who eat their own hair.

trichoesthesia Same as trichesthesia.

trichoid Resembling hair.

trichology The study of diseases of the hair.

trichomonas vaginitis Inflammation of the vagina with discharge; caused by infection with *Trichomonas vaginalis*. A common condition lending itself to cure but having a tendency to recur.

trichomycosis A fungus infection of the hair.

trichophagy Eating hair.

trichophytobezoar A ball of food and hair which collects in the stomach and does not pass on through the intestines; seen in some children who eat hair and in some mental patients.

trichophyton Fungus which attaches to hair.

trichophytosis Fungus infection of hair, often occurring in the scalps of children, causing dermatitis and hair loss.

trichosis Any hair disease.

Trichotine douche A vaginal medication, helpful in removing mucus and discharge.

trichuriasis Infestation with roundworms (nematodes).

Tricofuron suppositories Vaginal suppositories helpful in the treatment of trichomonas or monilia infections.

tricuspid Having three cusps, as the *tricuspid valve* of the heart.

triethylenemelamine (TEPA) An agent used in the treatment of leukemia; a chemical related to nitrogen mustard.

trifacial nerve The trigeminal nerve.

trifocal lenses Eyeglasses with three prescriptions; for near, intermediate, and far vision.

trigeminal nerve The fifth cranial nerve, supplying the face.

trigeminal neuralgia Neuritis of the trigeminal (fifth cranial) nerve, characterized by severe pain in the face occurring in sudden paroxysms. Tic douloureux.

trigger finger A dislocation of a tendon so that the flexion or extension of a finger is momentarily halted.

trigger point A spot on the body

that, when touched or pressed, calls forth a painful response.

triglyceride A fatty acid compound present in all people; consistently elevated levels of triglycerides may be conducive to premature arteriosclerosis.

trigone The triangular zone at the base of the urinary bladder, bounded by the entrance of the two ureters from the kidneys and the exit to the urethra.

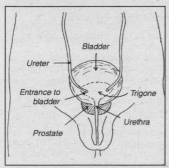

Trigone of the bladder

trigonitis Inflammation of the base of the urinary bladder.

trimester A three-month period, as the first, second or third *trimester* of pregnancy.

trimethadione A medication used to control convulsions and petit mal in epilepsy.

trimetrexate An anti-cancer drug; also a drug that may help patients with pneumocystis pneumonia (*PCP*).

Tri-Norinyl 21-Day Tablets An oral contraceptive drug.

triorchid A birth deformity in which there are three testicles.

Trip A "trip." Slang expression for the sensations experienced from LSD or marijuana.

tripara Having borne three children.

triphammer pulse A strong, hard-beating pulse. Also called water-hammer pulse.

triple coverage The use of three different types of antibiotics to act against any combination of gram-positive, gram-negative, aerobic, and anaerobic bacteria. (Penicillin-Gentamicin-Flagyl are often prescribed for this purpose.)

triplet One of three infants born at the same time.

triple vaccine *See* DPT.

trisomy A cell containing an extra (47th) chromosome.

trismus Lockjaw; severe spasm of the muscles of the jaw. This can be caused by any infection in the lower jaw or cheek.

triturate To pound into a fine powder, as in preparing prescriptions.

trocar A sharply pointed surgical instrument used to puncture a cavity so as to remove fluid, blood, pus, etc.

trochanter The prominence of the thighbone (femur) which can be felt below the hip region on the outer aspect of the upper thigh.

troche A lozenge, used for inflamed throat.

trochlear nerve The fourth cranial nerve which supplies the muscle going to the upper, outer portion of the eyeball.

trophedema A localized swelling of a part of the body due to damage to nerve or blood supply to the area.

trophic Pertaining to nutrition; a *trophic ulcer* is one caused by lack of adequate nourishment being brought to the area.

trophology The science of nutrition.

trophoneurosis Any condition due to disturbance of the nerves which are connected to the diseased region.

tropical disease One encountered in the tropics. With increased communication and travel, many of these diseases have become prevalent in temperate climates.

tropism The uncontrolled attraction or rejection of a substance or organism to another substance or organism. Phototropism is the involuntary turning of a plant toward the sunlight.

truncated Shortened; having excess parts cut off.

truss A support, worn to keep in a hernia.

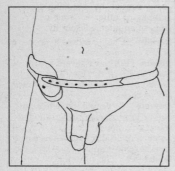

Truss

Trypanosoma A parasite which looks, under a microscope, something like a tadpole. It causes many serious diseases such as African sleeping sickness, Chagas' disease, etc. It is transmitted by insect bites.

trypanosomiasis African sleeping sickness.

tryparsamide An arsenic preparation used in the treatment of trypanosome infestations and syphilis of the nervous system.

trypsin An intestinal enzyme (body chemical) which digests proteins.

trypsinogen The enzyme trypsin before it is secreted by the pancreas into the intestinal tract.

tryptophan An essential amino acid.

tsetse fly The African fly which sometimes carries the causative agent of African sleeping sickness. *See Trypanosoma.*

TSH Abbreviation for thyroid stimulating hormone.

tsp An abbreviation for teaspoonful.

TSS Abbreviation for *toxic shock syndrome.*

tsutsugamushi fever A rickettsial disease transmitted by the bite of an infected insect. Its symptoms are fever, rash and severe headache. Seen mostly in Japan. Also called *scrub typhus fever.*

tubal ligation An operative procedure to close the fallopian tubes, thus preventing pregnancy.

tubal pregnancy Ectopic pregnancy. Pregnancy taking place in the fallopian (uterine) tubes.

tube, drainage A rubber, plastic or glass tube inserted into the body to drain off fluid.

    endotracheal A tube inserted through the nose or mouth to obtain a clear airway to the lungs.

    Levin A hollow tube inserted through the nose down into the stomach.

    Miller–Abbott A tube with two passageways, inserted into the small intestines in order to drain out fluid or intestinal contents from obstructed bowel.

    Sengstaken–Blakemore A tube inserted into the esophagus and stomach in order to stop bleeding from varicose veins of the esophagus.

    Wangensteen A tube connected to an apparatus that sucks excess fluid out of the small intestines.

tubercle The inflammatory reaction caused by the tuberculosis germ.

tubercle, Darwin A small projection of cartilage in the upper portion of the ear.

tubercular Having many tubercles.

tuberculid Skin conditions seen in people who have tuberculosis of the lungs or other organs.

tuberculin test A skin test to determine the presence of tuberculosis.

tuberculoma A mass, appearing like a tumor, caused by tuberculous infection with breakdown of tissue into puslike, dead material.

tuberculosis Any infection caused by *Mycobacterium tuberculosis*. Infection of the lungs is the most common type. Newer drugs are able to control most cases if the diagnosis is made early.

active That which is causing symptoms such as fever, weight loss, coughing, etc.

arrested That which was once active but has been brought under control to an inactive state.

avian That type found in birds.

bovine That type found in cattle. It can be transmitted to man through infected milk.

disseminated That which has spread throughout the whole body.

extrapulmonary That which occurs outside of the lungs, as in the bones, intestines, nervous system, etc.

inactive That which has healed and causes no symptoms.

open That which can be caught by others through coughing of sputum containing the tuberculosis germ.

primary The first infection, almost always in childhood, with the tuberculosis germ. It usually heals without causing illness. Such *primary tuberculosis* usually affects the lung and heals leaving a calcified scar which can be seen on X ray.

pulmonary Lung tuberculosis.
tuberculous Infected with tuberculosis.
tuberosity A jutting-out area on a bone.
tuboplasty Plastic reconstruction of a closed fallopian tube, carried out in some cases of female sterility.
tubovarian Referring to the fallopian tube and the ovary, as a *tubovarian infection*.

disease Inflammation involving both the fallopian tube and adjacent ovary.

tubule A small tube, usually referring to a tube-shaped structure when viewed under the microscope; the *tubules* of the kidneys.

Tucks A medicated pad used to cleanse the anus, especially after defecation.

tularemia A severe infectious disease caused by handling infected rabbits or other rodents, or by the bite of an infected deer fly.

tumefacient Causing swelling of a part.

tumefaction A swelling.
tumescence A swelling.
tumor A swelling. More particularly, the term refers to a growth, either cancerous or non-cancerous.

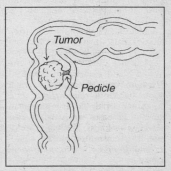

Pedicle of a tumor

benign One that is not malignant; non-cancerous.

Brown-Pearce A markedly malignant skin cancer.

carcinoid One that appears considerably like a cancer but is composed of a different type of cell (argentaffin cells); found in the intestinal tract. It may remain localized indefinitely or may spread.

chromaffin A tumor derived from cells of the medulla (center) of the adrenal gland; a pheochromocytoma.

dermoid A congenital tumor arising from tissues that go to form skin, teeth, and hair; thus, a dermoid cyst of an ovary may actually contain teeth or hair or other elements of the dermis.

desmoid A tumor frequently found in the abdominal muscles of women who have recently borne children. It is composed mainly of fibrous tissue.

Ewing's A malignant tumor of bone, usually occurring in children and adolescents. The bones of the extremities are the most frequent sites.

fibroid One containing large amounts of fibrous tissue, such as a fibroid tumor of the uterus.

glomus An extremely painful, pea-sized tumor often occurring beneath a fingernail; or beneath the skin. Composed of nerve tissue.

granulosa cell An ovarian tumor arising from a follicle from which an egg has been expelled.

Hürthle cell A tumor of the thyroid gland composed of special (Hürthle) cells. Some are benign; others malignant.

Krukenberg A malignant tumor of the ovaries secondary to a cancer elsewhere within the abdomen, usually the stomach.

malignant Cancer, sarcoma, leukemia, etc. A tumor that has a tendency to spread and has a tendency to return after surgical removal.

mixed One composed of two or more different kinds of tissue, such as a mixed tumor of a salivary gland. Usually nonmalignant.

phantom False pregnancy; enlargement of the abdomen in a hysterical individual who imagines he or she has a tumor.

Schminke A special kind of tumor arising from tonsil tissue within the throat.

Schwann's A tumor composed of nerve and fibrous tissue.

theca cell An ovarian tumor arising from theca cells.

Warthin's A benign tumor of the parotid gland beneath the angle of the jaw.

Wilm's A malignant tumor of the kidney seen in newborn children and infants.

tumoricidal Something that can kill a tumor.

tumorous Having the characteristics of a tumor or growth.

tunic A membrane covering an organ or structure.

tunica vaginalis The covering membranes of the testicle.

tuning fork A vibrating instrument used to test the senses, especially that of bone conduction.

tunnel disease *See* caisson disease.

tunnel vision Loss of peripheral vision with preservation of vision directly in front of the eyes.

T.U.R. Abbreviation for transurethral resection of a portion of the prostate gland.

turbid Cloudy, as turbid urine.

turbinate The bony ledges within the nose.

turbinectomy Removal of the turbinate bones in the nose.

turgid Swollen as a result of having excess blood in an organ or part.

Turner's syndrome *See* syndrome.

tussal Pertaining to coughing.

tussis A cough.

TVB Abbreviation for total blood volume.

Tweens Chemicals that have the property of emulsifying (breaking down) fat; sometimes given to those who are unable to properly digest and absorb fats from the intestinal tract.

twilight sleep The state produced by injection of morphine and scopolamine. This is sometimes used as the sole anesthesia in obstetrical delivery.

twin One of a pair born at the same time.

    conjoint Siamese twins. Twins joined at some part of their bodies.

    dissimilar Fraternal twins.

    fraternal Twins originating from two separate eggs. They may not look at all alike. They may be of the same or opposite sex.

identical Twins originating from a single egg. They are of the same sex and they look alike.

Siamese Twins whose bodies are joined together.

unequal Twins only one of whom is fully developed at birth.

twinge A sudden, sharp pain.

tylectomy Lumpectomy, removal of a tumor.

Tylenol Some forms of this medication have other drugs added for the specific treatment of conditions such as allergies, sleeplessness, colds, sinus infections, etc.

tympanic membrane The eardrum.

tympanic nerve The nerve supplying the middle ear, eustachian tube and the mastoid bone.

tympanites Distention of the abdomen due to excess gas in the intestines.

tympanitic Sounding like a drum when tapped with the examining fingers of the physician.

tympanitis Inflammation of the middle ear and eardrum.

tympanoplasty A plastic operative procedure to repair a damaged eardrum.

tympany The drumlike tone heard when tapping with the fingers on a distended abdomen.

typhlitis Inflammation of the cecum, the first portion of the large intestine located in the right lower part of the abdomen.

typhoid fever A disease caused by *Salmonella typhosa*. It enters the body through infected water, milk, food, seafood or by contagion from a person harboring the typhoid germs. It causes high fever, ulcers of the intestine, diarrhea, headache, weakness, hemorrhages, etc. It takes six to eight weeks to subside and is often accompanied by complications and relapses. Protection against this disease can be obtained by a series of typhoid vaccinations.

typhus fever A disease caused by *Rickettsia*. It has no relation to typhoid fever and is often caused by the bite of infected body lice. Seen in epidemic form, especially when hygienic precautions are at a low ebb, as during wartime. It is characterized by high fever, headache, a body rash, mental confusion, with sudden recovery in about two weeks. In severe cases, death ensues. Protection against this disease can be obtained through vaccination.

typical Following the usual pattern; the opposite of atypical.

typing Determining the blood group prior to giving a transfusion.

tyrosine A protein breakdown product (amino acid) found in the casein of milk.

U

U Symbol for uranium.

ulcer An absence of the normal lining of a body surface limited to a particular area, such as *ulcer* of the stomach or of the skin. The base of the ulcer is usually inflamed and raw.

Curling's An ulcer of the stomach or duodenum occurring in people who have sustained severe skin burns.

decubitus Bedsores usually seen over the base of the spine where contact has taken place with the mattress. Seen mostly in chronically ill people.

diabetic Ulcers of the feet or legs seen in diabetics who have not taken care of themselves and who have poor healing powers.

diphtheritic An ulcer in the throat which appears after a diphtheritic membrane has become detached. Seen very rarely today.

duodenal One located in the first portion of the small intestine, the duodenum.

esophageal One located in the esophagus (food pipe).

gastric One located in the stomach.

indolent One that shows little tendency to heal.

kissing An ulcer which faces another ulcer, as on both sides of the duodenum.

marginal An ulcer which forms at the junction of the stomach and small intestine following an operation for ulcer.

penetrating One which extends deeply into the tissues.

peptic An ulcer occurring in

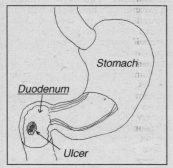

Ulcer of the duodenum

the esophagus, stomach or duodenum.

perforated One which has ruptured through the wall of the stomach or duodenum.

rodent A skin cancer, with ulcer formation, most commonly seen on the side of the nose, cheek or face.

serpiginous One which has undermined edges and is extending out sideways into adjoining tissues.

stasis An ulcer in the vicinity of varicose veins of the leg, caused by poor circulation through the varicosities.

stomal Same as marginal ulcer.

trophic One caused by lack of blood supply to a part.

varicose An ulcer of the leg associated with varicose veins.

ulcerate To form an ulcer.

ulcerative colitis A specific form of colitis, chronic in nature, associated with bloody diarrhea, ulcerations of

388

the large bowel, anemia, and weight loss.

ulcerogenic Ulcer-producing.

ulcus An ulcer.

ulitis Inflammation of the gums; gingivitis.

ulna The long bone of the inside of the forearm, lying next to the radius.

ultrafiltration Filtration through an exceptionally fine filter which can separate out all the solid particles from a solution except viruses.

ultramicroscope An exceptionally high-powered microscope.

ultramicroscopic Too small to be seen under a microscope, as certain viruses.

ultrasonic Referring to sound waves which are of such high frequency that they cannot be heard.

ultrasonic lithotresis The breaking up of stones by high-frequency sound waves. This technique has been used for stones in the kidney, ureters, and gall bladder.

ultrasonography *See* sonography.

ultrasound tests *See* sonography.

ultraviolet radiation Sunlight; light rays that are beyond the violet end of the visible spectrum.

umbilectomy Surgical removal of the navel; done sometimes for large hernias of the navel.

umbilical cord The cord going from the embryo's navel to the placenta of the uterus.

umbilical hernia One that takes place through the navel.

umbilicus The navel.

unciform Shaped like a hook.

uncinariasis Hookworm infestation of the intestinal tract. *See also* hookworm disease.

unconditioned reflex An instinctive response, as opposed to one that is conscious and not inborn. (To take one's hand away from a hot stove is an example of an *unconditioned reflex.*)

unconscious Asleep, or in coma, or under anesthesia. Unconscious thinking is that of which we are not

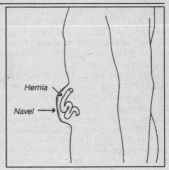

Umbilical (navel) hernia

aware and cannot consciously control.

unction An ointment or salve.

undecylenic acid An acid frequently used as an ingredient of ointments for the treatment of psoriasis or fungus infections of the skin.

undescended testicle A testicle which has not come down into the scrotum. This is a birth deformity which may require surgical correction.

undifferentiated Immature primitive; a term often applied to the microscopic appearance of rapidly growing cancer cells.

undulant fever Brucellosis; Mediterranean fever; Malta fever. An infection with a germ known as brucella, associated with recurrent fever, weakness and anemia. Often caused by drinking infected goat or cow's milk.

unguentum A salve or ointment.

uni- A prefix signifying one or single.

Unicap Trademark for a multivitamin medication.

unicentric Referring to a growth that has one point of origin, as opposed to multicentric.

uniform Having the same shape.

unilateral One side of the body, as distinguished from bilateral.

unilocular Referring to one pocket, as an abscess having but one cavity.

union The healing of tissues, as fractured bones which have knit or a surgical wound that has united.

United States Pharmacopeia The official publication listing all bona fide drugs and medications.

United States Public Health Service (USPHS) The Department of Health and Human Services concerned with scientific research, domestic and insular quarantine, administration of government hospitals, publications and statistics, etc.

univalent antibody An incomplete antibody, usually not functioning adequately.

Unna boot A semisolid pastelike covering composed of zinc oxide, glycerin, etc., used to promote the healing of leg ulcers.

unphysiologic Referring to abnormal function of a part or organ.

unsaturated Denoting a solution that can absorb more of an active ingredient; the opposite of saturated.

unsaturated fats Fats derived mainly from vegetables, nuts, and fish. They are low in cholesterol content and are therefore recommended for people with arteriosclerosis or high blood pressure.

ununited Referring to an unhealed, *ununited* fracture of a bone.

upper endoscopy Viewing the lumens (insides) of the esophagus, stomach, and duodenum passing an instrument through the mouth.

upper respiratory infections Those affecting the nose, throat, sinuses, larynx, trachea, or bronchial tubes, but not the lungs.

urachus A structure seen in the embryo extending from the bladder to the navel. Normally, this structure degenerates by the time the child is born.

uranium (U) An element having radioactive properties.

uranoplasty An operation to repair a cleft palate in the roof of the mouth.

urea A carbon compound found normally in the blood and urine. It represents the waste product of protein metabolism. An excess in the blood is known as uremia.

Urea Nitrogen 6-20 mg/dL Elevated quantities may indicate a possibility of faulty kidney function.

Urecholine A medication which stimulates the muscle of the urinary bladder to contract; used postoperatively when there is difficulty in spontaneous urination.

uremia A serious illness caused by the inability of the kidneys to eliminate waste products of metabolism. Unless kidney function is restored, death from uremic poisoning will ensue.

ureter The tube leading from the kidney to the bladder.

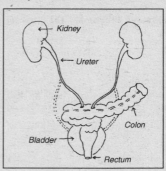

Implantation of the ureters

ureteral implantation operation A surgical procedure in which the ureters are transplanted into the bowel. Performed when the patient has a bladder malignancy necessitating its removal.

ureteritis Inflammation of the ureter; a rare condition.

ureterocele A bulging and ballooning out of the ureter located near its entrance into the urinary bladder.

ureteroileostomy An operation in which the ureter from the kidney is implanted into the ileum (small intestine); performed in some cases when it has been necessary to remove the urinary bladder.

ureterolithiasis A stone in the ureter, the hollow tube connecting the kidney and the bladder. These stones originate in the kidney and are washed down with the urine.

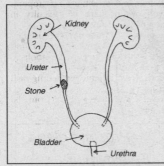

Kidney

Ureter →

Stone

Bladder

← Urethra

Ureter and stone

ureterolithotomy Surgical removal of a stone from a ureter, the tube leading from the kidney to the bladder.

ureteroscopic ultrasonic lithotrypsy A procedure for breaking up stones in the ureter by means of ultrasound waves.

ureterostomy An operation in which the ureter is brought out onto the skin surface.

ureterotomy A surgical incision into the ureter, usually performed to remove a stone.

uretero-ureterostomy A surgical procedure in which a ureter from one kidney is sutured to the ureter of the other kidney.

ureterovesical Referring to the ureter from the kidney and the urinary bladder.

urethane A carbon compound sometimes used in treating certain types of leukemia.

urethra The tube leading from the urinary bladder to the outside.

urethritis Inflammation of the ure-

thra, the outlet from the bladder to the outside.

urethrocele Overgrowth of the fibrous tissue surrounding the urethra (the outlet from the bladder).

urethroplasty A plastic operation upon the urethra, the outlet from the bladder.

urethroscope An illuminated instrument which, when inserted into the urethra, permits the examiner to view its contours and lining.

urgency Frequent desire to urinate.

uric acid A normal chemical constituent of the blood. When present in excessive amounts it may be associated with gout.

uricemia Excess uric acid in the blood, a constant finding in individuals suffering from gout.

urinalysis Examination of the urine.

urinary frequency *See* frequency.

urinary incontinence *See* incontinence.

urine The liquid excreted by the kidneys. Normally it has a clear amber color. Its specific gravity varies from 1.005 to 1.030. It ordinarily contains urea, chlorides, and other chemicals. Urine does not normally contain sugar, albumin, pus, blood, bacteria, acetone or casts.

urinometer An instrument which determines the specific gravity (degree of concentration) of urine.

urobilin Bile pigments excreted in the urine.

urobilinogen A substance which goes into the formation of urobilin.

urogastrone A hormone normally present in urine which, when extracted and refined, has the power to slow down stomach activity and secretion.

urogenital Referring to the organs responsible for reproduction and urination; genitourinary.

urogenital tract The urinary and genital organs (kidney, ureter, bladder, prostate, penis, urethra, etc.).

urography X-ray visualization of the urinary tract by use of opaque dyes.

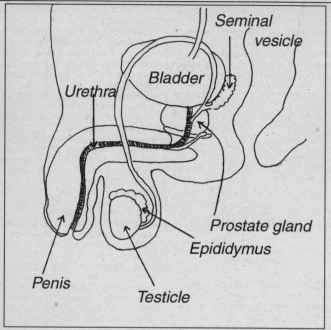

Urethra

urokinase A substance injected to help dissolve a blood clot, as after a coronary thrombosis.

Urologist A physician who specializes in diseases of the urogenital system.

urosepsis An infection within the urinary system, resulting in high fever, chills, etc.

urticaria Hives. An allergic condition of the skin characterized by the formation of large blotches or welts which itch intensely.

U.S.P. *See* United States Pharmacopeia.

U.S.P.H.S. United States Public Health Service.

uterine Pertaining to the womb (uterus).

uterine cavity The hollow space within the uterus.

uterine tubes Fallopian tubes, one on either side of the uterus, connecting the cavity of the uterus to the abdominal cavity.

uterogestation Pregnancy within the womb.

uterography X-raying the cavity of the uterus and fallopian tubes after injection of opaque dyes into the cervix.

uteropelvic Referring to the uterus and the ligaments which hold it in place.

uterosacral Pertaining to the uterus and the sacrum (the bones upon which we sit).

uterus The womb. The female organ in which the embryo develops.

   bicornuate One which has not developed fully and therefore has two parts, or horns.

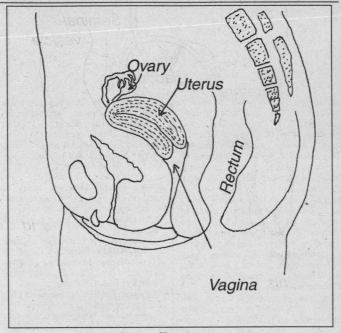

Uterus

didelphys A uterus divided into two separate compartments due to failure of fusion during development.

infantile A small, undeveloped uterus.

retroverted One tipped backwards toward the sacrum.

utricle A small sac.

uvea That part of the eye containing the iris and blood vessels.

uveitis Inflammation of the uvea of the eye.

uveoparotitis An inflammation of the uvea of the eye and the parotid gland (salivary gland) in the angle of the jaw, associated with fever. Cause unknown.

uvula The cone-shaped piece of tissue which hangs down from the soft palate in the back of the mouth.

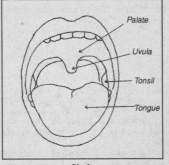

Uvula

uvulectomy Surgical removal of an elongated uvula.

uvulitis Inflammation of the uvula.

V

vaccinate To immunize against a disease; as to inoculate against smallpox.

vaccination The giving of a vaccine to prevent the onset of a disease. The effect of the *vaccination* is to cause the body to manufacture antibodies which prevent the onset of the disease.

vaccine Killed, or markedly weakened, bacteria in solution, given to build up body resistance against the bacteria. Repeated injections often confer immunity to specific diseases.

    autogenous A vaccine prepared from the patient's own bacteria. These killed bacteria are then injected over a period of time and they cause the body to form antibodies. This form of treatment is only occasionally effective.

    BCG A vaccine to protect against tuberculosis. It is taken by mouth, not injected. (There is some doubt as to the effectiveness of this type of vaccination.)

    cholera A vaccine to protect against cholera. It is given by injection and has proven most effective in protecting against this disease.

    cowpox The vaccine given to prevent smallpox.

    hepatitis Used to protect against Types A and B.

    influenza, Type A Monovalent; used to protect against Asian flu.

    influenza, polyvalent Used to protect against several types of influenza.

    live One prepared from living bacteria in such a weakened state that they are incapable of causing disease but will stimulate the body to produce antibodies against them.

    measles An effective vaccine to protect against measles. (Must be given with care to children who are allergic to eggs.) *See* Immunization Table in Health Manual.

    multivalent A vaccine containing several different types of bacteria in order to protect against several conditions, such as typhoid, paratyphoid A and paratyphoid B vaccine.

    mumps An effective vaccine to protect against mumps. (Must be given with care to children who are allergic to eggs.) *See* Immunization Table in Health Manual.

    paratyphoid A vaccine to protect against paratyphoid fever.

    pertussis Whooping cough vaccine. It is given by a series of injections and is successful in protecting against whooping cough in the great majority of cases.

    plague An effective vaccine to protect against bubonic plague. *See* Immunization Table in Health Manual.

    poliomyelitis Vaccine to protect against infantile paralysis.

    polyvalent Vaccine made from several different groups of the same bacteria.

    rabies A vaccine given in many doses over a period of two to three weeks in order to protect against rabies. Rabies, or hydrophobia, results from a dog or other animal bite from a rabid animal.

    Rocky Mountain spotted fever A vaccine prepared from the infected bodies of the ticks (lice) which cause the disease.

Sabin An oral vaccine for prevention of infantile paralysis.

Salk Infantile paralysis vaccine. It is effective in 80-85 percent of cases.

smallpox A vaccine which prevents smallpox. It is prepared from cows infected with cowpox. (This vaccine is seldom used today since smallpox has been eradicated.)

staphylococcus One prepared from killed staphylococcal germs; sometimes effective in protecting against the formation of staphylococcal boils and abscesses.

T.A.B. Also called *triple vaccine*. It protects against typhoid fever, paratyphoid A and B fever.

whooping cough A moderately good protection is afforded through this vaccine.

yellow fever An excellent protection is afforded through this vaccine.

vaccinia A virus disease of cattle which, when used to inoculate man, induces immunity to smallpox. When the arm reddens, swells, becomes painful and the vaccination area forms the typical pustular appearance, it is probable that the vaccination was successful.

typhus An effective vaccine to protect against typhus fever. *See* Immunization Table in Health Manual.

vacuolar Relating to a vacuole (a clear space within a cell).

vacuum A space from which all air has been withdrawn. Such a space must be airtight.

vagal Referring to the vagus nerve, the largest nerve in the body.

vagal attack Fainting, secondary to sudden stimulation of the vagus nerve. *See* vagus nerve.

vagal episode A feeling of dying, supposedly caused by excess stimulation of the vagus nerve with resultant spasm of blood vessels.

vagina The female mucous membrane canal leading from the vulva to the cervix of the uterus. The canal in which copulation takes place.

vaginal hysterectomy Removal of the uterus through incisions made in the vagina.

vaginectomy Surgical removal of the vagina.

vaginismus Spasm of the vagina; sometimes so severe as to prevent entrance of the male organ. It is usually a functional disorder, not due to an actual disease process.

vaginitis Inflammation of the vagina.

atrophic Inflammation occurring in older women. Also called *senile vaginitis*. (It is thought to be caused by lack of female sex hormone.)

gonorrheal Inflammation of the vagina caused by the gonococcus germ.

trichomonas vaginalis One of the most common forms of genital irritation; caused by a fungus infection. Also called *leukorrhea*.

vaginoplasty Surgical repair of a torn vagina. Usually performed upon women who have received tears during childbirth.

vagotomy Cutting the vagus nerve. An operation sometimes performed to relieve the symptoms of an ulcer of the stomach or duodenum. It may be performed either through the chest or abdomen.

vagovagal reaction An episode characterized by low blood pressure and a lower than normal heart rate.

vagus nerve The tenth cranial nerve. The largest nerve in the body, supplying the heart, lungs and the abdominal organs.

valence The specific ability of an atom to combine with other atoms. For instance, two hydrogen atoms customarily combine with one oxygen atom to form H_2O, water.

valerian A strong-smelling compound given to calm hysterical, emotionally disturbed people.

valgus The turning out of the foot.

valine An essential amino acid.

Valium A valuable tranquilizer medication.

valley fever San Joaquin Valley

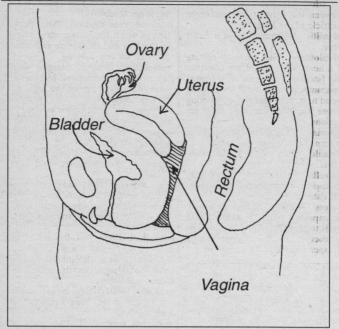

Vagina

fever, coccidioidomycosis. A chronic lung infection found in the San Joaquin Valley in California.

Valsalva's maneuver Blowing out a collapsed eustachian tube (from the throat to the ear) by closing the mouth and nose, and then forcefully expelling air from the lungs.

valve An anatomical fold in an organ or blood vessel which permits the contents of the vessel or organ to pass through but which prevents backflow.

    aortic One situated in the left ventricle of the heart. It allows blood to flow out into the aorta but prevents it from backing up into the heart after it has been expelled.

    bicuspid The mitral valve, between the left atrium (auricle) and left ventricle of the heart.

    Houston's Folds of mucous membrane in the rectum.

    ileocecal The valve between the end of the small intestine (ileum) and the beginning of the large intestine (cecum).

    mitral (bicuspid) The valve located between the left atrium and ventricle of the heart. It is this valve which often closes down because of disease caused by rheumatic fever. This valve is often cut surgically to relieve its contraction and deformity.

    pulmonary The one located at the exit of the right ventricle of the heart.

    pyloric The fold of mucous membrane between the end of the stomach and the beginning of the duodenum.

tricuspid The valve located between the right atrium and right ventricle of the heart.

valvulitis Inflammation of a heart valve.

valvulotomy The surgical cutting of a heart valve to relieve constriction (stenosis), as in mitral stenosis.

Vancomycin An antibiotic drug found to be very useful in combating severe staphylococcal and other infections.

vaporize To heat a substance so as to turn it into steam or vapor.

variable That which is not constant.

varicella Chickenpox. A highly contagious virus disease with characteristic skin eruption.

varices Varicose veins; enlarged, incompetent veins in which blood tends to stagnate.

varicocele Varicose veins along the spermatic cord and scrotum.

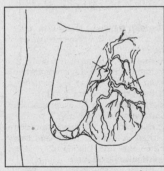

Varicocele

varicocelectomy The surgical removal of a varicocele, performed only when the veins are very large and the patient has pain in the area.

varicose ulceration An ulceration of the skin in the region of varicose veins in the legs, caused by poor venous circulation.

varicose vein An enlarged vein resulting from a breakdown of its valves. Blood tends to stagnate

within such a vein, often necessitating surgical removal.

varicose vein ligation An operation in which the incompetent veins in the legs and thighs are dissected out, tied off and severed.

varicosities Dilated, enlarged veins whose valves are damaged. Most common site is the veins of the legs.

variola Smallpox.

Varivax *See* chickenpox vaccine.

varix A varicose vein.

varus A turned-in foot deformity; bowleggedness.

vasa brevia Blood vessels traveling between the stomach and the spleen.

vas deferens The tube carrying sperm from the testicles to the glands where they are stored (seminal vesicles) in preparation for ejaculation.

vascularization The formation of new blood vessels in a structure.

vascular system Blood vessel system. *See* Manual for important arteries and veins.

vascular bed All the blood supply of a part of the body or organ of the body.

vascular surgery The branch of surgery that confines itself to disorders of the arteries and veins.

vasculitis Inflammation of a blood vessel.

vasectomy Surgical cutting of the tube which transports sperm. (If this is done on both sides, the male becomes sterile but will maintain his potency.) Cutting the vas deferens.

Vaseline A trade name for petroleum jelly; used as a lubricant.

Vasocidin Eyedrops containing antibiotics, excellent for clearing up conjunctivitis.

vasoconstriction The narrowing and contraction of blood vessels.

vasodepressor A medication that lowers the blood pressure.

vasodilatation Enlargement or dilation of blood vessels.

vasodilator A drug that causes blood vessels to dilate.

vasomotor mechanism That which regulates the contraction or dilatation of blood vessels.

vasopressor An agent which causes constriction of blood vessels and a rise in blood pressure.

vasospasm Marked contraction and narrowing of a blood vessel or a segment of a blood vessel.

Vasotec A proprietary drug used to reduce blood pressure.

vasovagal reaction An acute attack caused by excessive vagus nerve activity in the neck region. It is accompanied by sudden loss of consciousness and an abrupt drop in blood pressure.

vasovasostomy An operation to restore the continuity of the vas deferens, after it had been previously cut during vasectomy.

VD *See* venereal disease.

VDRL An abbreviation for a test for the presence of syphilis.

vector An insect or other form of animal life which acts as a "go between" in the transmission of germs to humans.

vegetarian One who eats only fruit, vegetables, nuts, etc.

vegetative nervous system Same as *autonomic nervous system*. It supplies the internal organs, glands and the muscles over which there is no voluntary control.

vehicle A substance, usually a liquid, used as a mixer with an active drug. The vehicle itself usually has no treatment value.

veins The blood vessels which transport blood from the tissues back to the heart.

vellicate To twitch; as a muscle twitch.

Velpeau bandage A bandage that holds an arm immobile to the chest wall.

vena cava, inferior The large vein in the abdomen which transports blood back to the heart from structures and organs located below the diaphragm.

superior The large vein above

the heart which transports blood from the head, neck and upper extremities.

venereal disease Disease acquired through sexual intercourse, such as syphilis and gonorrhea.

venery Intercourse.

venesection Removing blood from a vein; blood letting.

venipuncture Placement of a needle into a vein.

venogram X ray of the course of a vein, usually performed after the injection of an opaque substance into the vein.

venom Poisons transmitted to man by snake bites or insect stings.

venostasis Stoppage of the flow of blood through a vein, as when pressure is placed over large varicose veins.

venous thrombosis Clotting of a vein.

venter Latin for *belly*.

ventilate To supply oxygen to the lungs.

Ventolin inhaler Helpful in relieving spasms of the bronchial tubes of the lung.

ventral The front of the body; the abdominal region. (A *ventral hernia* is one in which there is a protrusion through the abdominal wall.)

ventricle A cavity or pouch. The heart ventricles are the lowermost heart chambers. Brain ventricles are located within the brain and carry the cerebrospinal fluid.

ventricular fibrillation Heart irregularity orginating in the ventricles. If continued for any length of time, it results in ineffectual heart contractions and death.

premature contractions A heart beat coming on before the next expected beat. Such a premature contraction may originate from a point in the ventricle, although most such beats originate in the atrium of the heart.

septal defect A birth deformity in which there is an abnormal opening between the left and right ventricles of the heart.

standstill Heart stoppage due to failure of the ventricles (the large muscular chambers) to contract.

ventriculography A method of demonstrating the ventricles of the brain by X ray.

ventriculo-peritoneal shunt An operation to relieve hydrocephalus, performed by placing a polyethylene tube between the ventricle of the brain and the abdominal cavity. *See* hydrocephalus.

ventriculotomy An operation in which the ventricle of the heart is opened.

venule A small vein.

vermicide A medication given to kill worms.

vermifuge A medication taken to kill worms in the intestines.

vermin Lice.

vernix caseosa The coating, consisting of old skin cells and oily matter, on a newborn child's body. (It is thought to have certain protective properties and is not washed off.)

verruca Warts.

version Altering the position of the fetus in the uterus prior to childbirth, done on occasion to facilitate delivery.

vertebra One of the bones forming the spinal column.

vertebrate Any animal having a spinal column.

vertex The top of the skull.

vertex presentation The most common position of the unborn child during labor, that is, with the back of the head presenting at the vaginal outlet.

vertigo Dizziness, especially the feeling that one's surroundings are whirling.

verumontanum A small depression deep in the male urethra (the tube leading from the bladder to the outside). It represents a primitive tissue area in the early life of the embryo before its sex is determined.

vesical Relating to the urinary bladder.

vesication Blister formation.

vesicle A small blister.

vesicovaginal fistula A false opening between the urinary bladder and the vagina, as a result of injury during childbirth or as a result of surgery.

vesiculation Blistering.

vesiculitis An inflammation of the seminal vesicles, the glands at the base of the prostate which store semen (the fluid containing sperm).

vestibular Referring to the vestibule of the ear.

vestige An anatomical part which represents a primitive structure; the coccyx represents the *vestige* of a tail.

viable Able to live; a term applied to an embryo within the uterus.

Viagra *See* sildenafil.

Vibramycin A synthetic antibiotic, effective in the treatment of many different kinds of bacteria. *See* doxycycline.

vibrion septique A germ which can cause gas gangrene, a most dangerous type of infection often seen in war wounds or accidents in the street.

vibrissae The hairs in the nose.

vicarious menstruation The passage of blood from some other part of the body than the vagina occuring during the menstrual period. (Nosebleed during the menstrual period.)

Vicryl An absorbable suture material, used in much the same way as catgut.

Videx *See* ddl.

villous adenoma A warty growth, often in the rectum or colon, characterized by many shaggy projections which protrude from the mucous membranes.

villus A stalklike growth of tissue originating from a mucous membrane.

Vincent's angina Ulceration of the back of the throat, tonsil region, high fever, and severe toxicity as a

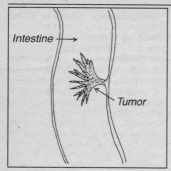

Villous tumor

complication of a trench mouth infection.

vincristine A powerful chemotherapeutic agent, especially useful in the treatment of acute leukemia.

Vinethene Vinyl ether; a general anesthetic agent, particularly useful when a short anesthesia is all that is necessary.

Vinyl ether *See* Vinethene.

Vioform-Hydrocortisone Ointment A patented medication used to combat various skin disorders.

violaceous Purplish; a term used in denoting a purplish discoloration of the skin.

viosterol Vitamin D_2. It is given to prevent or treat rickets in infants.

viral hepatitis Inflammation of the liver caused by a virus. Symptoms include jaundice, dark urine, clay-colored stool, weakness, loss of appetite, fever, headache, and malaise.

viral infections Infections caused by viruses rather than bacteria. They are rarely pus-forming. Most of the diseases of childhood are viral in origin as are certain types of pneumonia, hepatitis, and meningitis.

viral particles Small particles of dead virus, sometimes seen when examining tissues through an electron microscope. They are thought to represent the existence of a previous viral infection.

Virchow lymph node An enlarged lymph node in the left side of the neck, occasionally seen when a cancer has spread from the lung or from an abdominal organ.

viremia Infection of the blood stream with a virus.

virgin A person who has never experienced sex relations.

virile Masculine appearing.

virilism A pseudohermaphrodite who is in actuality a female but who has external genitals having many characteristics of the male.

virility Ability to have offspring and ability to perform the sex act.

Virilon A patented drug for intramuscular injection, composed of the male sex hormone testosterone.

virology The study of diseases caused by viruses.

virulent Able to cause disease; a powerful germ.

virus An organism, smaller than bacteria, capable of causing various infectious or contagious diseases. It can grow while living in the human body.

vis a tergo The force which pushes forward, as the force of the contractions of the uterus in expelling the child; a Latin term.

viscera Organs, such as those in the chest or abdominal cavities.

visceroptosis A condition in which internal organs, especially those within the abdomen, have dropped in position.

viscid Sticky; thick, as a syrupy fluid.

viscoidosis *See* Cystic fibrosis. Mucoviscoidosis.

viscosity The quality of being thick and sticky, as a viscid substance which flows with difficulty.

viscous Semifluid.

viscus Any internal organ, such as the stomach, intestine, liver, etc.

visual field That which can be seen when the eyes look straight forward without moving.

visualization The act of making something visible which is ordinarily not visible, such as *visualizing* internal organs by means of X rays.

vital Relating to life; alive.

vital capacity The amount of air that can be breathed out after inhaling as much air as possible; a guide to lung efficiency.

Vitallium A metal alloy containing chromium and molybdenum. It is inert in the body and is therefore used as graft material or as a bone support or replacement.

vital signs Those signs necessary to sustain life, such as heart action, blood pressure, respiration, temperature, etc.

vitamins Organic compounds or chemicals, found in various foodstuffs, necessary for the maintenance of normal life. Deficiencies may cause diseases such as beriberi, scurvy, pellagra, rickets, etc. *See* Vitamin Table in Manual.

A deficiency In the young it leads to inadequate growth. In all people, it interferes with accuracy of vision and increases susceptibility to infection. Xerophthalmia, a dryness and inflammation of the conjunctiva (membrane covering the eyeball) is caused by vitamin A deficiency.

B_1 deficiency (beriberi) Thiamine deficiency. Characterized by numbness, tingling and burning in the feet and muscle tenderness in the legs. Severe cases may show swelling in the legs, heart enlargement and circulatory collapse.

B_2 deficiency Vitamin B_2, or riboflavin, deficiency causes cracking of the skin at the corners of the mouth, chapped hands and dry scaling of the skin of the body. Severe deficiency may result in irritation of the eyes.

B_6 deficiency Clinically, its deficiency occurs almost exclusively in infants. When it does take place, it may cause convulsions, stunted growth and severe anemia.

B_{12} deficiency This may cause severe anemia and associated nerve symptoms.

C deficiency Scurvy is caused by vitamin C deficiency. It is characterized by irritability, hemorrhage from the gums and into joints, a severe anemia and eventual heart failure. It is seen most often in infants with inadequate vitamin C intake.

D deficiency This deficiency causes rickets in children, with improper formation and deformity of the bones. Knockknees, bowlegs and pigeon chest are common deformities caused by this vitamin deficiency.

K deficiency Lack of this vitamin results in failure of the blood-clotting mechanism with resultant hemorrhages. Brain hemorrhage in newborns can occur because of vitamin K deficiency. In cases of jaundice there is often a vitamin K deficiency with hemorrhage from mucous membranes.

niacin deficiency Lack of niacin (nicotinic acid) causes pellagra with its mental deterioration, inflammation of the tongue and mouth, diarrhea and a characteristic rash over the exposed surfaces of the body. (Seen frequently among alcoholics.)

vitiation A change that reduces efficiency.

vitelline duct The primitive portion of the developing embryo which eventually goes to form the umbilical cord which attaches the embryo to the mother's uterus.

vitiligo A skin condition, of unknown cause, characterized by patchy loss of pigment, resulting in a "piebald" appearance.

vitrectomy An operative procedure in which blood secondary to a hemorrhage is washed out of the vitreous of the eye in order to restore vision.

vitreous humor The jellylike transparent substance filling the inside of the eyeball.

viviparous Giving birth to live offspring, as in humans; unlike ovipa-

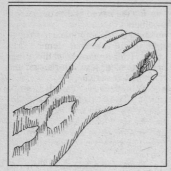

Vitiligo

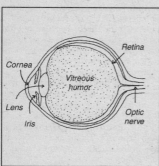

Vitreous humor

rous animals, which bring forth offspring as eggs.

vivisection Surgery upon animals for the purpose of research.

Vivonex Trademark for a combination of nutriments given intravenously as a temporary replacement of one's dietary needs; used frequently in hyperalimentation. *See* hyperalimentation.

vocal cords The two bands of tissue in the larynx which make speech possible. The expansion and contraction of these cords, as air passes between them, create the sounds we know as speech.

void To pass urine.

volar Pertaining to the palm or sole surfaces.

volatile A substance which is easily converted into a vapor, such as ether.

volemic Referring to the volume of blood or plasma which is circulating throughout the body.

volitional Voluntary.

Volkmann's contracture Deformity and permanent contraction of the muscles of the arm caused by insufficient blood supply. This condition usually has its onset after the too tight application of a plaster cast to the elbow region.

voluntary muscle Muscles that a person can control himself or herself.

volvulus A twist of the bowel sometimes leading to gangrene. It may be brought on by an adhesion or by a tumor within the bowel. (Immediate surgery is necessary for this condition.)

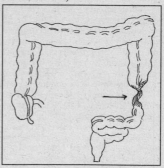

Volvulus

vomer bones The bones separating the two sides of the nose.

vomit To throw up the contents of the stomach.

    coffee-ground Vomit denoting the presence of blood.

    fecal Vomit containing stool, indicative of intestinal obstruction.

    projectile Vomiting with great force.

von Recklinghausen's disease A hereditary disease characterized by the formation of small tumors along the course of nerves. The tumors are superficial, being located beneath the skin, and may number a few, or hundreds. The condition is usually benign although the tumors tend, over the years, to increase in size and number.

voracious Having an abnormal appetite for food.

voyeur A person who obtains gratification from watching others perform sex acts.

voyeurism Sexual gratification from viewing the naked bodies or sex acts of others.

vulnerable Susceptible.

vulva The external female sex organ. It is composed of the major and minor lips, the clitoris, and the opening the vagina.

vulvectomy The surgical removal of the vulva, carried out when these parts are affected with cancer.

vulvitis Inflammation of the vulva, the external female sex organs.

vulvovaginitis Inflammation of both the vulva and the vagina.

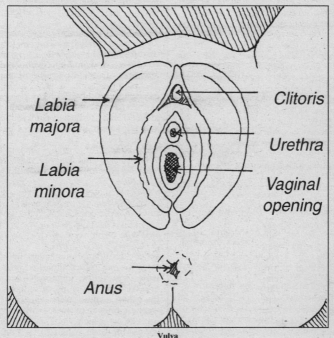

Vulva

W

walking iron A metal attachment to a leg cast which permits the patient to walk while still in the plaster.

walleye A condition in which one or both eyes are off center and point in an outward direction. (Divergent strabismus.)

wandering pacemaker The "pacemaker" is the point of origin, located in the atrium (auricle), of the impulse which stimulates the heart to beat. When the impulses originate from other sites, there is said to be a "wandering pacemaker."

ward A hospital room, usually large, in which there are several patients. "Ward" patients are frequently patients who pay no fee for the services they receive.

Warfarin An anticoagulant medication; often given to forestall further blood clotting in those who have sustained a thrombosis of a vessel.

warm blooded Maintaining a constant body temperature despite marked changes in the temperature of the environment. Homothermal.

wart An overgrowth of skin localized in a rounded area; not caused by contact with frogs.

Warthin's tumor *See* tumors.

Wassermann test A blood test for syphilis. A positive Wassermann result means that the patient has syphilis; a negative one, that syphilis does not exist.

water balance The mechanism whereby there is a balance between the amount of fluid taken into the body and the amount of fluid excreted.

"water on the brain" A nonmedical phrase for *hydrocephalus*.

waters, bag of The fluid surrounding the embryo in the uterus. When the bag of waters breaks, labor usually commences.

wave, brain A tracing of brain activity, as seen on electroencephalography.

    electrocardiographic A tracing of heart activity, as seen on electrocardiography.

    fluid A sign of fluid within the abdomen. Tapping one side of the abdomen transmits a wave which can be felt on the other side.

    P,Q,R,S,T,U Various tracings of heart activity during contraction and relaxation, as seen on an electrocardiogram.

wax, bone A specially prepared compound to plug the bone marrow after surgery involving the cutting of bone.

WBC White blood cell. There are many different types such as leukocytes, lymphocytes, monocytes, eosinophils, basophils, etc.

WDWN Abbreviation for *well-developed, well-nourished*.

wean To discontinue breast feeding. This may be accomplished gradually by alternating bottle and breast feedings, or by introducing the use of a cup or glass.

webbed fingers or toes Birth deformity in which there is a thin membrane connecting two or more fingers or toes, giving them the appearance of a duck's feet.

wedge pressure The pressure reading when a central venous catheter is advanced into a vessel in the lung. Used to measure the pressure in the left atrium (auricle) of the heart. *See* central venous catheter.

weightlessness The sensation that is felt at zero gravity.

Weil's disease Jaundice caused by infection with a spirochete germ. It lasts for several weeks and then clears up.

Welch, William H. (1850–1934) An eminent American physician, the founder of Johns Hopkins Medical College and the discoverer of the cause of gas gangrene.

wens Sebaceous cysts, located just beneath the skin, seen most frequently in the scalp.

Wertheim operation Surgical removal of the entire uterus, tubes, ovaries and the ligaments and tissues surrounding them. A radical operation performed to cure cancer of the cervix or uterus.

"wet brain" A term applied to swelling and excessive fluid about the brain secondary to alcoholism. Patients so affected show mental deterioration.

wet nurse A woman who breast feeds another woman's infant.

Wharton's duct The tube leading from the submaxillary (salivary) gland to the mouth. It transports saliva.

wheal The individual hive seen on the body surface in some allergic conditions such as urticaria. They itch and have a tendency to appear and disappear.

wheat germ oil A rich source of vitamin E. (Improved fertility has been erroneously attributed to this substance.)

wheeze Noisy or difficult breathing, usually due to spasms or mucus collection within the trachea and bronchial tubes.

whiplash injury A sprain of the muscles and tendons of the back of the neck, caused by a sudden blow from the rear such as when the rear of one's automobile is smashed into.

Whipple's disease A rare condition occurring in males in which the lining of the intestines and the absorptive channels leading from the intestines become filled with fat. Also called *intestinal lipodystrophy*.

Whipple procedure An operation in which the duodenum and pancreas are removed to eradicate cancer of the pancreas, duodenum or the terminal portion of the common bile duct.

white leg *See* phlegmasia alba dolens.

whites A slang expression for the whitish discharge from the vagina; leukorrhea.

whitlow An infection, containing pus, of the finger tip; a felon; a paronychia.

WHO World Health Organization

whooping cough Pertussis. A contagious disease lasting several weeks, characterized by paroxysms of severe coughing and a whooping sound on deep respiration.

Widal test A blood test for typhoid fever. It becomes positive about ten days to two weeks after the onset of symptoms.

Wilm's tumor A malignant tumor of the kidneys seen in children.

wiring An orthopedic procedure using wire to fasten broken bones together.

Wirsung's duct The tube leading from the pancreas to the intestines. It transports the pancreatic digestive juices.

wisdom teeth Third molars, the last teeth in the upper and lower jaws.

witch hazel A soothing application applied to irritated skin surfaces; it is an extract of a leaf.

witch's milk Milk secreted from the breasts of some newborns. It disappears soon after birth.

withdrawal 1. The interruption of intercourse before climax; coitus interruptus. 2. The stoppage of alcohol or drugs in an addict.

withdrawal bleeding Vaginal bleeding which takes place after hormone therapy has been discontinued.

WNL Abbreviation for *within normal limits*.

Wolffian duct The primitive duct of the kidney in the embryo which goes to form the *ureter* and the duct leading from the testicle.

womb The uterus.

Wood's light An ultraviolet light that is used to diagnose certain fungus infections of the scalp and hair.

wound, blowing One in which air enters and exits on breathing; a wound involving the chest cavity.

    contused A bruise; an injury to the body not involving a break in the skin.

    incised A surgical wound, made with a knife.

    open One in which the tissues beneath the surface are freely exposed.

    penetrating One that extends into the body but there is no point of exit.

    perforating A wound that has both a point of entrance and a point of exit.

    puncture One caused by a thin, sharp object.

    sucking A chest wound that sucks air.

writer's cramp Spasm of the muscles of the hand and arm in people who do a great deal of writing. It is thought to be of neurotic origin.

wryneck Torticollis. A spasm or contraction of the muscles on one side of the neck, causing the head to be held in an abnormal, tilted position.

Wuchereria (filariasis) *See* filariasis.

Wyanoid suppositories Rectal suppositories used to relieve symptoms of hemorrhoids, fissure or other anal conditions.

X

Xanax A drug indicated for people who are subject to attacks of anxiety or panic.

xanthelasma A benign, yellow-colored, flat growth on the eyelids. It is made up of flatlike cells having a yellow color.

xanthochromia A yellowish discoloration of the spinal fluid caused by a recent brain hemorrhage.

xanthoma A benign tumor, yellowish in color, of the skin composed of cells having many of the characteristics of fat cells. (Lipoid cells)

xanthomatosis A deposit of yellow-colored xanthoma cells throughout the tissues and organs of the body. Also called *lipoidosis* or *Schüller-Christian disease*.

xanthopsia A yellow-colored vision sometimes seen by jaundiced patients.

xanthosis Yellow color of the skin due to food eaten (carrots, squash, etc.) or medications taken (atabrine for malaria). The condition lasts only a short time.

X chromosome A gene found in the male sperm. When an egg is fertilized by a sperm which possesses the X chromosome, the child develops as a female.

xenogenic A condition arising from the introduction of some outside (foreign) substance into the body.

xenograft A heterograft; one taken from an animal and grafted onto a human.

xenology The study of parasites and their relationship to the animals or people they infest.

xenophobia Fear of strangers.

xero- Prefix meaning dry.

xeroderma Excessive dry skin. Skin having the appearance of scaly fish skin.

xerogram An X ray recorded on a specially sensitized paper rather than on an X-ray film.

xerography An instrument for recording X-ray images on a selenium-coated metal plate. It produces a bas-relief effect, accentuating boundaries between tissues of varying densities. (Recently used in addition to mammography as a means of detecting presence or absence of a breast tumor.)

xeromammogram An X ray of the breast, recorded upon a specially prepared paper. It gives greater detail of the breast than the ordinary mammogram.

xeromenia Having all the symptoms such as cramps, bloating, etc., of menstruation without any actual flow of blood.

xerophthalmia A thickening of the conjunctiva of the eye secondary to vitamin A deficiency. If unchecked, it will interfere with normal vision.

xerosis Dryness of the skin or conjunctiva of the eye.

xerostomia Dry mouth caused by insufficient secretion of saliva.

xiphisternum The downward projection of bone at the end of the breastbone.

xiphoid The lowermost extent of the breastbone.

X-linked A reference to the X-sex chromosome.

X rays Light rays of short length which are passed by an electric generator through a glass vacuum tube

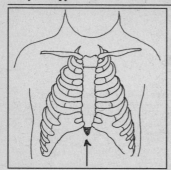

Xiphoid cartilage of the sterum

(the X-ray tube). Such rays have special penetrative powers through body tissues. Also called *roentgen rays*.

X-ray therapy Radiation therapy; treatment with X rays.

XX chromosomes The normal complement in the female.

XXY chromosomes An abnormal chromosome complement in males; characteristic of Klinefelter's syndrome. *See* syndrome.

XY chromosomes The normal complement in the male.

xylene A benzene compound used as a solvent, e.g., in laboratories to clean the lenses of microscopes.

Xylocaine A patented local anesthetic agent having the same usages as procaine or Novocain.

Y

yaws A tropical infection caused by a germ resembling the germ of syphilis. It is not, however, a venereal disease.

Y chromosome A gene found in the male sperm. When an egg is fertilized by a sperm which possesses the Y chromosome, the child develops as a male.

yellow fever An acute infectious disease caused by a virus which gets into the body through the bite of an infected mosquito (*Aedes aegypti*). It is characterized by chills, fever, aches and pains, jaundice, vomiting, hemorrhage from mucous membranes, kidney damage, uremia and in many cases death. Protection against the disease can be obtained through vaccination.

yellow jack Yellow fever.

yellow jaundice Same as jaundice.

yolk sac A primitive sac in embryos, lasting only during the early stage of development. Early blood cells are formed in the yolk sac.

Y-plasty An operation performed at the junction of the ureter (tube from the kidney) and the pelvis of the kidney in order to correct an obstruction of the outflow of urine from the kidney.

yttrium-90 A radioactive substance, occasionally implanted in the pituitary gland to destroy its function.

Z

Zantac A proprietary drug that lowers the amount of hydrochloric acid secreted by the stomach. Very useful in the treatment of peptic ulcers.

Zeiss' gland Oil secreting glands of the skin.

zinc oxide A medication, usually used in ointment form, which relieves many skin irritations.

zinc peroxide A chemical which liberates oxygen, sometimes instilled into wounds caused by anaerobic (those that die when exposed to air) bacteria.

Zoladex A medication indicated for the treatment of advanced cases of prostate cancer.

Zollinger-Ellison syndrome *See* syndromes.

Zoloft A drug that may help to relieve mental depression.

Zondek, Bernhard (1891-1966) The co-discoverer of the Ascheim-Zondek test for pregnancy.

zone A region; an area.

    anacoustic The region of silence in space, about 100 miles above the earth's surface.

    comfort The temperature range that is most equable to the body; between 28° and 30° Centigrade.

    erogenous An area which, when stimulated, excites sexual feelings.

    language An area in the front portion of the brain that controls speech; the word center. It is on the left side of the brain in a right-handed person and on the right side in a left-handed person.

    trigger An area of extreme irritability which, when stimulated, will bring on an attack of a disease,

such as an epileptic convulsion, an attack of neuralgia, etc.

zoology The science and study of animal life.

zoonoses Diseases of animals which can be transmitted to man, such as rabies, bovine tuberculosis, etc.

zoophilism An extraordinary love for animals.

    erotic The deriving of sexual pleasure from fondling animals.

zoophobia An inordinate fear of animals.

zooplasty The procedure for grafting tissue from an animal to a human.

zoosadism Sexual pleasure derived from hurting animals.

zoster Herpes zoster or "shingles."

Zosyn A powerful antibiotic for the treatment fo severe infections; contains pipericillin and other ingredients.

Zovirax Ointment An ointment used in treating cases of herpes, especially those located in the genital area.

Z-plasty A plastic operation in which skin is cut in the shape of the letter Z, in order to cover a raw surface.

zygoma The cheekbone.

zygomatic Pertaining to the cheek region.

zygote A term referring to the fertilized egg before it starts to divide and multiply.

Zyloprim (allopurinal) A drug which reduces blood uric acid, used to prevent attacks of gout.

zymase The chemical (enzyme) in yeast which causes fermentation and alcohol formation.

410

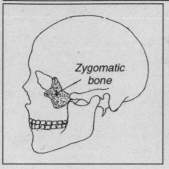

Zygoma

zymology The study of the processes involved in fermentation.
zymosis A condition caused by infection.

Health Manual

CONTENTS

1. BLOOD VESSELS

A. *Important Arteries**

Name of Artery	Origin of Artery	Major Areas or Organs Supplied
Acetabular (*Articular*)	Obturator, in pelvic region.	Hip joint and head of thigh bone (femur).
Acromial	Scapular and thoraco-acromial, in neck and shoulder regions.	Muscles about shoulder (deltoid) and upper back.
Alveolar	Internal maxillary, in the face.	Gums, teeth, and muscles which control chewing.
Anastomotic		This is a term used to describe an artery which communicates with another artery (as a channel connects two bodies of water).
Angular	External maxillary, in the face.	The muscles which control facial expressions and open and close the eyes.
Aorta, Abdominal	From aorta, in the chest.	The abdominal wall, diaphragm, organs within the abdomen, thighs and legs.
Aorta, Arch	Ascending aorta, or part closest to the heart.	It gives off branches which go to the head, neck and arms.
Aorta, Thoracic (*descending*)	The aorta in the chest, just beyond the arch.	The chest wall, lungs, esophagus and diaphragm.
Appendicular	Ileocolic, in the right lower abdomen.	The appendix and cecum (beginning of large intestine).
Auditory	Cerebellar, in the base of the brain.	The inner ear.

*Arteries carry blood from the heart, out to the tissues.

Name of Artery	Origin of Artery	Major Areas or Organs Supplied
Auricular	Carotid and maxillary, in neck and face.	The outer and middle ear, muscles at base of skull and side of neck, parotid (salivary) gland, and scalp.
Axillary	Subclavian, in the root of the neck.	The chest muscles (pectorals) and shoulder and upper arm muscles.
Basilar	The two vertebral arteries which ascend from the neck into the skull.	The base of brain, cerebellum, and inner ear.
Brachial	Axillary, in the base of the neck.	Muscles of shoulder, upper arm, forearm, and hand.
Bronchial	Thoracic aorta.	The lungs, bronchial tubes, and esophagus.
Buccal	Internal maxillary, in the face.	Some muscles responsible for chewing, gums, and membrane lining mouth.
Common Carotid	On right side, from the innominate artery. On left side, from arch of aorta.	The neck and head.
External Carotid	Common carotid, in the neck.	The front portion of the neck, face, ear, and scalp.
Internal Carotid	Common carotid, in the neck.	The front part of the brain, eye, nose, and forehead.
Celiac	Abdominal aorta.	The esophagus and abdominal organs such as stomach, duodenum, gallbladder, pancreas, spleen, etc.
Cerebellar	Basilar, in the base of the brain.	The base of brain and cerebellum.
Cerebral	Internal carotid and basilar arteries.	Most of brain, except its base.
Cervical	From arteries in the base of the neck.	Muscles of neck, shoulder, and head.
Choroid	Internal carotid, in the neck.	Parts of brain, optic (eye) tract, choroid plexus of ventricles.

Name of Artery	Origin of Artery	Major Areas or Organs Supplied
Ciliary	Ophthalmic.	The colored portion of eye (iris) and membrane of eye (conjunctiva).
Circumflex, femoral	The deep femoral artery in the upper thigh and groin.	Muscles of thigh and hip region.
Circumflex, humeral	Axillary.	Muscles of shoulder region and upper arm.
Circumflex, iliac	External iliac, in the pelvis.	Muscles of the lower back, lower abdominal wall and thigh.
Circumflex, scapular	Subscapular, in shoulder region.	The shoulder joint, muscles in upper back and back of upper arm.
Colic, left	The inferior mesenteric, in abdomen.	The left side of transverse colon and upper part of descending colon.
Colic, middle	Superior mesenteric, in abdomen.	Most of right (ascending) colon and right side of transverse colon.
Colic, right	Superior mesenteric, in abdomen.	The ascending colon.
Conjunctival	Ciliary and palpebral arteries in eye region.	The conjunctiva (lining membrane of the eyes).
Coronary, left	Left aortic sinus of the heart.	The left auricle (atrium) and both ventricles of heart.
Coronary, right	Anterior aortic sinus of the heart.	The right auricle (atrium) and parts of ventricles of heart.
Cystic	Right hepatic artery in upper abdomen.	The gallbladder.
Dental	Internal maxillary, in face.	The gums and teeth.
Digital	Main arteries of hands or feet.	The fingers or toes.

Name of Artery	Origin of Artery	Major Areas or Organs Supplied
Dorsal pedis	Anterior tibial artery in the leg.	The front portion of foot. (Adequacy of circulation in foot is determined by feeling its pulsations.)
Epigastric, deep	External iliac artery in the pelvis.	Muscles and skin of lower abdomen; cord going to genitals.
Epigastric, superior	Internal mammary, in chest.	Muscles and skin of upper abdomen and diaphragm.
Esophageal	Aorta in chest.	The esophagus (food pipe).
Facial (*External maxillary*)	External carotid, in neck.	The throat, muscles which control chewing, muscles of facial expressions, tonsils, lymph glands and skin of neck, etc.
Femoral	External iliac, in groin.	The genitals, lower abdomen, and thigh muscles and bones.
Frontal	Ophthalmic artery.	The muscles and skin of forehead.
Gastric, left	The celiac artery in upper abdomen.	The lower end of esophagus and upper and inner (lesser curvature) sides of stomach.
Gastric, right	Hepatic artery, in upper abdomen.	The lower portion (pylorus) of stomach.
Gastric, short	Splenic (spleen) artery, in upper abdomen.	The greater curvature of stomach.
Gastroduodenal	Hepatic artery in the upper abdomen.	The lower portion of stomach (pylorus), duodenum, pancreas, and bile duct.
Gastro-epiploic	From splenic and hepatic arteries.	The greater curvature of stomach.
Genicular	Femoral and popliteal arteries, in knee region.	The knee joint and some of the muscles in lower thigh.
Gluteal	Internal iliac, in the pelvis.	The muscles of buttocks, prostate gland, and seminal vesicles, some of the muscles of upper part of back of thigh.
Hallucis	Dorsalis pedis and	Big toe and second toe.

	plantar arteries in the foot.	
Hemorrhoidal	Arteries in abdomen, such as internal iliac, inferior mesenteric, etc.	The lower portion of descending colon, rectum and anus; muscles regulating rectal function.
Hepatic	Celiac artery in upper abdomen.	The liver, gallbladder, stomach, pancreas, and omentum.
Ileocolic	Superior mesenteric artery in upper abdomen.	The last part of small intestine, the appendix, cecum, and ascending colon.
Iliac, common	Abdominal aorta.	The organs within pelvis, genitals, and lower limbs.
Iliac, external	Common iliac, in pelvis.	Muscles of thigh and leg.
Iliac, internal	Common iliac, in pelvis.	The organs within pelvis, genitals, and anal region.
Iliolumbar	Internal iliac, in pelvis.	The muscles in back of abdominal cavity.
Infraorbital	Internal maxillary, in face.	The muscles which manipulate the eyeball; the tear gland; some of the upper teeth.
Innominate	Arch of aorta, in upper chest.	The right shoulder region, right arm, right side of neck and head.
Intercostal, of Aorta	Descending aorta, in chest.	The chest wall, rib cage, muscles of upper back, breasts, spine, and part of abdominal wall.
Interosseous	Ulnar artery in arm.	Many of the muscles, tendons, bone, and skin of forearm.
Intestinal	The superior mesenteric artery in upper abdomen.	The small intestines.
Labial	External maxillary, in face.	The upper and lower lips.

Name of Artery	Origin of Artery	Major Areas or Organs Supplied
Laryngeal	Inferior and superior thyroid arteries in neck.	The larynx and surrounding muscles.
Lingual	External carotid, in neck.	The tongue, mouth, and surrounding structures.
Lumbar	Abdominal aorta.	There are four pairs which supply muscles in back of abdomen.
Malleolar	Tibial arteries, in leg.	The ankle and back portion of foot.
Mammary, internal	Subclavian, beneath collarbone.	The anterior chest region beneath breastbone, ribs, coverings of the heart and lungs, breasts, etc.
Masseteric	Internal maxillary, beneath jaw.	The masseter muscle which helps in act of chewing.
Maxillary, external	External carotid, in neck.	Muscles of face, muscles which control chewing, skin of face, glands of neck, tonsils, etc.
Maxillary, internal	External carotid, in neck.	Most of face, jaws, skull, teeth, roof of mouth, muscles around eyes, nose, etc.
Mediastinal	Internal mammary, in the chest.	The mediastinum (tissue lying beneath breastbone).
Meningeal	Internal carotid and maxillary arteries, in neck and head.	The skull and coverings of brain.
Mental	Inferior alveolar artery.	The chin and lower lip.
Mesenteric, inferior	Abdominal aorta.	The transverse colon, (large bowel), descending colon, and upper portion of rectum.

Name of Artery	Origin of Artery	Major Areas or Organs Supplied
Mesenteric, superior	Abdominal aorta.	The duodenum and all of small intestine, appendix, and ascending colon.
Metacarpal	Radial artery, in forearm, near wrist.	The thumb and fingers.
Metatarsal	Arteries in arch of foot.	The toes.
Musculophrenic	Internal mammary, in chest.	Muscles of upper abdominal wall, diaphragm, and lower ribs,
Nasal	The ophthalmic and palatine arteries.	The nose and tear sac, and sinuses.
Nutrient	———	A term for the arteries which supply bones and bone marrow.
Obturator	Internal iliac artery in pelvis.	The urinary bladder, pubis, hip joint, and muscles in pelvis regions and thigh.
Occipital	External carotid, in neck.	The muscles in back of neck, back portion of ears and scalp, etc.
Ophthalmic	Internal carotid, in neck.	The tissue about eye, eye itself, sinuses, and portion of front of skull.
Ovarian	Abdominal aorta.	The ovary, fallopian tube, and tissues about uterus.
Palatine	Maxillary arteries.	The soft and hard palates and gums, parts of throat and tonsils.
Palpebral	The ophthalmic and the lacrimal arteries.	The eyelids, membrane covering eye, and tear sac.
Pancreaticoduodenal	The superior mesenteric and gastroduodenal arteries in the upper abdomen.	The pancreas, duodenum, and bile duct.
Penis	Internal pudendal artery.	The penis.

Name of Artery	Origin of Artery	Major Areas or Organs Supplied
Perineal	Internal pudendal artery.	The base of penis and superficial tissues beneath it.
Peroneal	Posterior tibial artery in back of leg.	The muscles of back of leg, leg, ankle joint and parts of foot.
Pharyngeal	External carotid, in neck.	Muscles of neck and parts of membranes of skull.
Phrenic	Aorta in chest.	The esophagus, spleen, adrenal glands, and diaphragm.
Plantar	Posterior tibial and dorsalis pedis arteries.	The sole and muscles of foot.
Popliteal	Femoral artery in thigh.	The muscles and bones of thigh and leg.
Profunda femoris	Femoral artery in thigh.	The muscles of thigh, hip joint, and thigh bone (femur).
Pudendal	Femoral and internal iliac arteries.	The muscles of inner thigh, muscles of anus, penis, lips of vagina, etc.
Pulmonary	Right ventricle of heart.	The lungs.
Radial	Brachial artery in upper arm.	Many of the muscles and other structures of forearm and hand.
Renal	Abdominal aorta.	The kidney and adrenal gland.
Sacral	Abdominal aorta and internal iliac arteries.	The rectum and sacral canal.
Scapular arteries	Subscapular and thyro-cervical vessels in neck.	Muscles extending from head to shoulders, collarbone, scapula (wingbone) and its attached muscles, etc.
Sciatic	Internal iliac artery.	The buttocks, hip region, and area about the anus.
Scrotal	Pudendal and perineal arteries in genital region.	The scrotum (sac covering testicles).

Name of Artery	Origin of Artery	Major Areas or Organs Supplied
Sigmoidal	Inferior mesenteric artery in abdomen.	The sigmoid colon in lower left portion of abdomen.
Spermatic	Abdominal aorta and inferior epigastric arteries.	The ureter from kidney, cord to and from the testicles, and ligaments of uterus in female.
Sphenopalatine	Internal maxillary, in face.	The back of nose and sinuses.
Spinal	Vertebral artery.	The spinal cord.
Splenic (*lineal*)	Celiac artery in upper abdomen.	The spleen, pancreas, and part of stomach.
Subclavian	On right, from innominate artery; on left, from arch of aorta.	Muscles of neck, arms, brain and skull, lining of heart and lungs, bronchial tubes, etc.
Sublingual	Lingual artery, in neck.	The muscles beneath chin and sublingual gland.
Submental	External maxillary, in neck.	Muscles beneath chin, muscles of facial expression and submaxillary (salivary) gland.
Subscapular	Axillary artery, near armpit.	Muscles around shoulder joint, back of arm, back below shoulder.
Supraorbital	Ophthalmic artery in head.	The orbit, sinuses, muscles about eye and upper eyelid.
Suprarenal	Renal artery, which also supplies kidney and abdominal aorta.	The suprarenal (adrenal) gland.
Suprascapular	Thyrocervical vessel in neck.	Muscles and bones of neck, collarbone, shoulder blade, back, etc.
Tarsal	Dorsalis pedis artery, in foot.	Muscles supplying toes and skin of part of foot.
Temporal	External carotid and internal maxillary arteries in neck.	Skin and muscles of face, eye and temple region, parotid (salivary) gland at angle of jaw.

Name of Artery	Origin of Artery	Major Areas or Organs Supplied
Testicular	Internal spermatic artery alongside cord in groin.	The testicle.
Thoracic, lateral	Axillary artery near armpit.	Muscles of front and back of chest.
Thoraco-dorsal	Subscapular artery.	Muscles of side and back of chest.
Thymic	Internal mammary, in chest.	The thymus gland lying beneath breastbone in chest.
Thyroid	External carotid and thyrocervical, in neck.	Muscles in front and sides of neck, thyroid gland, trachea, esophagus, larynx, etc.
Thyrocervical trunk	Subclavian artery in neck.	The thyroid gland, trachea, esophagus, muscles of neck, etc.
Tibial, anterior	Popliteal artery, in back of knee.	Most muscles of leg, especially those in front of leg, ankle region, some skin areas of leg.
Tibial, posterior	Popliteal artery, in back of knee.	The muscles of back of leg, knee region, sole and back portion of foot.
Tympanic	Middle meningeal, pharyngeal, internal maxillary, etc.	The tympanic cavity of ear.
Ulnar	Brachial, in upper arm.	Many of muscles of forearm, bone of forearm, and part of hand.
Uterine	Internal iliac, in pelvis.	The uterus and ligaments surrounding it, the fallopian tubes.
Vaginal	Internal iliac, in pelvis.	The vagina, bladder, and rectum.
Vasa brevia	Splenic artery, in upper abdomen.	The greater curvature of stomach.
Vesical	Internal iliac, in pelvis.	The prostate gland, seminal vesicles, bladder, and part of ureters.

| Volar arches | Radial and ulnar arteries in hand. | The muscles and tendons of hand, joints, and fingers. |
| Zygomatico-orbital | Temporal artery, in face. | The muscle surrounding orbit, outer side of orbit. |

B. Important Veins*

Name of Vein	Area or Organ Blood Drainage from:	Vessel or Structure Blood Carried to:
Anterior jugular	Front part of neck.	External jugular vein, in neck.
Azygos	Right side of chest wall and back.	Superior vena cava in upper chest.
Basilar	Back part of base of brain.	Vertebral veins in back of neck.
Basilic	Part of hand, forearm and upper arm (inside of arm).	Axillary vein in armpit.
Cavernous sinus†	Ophthalmic vein in back of eye.	Petrosal sinuses in base of brain.
Cephalic	Thumb side of hand and forearm.	Axillary vein in armpit.
Common facial	Side of face and jaw.	Internal jugular, in neck.
Coronary sinus	Heart.	Right atrium (auricle) of heart.
Coronary, of Stomach	Stomach.	Portal vein leading to liver.
Diploic	Bones of skull.	Veins (sinuses) of skull and veins above eyes.

*This list does not include those veins which accompany arteries and have the same names, or travel the same course. (Veins carry blood back toward the heart.)

†A "sinus" is a large channel containing venous blood.

Name of Vein	Area or Organ Blood Drainage from:	Vessel or Structure Blood Carried to:
Emissary	Veins within skull.	Veins in back of head (occipital) and in the ear region (posterior auricular).
External jugular	Side of neck.	Subclavian vein in neck.
Great cardiac	Ventricles of heart.	Coronary sinus of heart.
Great cerebral	Veins within brain.	Straight sinus within skull.
Great saphenous	Inner side of leg and thigh.	Femoral vein just below groin.
Hemiazygos	Left side of back and chest.	Azygos vein in chest.
Hemorrhoidal	Rectum and lower bowel.	Portal vein leading to liver.
Hepatic	Liver.	Inferior vena cava, which empties into heart.
Inferior petrosal sinus	Venous channels within skull.	Internal jugular vein in neck.
Inferior sagittal sinus	Cerebral portion of brain.	Straight sinus of brain.
Inferior vena cava	Abdomen, thighs and legs.	Right atrium (auricle) of heart.
Innominate	Head and neck.	Superior vena cava which empties into heart.
Inter-cavernous sinuses	Two cavernous sinuses within skull.	They cross drain into each cavernous sinus.
Internal cerebral	Inner portion of brain.	Great cerebral vein within skull.
Internal jugular	Neck, face and brain.	Innominate vein.
Internal vertebral veins	Spinal cord and spine.	Intervertebral veins lying between in the vertebrae.

Name of Vein	Area or Organ Blood Drainage from:	Vessel or Structure Blood Carried to:
Middle cardiac	Posterior portion of heart.	Coronary sinus of heart.
Occipital sinus	Cerebellar portion of the brain toward the base of skull.	Sinuses at base of brain.
Parumbilical	Area around navel.	Portal vein leading to liver.
Portal	Organs within abdomen, including intestines.	Liver.
Posterior, of left ventricle	Left ventricle of heart.	Coronary sinus of heart.
Prostatic	Prostate gland.	Pudendal plexus in pelvis.
Pudendal plexus*	Penis.	Vesical veins from bladder.
Pyloric	Stomach.	Portal vein leading to liver.
Small saphenous	Foot and back of leg.	Popliteal vein in back of knee.
Superior ophthalmic	Area about the eye and bridge of nose.	Cavernous sinus within brain.
Superior petrosal sinus	Upper portions (cerebrum) of brain.	Transverse sinus within brain.
Superior sagittal sinus	Upper portions (cerebrum) of brain.	Transverse sinus within brain.
Superior vena cava	Head, neck, chest wall and arms.	Right atrium (auricle) of heart.
Transverse sinus	Brain.	Internal jugular vein leading to neck.
Vesical plexus*	Bladder and prostate gland.	Hypogastric vein in pelvis.
Vorticose	Eyeball	Ophthalmic vein.

*A "plexus" is a group of connecting, interlacing veins; a network.

2. IMPORTANT BONES

Name of Bone	Description, Location, and Connection
Astragalus (*talus*)	Located just below tibia and fibula (leg bones) in ankle. It connects with the heel bone (calcaneus).
Atlas	First vertebra lying just beneath skull.
Axis	Second vertebra in neck, lying just below atlas.
Calcaneus (*os calcis*)	Heel bone, the largest bone of the foot.
Calvarium	Bones which form top of skull.
Capitate	Largest bone in wrist, located toward center of wrist joint.
Carpal	Eight small bones of wrist: greater multangular, lesser multangular, lunate, capitate, hamate, navicular, triquetrum and pisiform bones.
Clavicle (*collarbone*)	Collarbone extending from sternum (breastbone) to shoulder tip.
Coccyx	Tailbone, the last vertebrae at base of spine.
Concha	A shell-shaped, small bone located along the outer side of nasal cavity.
Costal (*ribs*)	There are 12 bones on each side, arising from the spinal column.
Coxae	The hipbone. It joins with sacrum and other hipbone to form the bony pelvis. The coxae is composed of 3 fused bones: ilium, ischium, and pubis.
Cranium	The skull. It is composed of occipital bone, 2 parietal bones, 2 temporal bones, 2 frontal bones, sphenoid and ethmoid bones.
Cuboid	A cube-shaped, small bone of the foot.
Cuneiform	A general term for some of the small bones of foot or hand.
Ethmoid	A small bone located in front of the base of the skull forming part of the orbit and nose. Within it are spaces, making up the ethmoid sinuses.
Facial	There are 10 small bones which fuse to make up the bony structure of the face: nasal, zygoma,

Name of Bone	Description, Location, and Connection
	maxilla, vomer, palatine, lacrimal, nasal concha, ethmoid, sphenoid and mandible (jawbone).
Femur	The thighbone, extending from hip to knee.
Fibula	Outer bone of leg, extending from knee to ankle. (It does not bear weight.)
Foot	These consist of the 7 tarsal bones (calcaneus, talus, cuboid, navicular and 3 cuneiforms), 5 metatarsal bones and the bones of the 5 toes.
Frontal	Bones of the forehead, parts of the orbit and nose.
Humerus	Arm bone, extending from shoulder to elbow.
Hyoid	The thin U-shaped bone beneath the chin and above the larynx.
Ilium	Part of hipbone, into which the femur fits.
Incus	The anvil. One of 3 small bones of middle ear, adjacent to eardrum.
Inferior turbinate	Same as concha (inferior nasal bone).
Innominate	An old term for hipbone (coxae).
Ischium	Part of hipbone.
Lacrimal	A small bone of the skull located in front inner part of orbit.
Malar	The cheekbone; the zygoma.
Malleus	The hammer. One of 3 small bones of middle ear, adjacent to eardrum.
Mandible (*inferior maxilla*)	The jawbone. It is attached to the skull at the temporomandibular joint in front of the ear.
Maxilla	The upper jawbone. It makes up part of the face, orbit, nose, etc.
Metacarpal	The 5 bones of the hand to which the finger bones are attached.
Metatarsal	The 5 bones of the foot to which the toe bones are attached.

Name of Bone	Description, Location, and Connection
Nasal	The bones of the nose.
Navicular	Small bones of the hand and foot; shaped like a boat.
Occipital	The back and part of base of skull.
Palatine	An irregularly shaped bone making up part of the hard palate, nose and orbit.
Parietal	This bone makes up part of the side and top of the skull.
Patella	The kneecap.
Pelvis	The bony pelvis is made up of the hipbones, sacrum, and coccyx.
Phalanges	The bones of fingers and toes.
Pubis	The bone in front of pelvis.
Radius	The long bone on outer (thumbside) side of forearm, extending from elbow to wrist.
Ribs	There are 12 ribs on each side, arising from the spinal column in the back.
Sacrum	Five fused vertebrae in the lower back which make up back part of bony pelvis.
Scapula	The shoulder blade (wingbone). It connects with the collarbone and humerus of upper arm.
Sesamoid	Small, irregularly shaped bones (which develop in adult life) in tendons or sites where muscles or tendons rub against larger bones. They are seen most often in hands or feet.
Skull	It is composed of the occipital, 2 parietal, 2 temporal, 2 frontal, the sphenoid and ethmoid bones.
Sphenoid	An irregularly shaped bone making up the front portion of the base of the skull and parts of the orbit and nose.
Stapes	The stirrup. One of 3 small bones of middle ear adjacent to eardrum.
Sternum	The breastbone. Cartilages of ribs and collarbone are attached to the sternum.

Name of Bone	Description, Location, and Connection
Talus	The same as the astragalus.
Tarsal	The same as the foot bones.
Temporal	The bone forming the front portion of side of skull and part of base.
Tibia	The large inner bone of the leg extending from knee to ankle. (It is responsible for weight bearing.)
Turbinate	Three bones located on outer side of the nasal cavity.
Tympanic	Three small bones of middle ear: the incus, malleus, and stapes.
Ulna	The long bone on the inner side of forearm, extending from elbow to wrist.
Vertebrae	The spinal column, or backbone. There are 33 vertebrae: 7 in neck, 12 in chest (thoracic), 5 in lower back (lumbar), and 9 making up the sacrum and coccyx.
Vomer	This bone forms the back segment of the nasal septum separating the two sides of the nose.
Wrist	The same as the carpal bones.
Zygoma	The cheekbone; the malar bone.

3. IMPORTANT MUSCLES

Name of Muscle	Origin and Termination	Function
Abductor 5th finger and 5th toe	Small muscles arising from the back portion of hand and foot and extending to base of little finger or little toe.	Pulls little finger and/or little toe away from other fingers and/or toes.
Abductor hallucis	Extends from heel bone to base of big toe.	Bends big toe and pulls it away from other toes.
Abductor pollicis brevis	Extends from small hand bones to base of thumb.	Bends thumb and pulls it away from other fingers.

Name of Muscle	Origin and Termination	Function
Abductor pollicis longus	Extends from muscles and tendons of forearm to base of thumb.	Straightens (extends) the thumb and pulls it away from other fingers.
Abductor brevis	Extends from pubic bone to thighbone (femur).	Pulls thigh toward midline (in an inward direction).
Abductor hallucis	Extends from bones of foot to base of big toe.	Pulls big toe toward other toes.
Adductor longus	A larger muscle than adductor brevis, arising from the pubic bone and extending to femur.	Pulls thigh toward midline (in an inward direction).
Adductor magnus	Extends from pubic bone and ischium to femur.	Pulls thigh toward midline and extends (straightens) hip joint.
Adductor pollicis	Extends from small bones of hand to base of thumb.	Brings thumb toward other fingers and puts it in a position to grasp objects.
Anconeus	Extends from humerus in upper arm to ulna in forearm.	Straightens elbow joint.
Aryepiglottic	From the arytenoid cartilage to the epiglottis (structure which closes windpipe when swallowing)	Closes entrance to larynx.
Arytenoid	From one arytenoid cartilage to other.	Closes larynx.
Auricularis	Extending (when present) from covering membrane of skull to outer ear.	Moves outer ear. (This muscle is rarely developed and represents a vestige of our primitive past.)
Biceps brachii	Extends from scapula and humerous in upper arm to bones and tissue of forearm.	Powerful muscle which flexes upper arm.

Biceps femoris	Extends from femur and ischium to fibula and fibrous tissues below knee.	Flexes knee joint and extends (straightens) hip joint.
Brachialis	Extends from humerus in upper arm to ulna in forearm.	Flexes (bends) elbow joint.
Brachio-radialis	From humerus in upper arm to radius in the forearm.	Flexes (bends) elbow joint.
Buccinator	Extends from upper and lower jaw bones to muscles about mouth.	Pulls back angles of mouth and tightens cheeks.
Bulbo-carvernous	Extends from perineum (a point below the genitals) to penis.	Compresses urethra (tube passing through penis).
Ciliary	Extends from membrane around iris to ciliary process of iris in eye.	Opens and closes pupil of eye.
Coccygeus	From ischium (bone upon which one sits) to coccyx at base of spine.	Helps to close diaphragm of pelvis (muscles surrounding rectum).
Constrictor, of pharynx	Extends from cartilages and ligaments of neck to pharynx (throat).	Constricts the muscles of the throat.
Coraco-brachialis	From shoulder blade (scapula) to humerus in upper arm.	Pulls upper arm toward body and bends it.
Cremaster	From muscles of lower abdomen to pubis.	Pulls testicle up toward abdomen.
Crico-arytenoid	From cricoid cartilages to arytenoid cartilages in neck.	Opens and closes vocal cords.
Cricothyroid	Extends from cricoid cartilage to thyroid cartilage ("Adam's apple").	Tightens vocal cords.

Name of Muscle	Origin and Termination	Function
Dartos	Located beneath skin of scrotum.	Tightens skin of scrotum (sac of testicles).
Deltoid	Extends from collarbone and scapula, over the shoulder, to humerus in upper arm.	Lifts upper arm away from body.
Diaphragm	Extends across body and separates chest cavity from abdomen cavity.	The muscle of breathing, particularly breathing in.
Digastric	Extends from lower jaw to hyoid cartilage in neck.	Lifts up hyoid bone.
Erector clitoris	From ischium of pelvis to tissues around the clitoris.	Causes erection of clitoris.
Erector penis	From ischium of pelvis to tissues around base of penis.	Aids in erection of penis.
Erector pili	From deep layer of skin to hair follicles.	Makes hair stand on end.
Extensor carpi radialis	From humerus to bones of wrist.	Extends (straightens) wrist.
Extensor carpi ulnaris	From humerus in upper arm to bones of wrist.	Extends (straightens) wrist.
Extensor digitorum, of feet	From heel bone to toes.	Straightens toes.
Extensor digitorum, of hands	Extends from humerus in upper arm to tendons of fingers on back of hands.	Straightens wrist and fingers.
Extensor hallucis	Extends from fibula bone of leg and heel bone to base of big toe.	Straightens big toe and helps to bend ankle upward.
Extensor pollicis	Extends from radius and ulna bones of forearm to thumb.	Straightens thumb and pulls it away (abducts) from other fingers.

Name of Muscle	Origin and Termination	Function
Flexor carpi radialis	Extends from humerus to bones in front of the wrist.	Bends wrist.
Flexor carpi ulnaris	From humerus and ulna to bones in front of the wrist.	Bends wrist.
Flexor digitorum, of feet	Extends from tibial and heel bone to toes.	Bends toes.
Flexor digitorum, of hands	From ulna in forearm to fingers.	Flexes (bends) fingers.
Flexor hallucis	From fibula in leg and bones of foot to base of big toe.	Flexes big toe.
Flexor pollicis	From radius bone in forearm and bones of wrist to thumb.	Flexes thumb.
Gastrocnemius	Extends down leg from femur to heel bone.	Bends ankle in a downward direction and helps to flex knee.
Gemellus	From ischium of pelvis to femur bone of thigh.	Turns femur in an outward direction.
Genioglossus	Extends from lower jawbone to tongue.	Sticks out and returns tongue.
Glosso-palatine	From soft palate to tongue.	Lifts up tongue.
Gluteus maximus, medius and minimus	From bones of pelvis to upper, outer part of femur (thigh bone).	These muscles straighten the hip joint and pull thighbone away from body.
Gracillis	From pubic bone down to tibia in leg.	Pulls thighs toward midline of body.
Hamstring	Three large muscles extending down back of thigh, from ischium to tibia below knee.	Flexes (bends) knee joint.
Iliacus	Extends from pelvis bones to femur in thigh.	Flexes hip joint.

Name of Muscle	Origin and Termination	Function
Iliocostal	From ribs to vertebral column.	Straightens spinal column and bends trunk sideways.
Iliopsoas	From lumbar vertebra in back to thigh-bone.	Flexes trunk.
Infraspinatus	Extends from shoulder blade to upper arm.	Rotates arm in an outward direction.
Intercostal	Extends from one rib to another.	Aid in breathing in and out.
Interossei	Extends from bones of hands and/or feet to tendons of hands and/or feet.	Brings fingers or toes close to one another.
Latissimus dorsi	Extends from spine and ribs to humerus in upper arm.	Brings arms close to body. Aids in breathing.
Levator ani	From fibrous tissue and bones of pelvis, it forms a sling and goes to the coccyx and perineum (a point behind the genitals).	Holds up pelvis organs.
Levator scapulae	Extends from spinal column in neck to shoulder blade.	Lifts up shoulder.
Lingual	Extends from base to tip of tongue.	Changes shape of tongue.
Longissimus	Extends up back near spine.	Straightens spine.
Longitudinal, of tongue	Same as lingual muscles.	Changes shape of tongue.
Longus capitis	Extends from vertebrae in neck to base of skull.	Bends (flexes) head.
Longus colli	Vertebra of neck and chest, up and down spine.	Bends (flexes) spine in neck region.

Name of Muscle	Origin and Termination	Function
Lumbrical, of hands and toes	Extend from flexor tendons of hands and/or toes to extensor tendons.	Flex and extend fingers.
Masseter	Extends from cheekbone to lower jawbone.	Closes mouth; called "the muscle of chewing."
Mylohyoid	Extends from lower jaw to hyoid bone in neck.	Lifts floor of mouth.
Nasalis	Maxillary bone of face to bridge.	Alters expression of face.
Oblique, abdominal	Extends from lower ribs to midline of abdomen and pubis.	These muscles support abdominal wall.
Oblique, of eye	Extends from orbit to outer membrane (sclera) of eyeball.	Rotates eyeball.
Obturator	Extends from bones of pubis to femur (thighbone).	Rotates thigh outward.
Omohyoid	Extends from upper border of shoulder blade to hyoid bone in neck.	Lowers hyoid bone and floor of mouth.
Opponens pollicis	Extends from bones of hand to base of thumb.	Rotates thumb so that it faces other fingers.
Orbicularis oculi	Extends from orbit to skin about eyes.	Closes eyes.
Orbicularis oris	Lies beneath skin of mouth.	Brings mouth into a "kissing" shape.
Palmaris	Extend down front of forearm to palm of hand.	Help to flex wrist and to make "hollow of the hand."
Pectineus	Extends from pubic bone to femur (thighbone).	Pulls thigh toward midline of body and flexes hip.

Name of Muscle	Origin and Termination	Function
Pectoral	Extend from collar-bone, breastbone and ribs to shoulder blade and humerus of arm.	Rotate arm inward, bring shoulder forward and pull arm close to body.
Peroneus	Extend from bones of leg (tibia and fibula) to bones of foot.	Bend foot outward, flex and extend ankle.
Pharngo-palatine	Extends from soft palate to back of throat.	Helps the act of swallowing.
Piriformis	Extends from sacrum and other bones of pelvis to femur (thighbone).	Turns thigh in an outward direction.
Plantaris	Extends, when present, from lower end of femur (thighbone) to heel.	Bends ankle in a downward direction.
Platysma	Tissues beneath skin of neck.	Helps in altering expressions of face.
Popliteus	Outer, lower portion of femur to tibia in upper leg.	Turns knee inward and helps in bending knee joint.
Pronator	Extend from lower end of humerus (upper arm bone) and ulna to radius in forearm.	Rotate forearm so that palm of hand faces down.
Psoas	Extends from vertebrae in lower back to femur in thigh.	Flex (bend) trunk and hip.
Pterygoid	Extend from face and upper jaw to lower jaw.	Aid in chewing and in clenching teeth.
Quadratus femoris	Extends from ischium (bone upon which one sits) to upper thigh (femur).	Rotates thigh outward and pulls thigh toward midline of body.

Name of Muscle	Origin and Termination	Function
Quadratus lumborum	Extends from hipbone and vertebra to last rib in lower chest.	Bends spine in a sideward direction.
Quadriceps femoris	General term for the vastus and rectus femoris muscles.	*See* Rectus femoris muscles; *also* Vastus muscles.
Rectus abdominis	Extends from bottom of breast bone and lower ribs to pubis.	Bends spine forward; supports abdominal wall.
Rectus capitis	Extend from vertebra in neck to skull.	Bend head forward and backward.
Rectus femoris	Extends from hipbone down front of thigh, over knee to upper leg.	Straightens knee.
Rectus oculi	Extend from orbit to eyeball.	Rotate eye in various directions.
Rhomboid	Extend from vertebra in neck to scapula near midline.	Squares shoulders by drawing shoulder blades backward.
Risorius	Extends from tissue beneath skin of face to corners of mouth.	Alters facial expressions and draws corners of mouth out and down.
Sartorius	Extends from hipbone to tibia in leg.	Bends knee and hip joints and rotates thigh outward.
Scalene	Extend from vertebra in neck to first and second ribs.	Bend head and neck sideways.
Semi-membranosus	Ischium (bone upon which one sits) to tibia in leg.	Bends knee and straightens hip.
Semispinalis	Extend from vertebrae in neck and upper chest upward to base of skull.	Bend head backward and rotate spine in neck region.
Semi-tendinosus	Ischium (bone upon which one sits) to tibia in upper leg.	Bends knee and straightens hip.
Serratus	Extends from spine in chest and lower back to ribs.	Elevates ribs and thus aids in breathing.

Name of Muscle	Origin and Termination	Function
Soleus	Extends from tibia and fibula in upper leg to heel (calcaneus).	Bends ankle down.
Sphincter ani	Extends from coccyx at base of spine around anus.	Constricts anus.
Sphincter pupillae	Surrounds pupil of eye.	Contracts pupil.
Sphincter urethrae	Extends from pubic bone to midline.	Tightens urethra (passageway from bladder).
Sphincter vaginae	Extends around vaginal opening.	Constricts vaginal opening.
Spinalis	Extend from vertebrae in neck, chest, and back to other vertebrae in neck, chest, and back.	Straighten head and spine.
Splenius	Extend from vertebrae in the chest and neck to back of head.	Straighten head and spine.
Stapedius	A tiny muscle extending from stapes in middle ear to eardrum.	Moves stapes (one of 3 small bones in middle.)
Sternocieido-mastoid	Extends from upper end of breastbone and collarbone to mastoid region of skull.	Bends head forward.
Sternohyoid	Extends from upper end of breastbone to hyoid bone beneath chin.	Pulls hyoid bone downward.
Sterno-thyroid	Extends from upper end of breastbone (sternum) to thyroid cartilage	Pulls larynx (voicebox) downward.
Styloglossus	Extends from styloid bone (part of skull in front of mastoid bone) to tongue.	Lifts up tongue.

Name of Muscle	Origin and Termination	Function
Subscapularis	Extends from scapula (shoulder blade) to humerus (in upper arm).	Rotates arm inward.
Supinator	Extends from humerus, in upper arm, and ulna to radius in forearm.	Rotates forearm so that palm of hand faces up.
Supraspinatus	Extends from scapula to humerus.	Draws upper arm away from body.
Temporal	Extends from temple to lower jaw.	Closes mouth.
Tensor fascia latae	Extends from crest of hip, down along outside of thigh, to leg.	Draws leg away from body and bends hip joint.
Teres major	Extends from outer border of scapula to humerus.	Rotates arm inward and draws arm toward body.
Teres minor	Extends from outer border of scapula to humerus.	Rotates arm outward.
Thyro-arytenoid	Extends from thyroid cartilage to arytenoid cartilage in larynx.	Separates vocal cords.
Thyro-epiglottis	Extends from thyroid cartilage to epiglottis (the structure which shuts off larynx and trachea).	Shuts off larynx and trachea.
Thyrohyoid	Extends from thyroid cartilage to hyoid bone in neck.	Draws hyoid bone downward and thyroid cartilage upward.
Tibialis anterior	Extends from tibia, in front of leg, down to bones of foot.	Bends foot upward and inward.
Tibialis posterior	Extends from tibia and fibula, in back of leg, down to bones of foot.	Bends foot downward and inward.

Name of Muscle	Origin and Termination	Function
Transversus abdominis	Extends from lower six ribs and crests of hip across abdomen to midline.	Aids in bending spine forward; helps to support abdominal wall.
Trapezius	A large muscle extending from base of skull and vertebrae in neck to the collarbone, shoulder blade, and tip of shoulder.	Raises shoulder and pulls shoulder blade (scapula) backward.
Triceps brachii	Extends from upper end of humerus, in upper arm, to ulna bone in forearm.	Straightens elbow.
Vastus	Extend down entire front of thigh to kneecap and tibia in leg.	Straightens knee.

4. IMPORTANT NERVES

Name of Nerve	Distribution and Function
Abducens (6th cranial)	Arises from brain and supplies eye muscle which turns eyeball in an outward direction.
Accessory (11th cranial)	Arises from base of brain and supplies muscles which control throat, voice box (larynx), and muscles in neck and shoulders.
Acoustic (8th cranial)	Arises from brain and supplies organ of hearing in inner ear. Disease of this nerve results in loss of hearing.
Alveolar	These nerves supply sensation to teeth, and also supply muscles which work lower jaw.
Ampullary	These are branches of nerves supplying inner ear. Damage to these nerves may result in loss of sense of balance (equilibrium).
Auditory (8th cranial)	Same as acoustic nerve.
Auricular	A branch of the vagus (10th cranial) which supplies sensation to outer ear.
Axillary	Arises from spinal cord in neck and supplies muscles and skin of shoulder region.
Bell, nerve of	Also called "long thoracic nerve." Arises from spinal cord in neck and supplies muscle which controls movements of scapula (wingbone in back).

Name of Nerve	Distribution and Function
Buccinator	Arises from the mandibular nerve and supplies sensation to cheek.
Cardiac	A group which supply heart. (Peculiarly, if these nerves are damaged or severed, the heart continues to function without them.)
Carotid	In neck, arising from sympathetic nerves and supplying the glands in head.
Cervical	There are 8 pairs of cervical nerves. They supply muscles of neck, shoulders and arms. They also are responsible for sensation in skin in these regions.
Chorda tympani	Filaments from this nerve supply sensation of taste to tongue. It also supplies salivary glands beneath chin.
Cilliary	These nerves go to muscle of iris, controlling contraction and dilation of pupil. Branches also supply eyeball.
Cranial	There are 12 pairs of cranial nerves, all arising from the brain: 1. Olfactory; 2. Optic; 3. Oculomotor; 4. Trochlear; 5. Trigeminal; 6. Abducens; 7. Facial; 8. Acoustic; 9. Glossopharyngeal; 10. Vagus; 11. Accessory; 12. Hypoglossal.
Cutaneous	Located in every area of body. They supply sensation to skin.
Digital	Supply sensation to skin of fingers and toes. Arises
Facial (7th cranial)	from brain and supplies muscles of face and of facial expression.
Femoral	A large nerve arising from spinal cord in lower back and supplying muscles of hip and thigh. Also supplies skin sensation to these areas.
Genitofemoral	Arises from spinal cord in lower back and supplies sensation to skin of thigh, and over testicles and/or around lips of vagina.
Glossopharyngeal (9th cranial)	Arises from brain and supplies muscles of palate and throat, tongue, etc. Also supplies sensation to tongue. Branches go to parotid (salivary) gland.
Gluteal	Arise from spinal cord in lower back and supplies muscles of buttocks.
Hemorrhoidal	Supplies muscle and skin about anus.

Name of Nerve	Distribution and Function
Hypogastric	Supplies uterus and other organs in pelvis.
Hypoglossal (*12th cranial*)	Arises from brain and supplies muscles of tongue.
Iliohypogastric	Arises from spinal cord in lower back and supplies muscles of lower abdomen. Also supplies sensation to skin of lower abdomen and buttocks.
Ilioinguinal	Arises from spinal cord in lower back and supplies muscles of lower abdomen. Also supplies sensation to lower abdomen, to scrotum (skin over testicles), and to skin about lips of vagina.
Infraorbital	Supplies sensation of skin of face beneath eyes, to floor of nose and to upper teeth.
Interosseous	These are branches of the radial and median nerves in the forearm. They supply muscles of forearm.
Labial	Supply sensation to lips of face.
Lacrimal	Supplies sensation to skin around outer portion of eye.
Laryngeal	A group of nerves originating from the vagus nerve and supplying muscles of larynx, esophagus (food-pipe), trachea (windpipe) and base of tongue.
Lingual	Supplies sensation to floor of mouth and to part of tongue.
Lumbar	Five pairs of nerves arising from spinal cord in lower back. They supply the muscles of lower back and abdomen, organs in pelvis, and sensation to skin of lower abdomen and legs.
Mandibular	A branch of 5th cranial nerve (trigeminal). It supplies muscles of chewing; also, sensation to the lower teeth.
Maxillary	A branch of 5th cranial nerve (trigeminal). It supplies sensation to skin of upper face, cheeks, palate, and upper teeth.
Median	A large nerve arising from spinal cord in lower neck. It supplies many muscles of forearm and sensation to wrist and hand.
Mental	Supplies sensation to skin of lower lip and chin.

Nasal	A group of nerves supplying sensation to skin of nose.
Nasociliary	Supplies sensation to eyeball, skin, and mucous membranes of eyes and eyelids.
Nasopalatine	Supplies sensation to lining membrane of nose and hard palate.
Obturator	Arising from spinal cord in lower back, they supply muscles on inner side of thigh. Also, sensation to skin over thigh, knee, and hip region.
Occipital	Three nerves which originate from spinal cord in upper part of neck and supply sensation to back of neck, back of ear, and back of scalp.
Oculomotor (*3rd cranial*)	Arises from brain and supplies several muscles which move the eyeball.
Olfactory (*1st cranial*)	Arises from brain and goes to mucous membrane of nose. It is responsible for sense of smell.
Ophthalmic	A branch of trigeminal (5th cranial nerve) which supplies sensation to forehead, eyeball, and sinuses.
Optic (*2nd cranial*)	Arises from brain and supplies the retina of eye. Disease or damage to this nerve will cause loss of sight.
Palatine	A group of nerves which give sensation to membranes of soft palate, tonsils, and back of mouth.
Palpebral	A pair of nerves which supply sensation to eyelids.
Peroneal	A group of nerves which supply many muscles of knee region and leg. They are also responsible for skin sensation in leg, ankle, and foot.
Petrosal	A group of nerves supplying parotid (salivary) gland at angle of jaw, and also parts of the palate.
Phrenic	Arises from spinal cord in neck and supplies the diaphragm, which separates chest from abdominal cavity. Paralysis of a phrenic nerve leads to paralysis of diaphragm on that side.
Plantar	Two nerves which supply those muscles of the foot which move toes.
Pneumogastric	*See* Vagus Nerve. (An old term for vagus nerve.)

Name of Nerve	Distribution and Function
Popliteal	The main nerve from which peroneal and tibial nerves originate. It is located in back of knee.
Pterygoid	A group which sends branches to jaw joint and muscles which move jaws.
Pudendal	Arises from spinal cord in lower (sacral) back and supplies the penis (or clitoris) and region between genitals and anus (perineum).
Radial	A large nerve originating from spinal cord in neck and supplying various muscles in upper arm and forearm. Also supplies sensation to parts of forearm, hand, thumb, and index fingers.
Recurrent laryngeal	A branch of the vagus nerve which supplies the larynx. Damage or disease of this nerve will cause partial vocal cord paralysis and hoarseness.
Sacral	Five pairs of nerves arising from the lowest portion of spinal cord. Branches supply organs in pelvis, muscles of thighs and legs, and sensation to these areas.
Scapular	Arises from spinal cord in neck and supplies muscles which control movement of scapula (wingbone).
Sciatic	One of the largest nerves in the body, arising from spinal cord in lower back and descending back of thigh. It supplies many muscle and skin areas of thigh and leg.
Scrotal	These nerves supply sensation to skin of scrotum.
Sphenopalatine	Same as nasopalatine nerves.
Spinal	Thirty-one pairs of nerves arising from spinal cord. (Many have special names and are listed under those names.)
Splanchnic	These supply organs such as the stomach, gallbladder, liver, pancreas, intestines, etc. They form "plexuses" or groups of nerves, such as the celiac plexus, cardiac plexus, etc. They help to regulate function of above-named organs.
Supraclavicular	Nerves arising from the spinal cord in neck which supply sensation to skin of neck, shoulder, and chest wall.
Supraorbital	A branch of the frontal nerve which supplies sensation to upper eyelid and part of forehead.

Name of Nerve	Distribution and Function
Thoracic	Twelve pairs of nerves arising from spinal cord in chest. They supply muscles and skin of back, the arms, and the abdominal wall.
Thoracic, lateral anterior	Arises from spinal cord in neck and supplies chest muscles (pectorals).
Thoracic, long	Also called the "Nerve of Bell." Arises from spinal cord in neck and supplies muscles (serratus anterior) which controls movement of scapula (wingbone).
Thoracodorsal	Arises from spinal cord in neck and supplies the large muscle (latissimus dorsi) which lifts up upper arm.
Tibial	Branches of sciatic nerve, which supply skin and many of the muscles of left leg and foot.
Trigeminal (*5th cranial*)	Arises from brain and divides into 3 branches; the ophthalmic, maxillary and mandibular nerves. They supply muscles and skin of face and jaws. (Inflammation of branches of this nerve is called *tic douloureux.*)
Trochlear (*4th cranial*)	Arises from brain and supplies a muscle of the eyeball, the superior oblique muscle.
Tympanic	A branch of glossopharyngeal (9th cranial nerve) which supplies sensation to middle ear and mastoid region.
Ulnar	A large nerve of the arm which supplies many of the muscles of forearm and hand. It also supplies sensation to skin in region of ring and little fingers, and certain areas of wrist and elbow.
Vagus (*10th cranial*) (*Pneumogastric nerve*)	Arises from brain and sends branches to supply muscles of throat, larynx, and heart. Also supplies branches to lungs and abdominal organs, the mucous membranes of intestines, stomach, etc., thus influencing secretions. (Cutting the vagus nerve, as it enters the abdominal cavity, reduces the amount of acid secreted by the stomach.)
Zygomatic	These nerves supply sensation to skin over cheekbone and part of temple.

5. IMPORTANT ORGANS

Name of Organ	Location	Major Function
Adenoids	High up in back of throat behind nose.)	Unknown. (They frequently are enlarged in children and obstruct nasal breathing.)
Adrenal glands (*Suprarenal*)	Located just above kidneys in loin.	Essential to life and for hormone secretions such as adrenalin, cortisone, etc. Regulates chemistry of essential body chemicals such as sodium, chlorides, potassium.
Anus	Outlet of intestinal tract.	Its muscles control bowel evacuation.
Appendix	In right lower part of abdomen, near begining of large intestine.	None. (It is a vestige of man's primitive past.)
Bladder (*Urinary*)	In lower abdomen, in midline above pubic bones.	Acts as reservoir for urine which has been excreted by kidneys.
Bone marrow	Inside of bones.	Manufactures blood cells.
Brain	Within the skull.	Control of mental and nerve activities.
a. Cerebrum	Upper portion of brain.	Higher brain functions, such as thought processes, movements, etc.
b. Cerebellum	Below cerebrum.	Controls muscle reflexes, equilibrium, etc.
c. Pons	Below cerebellum, at base of brain.	Receives and transmits impulses from cerebrum.
d. Medulla (*medulla oblongata*)	Below pons, extending to spinal cord.	Transmits impulses received from higher brain centers.
Bronchial tubes	In chest, extending from trachea (windpipe) into lungs.	These are the tubes through which air moves in and out of the lungs.
Breasts	Chest wall.	Female: To secrete milk. Male: None.

Name of Organ	Location	Major Function
Cervix of uterus	In vagina; lowermost portion of uterus.	Acts as barrier to infection; acts as passageway for sperm to enter uterus; dilates at child-birth to allow exit of unborn child.
Colon	In abdomen.	Absorbs water from stool; propels stool on toward anus.
a. Cecum	In right lower part of abdomen, connecting with small intestine.	
b. Ascending	Extends up right side of abdomen, from cecum to transverse colon.	
c. Transverse	Across abdomen from ascending to descending colon.	
d. Descending	Down left side of abdomen to sigmoid colon.	
e. Sigmoid	In left lower part of abdomen, from descending colon down to rectum.	
f. Rectum	In pelvis extending from sigmoid colon down to anus.	
g. Anus	Last inch of bowel.	
Duodenum	In upper midabdomen, extending for 8–10 inches from stomach to jejunum (part of small intestine).	Receives food from stomach and propels it on; receives bile from liver and gallbladder; receives digestive juices from pancreas; secretes digestive juices of its own.
Esophagus (*food pipe*)	Extending from throat to stomach.	Transports swallowed food to stomach.
Fallopian tubes (*uterine tubes*)	Extend outward from uterus for 3–4 inches to ovaries.	Transports egg from ovary to uterus. Fertilization of egg takes place within fallopian tube.

Name of Organ	Location	Major Function
Gallbladder	In upper right part of abdomen beneath ribs.	Stores and concentrates bile received from liver, and expels it into bile ducts, which carry it to intestinal tract.
Heart	In chest, extending slightly to right of midline, but mostly to left of midline.	Pumps blood throughout body.
Ileum	In midabdomen, extending from jejunum to cecum (large intestine) in right lower part of abdomen.	Absorbs food; absorbs water from intestinal contents; aids in digesting foods; propels contents on to large intestine.
Jejunum	In midabdomen, extending from duodenum down to ileum.	Absorbs food; absorbs water from intestinal contents; aids in digesting foods; propels contents onward.
Kidneys	In back, on both sides, below level of ribs in loins.	Filters, excretes and reabsorbs and thus helps to control balance of blood constituents.
Larynx	In neck, behind Adam's apple.	Controls act of speaking.
Liver	In abdomen, beneath diaphragm, more on right than on left.	Manufactures bile, controls metabolism of proteins, stores fat and sugar, and purifies the blood.
Lungs	In both sides of chest cavity.	Lungs are the organs of respiration. They extract oxygen from air which is inhaled and they get rid of cabon dioxide with air which is exhaled.
Ovaries	In pelvis, on each side of uterus, adjacent to fallopian tubes.	Produce an egg each month which when fertilized, forms an embryo. Manufacture female hormones which are secreted into blood stream.
Pancreas	In upper midabdomen just below level of stomach, near duodenum.	Manufactures insulin, which controls sugar metabolism. Manufactures juices which help to digest foods.
Parathyroid glands	Four small glands located behind thyroid in neck.	Manufacture a hormone which controls metabolism of calcium and phosphorus. (Their removal may lead to convulsions and eventual death.)

Name of Organ	Location	Major Function
Penis	In genital region, below pubis.	Male organ of intercourse; also acts as conveyor of urine from bladder.
Pharynx	Behind nose and mouth.	Commonly called the throat, it is the passageway for food and drink and also for air which is breathed.
Pituitary gland	At base of skull in a hollowed-out place in the bone (the sella turcica).	A most important gland whose hormone secretions, directly or indirectly, control metabolism. It is responsible for growth and for proper thyroid, adrenal, and ovarian gland function.
Prostate gland	Located around bladder outlet in males.	It secretes fluid in which sperm are transported during ejaculation.
Pylorus	That part of stomach adjacent to duodenum.	Its strong muscle fibers regulate outflow of stomach contents into duodenum (beginning of small intestine).
Rectum	In pelvis; the continuation of descending and sigmoid colon.	It conveys stool toward outlet of intestinal tract.
Seminal vesicles	Located just above prostate gland in male pelvis.	Store semen (with contained sperm) for discharge through the ejaculatory ducts when orgasm takes place.
Spinal cord	Within spinal canal of vertebra column, extending from base of brain to the lower back region.	This structure contains the nerves which travel from and to the brain and thus are responsible for sensation and movements.
Spleen	In upper left part of abdomen, just beneath diaphragm.	In the unborn child, it manufactures blood cells. In the fully formed human, it destroys old, worn-out blood cells.
Stomach	In left upper part of abdomen.	It churns undigested food and initiates digestion. It manufactures hydrocholoric acid which helps to break down large food particles.

Name of Organ	Location	Major Function
Testicles	Below penis in scrotal sac.	They manufacture sperm which are conveyed by the vas deferens to the seminal vesicles. They secrete male sex hormone into bloodstream.
Thymus gland	In upper front part of chest, beneath breastbone.	Its function is not known. After the second year of life it degenerates.
Thyroid gland	On both sides of trachea (windpipe) in front of neck.	Manufactures the hormone thyroxin, which controls metabolism.
Tongue	Occupies floor of the mouth.	An organ of taste; assists chewing and swallowing; aids in the act of speaking.
Tonsils	On both sides of the mouth, behind tongue.	Function unknown. (Some think it is helpful in preventing bacteria from entering the body.)
Trachea (windpipe)	Extends from larynx in neck to bronchial tubes in chest.	Conveys air into and out of lungs.
Ureters	Extend from kidneys to bladder, behind abdominal organs.	Convey urine from kidneys to bladder.
Urethra	A tube extending from bladder to outside. In male, it courses through penis. In female, it is located just above vaginal opening.	Conveys urine from bladder to outside.
Uterus	In pelvis, just behind bladder and in front of rectum.	The organ (the womb) within which the embryo develops.
Vagina	The membranous canal located in front of rectum and below urethra.	The female organ of intercourse leading to the cervix (entrance to the uterus). It is also through this canal that the newborn child is delivered.

II. ANTIDOTES AND EMERGENCY MEASURES FOR POISONING

Many household products and medications, although not true poisons, may be very dangerous if taken internally. It is extremely important to always take special precautions to keep these items out of a child's reach. Every item in the medicine chest must be plainly labeled. This can be done easily by attaching a piece of adhesive tape to the container and writing the name in large letters. *See also* SECTION XIV—THE MEDICINE CHEST, PRECAUTIONS.

All first-aid measures are essentially only emergency measures—UNTIL the doctor arrives. Therefore, if at all possible, it is best to have one person begin the first aid while somebody else summons a doctor. When a doctor is not available, call the police for help.

For GAS POISONING, good rules in an emergency are:
1. Provide fresh air—open all doors and windows and bring the person to the fresh air. Be careful that there is a minimum of exertion on his part.
2. Prevent chilling.
3. Loosen all tight clothing, belts, collars, etc.
4. Keep the person as quiet as possible.
5. Do NOT give alcohol in any form.
6. If the person is unconscious or has stopped breathing, apply artificial respiration.

For SWALLOWED POISONS, good rules in an emergency are:
1. Find the poison container. Most containers of poisonous substances have printed directions pasted on them.
2. If the poisoned person is fully conscious, induce vomiting. This should be done only when the person is not in a stuporous condition and there are no convulsions. Also, make sure that the poison swallowed is not a corrosive substance or kerosene, gasoline, etc.
3. When vomiting and retching begin, place the person facedown, with head lower than the rest of the body, so that the vomit will not enter the lungs and cause further damage.
4. Save the poison container, or some of the vomit, for the doctor's inspection. This may help him to decide on the appropriate treatment.

Substances	Procedures*

Acids
  Sulfuric
  Nitric
  Hydrochloric
  Chromic
  Carbolic
	1. Cause vomiting.†
	2. Give milk, raw eggs, Jell-O, gelatin.
	3. Gargle with solution of bicarbonate of soda.

*Adapted from "Poisons," a chart compiled by U.S. Vitamin and Pharmaceutical Corp.
†To cause vomiting: 1. Add baking soda or salt to drinking water. 2. Give large quantities of warm water. 3. Put finger in back of throat and tickle.

Substances	Procedures
Alcohol	1. Cause vomiting. 2. Have stomach washed out, preferably at hospital. 3. Keep body warm. 4. Give several cups of black coffee.
Alkalies	1. Give vinegar diluted in water, wine, lemon or apple juice. 2. Cause vomiting. 3. Have stomach washed out as soon as possible. 4. Give milk.
Ammonia	1. Inhale hot vapors. 2. Inhale a dilute vinegar solution.
Arsenic	1. Cause vomiting.* 2. Have stomach washed out at nearest hospital. 3. Give milk.

Barbiturates
  Phenobarbital
  Seconal
  Amytal
  Luminal, etc.
	1. Cause vomiting.
	2. Have stomach thoroughly washed out as soon as possible.
	3. Apply artificial respiration.†
	4. Give laxative.
	5. Give strong coffee.

Belladonna *(Atropine)*	1. Cause vomiting. 2. Give strong coffee. 3. Give charcoal tablets. 4. Sponge body with cold water.
Botulism *(and other food poisoning)*	1. Cause vomiting. 2. Have stomach washed out as soon as possible. 3. Give enema with soap suds and water. 4. Give large dose of castor oil. 5. Give charcoal tablets.
Bromides	1. Give strong coffee. 2. Have stomach washed out.
Carbon monoxide *(or stove gas)*	1. Take patient to fresh air. 2. Apply artificial respiration. 3. Call police or fire department for oxygen. 4. Keep person lying down and quiet. 5. Keep person warm.
Carbon tetrachloride	1. Apply artificial respiration, if breathing is poor. 2. Have stomach washed out. 3. Give strong coffee.

*To cause vomiting: 1. Add baking soda or salt to drinking water. 2. Give large quantities of warm water. 3. Put finger in back of throat and tickle.

†For artificial respiration method, *see* First Aid, Artificial Respiration, p. 487.

Substances	Procedures
Chloral hydrate	1. Give oxygen. 2. Apply artificial respiration. 3. Give black coffee, strong. 4. Sponge head with cold water.
Chlorine gas	1. Inhale warm steam. 2. Breathe weak ammonia fumes.
Chloroform	*See* Narcotic poisoning.
Cocaine	1. Cause vomiting. 2. Have stomach washed out. 3. Apply artificial respiration, if necessary. 4. Give any available barbiturate such as phenobarbital, amytal, etc.
Copper	1. Cause vomiting. 2. Have stomach washed out. 3. Give white of egg every 4 hours. 4. Give charcoal tablets. 5. Give milk.
Corrosive sublimate	*See* Mercury poisoning.
Cyanide	1. Cause vomiting. 2. Have stomach washed out as soon as possible. 3. Apply artificial respiration. 4. Obtain oxygen from police or fire department as soon as possible. 5. Give strong coffee.
Digitalis	1. Cause vomiting.* 2. Give charcoal tablets. 3. Give small doses of alcoholic beverage. 4. Give tea or coffee. 5. Rest in bed.
Ether	*See* Narcotic poisoning.
Illuminating gas	*See* Carbon monoxide poisoning.
Insulin	1. Give sugar or any available candy. 2. Give orange juice, grape juice.
Iodine	1. Cause vomiting. 2. Have stomach washed out. 3. Give flour or starch in a paste or solution. 4. Give white of raw egg.

*To cause vomiting: 1. Add baking soda or salt to drinking water. 2. Give large quantities of warm water. 3. Put finger in back of throat and tickle.

Substances	Procedures

5. Give milk.
6. Give bicarbonate of soda solution.
7. Give laxative.

Kerosene

Give milk and water.

Lead

1. Cause vomiting.
2. Have stomach washed out as soon as possible.
3. Give dose of epsom salts.
4. Give white of raw egg and milk.
5. Give charcoal tablets.

Lysol

1. Cause vomiting.
2. Give milk.
3. Give raw eggs, Jell-O, gelatin.
4. Gargle with solution of bicarbonate of soda.

Meat poisoning

1. Cause vomiting.
2. Have stomach washed out as soon as possible.
3. Give enema with soap suds and water.
4. Give large dose of castor oil.
5. Give charcoal tablets.

Mercury

1. Wash out the mouth with sodium perborate solution or other available mouth wash.
2. Cause vomiting.
3. Have stomach washed out as soon as possible.
4. Give white of eggs and milk.
5. Give sugar.
6. Give bicarbonate of soda.

Methyl alcohol

See Wood alcohol poisoning.

Morphine

1. Cause vomiting.
2. Have stomach washed out.
3. Give strong tea or coffee.
4. Give charcoal tablets.
5. Apply artificial respiration.*

Mushrooms

1. Cause vomiting.
2. Have stomach washed out as soon as possible.
3. Give starch or flour paste.
4. Give charcoal tablets.
5. Give strong tea.

Narcotics

1. Apply artificial respiration.
2. Cause vomiting.
3. Give strong coffee or tea.
4. Give charcoal tablets.

*For artificial respiration method, *see* First Aid, Artificial Respiration p. 487.

Substances	Procedures
Nicotine	1. Have stomach washed out. 2. Give any sedative medication available. 3. Give charcoal tablets.
Opium	*See* Morphine poisoning.
Phenol	*See* Acid poisoning.
Phosphorus	1. Cause vomiting.* 2. Have stomach washed out as soon as possible. 3. Give large dose of epsom salts. 4. Give dose of bicarbonate of soda. 5. Do *NOT* give milk or eggs.
Poison ivy or Poison oak	1. Wash thoroughly with soap and water immediately after contact. 2. Wash with rubbing alcohol to relieve itching.
Snake bite	1. Immediate sucking out of wound. 2. Criss-cross incision with knife in area of bite. 3. Place tourniquet above the site of the bite. Release every 20 minutes for a few minutes in order to permit some circulation to return. 4. Keep patient as quiet and still as possible.
Strychnine	1. Cause vomiting. 2. Have stomach washed out as soon as possible. 3. Give any sedative available. 4. Give moderate dose of alcoholic beverage. 5. Apply artificial respiration if breathing is poor.†
Sulfur	1. Apply artificial respiration. 2. Give salt water to drink.
Tobacco	*See* Nicotine poisoning.
Wood alcohol (methyl alcohol)	1. Cause vomiting. 2. Have stomach washed out. 3. Keep body warm. 4. Apply artificial respiration if necessary. 5. Give strong coffee.
Zinc	1. Cause vomiting. 2. Have stomach washed out. 3. Give white of egg and milk. 4. Give strong tea.

*To cause vomiting: 1. Add baking soda or salt to drinking water. 2. Give large quantities of warm water. 3. Put finger in back of throat and tickle.

†For artificial respiration method, *see* First Aid, Artificial Respiration, p. 487.

III. BLOOD

1. CHEMICAL ANALYSIS

	Normal	Abnormal
Urea nitrogen	12.0 to 15 milligrams per 100 cc.	Increased amounts may indicate kidney disease (nephritis, etc.).
Glucose-sugar	80 to 120 milligrams per 100 cc.	Increased amounts may indicate presence of diabetes mellitus.
Uric acid	4 to 8 milligrams per 100 cc.	Increased amounts may indicate presence of gout.
Nonprotein nitrogen	25 to 45 milligrams per 100 cc.	Increased amounts may indicate kidney or genitourinary disorder.
Creatinine	1 to 2.5 milligrams per 100 cc.	Increased amounts may indicate inability of kidneys to excrete urine (as in obstruction due to markedly enlarged prostate gland.)
Cholesterol	130 to 240 milligrams per 100 cc.	a) Increased amounts may indicate a tendency toward premature hardening of arteries. b) Increased amounts are also seen in some pregnant women and in disorders of the thyroid gland.
Triglyceride	less than 165 mg/dL*	When high, is a risk factor for heart disease.
Calcium	9 to 11 milligrams per 100 cc.	Increased amounts may indicate overactivity or a tumor of parathyroid glands in neck.
Sodium	137 to 143 milli equivalents per liter	Decreased amounts may occur from excess vomiting or loss of body fluids, thus endangering normal body processes.

*dL: deciliter = $\frac{1}{10}$ of a liter

	Normal	Abnormal
Chlorides	585 to 620 milligrams per 100 cc.	Decreased quantities usually result from loss of salt from the body. Excessive loss is incompatible with normal body function.
Phosphorus	3 to 4.5 milligrams per 100 cc.	Variation in amounts may indicate function disorder of the parathyroid glands in the neck.
Potassium	4 to 5 milli equivalents per liter	Marked alterations occur in many disease states and may cause disturbance in heart function. Potassium quantities must be in balance with sodium quantities.
Magnesium	1.8 to 2.5 mg per decaliter	Decreased quantities can cause heart arrhythmias.
Bilirubin	0.1 to 0.25 milligrams per 100 cc.	Increased quantities may indicate jaundice, obstruction to normal flow of bile from liver, or liver disease.
Alkaline Phosphatase	1.5 to 4 units per 100 cc.	Increased quantities indicates obstruction to flow of bile or jaundice.
Icterus index	4 to 6 units	Increased reading indicates presence of jaundice.
Total protein	6.5 to 8.2 grams per 100 cc.	Decreased amounts are seen in debilitated states, in chronic illness.
Serum albumin: Globulin	1.5 to 2.5 grams per 100 cc. 2.5 to 3.0 grams per 100 cc.	A reversal so that the ratio is below 1, indicates poor protein metabolism.
pCO$_2$	35–45 mmHg	Increase indicates acidosis; decrease alkalosis.
pH	7.35–7.45	Increase indicates alkalosis; decrease acidosis.
pO$_2$ (*Arterial*)	95–104 mmHg	Increase indicates alkalosis; decrease acidosis.

	Normal	Abnormal
Amylase	80–160 Samagyi Units	Increase indicates pancreatitis.
SGOT	<40 I.U.	Increase may indicate liver disease, myocardial infarction, etc.

2. NORMAL AND ABNORMAL FINDINGS

	Normal	Abnormal
Red blood cells	4,200,000 to 5,500,000 per cubic millimeter	Lower counts indicate presence of anemia or blood loss.
White blood cells	5,000 to 8,000 per cubic millimeter	1. Increased numbers (up to 25,000) usually indicates presence of an infection. 2. Greatly increased numbers (from 25,000 to 100,000 or more) may indicate presence of leukemia. 3. Decreased numbers may indicate toxic poisoning of blood by a drug, or a poor response to an infection.
Hemoglobin	Female, 80–100% (12.8 to 15 grams) Male, 90–105% (14 to 17 grams)	Lower amounts indicates presence of anemia.
Coagulation time	4 to 6 minutes	Lack of coagulation (blood clotting), or markedly delayed coagulation time may indicate the presence of hemophilia.
Bleeding time	1 to 2 minutes	Prolonged bleeding time shows a bleeding tendency (not hemophilia), which may be due to liver disease, jaundice or disease of the spleen.
Prothrombin time	14 to 16 seconds	Extended prothrombin time shows a bleeding tendency, often caused by a liver disorder.

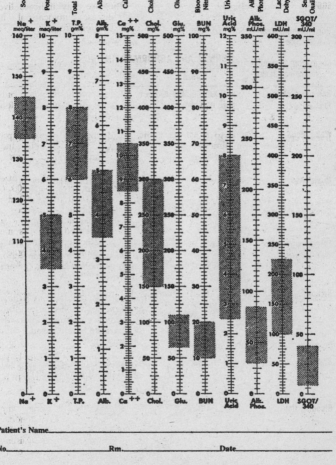

Patient's Name_____

No._____ Rm._____ Date_____

The above Chart records the 12 most frequently performed chemical tests of the blood. They are run through an automated analyzer which will give the results within a matter of minutes. The test is commonly referred to as an SMA-12 Channel Blood test. Shaded areas are within normal ranges.

NORMAL AND ABNORMAL FINDINGS (Concluded)

A. Differential White Cell Count

Leukocyte Count

	Normal	Abnormal
Polymorphonuclear leukocytes	68 to 70%	Increased percentage indicates an acute infection.
Segmented polymorphonuclear leukocytes	58 to 66%	Increased percentage indicates an acute infection.
Stab cells	3 to 15%	Increased percentage indicates an acute infection.
Juvenile cells	0 to 1%	Increased percentage may indicate presence of a blood disease, such as leukemia.
Myelocytes	None	Increased percentage may indicate presence of a blood disease.
Small lymphocytes	20 to 22%	Increased percentage may indicate presence of a chronic infection.
Large lymphocytes (*Monocytes*)	3 to 6%	Increased percentage may indicate presence of a subacute infection, such as mononucleosis (glandular fever).
Eosinophils	1 to 2%	Increased percentage may indicate presence of an allergic condition or presence of an infection with a parasite (tapeworm, other worms, etc.).
Basophils	0.5 to 1%	Increased percentage may indicate presence of a blood disease.

3. BLOOD PRESSURE

*Average Normal Pressures**

Age	Systolic Pressure	Diastolic Pressure
10 years	103	70
15 years	113	75
20 years	120	80
25 years	122	81
30 years	123	82
35 years	124	83
40 years	126	84
45 years	128	85
50 years	130	86
55 years	132	87
60 years	135	89

Systolic pressure is the force with which blood is pumped by the heart during the period of the heart's contraction; *diastolic pressure* is the force with which blood is pumped by the heart during dilatation or relaxation.

*Courtesy of U.S. Vitamin and Pharmaceutical Corp.

IV. CALORIC VALUES OF FOODS*

Food	Amount	Approximate Number of Calories	Food	Amount	Approximate Number of Calories
Cereals and Breadstuffs			Cream, heavy	1 tbsp.	60
Bran muffin	1 muffin	50	Cream, whipped	1 tbsp.	35
Biscuits	2 small biscuits	100	Egg	1 egg	75
Bun, cinnamon	1 small square	100	Milk	8 ounces	125
Cornflakes	½ cup	50	Skimmed milk	6 ounces	80
Cream of Wheat	½ cup	75	Malted milk	10–12 ounces	450–500
Farina	½ cup	70	Swiss cheese	1 small slice	60
Griddle cakes	4 cakes	225			
Hominy	⅔ cup	90	**Meats and Fish**		
Melba toast	1 slice	25	Bacon	1 slice	30
Oatmeal	½ cup	75	Bass	1 small piece	45
Pretzels	5 small sticks	20	Brook trout	1 small piece	45
Rice	½ cup	80	Caviar	1 tbsp.	25
Rye bread	1 slice	75	Haddock	1 small piece	50
Saltine cracker	1 cracker	15	Halibut	1 small piece	50
Shredded wheat	1 biscuit	100	Ham	1 average slice	100
Uneeda biscuit	1 biscuit	20	Hamburger	2 patties	85
Waffles	1 waffle	250	Lamb chop	1 medium size chop	160
White bread	1 slice	100	Liver, broiled	1 average slice	100
Popover	1	100	Oysters	6 large	50
Dairy Products			Pork chop	1 lean chop	100
American cheese	1 inch square	90	Roast beef	1 lean slice	85
Butter	1 tbsp.	95	Roast lamb	1 lean slice	95
Cheddar cheese	1 inch square	100	Round steak	1 lean slice	85
Buttermilk	8 ounces	75	Salmon, canned	½ cup	100
Cottage cheese	¼ cup	65			
Cream cheese	½ cake	95			

*Courtesy of Metropolitan Life Insurance Company and *The New Illustrated Medical Encyclopedia for Home Use*, Abradale Press, N.Y.

Food	Amount	Approximate Number of Calories	Food	Amount	Approximate Number of Calories
Tuna fish, canned	½ cup	100	Tomato, fresh	1 medium	20
			Turnips	¾ cup	35
Vegetables and Soups			Vegetable soup	1 cup	75
Artichoke	1 large	65	Water- cress	10 pieces	8
Asparagus	8 tips	20			
Avocado	½ pear	265	Olives, green	6	50
Beet soup	1 cup	90	Potato chips	10 large	100
Beets	¾ cup	50			
Brussels sprouts	⅔ cup	20	Potato salad with mayon- naise	½ cup	200
Cabbage, cooked	¾ cup	25	Popcorn	1½ cups	100
Carrots	¾ cup	40			
Cauli- flower	¾ cup	30	**Fruits and Nuts**		
Celery	3 stalks	15	Apple	1 small	55
Cucumber	10 slices	15	Apple- sauce	½ cup	85
Eggplant	½ cup	25			
Endive	10 stalks	15	Apricots, fresh	3 small	55
Green peas, canned	¾ cup	55	Banana	1 small	90
			Blue- berries	⅔ cup	50
Green peas, fresh	½ cup	95	Cherries	12	70
Lettuce	¼ small head	15	Cran- berries	⅔ cup	45
			Dates	4	100
Lima beans, fresh	¾ cup	115	Figs	3 dried	100
			Grape- fruit	½	40
Navy beans	⅓ cup	100	Grapes	24	90
Okra	½ cup	35	Lemon	1 medium	15
Onions	4 small	50	Orange	½ medium	25
Peppers	2 small	25	Orange juice	½ glass	50
Potato	¼ cup, mashed	50			
			Peach, fresh	1 medium	40
Pumpkin	½ cup	25	Pineapple	1 slice	40
Radishes	5 medium	8	Pear, fresh	1 medium	55
Rhubarb	¾ cup	15			
Scallions	3 small	50	Prunes	3 cooked	75
Spinach, cooked	½ cup	30	Water- melon	1½-inch thick slice	190
Spinach soup	1 cup	85			
Squash	½ cup	40	Almonds	15	100
String beans	½ cup	25	Cashew nuts	5	100

Food	Amount	Approximate Number of Calories	Food	Amount	Approximate Number of Calories
Peanuts	10	50	Sugar	1 tbsp.	50
Peanut butter	1 tbsp.	100	Soda	fountain size	325
Pecans	6	100	Syrup	¼	200
Walnuts	8	100	Cupcake, iced	1	250
Grape juice	½ glass	75			
			Beverages		
Desserts and Sweets			Carbonated sodas	6 ounces	80
Apple pie	3-inch cut	200	Club soda	8 ounces	5
Brownies	1 brownie	140	Gingerale	6 ounces	60
Cheese cake	2½-inch cut	275	Tea, plain	1 cup	0
Chocolate bar, plain	1	190	Coffee, plain	1 cup	0
Chocolate bar with nuts	1	250	Tea with cream and sugar	1 cup	75–90
Fudge	1-inch square	100	Coffee, with cream and sugar	1 cup	75–90
Custard pie	3-inch cut	360	Ale	8 ounces	130
Doughnuts	1	140	Beer	8 ounces	110
Fruit pie	3-inch cut	550	Gin	1½ ounces	120
Jellies and jams	1 tbsp.	100	Rum	1½ ounces	150
Lemon meringue pie	3-inch cut	300	Whiskey	1½ ounces	150
Maple syrup	1 tbsp.	70	Table wine	4 ounces	85–95
Mince pie	3-inch cut	300	Sherry	1 ounces	40
Milk sherbet	⅙ quart	250	Champagne	4 ounces	120
Pumpkin pie	1 average portion	400	Manhattan	1½ ounces	175
Fruit cake	1 medium portion	125	Martini	1½ ounces	150
Layer cake, iced	1 medium portion	340	Port	1 ounce	50
Ice cream	⅙ quart	225	**Miscellaneous**		
Ice cream soda	10 ounces	270	Fresh dressing	1 tbsp.	90
Sundae with nuts and whipped cream	fountain size	400	Brown gravy	¼ cup	80
			Mayonnaise	1 tbsp.	100

V. CEREBROSPINAL FLUID

	Normal	Abnormal
Color	Clear, colorless.	a) Cloudy indicates presence of infection (meningitis). b) Yellow indicates presence of brain hemorrhage. It may also indicate a tumor somewhere in brain or spinal cord.
Reaction	Slightly alkaline.	
Chlorides	120 to 130 milli equivalents per liter.	
Glucose	0.04 to 0.07 grams per 100 cc.	
Protein	Trace.	
White Cells	1 to 7 per cubic millimeter.	Increased numbers of cells indicates presence of an infection (meningitis, poliomyelitis, etc.).
Specific gravity	1.001 to 1.010.	
Blood	None.	Finding of blood indicates hemorrhage within the brain, as in fractured skull, cerebral accident (stroke), etc.
Manometric pressure	70–180 millimeters of water.	Increase indicates possible presence of a brain tumor, cyst, etc.

VI. CONTAGIOUS DISEASES

Disease	Cause	How Transmitted	Incubation Period	When Contagious?	Symptoms
Roseola (*Exanthem Subitum*)	Virus	Not definitely known.	7–17 days	Not known.	Fever for 3 days, followed by rash and swollen glands.
Mumps (*Parotitis*)	Virus	By direct contact, coughing, sneezing, etc.	12–24 days	As long as swelling of glands lasts.	Fever, pain and swelling of face and under the jaw.
Measles (*Rubeola*)	Virus	By direct contact, coughing, sneezing, etc.	10–14 days	A day before the rash and throughout its appearance	Fever, running nose and eyes, Koplik spots, cough, rash.
German measles (*Rubella*)	Virus	By direct contact, coughing, sneezing, etc.	14–21 days	2 days before and 3 days after rash appears.	Fever, symptoms of cold, enlarged glands in back of neck.
Chickenpox (*Varicella*)	Virus	By direct contact, coughing, sneezing, etc.	14–21 days	A day before appearance of rash and 6 days after.	Fever, pock rash, scabs, itching.
Whooping cough (*Pertussis*)	Pertussis Bacillus	By direct contact, coughing, sneezing, etc.	7–10 days	During coughing spells; usually about 4 weeks.	Onset like that of cold, then characteristic cough develops.

Disease	Cause	How Transmitted	Incubation Period	When Contagious?	Symptoms
Scarlet fever (*Scarlatina*)	Strepto-coccus	By direct contact, contaminated milk, clothing.	3–6 days	From onset of symptoms and a week thereafter.	Fever, sore throat, headache, vomiting, and characteristic rash.
Poliomyelitis (*Infantile paralysis*)	Polio Virus, Types I, II, III.	By direct contact possibly through food or water.	7–14 days	2 days before onset and 4–6 weeks thereafter.	Fever, headache, vomiting, sore throat, diarrhea, stiff neck, pains, paralysis.
Diphtheria	Diphtheria Bacillus	Contact with patient or carrier.	2–5 days	From onset of symptoms and 2 weeks thereafter.	Fever, sore throat, characteristic membrane in throat.
AIDS	HIV Virus	Contact with bodily fluids of carrier	Days to years	From onset.	*See AIDS.*

Disease	Rash Characteristics	Possible Complications	Treatment	Prevention or Immunization	Is Quarantine Necessary?	Is Second Attack Possible?
Roseola (*Exanthem Subitum*)	Looks like mild measles. Rash all over body.	Very rarely, convulsions.	None usually required	None	No	No
Mumps (*Parotitis*)	None	Inflammation of testicles, ovaries, pancreas, encephalitis.	Rest in bed, medicine to relieve fever and pain.	For adults, immune serum.	Yes, while swelling of glands persist.	No

Disease	Rash Characteristics	Possible Complications	Treatment	Prevention or Immunization	Is Quarantine Necessary?	Is Second Attack Possible?
Measles (*Rubeola*)	Starts on head, extends on to body. Purplish red spots.	Ear and gland inflammation, pneumonia, encephalitis.	Cough mixture, medicine to reduce fever, sponging.	Gamma globulin on exposure.	Yes, until rash disappears.	No
German measles (*Rubella*)	Appears as a light, mild measles rash.	None	None usually required.	When patient is pregnant, gamma globulin.	No	No
Chicken pox* (*Varicella*)	Individual blisters, scabs, crusts over face and body.	Occasional pneumonia, rarely encephalitis.	None usually, except to relieve fever and itching.	Chickenpox vaccine injection.	No	No
Whooping cough (*Pertussis*)	None	Pneumonia, encephalitis.	Antibiotic drugs and injections of immune serum.	Vaccine injections in early childhood.	Yes, for about 4 weeks.	No
Scarlet fever (*Scarlatina*)	Pinpoint scarlet rash on body; little or none on face.	Inflammation of ears, glands, kidneys, rheumatic fever.	Penicillin or other antibiotic drugs.	Penicillin for 3–4 days after exposure.	Yes, for 7–10 days.	No

*Aspirin and salicylate-containing medications may increase the likelihood of Reye's Syndrome. Consult your physician before using.

Disease	Rash Characteristics	Possible Complications	Treatment	Prevention or Immunization	Is Quarantine Necessary?	Is Second Attack Possible?
Poliomyelitis (*Infantile paralysis*)	None	Brain involvement (Bulbar). Paralysis of respiration, etc.	Respirator, if necessary. Orthopedic care for paralysis.	Polio vaccine.	Yes, 1 month.	Each type conveys its own permanent immunity.
Diphtheria	None	Inflammation of heart muscle, paralysis of palate, neuritis.	Diphtheria antitoxin, antibiotics	Diphtheria toxoid in early childhood.	Yes, until throat cultures are normal.	Yes, unless booster shots are given.

VII. DIETS

1. NORMAL ADULT DIET

(A total of approximately ten glasses of liquids should be consumed during each twenty-four hours.)

Breakfast	Lunch	Dinner
1 piece of any fruit, or several prunes or figs, or fruit juice.	1 meat or egg sandwich, or any meat, fish, vegetable or fruit salad, or 1 portion of meat.	1 portion of meat, fowl or fish.
1/2 cup of any cereal with sugar and milk or cream, or 2 eggs, any style.	1 or 2 vegetables.	1 or 2 vegetables. Green salad. 1 or 2 slices of bread with pat of butter.
1 slice of bread or toast with 1 pat of butter.	1 slice of bread with pat of butter.	Dessert: Fruit, cake, pie, ice cream, etc.
Tea, coffee or milk (sugar and milk or cream may be taken with tea or coffee).	1 piece of fruit or canned fruit, stewed fruit, etc.	Tea, coffee or milk.
	1 glass of milk, tea, or coffee.	

2. ELIMINATION DIET (for allergic persons)*

Foods	Include	Avoid
Breads	Quick bread, yeast bread, crackers—if made without eggs.	Bread or rolls containing eggs or nuts.
Cereals	All, except———	Chocolate-flavored cereals.
Soups	All	None
Meat, fish, eggs or cheese	Any meat or fowl except fresh pork. Cottage cheese.	Fresh pork, fish, seafood, eggs, all cheeses except cottage cheese.
Vegetables	All, except———	Corn, tomatoes.
Potato or substitute	Potato, hominy, rice, macaroni.	Noodles containing eggs.
Fats	Butter, cream, French dressing without pepper, lard, margarine, oil.	Salad dressings containing eggs or pepper.

*Courtesy of *The New Illustrated Medical Encyclopedia for Home Use,* Abradale Press, N.Y.

ELIMINATION DIET (for allergic persons)
(Concluded)

Foods	Include	Avoid
Fruits	All fruits, except——	Fresh strawberries, raspberries, huckleberries, blackberries, melon.
Desserts	Cakes, cookies, gelatin, puddings, ice cream—if prepared without eggs, chocolate, cocoa or nuts.	Baked custard, desserts containing eggs, chocolate, cocoa or nuts.
Sweets	Candy, jelly, sugar, honey, syrup.	Chocolate, nuts, candy containing eggs.
Beverages	Carbonated beverages, decaffeinated coffee, milk.	Cocoa, chocolate, coffee, tea.

3. GOUT DIET*
(Low Purine)

Foods	Include	Avoid
Breads	All	None
Cereals	All	None
Soups	Milk soups made with vegetables.	Bouillon, broth, consommé.
Meat, fish, eggs or cheese	Fish, fowl, shellfish, meats (except those listed), eggs, cheese.	Kidney, liver, meat extracts sweetbreads, roe, sardines, anchovies, gravy, broth, bouillon.
Potato or substitute	White potato, sweet potato, hominy, macaroni, rice.	Fried potato, potato chips.
Fats	Butter	None
Vegetables	All (except those listed)	Asparagus, beans, lentils, mushrooms, peas, spinach.
Desserts	Simple cakes, cookies, custard, gelatin, pudding, etc.	Mince pie.
Sweets	All	None

*Courtesy of *The New Illustrated Medical Encyclopedia for Home Use,* Abradale Press, N.Y.

3. GOUT DIET*
(Low Purine) (Concluded)

Foods	Include	Avoid
Beverages	Carbonated beverages, coffee, milk, tea.	None
Miscellaneous	Spices, cream sauces, nuts, salt, condiments.	Alcohol, gravy, yeast.

4. HIGH CALORIC
DIET FOR UNDERWEIGHT OR UNDERNOURISHED PEOPLE

Breakfast	Lunch	Dinner
Fruit juice with sugar or grapefruit with sugar	1 (or 2) meat or egg sandwich, or 1 large portion of meat or fowl.	1 plate of cream soup.
1 cup of cereal with cream and sugar.	2 vegetables with butter.	1 large portion of meat, fish or fowl.
2 scrambled or fried eggs.	1 potato, or portion of spaghetti or noodles.	1 potato, or portion of spaghetti or noodles.
2–3 slices of bread or toast with butter and jam.	2–3 slices of bread and butter.	2 vegetables with butter.
Tea or coffee with cream and sugar.	Dessert: Fruit, cake, pie, ice cream, etc.	2–3 slices of bread and butter.
	Milk with cream.	Green salad with Russian or Roquefort dressing.
		Dessert: Same as for lunch.

	Midday Snack	**Bedtime Snack**
	Malted milk, ice cream soda, eggnog, with cake or crackers.	Sandwich or delicatessen and milk, tea or coffee with cream and sugar.

5. LIQUID DIET

Broths, strained cream soups.
Tomato juice, carrot juice, fruit juice.
Raw eggs in beverages.
Custards, gelatins, junket, sherbet, ice cream.
Water, tea, milk, milk drinks, coffee, carbonated beverages.

*Courtesy of *The New Illustrated Medical Encyclopedia for Home Use,* Abradale Press, N.Y.

6. LOW CALORIC DIET FOR OVERWEIGHT PEOPLE

Breakfast	Lunch	Dinner
Orange juice or 1/2 grapefruit (no sugar)	Vegetable, meat, fish or fruit salad with juice of lemon and/or vinegar, or 1 portion of lean meat.	1 portion of boiled or broiled lean meat, fish or fowl.
1 boiled egg		2 vegetables such as: spinach, lettuce, tomato, celery, cucumber, cabbage, onion, peppers, asparagus, string beans, etc.
1 slice of toast	Dessert: 1 portion of fresh fruit or low-sugar canned fruit.	
1 cup of tea or coffee with saccharin and milk.	Tea, coffee, with saccharin and skimmed milk.	Dessert: Jell-O, fresh or stewed fruit.
		Tea, coffee or skimmed milk.

Avoid

Bread, rolls, crackers, butter, cream, cheese, beans, potato, noodles, spaghetti, cereals, sugar, nuts, cake, pie, pastry, ice cream, candy, gravies, sauces, fried foods, meat fats, etc.

7. LOW CARBOHYDRATE (SUGAR) DIET

Breakfast	Lunch	Dinner
1 portion of fruit, canned or stewed without sugar.	Meat, fish, seafood, vegetable or fresh fruit salad.	Clear soup.
2 soft or hard boiled eggs.	2 salt crackers	1 portion of any meat, fish, seafood or fowl.
1 slice of bread or toast.	Gelatin sweetened with saccharin.	Any 2 of the following vegetables: asparagus, string beans, water cress, celery, cucumber, cabbage, tomato, lettuce, eggplant, beets, carrot, endive.
Coffee or tea with saccharin, or milk.	Tea, milk or coffee.	
		Unsweetened canned fruit, or fresh fruit or gelatin.
		Tea, milk or coffee with saccharin.

Avoid

More than 1 slice of bread, potato, noodles, spaghetti, macaroni, lima beans, baked beans, corn, rice, gravies, sugar, cake, pie, pastry, ice cream, carbonated beverages, sweetened canned fruits, nuts, cream sauces, beer.

8. LOW FAT, LOW CHOLESTEROL, HIGH PROTEIN DIET*

Foods	Include	Avoid
Meat and other protein foods	Lean meats (trim off fat): veal, beef, ham, chicken, turkey, lamb. Non-oily fish: haddock, cod, halibut, fresh water fish, flounder, blue fish, bass. White of egg only.	Fried meats, fat meats, fresh pork, egg yolk, fish canned in oil, mackerel, herring, salmon, shad, brains, tuna, liver,† sweet-breads,† shell fish,† bacon,† kidney†
Fats	Margarine, corn oil, peanut oil, vegetable shortening used sparingly.	Butter, lard, suet and other animal fats.
Cereals	Any cereals (preferably whole grain), bread, wheat cakes made without eggs, macaroni, spaghetti, noodles made without eggs.	Noodles made with eggs, breads and hot breads made with eggs.
Dairy products	Skim milk, butter milk, cheese made from skim milk (nonfat cottage cheese).	Whole milk, cream, most cheeses, ice cream.
Fruits	Any fruit or juice.	Avocado.
Vegetables	Potatoes, baked without butter, or mashed with water or skim milk, any vegetable prepared without oil or fat.	None
Desserts and Sweets	Gelatin desserts, ices and sherbets, tapioca and rice puddings made with fruit and juices. Plain cookies, angel food and other cakes made without egg yolks and butter. Jams, jellies, honey, candy, made without butter or cream.	Rich desserts made with fat, cream, egg yolks. Rich candy made with butter. Ice cream, pastry, choco-late.

*Courtesy of U.S. Vitamin and Pharmaceutical Corp.
†Note: The following foods are of high nutritive value, but are omitted from the diet be-cause of their moderate cholesterol content. Any one (but not more than one) of these foods may be eaten once a day in amount not to exceed that suggested:

Liver—3 ounces	Lobster—3 ounces
Kidney—3 ounces	Canadian bacon—3 ounces
Sweetbreads—3 ounces	Peanut butter—1 tablespoon

Whole milk—1 glass (6 oz.)

8. LOW FAT, LOW CHOLESTEROL, HIGH PROTEIN DIET
(Concluded)

Foods	Include	Avoid
Beverages	Tea, coffee, cereal drinks, buttermilk, skim milk, soft drinks.	Whole milk, alcohol.
Soups, etc.	Clear broth, vegetable soup made without whole milk or fat.	Cream soups, gravies, cream sauce.
Miscellaneous	Salt, spices, vinegar, popcorn without butter, relishes, pickles, catsup, low fat yeast extracts.	Olives, mayonnaise, oily dressing, fried foods, potato chips, brewer's yeast.

9. LOW ROUGHAGE, LOW RESIDUE DIET*

Foods	Include	Avoid
Breads	White, enriched or fine rye bread, crackers, toast.	Whole wheat, graham, dark rye bread.
Cereals	Refined cereals, corn, rice, wheat, dry cereals prepared from cooked oatmeal.	Whole grain cereals.
Soups	Bouillon, broth.	Cream soups, vegetable soup.
Meat, fish, eggs or cheese	Bacon, tender meat, fish, fowl, canned fish, eggs, cheese.	Tough meat.
Vegetables	None.	All.
Potato or substitute	Potato, macaroni, noodles, refined rice.	Hominy, unrefined rice.
Fats	Butter, cream, margarine.	None.
Fruits	None.	All.
Desserts	Plain cakes, cookies, custard, gelatin, ice cream, pie, pudding, all without fruits or nuts.	Desserts containing fruits or nuts.

*Courtesy of *The New Illustrated Medical Encyclopedia for Home Use*, Abradale Press, N.Y.

9. LOW ROUGHAGE, LOW RESIDUE DIET
(Concluded)

Foods	Include	Avoid
Sweets	Hard candy, jelly, syrup, honey.	Candy containing fruits, jams or nuts.
Miscella-neous	Cream sauce, gravy, peanut butter, vinegar.	Nuts, olives, pickles, pop-corn, relish.

10. LOW SALT (Low Sodium) DIET*

Foods	Include	Avoid
Meat and meat substitutes	Lamb, beef, pork, veal, rabbit, liver, chicken, turkey, duck, goose, fresh cod, halibut, fresh salmon, fresh water fish, one egg daily.	Salted, canned, smoked meats, frankfurters, bacon, ham, sausage, liverwurst and other spiced meats, brain, kidney, tongue, salt or canned fish, haddock, shellfish (oysters, clams, lobster, shrimp), salt pork.
Vegetables	Fresh, frozen or specially canned without salt: asparagus, string beans, broccoli, brussel sprouts, cabbage, cauliflower, corn, cucumber, eggplant, endive, lettuce, mushrooms, okra, onions, parsnips, peas, peppers, potato, rutabaga, soybeans, squash, sweet potato, tomato, lima beans.	All canned vegetables and relishes, beets, beet greens, chard kale, celery, spinach, sauerkraut, rhubarb, potato chips, pickles.
Fruits	Any raw, cooked, canned fruit or juice, apricots, avocado, banana, blackberries, blueberries, cranberries, dates, grapes, grapefruit, lemons, oranges, peaches, pears, pineapple, plums, raspberries, strawberries . . . and other fresh and frozen fruits.	Dried fruits containing benzoate of soda, raisins, prunes.

*Courtesy of *The New Illustrated Medical Encyclopedia for Home Use,* Abradale Press, N.Y.

10. LOW SALT (Low Sodium) DIET
(Concluded)

Foods	Include	Avoid
Cereals and bread	Salt-free cereal: barley, farina, oatmeal, pettijohn's, ralston, rice, wheatena, puffed wheat or rice, shredded wheat, macaroni, spaghetti, noodles, yeast bread prepared without salt.	Most commercially prepared cereals, bread, crackers, pretzels, hot bread, etc. made with salt, baking powder or soda.
Desserts	Ice cream or puddings made with milk allowance, unsalted fruit pies, gelatin desserts, custards.	Those prepared with salt, baking powder or soda, or egg white.
Soups	Unsalted soups and broths, cream soups out of milk allowance.	Canned soups, and those made with bouillon cubes.
Dairy products	Whole milk 1 pt. per day (dialyzed milk may be used more freely, if available), unsalted cottage cheese— 1 oz. per day, unsalted butter, homemade ice cream, cream—1/3 cup per day.	All hard cheeses, all salted cheeses, salt butter, oleomargarine, buttermilk, commercial ice cream.
Beverages	Coffee, tea, cocoa, wine, fruit juices; beer and soft drinks—8 oz. per day.	
Fats	Lard, oil, vegetable fat.	Salted shortening, bacon fat, salad dressing.
Seasonings, condiments	Pepper, garlic, paprika, vinegar, herbs, dry mustard, onion, vanilla, lemon, cinnamon.	Catsup, chili sauce, prepared horse radish, pickles, relishes, steak sauce, salad dressings.
Miscellaneous	Sugar, syrup, candy, jam or jelly made without benzoate of soda, unsalted nuts, popcorn.	Olives, salted nuts and peanut butter.

11. DIET FOR PEOPLE WITH ULCER
OF STOMACH OR DUODENUM

Foods Permitted

Breads

White toast, crackers, rolls.

Cereals

Farina, cream of wheat, rice.

Soups

Cream soups, such as asparagus, tomato, beets, pea.

Meats, fish, eggs or cheese

Scraped beef, minced white meat of chicken, lamb chops, broiled liver, sweetbreads, fresh fish, salmon, eggs, cottage or cream cheese.

Vegetables

Cooked beets, asparagus, carrots, peas, beets, squash, string beans.

Potato, etc.

Baked or mashed potato, corn purée, lima bean purée, macaroni, noodles, rice.

Butter

Butter, margarine, cream.

Fruits

Avocado, banana, canned or stewed apples, apricots, cherries, peaches, pears. Dilute orange juice, prune juice, prune whip.

Desserts

Sponge cake, crackers, cookies, custard, jello, rice or bread pudding, ice cream, sherbet.

Sweets

Jellies, plain candies, sugar, honey.

Beverages

Milk, milk drinks, tea, decaffeinated coffee.

General Instructions

1. Eat, or drink milk every 2 to 3 hours.
2. Drink milk and eat lightly before retiring at night and if you wake up during the night.
3. Eat slowly and chew food thoroughly.
4. Adhere strictly to diet and *AVOID* the following: SMOKING; ALCOHOL; COFFEE; and mustard, chili sauce, horse radish, other spices and condiments. Also avoid gravies, hot sauces, nuts, pickles, etc.

VIII. DRUG DOSES*

Liquids

Apothecary doses	Metric System doses
1 quart	1000 cc.† ml††
1 pint	500 cc. ml
8 fluid ounces	240 cc. ml
3 ½ fluid ounces	100 cc. ml
1 fluid ounce	30 cc. ml
4 fluid drams	15 cc. ml
1 fluid dram	4 cc. ml
15 minims (drops)	1 cc. ml
1 minim (drop)	0.06 cc. ml

Solids

Apothecary doses	Metric System doses
1 ounce	30 grams
4 drams	15 grams
1 dram	4 grams
60 grains (1 dram)	4 grams
30 grains (1/2 dram)	2 grams
15 grains	1 gram
10 grains	0.6 grams
1 grain	60 milligrams (mg.)
¾ grain	50 mg.
½ grain	30 mg.
¼ grain	15 mg.
⅛ grain	10 mg.
1/10 grain	6 mg.
1/100 grain	0.6 mg.

*All equivalents are approximate.
† A cubic centimeter (cc.) is 1/1000 of a liter.
†† A milliliter is 1/1000 of a liter.

COMPARATIVE MEASURES

Liquids

1 teaspoonful	1 fluid dram	4 cc.
1 dessertspoonful	2 fluid drams	8 cc.
1 tablespoonful	1/2 fluid ounce	15 cc.
1 teacupful	4 fluid ounces	120 cc.
1 tumbler glassful	8 fluid ounces	240 cc.

Lengths

1 meter (M.)	39.37	inches
1 centimeter (cm.)	0.4	inches
2.5 centimeters	1.0	inch
1 millimeter	0.04	inches
25 millimeters	1.0	inch

IX. FIRST AID

1. CARDIOPULMONARY RESUSCITATION (CPR)
including ARTIFICIAL RESPIRATION*

a. Apply to all cases where breathing has stopped, from whatever cause. To determine this:
  1. Look to see if the chest is moving up and down.
  2. Listen to hear if there are breath sounds.
  3. Put your cheek next to the victim's mouth to note whether you feel his or her breath.

b. Stretch out the victim gently on his/her back and loosen any tight clothing around the neck or chest.

c. Lift up the chin and tilt head back as far as possible. This straightens out the windpipe and improves the airway to the lungs.

d. Pinch the nostrils closed while the heel of your hand presses on the forehead. This keeps the head tilted back.

e. Place your mouth tightly over the victim's mouth and give two full breaths. Do *not* release the fingers pinching the nostrils closed.

f. Take your mouth away to permit air to be expelled from the lungs.

g. Quickly, feel the neck next to the windpipe to note any pulsation. If no pulsations are felt, *closed cardiac massage* should be started immediately.

h. Also, if no pulsations are felt, send someone to call 911 and ask for Emergency Medical help.

i. To perform closed cardiac massage (which includes *artificial respiration*), kneel at the victim's side near the chest. Locate the spot where the two sides of the rib cage meet in the midline.

j. Place the heel of one hand on the breastbone above the spot where the two sides of ribs come together. Place the other hand on top.

k. Bring your shoulders directly over the victim's breastbone and press downward, keeping your arms straight. Push down the breastbone about 1½ to 2 inches. (In *infants and children*, only depress the breastbone for about 1/2 to 1 inch.) RELEASE IMMEDIATELY and REPEAT approximately 80 to 100 TIMES per MINUTE (*infants and children*, repeat 100 TIMES per MINUTE).

l. Do *NOT* remove your hands from the chest in between compressions.

m. Stop momentarily after 15 *compressions* and give two full breaths of mouth-to-mouth breathing. Pinch nose while so doing.

n. Continue until breathing and pulse resume! It can take several hours to revive someone.

o. When you tire, have someone substitute for you.

p. If the patient seems to have water or mucus in his throat or chest, tilt him upside down or on his side to permit such fluid to run out the mouth.

q. Wipe out patient's mouth with your fingers if mucus or other material collects there. (A nonbreathing person will never bite.)

r. If you are squeamish about direct mouth-to-mouth contact, you may

---

*The mouth-to-mouth method has replaced older methods, and is advocated by most medical organizations.

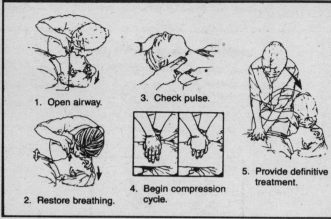

1. Open airway.
2. Restore breathing.
3. Check pulse.
4. Begin compression cycle.
5. Provide definitive treatment.

Artificial respiration (mouth to mouth breathing)

blow through an opened handkerchief. (This may not prove to be as effective as direct contact.)

s. Discontinue artificial respiration only when you are certain there is no pulse or heartbeat for several minutes. Listen carefully with your ear to patient's left chest region.

t. If patient is revived, keep him warm and do not move him until the doctor arrives, or at least for one-half hour.

2. BITES

A. Animal or Human Bites

1. Scrub wound thoroughly for 5–10 minutes with soap and plenty of water.
2. Apply a sterile gauze bandage, or if this is not available, use a clean handkerchief.
3. Take patient to a doctor who may give tetanus antitoxin, tetanus toxoid, or possibly, antibiotics. If the bite has been caused by a dog, cat, rat or other animal, your physician may recommend anti-rabies injections.
4. Do NOT pour strong antiseptics, such as iodine, on a wound caused by a bite.

B. Insect Bites

1. If a sting has been left in place, such as with a bee, wasp, etc., pluck it out. Do so gently, in order to avoid breaking the sting.
2. If a great deal of swelling is present, this indicates a marked sensitivity to the bite poison. In such cases, place a tourniquet

above the bite area so that the poison will be more slowly absorbed.

3. If the bite is caused by an insect which burrows under the skin, such as a chigger, or by one which attaches itself to the skin, such as a tick, wash the area thoroughly with soap and water. A drop or two of turpentine may dislodge a tick or kill a chigger. Cover with Vaseline so that the insect cannot breathe.

4. Antiallergic (antihistamine) medications may be prescribed by your physician to reduce the swelling and itching.

5. Do NOT scratch a bite area as it may lead to greater absorption of the poison or to infection.

6. If the bite has been caused by a black widow spider, treat as a snake bite.

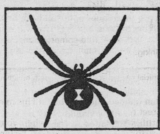

Black Widow Spider

C. Snake Bites

1. Treat all snake bites as if they have been caused by poisonous snakes, unless you are thoroughly familiar with the various types of snakes.

2. A tourniquet should be placed above the site of the bite. Do this immediately.

3. Crossed incisions *through* the skin should be made over the two fang marks. A penknife may be used. Do not wait to sterilize it. The incisions should be ¼ inch long.

4. The bite should be sucked out thoroughly. (No harm can come from swallowing, or taking into the mouth, the venom of a poisonous snake.)

5. The tourniquet should be loosened every 20 minutes for 2-3 minutes and then reapplied.

6. Suction to the wound should be repeated every 5 minutes for an hour.

7. Have victim lie down and keep quiet, so as to reduce circulation.

8. If ice, or running cold water, is available immerse the bitten area so as to reduce circulation.

9. Take victim to nearest hospital so that the appropriate antivenin can be administered.

10. If possible, kill the snake and take it to the hospital so that it can be identified. (Antivenin is effective only for the specific type of snake causing the bite.)

3. BLEEDING OR HEMORRHAGE

a. Have patient lie down flat.

b. Place sterile gauze pad, sanitary napkin, clean handkerchief, etc., directly over the wound.

c. Apply direct, firm pressure (with your fingers or hand) over the wound; continue pressure for 5–15 minutes.

d. If bleeding does not stop with prolonged direct pressure, and the wound is in the arm or leg, apply a tourniquet for 10–15 minutes. Release to see if bleeding has stopped. If not, reapply tourniquet and transport patient to nearest doctor.

e. Do NOT apply a tourniquet until you have first tried pressure upon arteries supplying the arm and leg. This will often stop the bleeding and make the use of a tourniquet unnecessary. (These pressure points are located on the inner side of the upper arm and just below the groin.)

f. Most bleeding, unless from a major vessel, will stop within a few minutes. Clean wound thoroughly with plain soap and water. If bleeding is too active, apply a tourniquet for 10 minutes in order to thoroughly cleanse the wound.

g. Bandage to stop bleeding should NOT be applied so tightly that it will interfere with circulation. If the patient feels it is too tight, or if the tissue below the bandage turns blue in color, cut the bandage down the middle and apply new bandage material more loosely *over* the original bandage.

h. Take patient to doctor for possible further cleansing and stitching of the wound.

i. Internal bleeding will usually evidence itself by the coughing up or vomiting of blood or "coffee ground" appearing material. Bleeding from the urinary tract will show itself upon passage of bloody urine. Bleeding from the intestinal tract will show itself by blood in the stool or by passage of back, tarry stools. Have such a patient:
   1. Lie flat.
   2. Breathe deeply.
   3. Transport him as soon as possible to a hospital.
   4. Do NOT attempt to give medicines to such patients.

j. Bleeding from areas where tourniquets can not be applied, such as the neck, should be treated by applying direct finger pressure over the wound. Keep pressure in place until doctor arrives.

4. BURNS

a. *First degree burns* extend only to the top layers of the skin. They can usually be self-treated by applying plain Vaseline or any other mild ointment which soothes the reddened area and prevents the skin from becoming too dry. (Sunburn, without blister formation, is the most common type of first degree burn.)

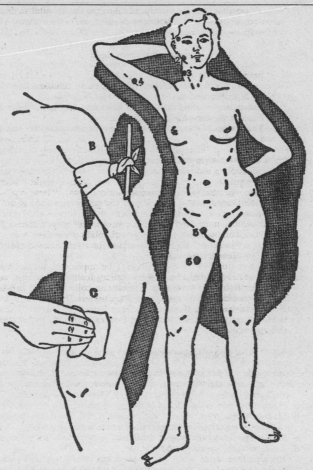

A. Pressure points
1. To stop bleeding from front of scalp
2. To stop bleeding from face
3. To stop jugular vein bleeding
4. To stop bleeding from arm and hand
5. To stop bleeding from thigh and leg
6. To stop bleeding from leg
B. Tourniquet applied to stop bleeding from arm and hand
C. Diagram showing direct pressure to stop local bleeding

b. *Second degree burns* extend deeper into the skin than first degree burns but do not involve the very deepest layer, the corium. They can be diagnosed by noting blisters and destruction of the top layers of skin.

    1. Such burned areas should be immediately placed under cold running water for 10–15 minutes and, if dirty, mild (soap) cleansing should be carried out.
    2. A clean, sterile gauze dressing should be applied.
    3. The patient should drink large quantities of fluids.
    4. Blisters should NOT be opened.
    5. The patient should be taken to a physician for further treatment.

c. *Third and Fourth degree burns* extend to or through all the layers of the skin. First aid should include:

    1. Place area under cold, running water.
    2. Gently clean away dirt. If clothes can be removed from the burned area, without pulling away tissue, this should be done.
    3. Do NOT put butter or ointments on deep burned areas.
    4. Patients should be given large quantities of fluids.
    5. If patient is in shock, he should be covered with blanket and transported, on a stretcher, to the nearest hospital.

d. *Chemical burns* should be flushed with cold running water to wash away the chemical. Cover the burned area with a sterile dressing. Patient should then be taken to a doctor.
e. *Eye burns* should be flushed with large amounts of water. The eye should then be covered with a sterile dressing and the patient taken to a physician.

5. CARBON MONOXIDE (GAS) POISONING

Carbon monoxide gas has no odor. It may originate from the exhaust of an automobile, or from defective stoves burning wood, coal or oil, etc.

a. Open all windows and doors to permit fresh air into the area.
b. Start artificial respiration if the patient is not breathing spontaneously or regularly. Continue as long as the heart is beating.
c. Encourage deep breathing of fresh air.
d. Keep patient lying down quietly.
e. Keep patient warm.
f. Notify the police or fire department, who will respond with emergency equipment.

6. CHOKING

a. Encourage coughing.
b. If a child, hold upside down and slap on back.
c. If obstructing object is not expelled, place both arms around victim's waist just below the rib cage. With a sudden inward and upward thrust, the grip on the victim is tightened as forcefully as possible.

Usually, this will force the offending object out of the windpipe. Repeat at least six or more times, if first thrust is not successful (Heimlich maneuver).

d. If victim becomes unconscious, open his mouth and insert your index finger as far back as possible to see if you can grab or dislodge the material causing the choking. (An unconscious person will *not bite* you!)

e. If the victim turns blue and cannot breathe at all, and if a doctor is not available—*and only when it is obvious that death will ensue*—an emergency tracheotomy may be performed. This is done by stabbing a hole with a knife into the windpipe below the Adam's apple. The hole is kept open, so that air can pass in and out of it, by twisting the knife blade.

f. If patient continues to choke, but is able to breathe, take him immediately to the nearest doctor or hospital.

g. If the offending object has not been coughed up, take patient to doctor even if the choking has subsided. Some foreign bodies go deep into the bronchial tubes, where they will eventually cause infection.

COLD. *See* Exposure, Frostbite.

7. CONVULSIONS AND "FITS"

a. Prevent further self-injury by protecting the patient, particularly the head.

b. Place patient on the floor or ground and give plenty of room for him to thrash about.

c. Loosen clothing around the neck and lift up the chin so that breathing is unobstructed.

d. Do NOT attempt to prevent tongue biting by placing anything in the patient's mouth. Keep your fingers away from patient's teeth, to avoid being accidentally bitten.

e. Do NOT throw cold water on these patients in an attempt to revive them.

f. Do NOT try to restrain their convulsive movements.

g. Most convulsions last only a few minutes. After recovery, comfort the patient, keep him quiet, and send for a physician.

h. Do not leave a patient alone, after he has emerged from a convulsion, for at least one-half hour. (They are often confused and it may take this length of time for them to fully regain their normal mental and physical senses.)

i. Search the patient's clothing for information. Epileptics and diabetics often carry instructions on what should be done for them.

j. Do NOT pick up a convulsing child and run for a doctor. It is better to keep him in his own bed.

k. Do NOT place a convulsing child in water. Keep him in bed.

8. DISLOCATIONS

a. Do NOT try to replace a dislocation yourself.

b. If a doctor is nearby, transport patient with as little movement of the joint as possible.

c. If you are a long distance from a hospital or doctor, bind the dislocated limb with a towel, bandage, etc., so that it does not move.
1. Gently tie dislocated ankle, knee or leg to the normal limb on the other side.
2. Bind the arm, in which there is a dislocation, to the chest and abdomen.

d. If neck dislocation is suspected, firmly pull on head and hold it in a straight position without permitting movement.

9. DROWNING. *See* also Cardiopulmonary Resuscitation.

a. If patient is breathing, place him on his abdomen with head turned to one side.

b. Do NOT place over a barrel or attempt to hold upside down. Water from the lungs will be brought up spontaneously if the patient is breathing.

c. If the patient is not breathing, place flat on his *back,* lift up the chin and commence artificial respiration.

d. If mouth-to-mouth breathing does not get air into the lungs, it indicates a severe spasm of the larynx. Continued spasm may require an emergency tracheotomy (*See* Choking) *but by other than a doctor, this should be done only when it is obvious that the patient is not getting air into the lungs and is dying.*

e. Continue artificial respiration as long as there is any pulse or heartbeat. This may mean hours!

f. Send for doctor, police or fire department, as soon as possible.

10. ELECTRIC SHOCK

a. Do NOT touch a person who is still in contact with an electric current. This may electrocute you.

b. Remove electric contact from patient, or the patient from electric contact, as quickly as possible.
1. Use a *dry* stick to shove away wire or to move the patient.
2. Cut off the source of current, such as an electric plug, if this is possible, or
3. Use an axe, with a wooden handle, to chop the wire bearing the current.
4. Do NOT attempt to remove a victim from his electric contact unless your body and hands are dry and you are standing on dry ground or on a dry surface.

c. If victim is not breathing, start mouth-to-mouth artificial respiration. Continue so long as there is any pulse or heartbeat.

d. Keep victim warm.

e. Send for doctor, police or fire department, for additional help in resuscitation.

f. Give first aid to any burned area on body. (*See* Burns)

11. EXPOSURE (COLD) *See* also Frostbite

a. Wrap patient in blankets.
b. Place in warm room.
c. Place in tub of warm (not too hot) water.
d. Dry body and place in warm bed.
e. Give warm drinks.
f. Do NOT give alcoholic beverage.
g. If necessary, start mouth-to-mouth artificial respiration.

12. FAINTING, DIZZINESS, AND VERTIGO

a. Place patient in a lying-down position with face up and head at body level or slightly lower.
b. Elevate legs to slightly above level of rest of body. (Use pillow, coat, blanket, etc.)
c. Loosen collar or any tight clothing that might interfere with breathing.
d. If breathing is shallow or stops, apply mouth-to-mouth method of artificial respiration.
e. Keep in lying-down position at least 15 minutes after regaining consciousness.
f. Do NOT throw cold water in face.
g. Examine head to make sure patient did not injure himself, if he fell during faint.
h. If patient has merely had dizziness, or vertigo, do not permit him to arise until the symptoms have completely disappeared.
i. If the fainting, dizziness or vertigo persists for more than a few minutes, call a physician.

13. FOREIGN BODIES

A. Eyes

1. Blink eyelids repeatedly to stimulate flow of tears which may wash out foreign body.
2. Do NOT rub eye. (This merely makes foreign body embed itself deeper.)
3. Wash out eye by dropping in drops of lukewarm water.
4. Draw down lower lid. If foreign body is embedded in lower lid, take moistened edge of clean handkerchief and gently wipe it off.
5. Bend up upper lid. If foreign body is embedded in upper lid, take moistened edge of clean handkerchief and gently wipe it off.
6. If foreign body is embedded in the pupil or in the colored portion of the eye, do NOT try to remove it. See a doctor.
7. If foreign body has been removed, irritation of the eye can be relieved by dropping in a drop or two of mineral oil or castor oil.

B. Ears

1. No lasting harm can come from a foreign body in the ear. Therefore, do NOT get excited or put a sharp instrument into the ear canal.
2. Have patient lie down and pour in sufficient mineral oil, castor oil or olive oil to fill the canal. Permit it to stay there a few minutes. This will usually float out or dislodge a foreign body.
3. If foreign body does not come out, take patient to a physician.

C. Nose

1. Stimulate sneezing by having patient sniff pepper or by tickling the opposite nostril. This will usually dislodge a foreign body.
2. If foreign body is not extruded, take patient to a physician.

D. Splinters

1. Only those splinters which protrude from the skin surface should be removed by nonmedical personnel.
2. Grasp firmly and withdraw slowly so as not to break.
3. Apply peroxide or alcohol to area, and cover with sterile bandage.
4. If splinter breaks off beneath the skin, take patient to a physician. Most foreign bodies become infected if permitted to remain in place.
5. Do NOT try to probe deep into the skin for a splinter. You may spread infection or push it deeper!

E. Dirt in Cuts or Lacerations (See *Lacerations, Abrasions and Contusions*)

F. Swallowed Foreign Bodies

1. Rounded objects such as marbles, nickles, dimes, buttons, etc., usually pass through the intestinal tract without causing any disturbance. Strain the stool daily and note its passage.
2. Open pins, needles, nails, if swallowed, may cause trouble but the majority of them do pass through uneventfully. However, see your doctor. He will X-ray the child and will advise further treatment, if necessary. Strain stool to note passage.
3. Do NOT give laxatives to children who have swallowed foreign bodies.
4. Give normal diet.
5. Call physician if child has trouble in breathing or has abdominal pain.

14. FRACTURES AND SEVERE SPRAINS

a. If medical aid is available, do NOT move the patient or the injured part. Permit NO weight-bearing!

b. Do NOT try to push back a broken bone if it protrudes from the skin.

c. Do NOT try to straighten a fracture yourself, if a physician will become available.

d. Keep the patient warm.

e. If patient must be moved, *splint* the broken bones before moving:

    1. An injured collarbone, shoulder or arm should be splinted by wrapping the arm securely to the body. Do NOT bend the arm if it is found in a hanging position. If found with elbow bent, then splint it in that position.

    2. Splint fractured leg in a straight position and then tie it to opposite leg, so as to prevent movement.

    3. A cane, umbrella, straight pieces of wood, etc., can be used as a splint. A torn shirt, or handkerchiefs, can be used as bandage material.

    4. Always pad with something, such as a piece of clothing, between the splint and the injured part of the body.

f. Transport patient in a lying-down position. A blanket or overcoat may be used as a stretcher if several people are available to carry the patient.

g. Give the same first aid to a sprain as you would to a fracture. A layman can not distinguish between a fracture and sprain.

h. Do NOT apply a tourniquet to limb unless there is uncontrollable bleeding.

i. If the fracture is accompanied by an open wound, cover such wound with a sterile dressing. If this is not available, use a clean handkerchief.

j. Broken Neck or Back:

    1. Do NOT move patient!

    2. Keep body straight.

    3. Do NOT lift the head or bend it forward!

    4. Keep patient lying down.

    5. If patient *must* be moved, place on stomach and transport on blanket, with head straight for back injury. Transport face up for neck injury.

15. FROSTBITE

a. Warm the patient gradually (room temperature).

b. Give warm liquids and food.

c. Thaw out frostbitten parts *slowly*.

d. Give medications to relieve pain (aspirin, etc.).

e. Start moving frostbitten part slowly.

f. Do NOT:

    1. Give alcohol to patient.

    2. Immerse frostbitten part in *hot* water.

    3. Rub frostbitten part.

    4. Apply snow.

g. Keep sterile dressing over frostbitten part, as skin may eventually break, leaving an open wound.

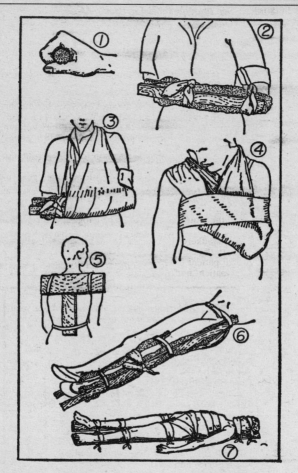

Splints

1. Bandage roll in hand for broken fingers or hand bones (metacarpals)
2. Splints of scrap wood padded with towels for broken forearm
3. Broken forearm supported by a sling
4. Sling and band for broken collarbone or dislocated shoulder
5. "T" board for broken collarbone
6. Splint of scrap wood or tree limbs padded with towels and bound with handkerchiefs and belts
7. Splints for severe back injury or high thigh break or broken pelvis

GAS POISONING. *See* Antidotes and Emergency Measures for Poisoning, Carbon Monoxide Poisoning; also Artificial Respiration.

16. HEAD INJURIES

a. Have patient lie flat on his back.

b. Keep patient warm.

c. Do not permit patient to get up and walk about.

d. If there has been loss of consciousness, patient should be transported to hospital for further observation.

e. If there is bleeding from an ear, it usually indicates a skull fracture.

f. If there is a cut on the head, apply a sterile dressing or clean handkerchief.

g. Do NOT give alcohol or any medication to relieve headache. This may mask symptoms.

h. Patient must be advised to consult a physician within the few hours after a head injury. Some injuries appear trivial at first but then develop into serious injuries within twenty-four hours.

i. Fractured Jaw:

    1. Close the mouth so that teeth come together as closely as possible.

    2. Tie a handkerchief or scarf so that it circles the head, from beneath the chin to the top of the head.

    3. Permit patient to remain in a sitting position.

    4. Urge patient not to attempt to move the jaw or to talk.

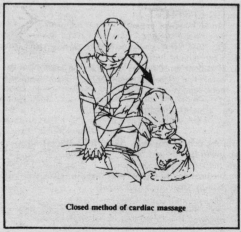

Closed method of cardiac massage

Closed method of cardiac massage (*illustration by George Cornell*)

17. HEART ATTACK

The most common signal of a heart attack is:
- Uncomfortable pressure, squeezing, fullness, or pain in the center of the chest behind the breastbone.

Other signals may be:
- Sweating
- Nausea
- Shortness of breath, or
- A feeling of weakness.

Sometimes these signals subside and return.

Actions for survival

- Recognize the "signals."
- Stop activity and sit or lie down.
- If signals persist 2 minutes or longer, call the local emergency number, usually 911. Until emergency assistance arrives:

a. Do not move patient!
b. Keep patient in semi-sitting position.
c. Open collar, loosen tie and belt.
d. Encourage deep breathing.
e. Give patient medication which he may have in his possession (if he has had previous attacks).
f. If heart stops beating, use "closed method" cardiac massage:
  1. Place patient flat on back.
  2. Kneel beside patient.
  3. Place heel of palm of right hand on patient's breastbone.
  4. Place left hand over your right hand and push down so that breastbone is depressed about 1 1/2 to 2 inches.
  5. Release.
  6. Repeat approximately 80 to 100 times per minute. If breathing has also stopped, commence mouth-to-mouth resuscitation.
  7. If someone else is also available, have him render mouth-to-mouth artificial respiration at the same time as you are conducting cardiac massage.
g. Do not permit a patient who has undergone obvious heart attack to move until he has been examined by a physician. (Pains which have subsided may return with greater intensity if the patient is allowed to exert himself.)

18. HEAT STROKE AND HEAT EXHAUSTION

a. Get patient out of the sun or out of the hot place.
b. Place him in cold water, or, of not possible, keep pouring cold water over him.
c. Wrap in cold, wet sheets or towels.
d. Give cold water to drink (4–5 glasses).
e. Give 1/2 teaspoonful of ordinary table salt with water every half hour for 3 or 4 doses.
f. Give an enema with iced water.
g. Keep patient quiet.
h. Call a doctor

HEMORRHAGE. *See* Bleeding and Hemorrhage.

19. LACERATIONS (CUTS), ABRASIONS, AND CONTUSIONS

a. If you are giving first aid, wash your own hands before touching someone's laceration or abrasion.

b. If possible, place injured part under running, tepid tap water for 5 minutes.

c. With absorbent cotton or sterile gauze, wash out wound for 5 minutes with soapsuds, using any plain soap.

d. If this is done, dirt and pieces of clothing will become dislodged. Wipe away any remaining dirt or clothing.

e. A deep abrasion (scratch or scrape) occurring in dirt or cinders must be scrubbed thoroughly to remove all visible dirt particles. This should be carried out, even if painful, in order to avoid subsequent infection or tetanus (lockjaw).

f. Most superficial wounds will stop bleeding spontaneously unless a large blood vessel has been severed. If marked bleeding and spurting continues, apply a tourniquet above the wound, being sure to release it every 15 minutes.

g. Cover wound with sterile gauze or clean handkerchief. Apply direct, steady pressure to stop bleeding.

h. Do NOT pour alcohol, iodine or other strong antiseptics on an open wound! Soap and water cleansing is much better as a safeguard against infection!

i. If tissues beneath the skin can be seen through the open wound, it is usually an indication that suturing (stitching) will be necessary. Take patient to a surgeon or nearest physician.

j. It is particularly important to get medical care for cuts and abrasions which originate outdoors, in dirty areas. Such wounds are more prone to infection. Wounds incurred in fields where cattle, horses, etc., are present, should be watched for tetanus. Tetanus antitoxin or toxoid is usually given in cases where wounds have resulted from rusty objects.

k. A severe contusion (bruise) should be treated by the application of steady pressure with the hand over the injured area. Ice or cold water should be applied for 20 minutes at a time, with a similar period of withdrawal of the application. Bruises more than a few hours old can no longer be helped by cold applications. Raise the injured part, such as a leg, to body level so that there will be less tendency for blood to gravitate to the area.

l. Pain, redness, heat, swelling or pink streaks leading away from a lacerated area are indications that infection has set in. See a doctor!

20. NOSEBLEED

a. Place patient in a sitting position.

b. Pack the bleeding nostril with a piece of clean absorbent cotton.

c. If there are nosedrops handy, moisten the packing with a few drops as this may help to contract the bleeding vessel.

d. Exert firm finger pressure against the bleeding nostril for at least 20 minutes.

e. Have patient bend head slightly forward during this maneuver. This will prevent blood from trickling down the back of the throat.

f. Leave cotton packing in place for 2–3 hours.

g. If bleeding does not stop, take patient to a doctor who will cauterize the bleeding point.

h. If bleeding is coming from the back part of the nose (only about 10% of cases) the above first aid will not help. Take such people to physicians as soon as possible. Do NOT panic; nosebleeds do not cause healthy people to hemorrhage seriously.

i. Do NOT place a cold key in the back of the neck. It won't help.

POISONING. *See* Section II: ANTIDOTES AND EMERGENCY MEASURES FOR POISONING

21. POISON IVY OR POISON OAK

a. Wash the skin thoroughly with soap and water immediately after contact.

b. Wash with rubbing alcohol to relieve itching.

PUNCTURE WOUNDS. *See* Stab Wounds.

22. RADIATION EXPOSURE

a. Get out of the radiation area as quickly as possible.

b. Cleanse *all* parts of your body in soap and water. Wash over and over again.

c. Discard all clothing, and all other objects, which were with you in an exposed area.

d. Contact the local authorities for further instructions.

23. SHOCK*

a. Place the patient on his back with his feet at a higher level than his head.

b. If there is active bleeding contributing toward the shock, measures should be taken to stop it. *See also* Bleeding.

c. Keep patient warm but do not overheat.

d. If there is severe pain (one of the greatest causes of shock) medication should be given as soon as possible to relieve it.

e. If there is a fractured bone (a frequent contribution toward shock), it should be splinted and immobilized at once.

f. If it can be ascertained positively that there has been no abdominal

---

*The diagnosis of shock can be made by noting the following symptoms and signs:

1. The skin is gray, cold and sweaty.
2. There may or may not be loss of consciousness.
3. Pulse is weak and rapid.
4. Breathing is rapid and shallow.
5. Pupils of the eyes are dilated.
6. Patient is excessively thirsty.
7. If conscious, patient is apprehensive and frightened.

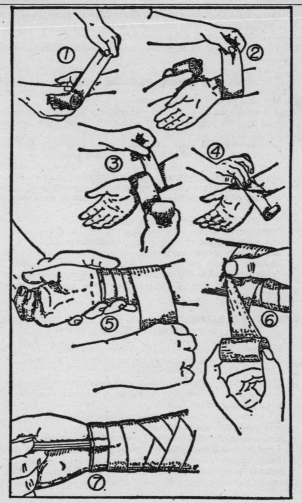

Bandaging
1–4. Steps in the bandage anchor
5. The roller bandage
6. Starting the "reverse" for the spiral reverse bandage for regions whose diameter changes
7. Testing for tightness

injury, and that the cause of the shock does not have anything to do with abdominal organs, then warm fluids may be given.

g. Do NOT give alcohol, tea or coffee!

h. Transport patient in lying-down position to the nearest hospital.

24. STAB WOULDS; PUNCTURE WOUNDS

a. Move the patient as little as possible.

b. If the stabbing object (a knife or pick) can be withdrawn easily, do so. This may prevent further injury to tissues when the patient moves.

c. Note carefully the angle and depth of the stabbing object so that you can report it accurately to the attending physician.

d. If the wound is in the chest, and air is being sucked into and blown out of the chest, cover the opening tightly. It can be plugged best with a sterile gauze dressing and adhesive tape. However, a clean handkerchief, Scotch tape, a tie, etc., can also be used to plug the opening.

e. Stop active bleeding. (*See* Bleeding for method)

f. If any internal organs are protruding through the wound, cover them with a sterile gauze dressing or a clean handkerchief.

g. Stab wounds always require expert care. Take patient to a doctor who will, in most instances, give tetanus antitoxin or toxoid.

h. Small puncture wounds should have their edges spread so as to promote some bleeding and prevent the sealing in of dirt, rust, etc.

25. SUFFOCATION OR STRANGULATION. See also Cardiopulmonary Resuscitation; Carbon monoxide poisoning; Choking.

a. Place patient in open air or throw open all windows.

b. Loosen anything tight around the neck, chest or abdomen.

c. Lift up the chin to improve airway.

d. Wipe away any secretions which may have collected in the mouth.

e. If foreign body is lodged in the throat, turn patient upside down and strike sharply on the back.

f. Put index finger in mouth and try to sweep out any foreign body which may be stuck in back of throat.

g. Encourage deep breathing and then a forceful cough.

h. Employ mouth-to-mouth breathing as described under Artificial Respiration.

i. Summon police or fire department, who will respond with Pulmotor and oxygen.

26. TOOTHACHE

a. Apply a hot water bag or ice bag to the side of the face, whichever gives most relief.

b. Take aspirin or other pain-relieving medications.

c. Call your dentist. You *will* be able to reach him at night if you try.

27. UNCONSCIOUSNESS. See also Fainting.

a. If patient is not breathing but has a pulse or heartbeat, apply mouth-to-mouth breathing.

b. Search the patient's clothing. You may find information that he is a diabetic, epileptic, heart patient, etc.

c. Keep patient lying flat on back with chin up.

d. Loosen tight clothing.

e. Check for possible head injury or bleeding.

f. Summon ambulance by telephoning the police.

g. Give nothing by mouth.

h. Do NOT throw cold water in face.

i. Keep patient warm. Cover with coat or blanket.

j. If patient is convulsing, do NOT try to put anything between his teeth. Keep your fingers away from his mouth.

X. IMMUNIZATION AND VACCINATION TABLES

Disease	Material used	When given	Number of injections	Spacing of injections	Reactions	Duration of immunity	Recall or booster injections	Remarks
Diphtheria	Diphtheria toxoid	Infancy and childhood, or on exposure	3	1 month	None to slight	Varies	1st booster—after 1 year; 2d and 3rd—2-year intervals; 4th and 5th-3-year intervals and on exposure to disease	All three (diphtheria, tetanus and whooping cough) may be combined in a single injection (in young children only)
Whooping cough	Pertussis vaccine	Infancy and childhood, or on exposure	3	1 month	Slight to moderate	Varies		
Tetanus	Tetanus toxoid	Infancy and childhood, or after injury	3	1 month	None to slight	Varies		
Smallpox	Cowpox virus	Given only when traveling to place where smallpox exists	1	—	Moderate	Several years	5-7 years and for foreign travel	—
Poliomyelitis	Salk polio vaccine	Infancy to 40 years or older	3-4	First two 1 month apart, third 7 months later	None	Unknown (probably long)	4th injection one year after 3d injection	Now used only occasionally
	Sabin polio vaccine	3, 4, 5 months of age	No injections; 3 oral doses	1 month	None	Probably permanent	Not necessary	—

X. IMMUNIZATION AND VACCINATION TABLES (Continued)

Disease	Material used	When given	Number of injections	Spacing of injections	Reactions	Duration of immunity	Recall or booster injections	Remarks
Typhoid fever	Typhoid, para-typhoid vaccine	When travel-ing to suspi-cious area	3	1-4 weeks	Moderate	1-3 years	Every 1-3 years	—
Mumps	Mumps vac-cine	During ado-lescence or adulthood	2	1 week	Bad if sen-sitive to eggs	Unknown	None	Not given to those sensitive to eggs
Infectious Hepatitis	Gamma glo-bulin	On exposure to case of in-fectious hep-atitis	1	—	None	4-6 weeks	None	—
Scarlet fever	Penicillin	On exposure to case of scarlet fever	3	Daily	None	4-6 weeks	Same proce-dure if reex-posed	May give peni-cillin only in adequate dosage
Rabies	Rabies vac-cine	Following sus-picious ani-mal bite	14	Daily	Slight	3-6 months	If bitten again after 3 months	May not need full series if ani-mal is found not infected
Cholera	Cholera vaccine	When travel-ing to suspi-cious area	2	7-10 days	Slight	Short	Every 6-12 months	—

X. IMMUNIZATION AND VACCINATION TABLES (Continued)

Disease	Material used	When given	Number of injections	Spacing of injections	Reactions	Duration of immunity	Recall or booster injections	Remarks
Typhus fever	Typhus vaccine	When traveling to suspicious area	2-3	1 week	Slight	Short	Every 12 months	—
Yellow	Yellow fever vaccine	When traveling to suspicious area	1	—	May be moderate	Long	Every 6 years	Must be careful of reactions in those sensitive to eggs
Plague	Plague vaccine	When traveling to suspicious area	2-3	1 week	Slight	Short	Every 6-12 months	—
Influenza	Influenza vaccine	During epidemics	2	1 week	Slight	Short	—	—
Rocky Mountain spotted fever	Rocky Mountain spotted fever vaccine	When exposed to ticks in suspicious areas	3	1 week	Moderate	Short	Annually	Must be careful of reactions in those sensitive to eggs
Measles	Measles vaccine	9 to 12 months of age	3	1 month	Moderate	Long	None	—

X. IMMUNIZATION AND VACCINATION TABLES (*Concluded*)

Disease	Material used	When given	Number of injections	Spacing of injections	Reactions	Duration of immunity	Recall or booster injections	Remarks
German measles	German measles virus	Childhood; adulthood for females of childbearing age	1	——	None	Unknown (probably long)	None	Woman should not be pregnant, nor become pregnant for 2 months
Chicken pox*	Varivax vaccine	12 months of age	1	——	Slight	Unknown	——	Avoid those with AIDS
Anthrax	Anthrax vaccine	To military personnel	Subcutaneous injections: time zero, 2, 4, 6 weeks and 6, 12, 18 months	Slight or mild	Unknown	Yearly	——	
AIDS	None available							

* Reye's Syndrome. See. pg. 479.

XI. INCUBATION PERIODS

(The interval of time between exposure to disease and development of symptoms)

Disease	Incubation Period
AIDS	Days—several years
Amebic dysentery	3–6 days
Chickenpox (Varicella)	14–21 days
Cholera	2–3 days
Common cold	1–3 days
Diphtheria	2–5 days
Encephalitis (Epidemic encephalitis)	Probably 3–7 days
German Measles (Rubella)	14–21 days
Gonorrhea	4–7 days
Grippe	1–3 days
Infectious Hepatitis (Catarrhal Jaundice)	2–6 weeks
Infectious mononucleosis (Glandular fever)	5–15 days
Influenza	1–3 days
Leprosy	Several months–several years
Malaria	5–10 days
Malta fever (Undulant fever, Brucellosis)	2 weeks–several months
Measles (Rubeola)	10–14 days
Meningitis (Epidemic meningitis)	2–4 days
Mumps (Epidemic parotitis)	12–24 days
Paratyphoid fever (Salmonella fever)	2–5 days
Plague (Bubonic plague)	3–8 days
Pneumonia (Lobar pneumonia)	2–4 days
Poliomyelitis (Infantile paralysis)	7–14 days
Rabies (Hydrophobia)	10 days–2 years
Rocky Mountain Spotted Fever (Rickettsial disease)	3–7 days
Roseola (Exanthem subitum)	7–17 days
Salmonella (Paratyphoid fever)	2–5 days
Scarlet fever (Scarlatina)	3–6 days
Smallpox	10–14 days
Syphilis (Lues)	20–30 days
Tetanus (Lockjaw)	5–10 days
Typhoid fever	10–14 days
Typhus fever	7–14 days
Whooping cough (Pertussis)	7–10 days
Yellow fever	3–6 days

XII. INFANT DEVELOPMENT*

1. BOYS' HEIGHTS AND WEIGHTS†

Age	Height in Inches	Weight in Pounds
At Birth	20⅝	7½
1 month	22½	10⅞
2 months	23⅝	12⅝
3 months	24½	14⅛
4 months	25⅜	15⅜
5 months	26⅛	16¼
6 months	26¾	17½
7 months	27¼	18¼
8 months	27¾	19
9 months	28¼	19⅝
10 months	28⅝	20¼
11 months	29	20¾
1 year	29½	21⅜

2. GIRLS' HEIGHTS AND WEIGHTS†

Age	Height in Inches	Weight in Pounds
At Birth	20½	7⅛
1 month	21⅞	10⅛
2 months	23⅛	11¾
3 months	24	13
4 months	24⅞	14¼
5 months	25½	15⅜
6 months	26⅛	16¼
7 months	26¾	17⅛
8 months	27¼	17¾
9 months	27⅝	18½
10 months	28⅛	19
11 months	28½	19½
1 year	28⅞	20

* Adapted from material prepared by U.S. Vitamin and Pharmaceutical Corp.
† It must be understood that heights and weights are only the *average*. There are wide variations of these figures within normal range.

3. MUSCULAR, MENTAL, AND CRANIAL‡

Age

3 months	Turns head in direction of sound.
4 months	Recognizes and grasps objects; holds head erect if trunk is supported.
7–8 months	Sits erect by himself.
9–10 months	Attempts to stand.
11–12 months	Stands with assistance; may say, "Mama" or "Papa."
12–13 months	Attempts to walk.
14–15 months	Walks.
End of 2nd year	Talks in short sentences.

‡ It must be understood that the above activities are only *average*. There are wide variations in these activities among normal babies.

XIII. LIFE EXPECTANCY TABLES

Expectation of Life (in Years) United States, 1979—81 to 1996

	National Center for Health Statistics						MetLife
Age	1979–81	1989–91	1992	1993	1994	1995	1996*
0	73.9	75.4	75.8	75.5	75.7	75.8	75.9
15	60.2	61.4	61.7	61.5	61.6	61.6	61.8
25	50.8	51.9	52.2	52.0	52.1	52.2	52.3
35	41.4	42.6	42.9	42.7	42.8	42.8	43.0
45	32.3	33.4	33.8	33.6	33.7	33.8	33.8
55	23.9	24.8	25.1	24.9	25.1	25.1	25.1
65	16.5	17.3	17.5	17.3	17.4	17.4	17.4
75	10.5	11.0	11.2	10.9	11.0	11.0	11.0
85	6.0	6.2	6.2	6.0	6.1	6.0	6.1

Male

0	70.1	71.8	72.3	72.2	72.4	72.5	72.8
15	56.5	57.9	58.3	58.1	58.3	58.4	58.8
25	47.4	48.7	49.1	48.9	49.1	49.2	49.5
35	38.2	39.6	40.0	39.8	40.0	40.1	40.4
45	29.2	30.7	31.1	31.0	31.2	31.3	31.5
55	21.1	22.3	22.7	22.6	22.8	22.9	23.0
65	14.2	15.1	15.4	15.3	15.5	15.6	15.7
75	8.9	9.4	9.6	9.5	9.6	9.7	9.9
85	5.1	5.3	5.3	5.2	5.2	5.2	5.4

Female

0	77.6	78.8	79.1	78.8	79.0	78.9	79.0
15	63.8	64.7	65.0	64.7	64.8	64.7	64.9
25	54.2	55.0	55.2	55.0	55.1	55.0	55.1
35	44.5	45.4	45.6	45.4	45.4	45.4	45.5
45	35.2	36.0	36.2	35.9	36.0	36.0	36.1
55	26.4	27.1	27.2	27.0	27.1	27.0	27.0
65	18.4	19.0	19.2	18.9	19.0	18.9	18.9
75	11.6	12.1	12.2	11.9	12.0	11.9	12.0
85	6.4	6.7	6.6	6.4	6.4	6.3	6.4

*Estimated.
Statistics from Metropolitan Life Insurance Co.

XIV. THE MEDICINE CHEST

1. CONTENTS (HOME MEDICAL SUPPLIES)

Adhesive bandages, 1 box
Adhesive tape, 1 roll of 1 inch
  1 roll of 2 inch
Alcohol, 1 bottle of rubbing (70 percent alcohol, to be used as a skin anti-
  septic instead of iodine, etc.)
Applicators, 1 dozen with cotton tips
Bandages, 1 roll of 1-inch-wide gauze
  1 roll of 2-inch-wide gauze
  1 three-inch-wide (Ace semi-elastic)
Bedpan
Bell (so patient may summon aid, if necessary)
Cotton, 1 large roll of sterile
Douche bag and attachments
Electric pad
Enamel basin (for preparing wet dressings; for bathing patient, etc.)
Enema bag and attachments
Flashlight
Gauze pads, 1 dozen sterile (paper-wrapped) 2x2
  1 dozen sterile (paper-wrapped) 4x4
Glass drinking tube
Hydrogen peroxide, 1 bottle (for use as a skin antiseptic)
Ice bag
Rubber pad (to go under sheets or to be used when wet dressings are
  being applied)
Rubber tubing, 1 two-foot-length (for possible use as a tourniquet)
Scissors, 1 pair (preferably bandage scissors)
Steam inhalator and electrical attachments
Thermometers, 1 mouth
  1 rectal
Tweezers, 1 pair (for splinter removal)
Urinal
Vaseline, 1 tube or bottle of sterile

2. MEDICINES*

Aspirin tablets, 1 bottle of 5 grain and Baby aspirins, 81 mg.
Tylenol tablets
Bicarbonate of Soda, 1 box of powdered
Bicarbonate of Soda tablets, 1 bottle of 10 grain
Boric acid, 1 box of powdered
Collyrium eyewash with eyecup, 1 bottle
Epsom Salts, 1 box of powdered
Milk of Magnesia, 1 bottle
Paregoric, 1 ounce bottle
Salt Tablets, 1 bottle of 5 grain
Sodium Perborate powder, 1 container (for mouth wash)
Talcum powder, 1 container of any bland type
Tincture of Benzoin, 1 bottle
Witch hazel, 1 bottle

3. PRECAUTIONS

1. Every medication and bottle must be clearly labeled.
2. If label is not easily read, throw medication away.
3. *All* medications, no matter how mild, must be kept out of children's reach!
4. Read every label *twice* before giving medication.
5. Any poison, or special medication, should be under lock and key. Do *not* keep such medications in your regular medicine cabinet where the whole family may get to it.
6. When in doubt as to the freshness of a medicine, throw it away.
7. Do *not* ever take a medication in the dark.
8. *Never* apply a hot, wet dressing unless it has been tested for intensity of heat by the patient himself. It is better too cool than too hot.
9. Do *not* go to sleep with an electric pad turned on.
10. Do *not* keep an icebag in place more than ½ hour at a time.

*Please note that powerful medications such as strong sleeping tablets, narcotics, strong antiseptics such as iodine, and other special medications are purposely omitted from this list. Such drugs should be kept apart from the family medicine chest.

XV. OBSTETRIC TABLES*

Date of Onset of Last Menstrual Period		Expected Date of Childbirth	
January	1	October	8
	2		9
	3		10
	4		11
	5		12
	6		13
	7		14
	8		15
	9		16
	10		17
	11		18
	12		19
	13		20
	14		21
	15		22
	16		23
	17		24
	18		25
	19		26
	20		27
	21		28
	22		29
	23		30
	24		31
	25	November	1
	26		2
	27		3
	28		4
	29		5
	30		6
	31		7
February	1		8
	2		9
	3		10
	4		11
	5		12
	6		13
	7		14
	8		15
	9		16
	10		17
	11		18
	12		19
	13		20
	14		21

*Adapted from chart prepared by U.S. Vitamin and Pharmaceutical Corp.

Date of Onset of Last Menstrual Period		Expected Date of Childbirth	
February	15		22
	16		23
	17		24
	18		25
	19		26
	20		27
	21		28
	22		29
	23		30
	24	December	1
	25		2
	26		3
	27		4
	28		5
March	1		6
	2		7
	3		8
	4		9
	5		10
	6		11
	7		12
	8		13
	9		14
	10		15
	11		16
	12		17
	13		18
	14		19
	15		20
	16		21
	17		22
	18		23
	19		24
	20		25
	21		26
	22		27
	23		28
	24		29
	25		30
	26		31
	27	January	1
	28		2
	29		3
	30		4
	31		5
April	1		6
	2		7
	3		8
	4		9
	5		10
	6		11

Date of Onset of Last Menstrual Period		Expected Date of Childbirth
April	7	12
	8	13
	9	14
	10	15
	11	16
	12	17
	13	18
	14	19
	15	20
	16	21
	17	22
	18	23
	19	24
	20	25
	21	26
	22	27
	23	28
	24	29
	25	30
	26	31
	27	February 1
	28	2
	29	3
	30	4
May	1	5
	2	6
	3	7
	4	8
	5	9
	6	10
	7	11
	8	12
	9	13
	10	14
	11	15
	12	16
	13	17
	14	18
	15	19
	16	20
	17	21
	18	22
	19	23
	20	24
	21	25
	22	26
	23	27
	24	28
	25	March 1
	26	2
	27	3

Date of Onset of Last Menstrual Period		Expected Date of Childbirth
May	28	4
	29	5
	30	6
	31	7
June	1	8
	2	9
	3	10
	4	11
	5	12
	6	13
	7	14
	8	15
	9	16
	10	17
	11	18
	12	19
	13	20
	14	21
	15	22
	16	23
	17	24
	18	25
	19	26
	20	27
	21	28
	22	29
	23	30
	24	31
	25	April 1
	26	2
	27	3
	28	4
	29	5
	30	6
July	1	7
	2	8
	3	9
	4	10
	5	11
	6	12
	7	13
	8	14
	9	15
	10	16
	11	17
	12	18
	13	19
	14	20
	15	21
	16	22
	17	23

Date of Onset of Last Menstrual Period		Expected Date of Childbirth	
July	18		24
	19		25
	20		26
	21		27
	22		28
	23		29
	24		30
	25	May	1
	26		2
	27		3
	28		4
	29		5
	30		6
	31		7
August	1		8
	2		9
	3		10
	4		11
	5		12
	6		13
	7		14
	8		15
	9		16
	10		17
	11		18
	12		19
	13		20
	14		21
	15		22
	16		23
	17		24
	18		25
	19		26
	20		27
	21		28
	22		29
	23		30
	24		31
	25	June	1
	26		2
	27		3
	28		4
	29		5
	30		6
	31		7
September	1		8
	2		9
	3		10
	4		11
	5		12
	6		13

Date of Onset of Last Menstrual Period   **Expected Date of Childbirth**

Date of Onset of Last Menstrual Period		Expected Date of Childbirth	
September	7		14
	8		15
	9		16
	10		17
	11		18
	12		19
	13		20
	14		21
	15		22
	16		23
	17		24
	18		25
	19		26
	20		27
	21		28
	22		29
	23		30
	24	July	1
	25		2
	26		3
	27		4
	28		5
	29		6
	30		7
October	1		8
	2		9
	3		10
	4		11
	5		12
	6		13
	7		14
	8		15
	9		16
	10		17
	11		18
	12		19
	13		20
	14		21
	15		22
	16		23
	17		24
	18		25
	19		26
	20		27
	21		28
	22		29
	23		30
	24		31
	25	August	1
	26		2
	27		3

Date of Onset of Last Menstrual Period		Expected Date of Childbirth
October	28	4
	29	5
	30	6
	31	7
November	1	8
	2	9
	3	10
	4	11
	5	12
	6	13
	7	14
	8	15
	9	16
	10	17
	11	18
	12	19
	13	20
	14	21
	15	22
	16	23
	17	24
	18	25
	19	26
	20	27
	21	28
	22	29
	23	30
	24	31
	25	September 1
	26	2
	27	3
	28	4
	29	5
	30	6
December	1	7
	2	8
	3	9
	4	10
	5	11
	6	12
	7	13
	8	14
	9	15
	10	16
	11	17
	12	18
	13	19
	14	20
	15	21
	16	22
	17	23

Date of Onset of Last Menstrual Period		Expected Date of Childbirth
December	18	24
	19	25
	20	26
	21	27
	22	28
	23	29
	24	30
	25	October 1
	26	2
	27	3
	28	4
	29	5
	30	6
	31	7

XVI. PULSE RATES*

	Average Beats per Minute
The Unborn Child	140 to 150
Newborn Infants	130 to 140
During first year	110 to 130
During second year	96 to 115
During third year	86 to 105
7th to 14th year	76 to 90
14th to 21st year	76 to 85
21st to 60th year	70 to 75
After 60th year	67 to 80

1. Pulse rates rise normally during excitement, following physical exertion and during digestion.
2. The pulse rate is generally more rapid in females.
3. The pulse rate is also influenced by the breathing rate.
4. Variation of one degree of temperature above 98° F. is approximately equivalent to a rise of 10 beats in pulse rate. *See also* Temperature—Pulse Relations.

*Adapted from chart prepared by U.S. Vitamin and Pharmaceutical Corp.

XVII. RESPIRATION: NORMAL BREATHING RATES*

Age	Number of Respirations per Minute
First year	25 to 35
12th to 17th year	20 to 25
Adulthood	16 to 18
Breathing rates tend to rise with the pulse rate.	

*Adapted from chart prepared by U.S. Vitamin and Pharmaceutical Corp.

XVIII. STOMACH (GASTRIC) CONTENT ANALYSIS

	Normal	Abnormal
Quantity	50 to 100 cc. after the giving of a test meal.	Decreased amounts are not significant.
Total acidity	50 to 100 degrees.	Increased amounts indicate hyperacidity.
Free hydrochloric acid	25 to 50 degrees.	Increased amounts indicate hyperacidity.
Lactic acid	Normally secreted in insignificant quantities.	Presence of measurable amounts may indicate stomach tumor.
Combined hydrochloric acid	10 to 15 degrees.	Increased amounts indicate excess acidity.
Blood cells	Present only in very small quantities, sometimes secondary to passage of stomach tube.	Large amounts may indicate presence of an ulcer or tumor.
Bile	May or may not appear in specimen removed.	When bile is present, it demonstrates that main bile duct is not obstructed.
Tumor cells	None	May be found on microscopic examination in some cases of cancer of the stomach.

XIX. TEETH

1. FIRST OR DECIDUOUS TEETH

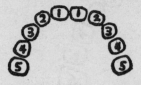

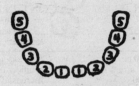

	Age of Appearance*
1. Central incisor teeth	6 to 8 months
2. Lateral incisor teeth	9 to 11 months
3. Eye teeth	18 to 20 months
4. First molar teeth	14 to 17 months
5. Second molar teeth	24 to 26 months

*The age at which teeth appear varies considerably from child to child.

2. FULL SET OF ADULT TEETH

Upper

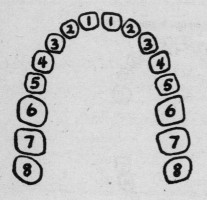

1. Middle incisor teeth
2. Lateral incisors
3. Canine teeth
4. Premolar teeth
5. Bicuspid teeth
6. Molar teeth
7. Molar teeth
8. Wisdom teeth

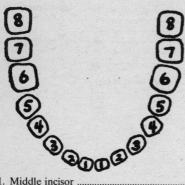

		Age of Appearance
1. Middle incisor	....	7 to 8 years
2. Lateral incisor	....	8 to 9 years
3. Canine teeth	....	12 to 14 years
4. Premolar teeth	....	10 to 12 years
5. Bicuspid teeth	....	10 to 12 years
6. Molar teeth	....	6 to 7 years
7. Molar teeth	....	12 to 16 years
8. Wisdom teeth	....	17 to 21 years

XX. TEMPERATURE*

1. NORMAL BODY TEMPERATURE*

Children: 99° F.
Adults: 98.6° F.
   a. Rectal thermometer readings tend to be up to one-half degree more
      than those recorded by mouth thermometers.
   b. Temperatures tend to be lowest on rising in the morning, and may rise
      as much as one degree toward evening.

2. CENTIGRADE AND FAHRENHEIT SYSTEMS

	Centigrade	Fahrenheit
Normal Body Temperature	37.0°	98.6°
Boiling Water (Sea Level)	100.0°	212.0°
Freezing Water (Sea Level)	0°	32.0°
Pasteurization of milk (30 minutes)	61.6°	143.0°

To convert Fahrenheit to Centigrade: Subtract 32 and multiply by 5/9.
To convert Centigrade to Fahrenheit: Multiply by 9/5 and add 32.

3. TEMPERATURE-PULSE RELATIONS

A variation of one degree of temperature above 98° F. is approximately
equivalent to a rise of 10 beats in pulse rate, thus:

Temp.	98° F.	corresponds with pulse of	60	per minute.
	99° F.	" " " "	70	" "
	100° F.	" " " "	80	" "
	101° F.	" " " "	90	" "
	102° F.	" " " "	100	" "
	103° F.	" " " "	110	" "
	104° F.	" " " "	120	" "
	105° F.	" " " "	130	" "

* Adapted from material prepared by U.S. Vitamin and Pharmaceutical Corp.

4. Comparitive Temperature Scales

CENTIGRADE	FAHRENHEIT
100	220
	210
90	200
	190
80	180
	170
70	160
	150
60	140
	130
50	120
	110
40	100
	90
30	80
	70
20	60
	50
10	40
0	30
	20
10	10
	0
20	10

XXI. URINE ANALYSIS

	Normal	Abnormal
Amount in 24 hours	1200–1500 cc. Between 1 and 1½ quarts)	Markedly decreased amounts, or failure to excrete urine, indicates: a) Kidney disease. b) Obstruction to outflow of urine from bladder, etc.
Color	Water color to amber.	a) Very dark urine may indicate marked concentration due to excessive perspiration or inadequate drinking of fluids. b) Dark, brownish urine may accompany jaundice. c) Reddish urine may indicate bleeding from kidney, ureter, bladder, prostate or urethra.
Specific gravity	1.017–1.020	Very low specific gravities (on repeated examinations) may indicate inadequate kidney function. Very high specific gravity indicates a concentrated urine.
Acidity	Slightly acid (pH 5.3)	Markedly acid or alkaline urine is often caused by the diet one follows or medications one takes. Acidity and alkalinity can be altered by changing diet or giving appropriate medication.
Albumin	None	Presence of albumin may indicate nephritis, nephrosis or other kidney disorders.
Sugar	None	Presence usually indicates diabetes.
Urea	30 grams in 24 hour specimen	
Uric acid	0.4 to 1.0 gram in 24 hour specimen	Marked alterations may indicate kidney or liver disease.
Ammonia	0.5 to 1.0 gram in 24 hour specimen	
Red blood cells	Very occasionally, cell is seen on microscopic examination.	A large number of red cells indicates bleeding from some point in the genitourinary tract.

	Normal	Abnormal
White blood cells	Very occasionally, cell is seen on microscopic examination.	A large number of white blood cells indicates an infection originating somewhere in the genitourinary tract.
Pus cells	None	A large number of pus cells indicates an infection in the genitourinary tract.

XXII. IMMUNIZATION SCHEDULE FOR CHILDREN

3 months:
  1st diphtheria, whooping cough, tetanus (DPT), combined in one injection.
  1st dose of oral polio vaccine.

4 months:
  2d DPT injection.
  2d dose of oral polio vaccine.

5 months:
  3d DPT injection.
  3d dose of oral polio vaccine.

9 months:
  Smallpox vaccination. (Infrequently given now.)

9–12 months:
  Measles vaccination.

12 months:
  Chicken pox vaccination.
  German measles vaccination.

15 months:
  Booster DPT injection.
  Booster dose of oral polio vaccine.

3½ years:
  Booster DPT injection.

6 years:
  Booster DPT injection.

9 years:
  Booster diphtheria and tetanus (combined)

12 years:
  Booster tetanus.
  Mumps vaccine.

BOOSTER INJECTIONS

Pertussis:
After exposure to a case of pertussis (whooping cough).

Diphtheria:
After exposure to a case of diphtheria.

Tetanus:
After injury from a rusty object or one contaminated by dirt. Such additional boosters may be advisable after any suspicious injury causing a puncture wound.

Smallpox vaccination:
Only if there is any suspicious case in the community. Also, before traveling to a foreign country where cases of smallpox have been reported recently.

XXIII. VITAMINS

Vitamin	Source	Body Function Effect	Deficiency Refults
A	Green leafy vegetables, milk, butter, eggs, liver, fishliver.	Essential to cell function of skin and cells lining the membrane of eye; also night vision.	Overgrowth of skin; disease of the eye called xerophthalmia; night blindness.
B₁ (Thiamine)	Yeast, potato, liver, grains, eggs, meat, vegetables.	Influential in stimulating growth; important for proper function of nerves; aids sugar metabolism.	Beriberi; heart disease; neuritis.
B₂ (Riboflavin)	Eggs, milk, liver, meats, cheese.	Important in metabolism of all body cells; promotes growth.	Overgrowth of skin (keratosis); cracking of skin in corners of the mouth (cheilosis); inflammation of the tongue (glossitis); fear of light (photophobia).
Nicotinic acis (Niacin)	Liver, wheat, yeast, meat.	Essential to good health; promotes growth; aids sugar metabolism; important for normal intestinal function.	Pellagra (skin disease); inflammation of tongue; nervous disorders.
B₆	Liver, cereals, fish, vegetables, yeast.	Important for proper protein metabolism; essential to cell function.	Nerve inflammation; skin irritation, such as seborrhea.
B¹²	Eggs, milk, liver, meats.	Important in fat and sugar metabolism; also in formation of blood; promotes growth.	Pernicious anemia; neuritis.

XXIII. VITAMINS (*Concluded*)

Vitamin	Source	Body Function Effect	Deficiency Refults
C (Ascorbic acid)	Citrus fruits (oranges, lemons, limes, grapefruits), potatoes, tomatoes.	Essential to function of blood vessels; healing of wounds; and function of connective tissue.	Scurvy with hemorrhages into tissues, from the gums, etc.
D	Fish livers (cod liver oil), milk, butter, eggs, sunlight.	Essential to bone metabolism and normal bone formation; also to calcium and phosphorus metabolism.	Rickets with bone deformities (bow-legs, pigeon chest, etc.); convulsions in infants (tetany).
Folic acid	Liver, yeast, green vegetables, (lettuce, etc.).	Important in formation of red blood cells.	Anemia accompanied by improperly formed red blood cells.
K	In intestinal tract of healthy persons on normal diet.	Necessary for normal blood clotting.	Hemorrhage, especially following surgery.

XXIV. WEIGHT CHARTS

1. BOYS—2 YEARS AND OLDER*

Height (Inches)	2 yrs.	3 yrs.	4 yrs.	5 yrs.	6 yrs.	7 yrs.	8 yrs.	9 yrs.	10 yrs.	11 yrs.	12 yrs.	13 yrs.	14 yrs.	15 yrs.	16 yrs.	17 yrs.	18 yrs.
33½	26½ lb.s																
36½		30¾ lbs.															
38			34 lbs.														
38				34 lbs.	34 lbs.												
39				35 lbs.	35 lbs.												
40				36 lbs.	36 lbs.												
41				38 lbs.	38 lbs.	38 lbs.											
42				39 lbs.	39 lbs.	39 lbs.	39 lbs.										

*Courtesy of U.S. Vitamin and Pharmaceutical Corp.

BOYS—2 YEARS AND OLDER

Height (Inches)	2 yrs.	3 yrs.	4 yrs.	5 yrs.	6 yrs.	7 yrs.	8 yrs.	9 yrs.	10 yrs.	11 yrs.	12 yrs.	13 yrs.	14 yrs.	15 yrs.	16 yrs.	17 yrs.	18 yrs.
43				41 lbs.	41 lbs.	41 lbs.	41 lbs.										
44				44 lbs.	44 lbs.	44 lbs.	44 lbs.	44 lbs.									
45				46 lbs.	46 lbs.	46 lbs.	46 lbs.	46 lbs.									
46				47 lbs.	48 lbs.	48 lbs.	48 lbs.	48 lbs.									
47				49 lbs.	50 lbs.	50 lbs.	50 lbs.	50 lbs.	50 lbs.								
48					52 lns.	53 lbs.	53 lbs.	53 lbs.	53 lbs.								
49					55 lbs.	55 lbs.	55 lbs.	55 lbs.	55 lbs.	55 lbs.							
50					57 lbs.	58 lbs.	58 lbs.	58 lbs.	58 lbs.	58 lbs.	58 lbs.						
51						61 lbs.	61 lbs.	61 lbs.	61 lbs.	61 lbs.	61 lbs.						
52						63 lbs.	64 lbs.	64 lbs.	64 lbs.	64 lbs.	64 lbs.	64 lbs.					

BOYS—2 YEARS AND OLDER

Height (Inches)	2 yrs.	3 yrs.	4 yrs.	5 yrs.	6 yrs.	7 yrs.	8 yrs.	9 yrs.	10 yrs.	11 yrs.	12 yrs.	13 yrs.	14 yrs.	15 yrs.	16 yrs.	17 yrs.	18 yrs.
53						66 lbs.	67 lbs.	67 lbs.	67 lbs.	67 lbs.	68 lbs.	68 lbs.					
54							70 lbs.	70 lbs.	70 lbs.	70 lbs.	71 lbs.	71 lbs.	72 lbs.				
55							72 lbs.	72 lbs.	73 lbs.	73 lbs.	74 lbs.	74 lbs.	74 lbs.				
56							75 lbs.	76 lbs.	77 lbs.	77 lbs.	77 lbs.	78 lbs.	78 lbs.	80 lbs.			
57								79 lbs.	80 lbs.	81 lbs.	81 lbs.	82 lbs.	83 lbs.	83 lbs.			
58								83 lbs.	84 lbs.	84 lbs.	85 lbs.	85 lbs.	86 lbs.	87 lbs.			
59									87 lbs.	88 lbs.	89 lbs.	89 lbs.	90 lbs.	90 lbs.	90 lbs.		
60									91 lbs.	92 lbs.	92 lbs.	93 lbs.	94 lbs.	95 lbs.	96 lbs.		
61										95 lbs.	96 lbs.	97 lbs.	99 lbs.	100 lbs.	103 lbs.	106 lbs.	

BOYS—2 YEARS OLD AND OLDER

Height (Inches)	2 yrs.	3 yrs.	4 yrs.	5 yrs.	6 yrs.	7 yrs.	8 yrs.	9 yrs.	10 yrs.	11 yrs.	12 yrs.	13 yrs.	14 yrs.	15 yrs.	16 yrs.	17 yrs.	18 yrs.
62										100 lbs.	101 lbs.	102 lbs.	103 lbs.	104 lbs.	107 lbs.	111 lbs.	116 lbs.
63										105 lbs.	106 lbs.	107 lbs.	108 lbs.	110 lbs.	113 lbs.	118 lbs.	123 lbs.
64											109 lbs.	111 lbs.	113 lbs.	115 lbs.	117 lbs.	121 lbs.	126 lbs.
65											114 lbs.	117 lbs.	118 lbs.	120 lbs.	122 lbs.	127 lbs.	131 lbs.
66												119 lbs.	122 lbs.	125 lbs.	128 lbs.	132 lbs.	136 lbs.
67												124 lbs.	128 lbs.	130 lbs.	134 lbs.	136 lbs.	139 lbs.
68													134 lbs.	134 lbs.	137 lbs.	141 lbs.	143 lbs.
69													137 lbs.	139 lbs.	143 lbs.	146 lbs.	149 lbs.

GIRLS—2 YEARS AND OLDER*

Height (Inches)	2 yrs.	3 yrs.	4 yrs.	5 yrs.	6 yrs.	7 yrs.	8 yrs.	9 yrs.	10 yrs.	11 yrs.	12 yrs.	13 yrs.	14 yrs.	15 yrs.	16 yrs.	17 yrs.	18 yrs.
33⅛	25⅛ lbs.																
36¼		29½ lbs.															
38			33 lbs.														
38				33 lbs.	33 lbs.												
39				34 lbs.	34 lbs.												
40				36 lbs.	36 lbs.	36 lbs.											
41				37 lbs.	37 lbs.	37 lbs.											
42				39 lbs.	39 lbs.	39 lbs.											
43				41 lbs.	41 lbs.	41 lbs.	41 lbs.										

GIRLS—2 YEARS AND OLDER

Height (Inches)	2 yrs.	3 yrs.	4 yrs.	5 yrs.	6 yrs.	7 yrs.	8 yrs.	9 yrs.	10 yrs.	11 yrs.	12 yrs.	13 yrs.	14 yrs.	15 yrs.	16 yrs.	17 yrs.	18 yrs.
44				42 lbs.	42 lbs.	42 lbs.	42 lbs.										
45				45 lbs.	45 lbs.	45 lbs.	45 lbs.	45 lbs.									
46				47 lbs.	47 lbs.	47 lbs.	48 lbs.	48 lbs.									
47				49 lbs.	50 lbs.	50 lbs.	50 lbs.	50 lbs.	50 lbs.								
48					52 lbs.	52 lbs.	52 lbs.	52 lbs.	53 lbs.	53 lbs.							
49					54 lbs.	54 lbs.	55 lbs.	55 lbs.	56 lbs.	56 lbs.							
50					56 lbs.	56 lbs.	57 lbs.	58 lbs.	59 lbs.	61 lbs.	62 lbs.						
51						59 lbs.	60 lbs.	61 lbs.	61 lbs.	63 lbs.	65 lbs.						
52						63 lbs.	64 lbs.	64 lbs.	64 lbs.	65 lbs.	67 lbs.						

GIRLS—2 YEARS AND OLDER

Height (Inches)	2 yrs.	3 yrs.	4 yrs.	5 yrs.	6	7 yrs.	8 yrs.	9 yrs.	10 yrs.	11 yrs.	12 yrs.	13 yrs.	14 yrs.	15 yrs.	16 yrs.	17 yrs.	18 yrs.
53						66 lbs.	67 lbs.	67 lbs.	68 lbs.	68 lbs.	69 lbs.	71 lbs.					
54							69 lbs.	70 lbs.	70 lbs.	71 lbs.	71 lbs.	73 lbs.					
55							72 lbs.	74 lbs.	74 lbs.	74 lbs.	75 lbs.	77 lbs.	78 lbs.				
56								76 lbs.	78 lbs.	78 lbs.	79 lbs.	81 lbs.	83 lbs.				
57								80 lbs.	82 lbs.	82 lbs.	82 lbs.	84 lbs.	88 lbs.	92 lbs.			
58									84 lbs.	86 lbs.	86 lbs.	88 lbs.	93 lbs.	96 lbs.	101 lbs.		
59									87 lbs.	90 lbs.	90 lbs.	92 lbs.	96 lbs.	100 lbs.	103 lbs.	104 lbs.	
60									91 lbs.	95 lbs.	95 lbs.	97 lbs.	101 lbs.	105 lbs.	108 lbs.	109 lbs.	111 lbs.
61									99 lbs.	100 lbs.	101 lbs.	105 lbs.	108 lbs.	112 lbs.	113 lbs.	116 lbs.	

GIRLS—2 YEARS AND OLDER

Height (Inches)	2 yrs.	3 yrs.	4 yrs.	5 yrs.	6 yrs.	7 yrs.	8 yrs.	9 yrs.	10 yrs.	11 yrs.	12 yrs.	13 yrs.	14 yrs.	15 yrs.	16 yrs.	17 yrs.	18 yrs.
62										104 lbs.	105 lbs.	106 lbs.	109 lbs.	113 lbs.	115 lbs.	117 lbs.	118 lbs.
63											110 lbs.	110 lbs.	112 lbs.	116 lbs.	117 lbs.	119 lbs.	120 lbs.
64											114 lbs.	115 lbs.	117 lbs.	119 lbs.	120 lbs.	122 lbs.	123 lbs.
65											118 lbs.	120 lbs.	121 lbs.	122 lbs.	123 lbs.	125 lbs.	126 lbs.
66												124 lbs.	124 lbs.	125 lbs.	128 lbs.	129 lbs.	130 lbs.
67												128 lbs.	130 lbs.	131 lbs.	133 lbs.	133 lbs.	135 lbs.
68												131 lbs.	133 lbs.	135 lbs.	136 lbs.	138 lbs.	138 lbs.
69													135 lbs.	137 lbs.	138 lbs.	140 lbs.	142 lbs.

MEN—25 YEARS OLD OR OLDER*
(Weight in pounds, with clothes)

Height		Small Frame	Medium Frame	Large Frame
(With shoes, 1 inch heels)				
Feet	*Inches*			
5	2	112–120	118–129	126–141
5	3	115–123	121–133	129–144
5	4	118–126	124–136	132–148
5	5	121–129	127–139	135–152
5	6	124–133	130–143	138–156
5	7	128–137	134–147	142–161
5	8	132–141	138–152	147–166
5	9	136–145	142–156	151–170
5	10	140–150	146–160	155–174
5	11	144–154	150–165	159–179
6	0	148–158	154–170	164–184
6	1	152–162	158–175	168–189
6	2	156–167	162–180	173–194
6	3	160–171	167–185	178–199
6	4	164–175	172–190	182–204

WOMEN—25 YEARS OLD OR OLDER*
(Weight in pounds, with clothes)

Height		Small Frame	Medium Frame	Large Frame
(With shoes, 2 inch heels)				
Feet	*Inches*			
4	10	92–98	96–107	104–119
4	11	94–101	98–110	106–122
5	0	96–104	101–113	109–125
5	1	99–107	104–116	112–128
5	2	102–110	107–119	115–131
5	3	105–113	110–122	118–134
5	4	108–116	113–126	121–138
5	5	111–119	116–130	125–142
5	6	114–123	120–135	129–146
5	7	118–127	124–139	133–150
5	8	122–131	128–143	137–154
5	9	126–135	132–147	141–158
5	10	130–140	136–151	145–163
5	11	134–144	140–155	149–168
6	0	138–148	144–159	153–173

For girls between 18 and 25, subtract 1 pound for each year under 25.

*Courtesy of the Metropolitan Life Insurance Company.

XXV. ABBREVIATIONS

1. DIPLOMATES IN SPECIALTIES

	Abbreviations
Diplomate American Board of Anesthesiology	D-A
Diplomate American Board of Dermatology	D-D
Diplomate American Board of Internal Medicine	D-IM
Diplomate American Board of Neurological Surgery	D-NS
Diplomate American Board of Ophthalmology	D-O
Diplomate American Board of Obstetrics and Gynecology	D-OG
Diplomate American Board of Otolaryngology	D-OL
Diplomate American Board of Orthopedic Surgery	D-OS
Diplomate American Board of Pathology	D-PA
Diplomate American Board of Preventive Medicine, Inc.	D-PM
Diplomate American Board of Physical Medicine and Rehabilitation	D-PMR
Diplomate American Board of Psychiatry and Neurology	D-PN
Diplomate American Board of Proctology	D-PR
Diplomate American Board of Plastic Surgery	D-PS
Diplomate American Board of Radiology	D-R
Diplomate American Board of Surgery	D-S
Diplomate of the Board of Thoracic Surgery	D-TS
Diplomate American Board of Urology	D-U
Licentiate American Board of Pediatrics	L-P
Diplomates certified by National Board of Medical Examiners	NB
Psychiatrists accredited by New York State Department of Mental Hygiene	QP

2. FELLOWS OF SPECIALTY COLLEGES

	Abbreviations
Associate Fellow of American College of Allergists	AFACAL
Fellow of American College of Allergists	FACAL
Fellow of American College of Angiology	FACA
Fellow of American College of Anesthesiologists	FACAn
Fellow of American College of Cardiology	FACC
Fellow of American College of Chest Physicians	FCCP
Fellow of American College of Gastroenterology	FACG
Fellow of American College of Obstetricians and Gynecologists	FACOG
Fellow of College of American Pathologists	FCAP
Fellow of American College of Physicians	FACP
Fellow of American College of Preventive Medicine	FACPM
Fellow of American College of Radiology	FACR
Fellow of American College of Surgeons	FACS
Fellow of International College of Surgeons	FICS

3. MEDICAL ASSOCIATIONS AND SOCIETIES

Name	Abbreviations	
Academy-International of Medicine	Ac-Intl Med;	AIM
Academy of Physical Medicine	APM	
Academy of Psychoanalysis	Ac Psychoan	
Academy of Psychosomatic Medicine	Ac Psychosom Med	
Aero Medical Association	Aero Med;	AeroMA; AMEL
American Academy of Allergy	Am Ac Alg;	AAA1
American Academy of Compensation Medicine, Inc.	Am Ac Comp Med	
American Academy of Dermatology and Syphilology	Am Ac Derm & Syph;	AADS
American Academy of General Practice	Am Ac GP	
American Academy of Neurology	AANeur;	Am Ac Neur
American Academy of Neurological Surgery	Am Ac Neur Sur;	AANS
American Academy of Ophthalmology and Otolaryngology	Am Ac Ophth & Otolar;	AAOO
American Academy of Orthopaedic Surgeons	Am Ac Orth Sur;	AAOS
American Academy of Pediatrics	Am Ac Ped;	AAPd
American Academy of Physical Medicine and Rehabilitation	Am Ac PM & Rehab	
American Academy of Tropical Medicine	AATM	
American Academy of Tuberculosis Physicians	Am Ac Tbc Phy;	AATP
American Association for Advancement of Science	AAAS	
American Association of Anatomists	Am Anat;	AAA
American Association of Blood Banks	AABB	
American Association for Cancer Research	Am Ca Res;	AACR
American Association for Forensic Science	AAFS	
American Association of Genito-Urinary Surgeons	Am G-U Sur;	AAGUS
American Association of Immunologists	Am Immun;	AAI
American Association on Mental Deficiency	Am Ment Def;	AAMD
American Association of Neuropathologists	Am Neuropath;	AAN
American Association of Obstetricians and Gynecologists	Am Obst & Gyn;	AAOG
American Association of Oral and Plastic Surgery	AAOPS	
American Association of Pathologists and Bacteriologists	Am Path & Bact;	AAPB
American Association of Physical Medicine and Rehabilitation	AAPMR	
American Association of Plastic Surgeons	AM Plast Sur	
American Association of Railway Surgeons	Am Rail Sur;	AARS
American Association for Research in Psychosomatic Problems	Am Psychosom	

Name	Abbreviations	
American Association for the Study of Neoplastic Disease	Am Neo Dis	AASND;
American Association for the Surgery of Trauma	Am Sur Traum;	AAST
American Association for Thoracic Surgery	Am Thor Sur;	AATS
American Association of University Professors	AAUP	
American Board of Legal Medicine	Am Bd Legal Med	
American Broncho-Esophagological Association	Am Broncho-Esoph;	ABEA
American Chemical Society	AChemS	
American Clinical and Climatological Association	Am Clin & Clim;	ACCA
American College of Allergists	ACA	
American College of Anesthetists	ACAnes	
American College of Cardiology	ACC	
American College of Chest Physicians	ACCP	
American College of Gastroenterology	ACG	
American College of Hospital Administrators	ACHA	
American College of Obstetrics and Gynecology	ACOG	
American College of Pathologists	ACPath	
American College of Physicians	ACP	
American College of Radiology	ACR	
American College of Surgeons	ACS	
American Congress of Physical Medicine and Rehabilitation	Am Cong PM & Rehab;	ACPMR
American Dermatological Association	Am Derm;	ADA
American Diabetes Association	ADiabA;	ADA
American Electroencephalographers Society	AEncephS	
American Epidemiological Society	Am Epidem;	AES
American Federation for Clinical Research	Am Fed Clin Res;	AFCR
American Gastro-Enterological Association	Am Gastroent;	AGEA
American Gastroscopic Society	Am Gastroscop	
American Geriatrics Society	Am Ger;	AGerA
American Goiter Association	Am Goiter;	AGA
American Group Psychotherapy Association	Am Group Psychother;	AGPA
American Gynecological Society	Am Gyn;	AGS
American Heart Association	AHA	
American Institute of Homeopathy	Am Inst Hom;	AIH
American Institute of Nutrition	AIN	
American Laryngological Association	Am Lar;	ALA
American Laryngological, Rhinological and Otological Society	Am Lar Rhin & Otol;	ALROS
American Medical Association	AMA	

Name	Abbreviations	
American Medical Women's Association	Am Med Wom;	AMWA
American Neurological Association	Am Neur;	ANA
American Nurses Association	ANA	
American Ophthalmological Society	Am Ophth;	AOS
American Orthopaedic Association	Am Orth;	AOA
American Orthopsychiatric Association	Am Or-	AOrPA
	thopsych;	
Amerian Otological Society, Inc.	Am Otol;	AOtS
American Otorhinologic Society for Plastic Surgery	Am Otorhin Plast Sur;	AOSPS
American Pediatric Society	Am Ped;	APdS
American Physiological Society	Am Physiol;	APS
American Physiotherapy Association	APhysthA	APA
American Proctologic Society	Am Proct;	APrS
American Psychiatric Association	Am Psych;	APA
American Psychoanalytic Association	Am Psychoan;	APsychoaA
American Psychological Association	APsychA	
American Psychopathological Association	Am Psycho- path;	APsychpthA
American Psychosomatic Society	APsychosomS	
American Public Health Association	Am Pub Health;	APHA
American Radium Society	Am Rad;	ARS
American Rheumatism Association	Am Rheum;	ARA
American Roentgen Ray Society	Am Roent Ray;	ARRS
American School Health Association	Am Sch Health	
American Society of Anesthesiologists, Inc.	Am Anest;	ASAnes
American Society of Bacteriologists	ASB	
American Society for Clinical Investigation	Am Clin In- vest;	ASCI
American Society of Cliniical Pathologists	Am Clin Path;	ASCP
American Society for the Control of Cancer	ASCC	
American Society for Experimental Patho- logy	Am Exp Path;	ASEP
American Society of Genetics	ASG	
American Society for the Hard of Hearing	ASHH	
American Society of Maxillo-Facial Sur- geons	Am Maxillo- Fac	
American Society of Parasitologists	ASP	
American Society for Pharmacology and and Experimental Therapeutics	ASPET	
American Society of Plastic and Recon- structive Surgery	Am Plast & Recon Sur;	
American Society for Research in Psychoso- matic Problems	ASRPP	
American Society for the Study of Allergy	ASSAl	
American Society for the Study of Arthritis	ASSArthr	
American Society for the Study of Sterility	Am Study Steril;	ASSS
American Society for Surgery of the Hand	ASSH	
American Society of Tropical Medicine	ASTM	

Name	Abbreviations	
American Society of Tropical Medicine and Hygiene	Am Trop Med & Hyg;	ASTMH
American Speech Correction Association	ASCA	
American Surgical Association	Am Sur;	ASA
American Therapeutic Society	Am Ther;	AThS
American Trudeau Society	Am Trudeau;	ATrudeauS
American Urological Association	Am Urol;	AUA
American Venereal Disease Association	Am VD	
Association for the Advancement of Psychotherapy	Adv Psychother	
Association of American Physicians	AAP	
Association of Life Insurance Medical Directors of America	Assn Life Ins Med Dir;	ALIMDA
Association of Military Surgeons of United States	AMSUS;	Milit Sur US
Association for Psychoanalytic Medicine	Assn Psychoan Med	
Association for Research in Nervous and Mental Disease	ARNMD;	Res Nerv & Ment Dis
Association for Research in Ophthalmology	ARO	
Association for the Study of Human Infertility	ASHI	
Association of Surgeons of Great Britain and Ireland	ASGBI	
British Association of Dermatology and Syphilology	BADS	
British Association of Radiology and Physiotherapy	BARP	
British Dermatological Association	BDA	
British Institute of Radiology	BIR	
British Laryngological, Rhinological and Otological Association	BLROA	
British Medical Association	BMA	
British Orthopaedic Association	BOA	
British Pediatric Association	BPA	
British Roentgen Society	BRS	
Canadian Association of Radiologists	CAR	
Canadian Medical Association	CMA	
Canadian National Committee for Mental Hygiene	CNCMH	
Canadian Ophthalmological Society	COphS	
Canadian Public Health Association	CPHA	
Canadian Society for the Study of Diseases of Children	CSSDC	
Canadian Tuberculosis Association	CTA	
Cardiac Society of Great Britain and Ireland	CSGBI	
Clinical Society of Genito-Urinary Surgeons	Clin G-U Sur;	CSGUS
College of American Pathologists	CAP	
Congress of Neurological Surgeons	CNS	
Endocrine Society	Ender	
Harvey Cushing Society	Cushing;	HCS

Name	Abbreviations	
Industrial Medical Association	Ind Med;	IMA
International Academy of Pathology	Intl Ac Paths	
International Academy of Proctology	Intl Ac Proct	
International Anesthesia Research Society	Intl Anest Res;	IARS
International Fertility Association	Internat Fertil	
International Leprosy Association	ILA	
International Society of Hematology	Intl Hematol;	ISH
International Society of Internal Medicine	Intl Int Med	
Investigative Dermatological Society	IDS	
James Ewing Society	Ewing Soc	
Medical Library Association	MLA	
National Committee for Mental Hygiene	NCMH	
National Eclectic Medical Association	Natl Ecl	
National Medical Association	NMA	
National Proctological Association	Natl Proct	
National Society for Crippled Children	NSCC	
National Tuberculosis Association	NTA	
Ophthalmological Society of the United Kingdom	OSUK	
Pan-American Medical Association	PAMA	
Pathological Society of Great Britain and Ireland	PSGBI	
Radiological Society of North America, Inc.	Radiol NA;	RSNA
Royal College of Obstetricians and Gynecologists (England)	RCOG	
Royal College of Physicians	RCP	
Royal College of Surgeons (Canada)	RCS	
Royal College of Surgeons (England)	RCS	
Royal Institute of Public Health and Hygiene (England)	RIPHH	
Royal Society of Medicine (England)	RSM	
Royal Society of Tropical Medicine and Hygiene (England)	RSTMH	
Society of American Bacteriologists	SAB;	Am Bact
Society of Clinical Surgery	SCS;	Clin Sur
Society for Experimental Biology and Medicine	SEBM;	Exp Biol & Med
Society for Investigative Dermatology	Invest Derm;	SID
Society of University Surgeons	Univ Sur	
Southern Surgical Association	SSA;	Southern Sur
William Alanson White Psychoanalytic Society	White Psychoan Soc	
World Medical Association	WMA	

4. MEDICAL TERMS

Name	Abbreviations
abdominal	abdom
academy	ac; acad
achievement age	A.A.
achievement quotient	A.Q.
administration	adminis; administr
admitting	admit
advisory	adv
aluminum	Al
Alienist	Alien
allergy	alg
American	Am
ammonium	NH_4
anatomy	anat
anesthesia	anes; anest
anterior pituitary gland	A.P.
anterior pituitary like	A.P.L.
Army of United States	AUS
arteriovenous	A.V.
arthritis	arthrit
Assistant	asst
Associate	Asso; Assoc
association	assn
Attending	att
atrioventricular	A.V.
auxiliary	aux
Bachelor of Surgery (Eng.)	ChB
Bacteriologist, bacteriology	bact
barium	Ba
basal body temperature	BBT.
basal metabolic rate	B.M.R.
before meals	a.c.
bicarbonate	HCO_3
biochemistry	biochem
bismuth	Bi
blood pressure	BP
Board	Bd
born	b
British thermal unit	BTU; B.Th.U.
bromsulphalein	BSP
calcium	Ca
cancer	ca
carbon	C
carbon tetrachloride	CCl_4
cardiography	Card; cardiog
cardiologist, cardiology	cardiol
cardiovascular disease	cardiovas dis
center	cent
centigram	cg

Name	Abbreviations
centimeter	cm
certified	c; cert; ct
cesium	Cs
chairman	chm
chemistry	chem
chemotherapy	chemother
chlorine	Cl
chloroform	$CHCl_3$
climatological	clim
clinical	clin
cobalt	Co
college	coll
communicable	commun
Consultant, consulting	cons
convalescent	conv
copper	Cu
cranial	cran
cubic centimeter	cc
cystoscopy	cystoscop
dead on arrival	doa
deficiency	def
dentist	D.D.S.
dermatology	derm
diabetes	diabet
diagnosis	diag
director	dir
disease, or diseases	dis
dispensary	disp
distilled water	aq.dest.
Doctor	Dr.
Doctor of Public Health	DPH
drop of water	min.
ear, eye, nose and throat	e,e,n & t
electrocardiography	electrocard; ECG; EKG
electroencephalography	EEG
electroshock therapy	ECS
electrotherapy	electrother
emeritus	emerit
encephalography	encephalog
endocrinology	endocrin
endoscopy	endoscop
epidemiology	epidem
esophagology	esoph
every hour	q.h.
experimental	exp
externe, externship	extern
extrasensory perception	ESP
eye and ear	ee
Fellow	F; Fell
fertility	fertil

Name	Abbreviations
fluid	fl
fracture surgery	fract sur
gastroenterology	gastroent; ge
gastro-intestinal	gas-int; gastro-int
general	gen
general practice	GP
genito-urinary	G-U
geriatrics	ger
gold	Au
graduate	grad
graduate nurse	RN
graduate pharmacist	Ph.G.
grain	gr
gram	g; gm
gynecology	gyn; gynec
hematology	hematol
hemoglobin	Hb
homeopathy	hom; homeop
honorary	hon
hospital	hosp
hydrochloric acid	HCl
hydrogen	H
hydrogen dioxide	H_2O_2
immunology	immun
iodine	I
industrial medicine	ind med
industrial surgery	ind sur
infant, infirmary	inf
infectious disease	infec dis
infectious mononucleosis	IM
Institute	inst
instructor	inst
intelligence quotient	I.Q.
Intern, internal	Int; Intern
internal medicine	int med
International	Intl; Internatl
intramuscular injection	I.M.; i.m.
intravenous	iv
junior	Jr
kilovolt	KV
kilowatt	KW
laboratory	lab
laryngology	lar; laryng
last menstrual period	L.M.P.
lead	Pb
lecturer	lect
left occiput anterior	L.O.A.
left occiput posterior	L.O.P.
left sacroposterior	L.S.P.
magnesium	Mg
malignant	malig

Name	Abbreviations
Master of Science	M Sc
maternity	mat
Medical Corps	MC
medicine, medical	med
member	mem
mental hygiene	ment hyg
mercury	Hg
metabolism	metab
Military	Milit
millicurie	mc
milliequivalent	mEq
milligram	mg
milligram-hour	mgh
milliliter	ml
millimeter	mm
minim	min
months	mos
National Formulary	N.F.
neoplastic disease	neoplast dis
Neurologist, neurology	Neur
neuropathology	neuropath
neuropsychiatry	neuropsych; neuropsy
neurosurgery	neurosur
New and Nonofficial Remedies	NNR
nitric acid	HNO_3
nitrogen	N
nonprotein nitrogen	N.P.N.
Obstetrician, obstetrics	obst
occupational disease	occupat dis
oncology	oncol
one drop	gt
one drop of water	min
ophthalmology	oph; ophth
oral surgery	oral sur
orthopedics, Orthopedist	Or; Orth
otolaryngology	otolar
otology	ot; otol
otorhinolaryngology	otorhinolar
ounce	oz
outpatient department	OPD
oxygen	O
ozone	O_3
parasitology	parasit
pathological, Pathologist, pathology	Path
pediatrics, Pediatrician	Ped; PD
peripheral vascular disease	periph vas dis
peroxide	H_2O_2
pharmacology, pharmacy	phar
phosphorus	p
phthisiology	phtisiol

Name	Abbreviations
physical medicine	phy med
physical medicine & rehabilitation	PM & Rehab
Physician	Phy; Phys
physiological, Physiologist, physiology	Physiol
physiotherapy	physiother
plastic	pl
plastic surgery	plast sur
polyclinic	poly
Post-graduate	P-G
potassium	K
pound	lb
prenatal	prenat
pressure, blood	BP
proctology, Proctologist	proct
Professor	Prof
Psychiatrist, psychiatry	Psy
psychoanalysis	Psychoa
Psychologist, psychology	Psych
Psychopathologist, psychopathology	Psychop
psychosomatic	psychosom
psychotherapy	psychother
Public Health	PH
pulmonary disease	pulmon dis
quart	qt
radiation therapy	radiat ther
radiography	radiog
Radiologist, radiology	R; Radiol
Radiotherapeutist, radiotherapy	Radiother
reconstructive	reconstruct
red blood cells	RBC
Registered nurse	R.N.
Resident, research	Res
respiratory quotient	R.Q.
reticuloendothelial system	RES
retired	ret
rheumatic, rheumatism	rheum
Rhinologist, rhinology	Rhin
rhinoplastic surgery	rhinoplas sur
right occiput anterior	R.O.A.
right occiput posterior	R.O.P.
Roentgenologist, roentgenology	roent
serology	serol
service	ser
skeletal	skel
society	soc
sodium	Na
sterility	steril
sulfur	S
Superintendent	Supt
Surgeon, surgery	Sur; Surg
Surgeon General's Office	S.G.O.

Name	Abbreviations
Syphilologist, syphilology	Syph
Therapist, therapy	Ther
thoracic surgery	thor sur
transfusion	transfus
traumatic	traum
tropical	trop
tuberculosis	TB Tbc
twice a day	b.d.
United States Army	USA
United States Navy	USN
United States Pharmacopeia	USP
United States Public Health Service	USPHS
Uranium	U
vascular disease	Vas Dis
venereal disease	VD
Veterans Administration	VA
water	HBO; Aq.
white blood cells	WBC
World Health Organization	WHO
X-ray technician	R.T.

1999
Guide to Health Insurance for People with Medicare

This booklet explains the Medicare program, but it is not a legal document. The official Medicare program provisions are contained in the relevant laws, regulations and rulings.

NOTICE

Listed [on page 609] are the addresses and telephone numbers of each of the state agencies on aging and the state insurance departments. They are available to assist you with any questions you may have about private insurance to supplement medicare, or so-called "medigap" policies. Suspected violations of the laws governing the marketing of these policies should generally be reported to your state insurance department since states are responsible for the regulation of insurance within their boundaries. There are also federal penalties for certain violations concerning medigap policies. It is, for example, a federal offense for an insurance agent to indicate that he or she represents the medicare program or any other federal agency in order to sell a policy. The federal toll-free telephone number for registering such complaints in 1-800-638-6833.

CONTENTS

WHAT MEDICARE DOES NOT PAY FOR
Custodial Care
Care Not Reasonable and Necessary Under Medicare Program Standards
Care Outside the United States
When Medicare Denies a Claim but You Do Not Have to Pay the Bill

MEDICARE MANAGED CARE PLANS

HEALTH INSURANCE AND COUNSELING (LISTED BY STATE)

NATIONAL HEALTH ORGANIZATIONS AND AGENCIES

ADOPTION:
Children's Aid Society
105 East 22nd Street—Main Office
New York, N.Y. 10010
(212) 949–4936

AGING:
The American Geriatrics Society
770 Lexington Ave. Suite 300
New York, N.Y. 10021
(212)308–1414

National Institute on Aging
1–800–222–2225
1–800–222–4225 (TTY)

ALCOHOLISM:
Alcoholics Anonymous World Services
875 Riverside Drive
New York, N.Y. 10021
(212)870–3400

American Council on Alcoholism
2522 St. Paul Street
Baltimore, MD 21218
1–800–527–5344

ALLERGY:
Allergy & Asthma Center
121 E 61st St
New York, N.Y. 10021–8143

Asthma and Allergy Foundation
1125 15th St. N.W. Suite 502
Washington, D.C. 20005
1–800–7–ASTHMA (278462)

ARTHRITIS:
Arthritis Foundation
1330 West Peachtree St.
Atlanta, Georgia 30309
1–800–283–7800

BIRTH CONTROL:
Planned Parenthood Federation of America
810 Seventh Avenue
New York, N.Y. 10019
1–800–230–PLAN(7526)

BRAIN:
National Foundation for Brain Research
1250 24th. St., NW, Suite 300
Washington, DC 20037
(202)293–5453

CANCER
American Cancer Society
1–800–ACS–2345

National Cancer Institute's
Cancer Information Center
1–800–4–CANCER

U-Me Breast Cancer Support Program
1–800–221–2141

Damon Runyon–Walter Winchell Cancer Fund
675 Third Avenue, 25th Floor
New York, N.Y. 10017
(212)697–9100

UNITED CEREBRAL PALSY:
United Cerebral Palsy
1660 L Street, NW. Suite 700
Washington, D.C. 20036
1–800–872–5827

CHILD ABUSE:
Childhelp's USA National
Child Abuse Hotline
1–800–4–A–CHILD

National Center for Missing
and Exploited Children
1–800–843–5678

CYSTIC FIBROSIS:
Cystic Fibrosis Foundation
6931 Arlington Road
Bethesda, MD 20814
1–800–FIGHT-CF (34448–23)

DIABETES:
American Diabetes Association
1660 Dyke Street
Alexandria, VA 22314
1–800–342–2383

DRUG ADDICTION:
Drug Addiction 24-Hour Information and Treatment Hotline
1–800–229–7708

Drug Abuse 24-Hour Assistance and Treatment Hotline
1–800–234–1253

EPILEPSY:

Epilepsy Education Association
4335 1C Irish Hills Drive
South Bend, Indiana 46614–3110
(219)273–4050

Epilepsy Society—Affiliate Epilepsy
Foundation of America
4351 Garden City Dr.
Landover, MD 20785
1–800–332–1000

EYES AND BLINDNESS:

American Foundation for the Blind
11 Penn Plaza, Suite 300
New York, N.Y., 10001
1–800–AFB–LINE (232–5463)

Tissue Banks International
815 Park Avenue
Baltimore, Maryland 21201
(410)752–3800

Foundation Fighting Blindness
Executive Plaza 1, Suite 800
11350 McCormick Road
Hunt Valley, MD 21031–1014
1-888-394-3937
TDD: 1–800–683–5551

HANDICAPPED:

NY State Office of Advocate For Persons With Disabilities
1–800–522–4369

HEALTH:

American Academy of Pediatrics
141 Northwest Point Boulevard
Elk Grove Village, Il 60007–1098
(847)228–5005

American Medical Association Education
and Research Foundation
515 North State
Chicago, IL 60610

American National Red Cross
8111 Gatehouse Rd.
Falls Church, VA 22042

American Pediatric Society
3400 Research Forest Dr. Suite B7
The Woodlands, TX 77381

American Public Health Association
1015 15th St., N.W.
Washington, D.C. 20005–2605

Centers of Disease Control & Prevention
Atlanta, GA
1–404–639–3311

National Health Council
1730 M St. N.W., Suite 500
Washington, D.C. 20036–4505

HEARING:
National Association of the Deaf
814 Thayer Ave.
Silver Spring, MD 20910–4500

HEART:
American Heart Association
1–800–242–8721

National Stroke Association
1–800–787–6537

HEMOPHILIA:
National Hemophilia Foundation
The Sotto Building
110 Greene St., Room 406
New York, NY 10012

HOSPICES:
Children's Hospice International
1–800–242–4453

Hospice Education Institute Hospicelink
1–800–331–1620

KIDNEY:
National Kidney Foundation
1–800–622–9010

LEUKEMIA:
Leukemia Society of America
600 Third Avenue
New York, NY 10016

LIVER:
American Liver Foundation
1–800–223–0179

LUNG:
    American Lung Association
    1–800–LUNG–USA

MENTAL HEALTH:
    National Clearinghouse on Family
    Support and Children's Mental Health
    1–800–628–1696

    National Depressive and Manic Depressive
    Association
    1–800–826–3632

    National Mental Health Association
    1–800–969–6642

MUSCULAR DYSTROPHY:
    Muscular Dystrophy Association
    1–800–572–1717

NERVE AND MUSCLE DISORDERS:
    National Multiple Sclerosis Society
    1–800–344–4867

NUTRITION:
    FDA Center For Food Safety
    and Applied Nutrition
    1–800-FDA–4010

OCCUPATIONAL SAFETY:
    U.S. Department of Labor
    Occupational Safety and Health Administration
    200 Constitution Ave., N.W.
    Washington, D.C 20210

OSTEOPOROSIS:
    National Osteoporosis Foundation
    1–800–223–9994

PARKINSON'S DISEASE
    National Parkinson Foundation
    1501 N.W. 9th. Ave.
    Miami, FL 33136–1494
    1–800–327–4545

POLIOMYELITIS:
    International Polio Network
    4207 Lindell Blvd. #110
    St. Louis, MO. 63108
    314–534–0475

PROSTATE:
Prostate Information Line
1–800–543–9632

REHABILIATION:
National Rehabilitation Information Center
1–800–34–NARIC

RESEARCH:
Gerontological Society of America
1030 15th St., N.W., Suite 250
Washington, D.C. 20005–1503

RETIREMENT:
American Association for Retired Persons
601 E St. N.W.
Washington, D.C. 20049

U.S. Department of Health and Human Services
200 Independence Ave., S.W.
Washington, D.C. 20201

SEXUALLY TRANSMITTED DISEASES:
National STD Hotline
1–800–638–8922

SPEECH AND HEARING:
American Speech-Language-Hearing
Association Helpline
1–800–638–8255

SPINAL INJURIES:
National Spinal Cord Injury Association
1–800–962–9629

National Spinal Cord Injury Hotline
1-800-526-3456

VETERANS:
Veterans Administration
1–800–827–1000

American Legion
1608 K Street, N.W.
Washington, D.C. 20006

X RAYS:
American Roentgen Ray Society
44211 Slatestone Court
Leesburg, VA 20176–5109

What is Medicare?

Medicare is a federal health insurance program for people 65 or older and certain disabled people. It is run by the Health Care Financing Administration of the U.S. Department of Health and Human Services. Social Security Administration offices across the country take applications for Medicare and provide general information about the program.

Fee-for-Service or Managed Care?

How do you want to receive your Medicare benefits? If you live in an area served by a managed care plan, you have a choice. You can choose to get your Medicare benefits either through the fee-for-service system or through a managed care plan such as a health maintenance organization (HMO).

If you choose fee-for-service, you can go to almost any doctor, hospital or other health care provider you want to. Generally, you are charged a fee each time you use a service. Medicare pays its share of the bill. You are responsible for paying the balance.

In managed care, you usually must get all of your care from the doctors, hospitals, and other health care providers that are part of the plan, except in emergencies. Depending on the plan, you may have to pay a monthly premium and make a copayment each time you go to the doctor or use other services.

The Two Parts of Fee-for-Service Medicare

Hospital Insurance (Part A)
- Hospital and skilled nursing facility, home health and hospice care.

Medical Insurance (Part B)
- Doctors' services, outpatient hospital services, durable med-

ical equipment, and a number of other medical services and supplies that are not covered by Part A.

Medicare Hospital Insurance is called Part A and Medicare Medical Insurance is called Part B.

Part A has deductibles and coinsurance, but most people do not have to pay premiums for Part A. Part B has premiums, deductibles, and coinsurance amounts that you must pay yourself or through coverage by another insurance plan. Premium, deductible and coinsurance amounts are set each year based on formulas established by law.

Who Can Get Medicare Hospital Insurance (Part A)?

Generally, people age 65 and older can get premium-free Medicare Part A benefits, based on their own or their spouses' employment. (Premium-free means there are no premium payments. Most people do not pay premiums for Medicare Part A.) You can get premium-free Medicare Part A if you are 65 or older and any of these three statements is true:

- you receive benefits under the Social Security or Railroad Retirement system.
- you could receive benefits under Social Security or the Railroad Retirement system but have not filed for them, or
- you or your spouse had Medicare-covered government employment.

If you are under 65, you can get premium-free Medicare Part A benefits if you have been a disabled beneficiary under Social Security or the Railroad Retirement Board for more than 24 months.

Certain government employees and certain members of their families can also get Medicare when they are disabled for more than 29 months. They should apply at the Social Security Administration office as soon as they become disabled.

Or, you may be able to get premium-free Medicare Part A benefits if you receive continuing dialysis for permanent kidney failure or if you have had a kidney transplant. People who can get Medicare because of kidney disease should contact their Medicare carrier to get a copy of *Medicare Coverage of Kidney Dialysis and Kidney Transplant Services*.

Check with Social Security to see if you have worked long enough under Social Security, Railroad Retirement, as a government employee, or a combination of these systems to be able to get Medicare Part A benefits. Generally, if either you or your spouse worked for 10 years, you will be able to get premium-free Medicare Part A benefits.

Who Can Get Medicare Medical Insurance (Part B)?

Any person who can get premium-free Medicare Part A benefits based on work as described above can enroll for Part B, pay the monthly Part B premiums and get Part B benefits. In addition, most United States residents age 65 or over can enroll in Part B.

Buying Medicare Part A and Part B

If you or your spouse do not have enough work credits to be able to get Medicare Part A benefits and you are 65 or over, you may be able to buy Medicare Parts A and B—or just Medicare Part B—by paying monthly premiums. Also, you may be able to buy Medicare Parts A and B if you are disabled and lost your premium-free Part A solely because you are working.

Enrollment in Medicare

Automatic Enrollment

If you are already getting Social Security or Railroad Retirement benefit payments when you turn 65, you will automatically get a Medicare card in the mail. If you are disabled, you will automatically get a Medicare card in the mail when you have been a disability beneficiary under Social Security or Railroad Retirement for 24 months.

The Medicare card will show that you can get both Medicare Hospital Insurance (Part A) and Medical Insurance (Part B) benefits. If you do not want Part B, follow the instructions that come with the card.

Some People Have to Apply

You may not automatically get a Medicare card in the mail. You will have to apply for Medicare benefits if:

- you have not applied for Social Security or Railroad Retirement benefits.
- government employment is involved, or
- you have kidney disease.

You should file your application during your initial enrollment period, to avoid late enrollment surcharges under Medicare Part B (unless you qualify for a special enrollment period. Your initial enrollment period is a seven-month period that starts three months before the month you first meet the requirements for Medicare. If you do not sign up for Medicare during the first three months of your initial enrollment period, there will be a delay in starting your Part B coverage. Your coverage will be delayed from one to three months after enrollment.

If you do not enroll for Medicare Part B at any time during your initial enrollment period, you will not have another chance to enroll until the next general enrollment period. A general enrollment period is held each year from January 1 through March 31 and if you enroll during this period you will not be able to get Medicare until July of that year. You may also be charged a premium surcharge for late enrollment.

The enrollment period requirements and surcharges for late enrollment described above for Part B also apply to people who buy Part A.

Your Medicare Card

The Medicare card shows the Medicare coverage you have—Hospital Insurance (Part A), Medical Insurance Part B), or both—and the date your protection started. If you do not have both parts of Medicare, see information on how you can get the part you don't have.

Your Medicare card also shows your health insurance claim number. Sometimes this claim number is referred to as your Medicare number. The claim number usually has nine digits and one or two letters. There may also be another number after the letter. Your full claim number must always be included on all Medicare claims and correspondence. When a husband and wife both have Medicare, each receives a separate card and claim number. Each spouse must use the exact name and claim number shown on his or her card.

It is important that you remember to:

- Use your Medicare card only after the effective date shown on it.
- Keep your card handy. And be sure to carry your card with you when you are away from home.
- Always show your Medicare card when you get care.
- Always write your complete health insurance claim number (including any letters) on all checks for Medicare premium payments or any correspondence about Medicare. Also, have your Medicare card available when you make a telephone inquiry.
- Immediately ask Social Security to get you a new card if you lose yours.
- Never let anyone else use your Medicare card.

Medicare Hospital Insurance (Part A)

What Part A Includes

Medicare Part A helps pay for four kinds of medically necessary care:

- inpatient hospital care,
- inpatient care in a skilled nursing facility following a hospital stay,
- home health care,
- hospice care.

There is a limit on how many days of hospital or skilled nursing facility care Medicare helps pay for in each benefit period. But, your Part A protection is renewed every time you start a new benefit period. Benefit periods are described below.

Skilled nursing facility care is the only type of nursing home care that Medicare covers. Medicare does not pay for care that is primarily custodial.

Benefit Periods

A benefit period is a way of measuring your use of services under Medicare Part A. A benefit period starts the first time you receive inpatient hospital care after your Hospital Insurance begins. A benefit period ends when you have been out of a hospital or other facility primarily providing skilled nursing or rehabilitation services for 60 days in a row (including the day of discharge). A benefit period also ends if you are in a skilled nursing facility but have not received skilled care for sixty consecutive days. After one benefit period has ended, another one will start whenever you again receive inpatient hospital care.

There is no limit to the number of benefit periods you can have for hospital and skilled nursing facility care.

Here are two examples of how the benefit period works:

- **Example 1:** Ms. Jones enters the hospital on January 5. She is discharged on January 15. She has used 10 days of her first benefit period. Ms. Jones is not hospitalized again until July 20. Since more than 60 days elapsed between her hospital stays, she begins a new benefit period, her Part A coverage is completely renewed, and she will again pay the hospital deductible.

- **Example 2:** Ms. Smith enters the hospital on August 14. She is discharged on August 24. She also has used 10 days of her first benefit period. However, she is then readmitted to the hospital on September 20. Since fewer than 60 days elapsed between hospital stays. Ms. Smith is still in her first benefit period and will not be required to pay another hospital deductible. This means that the first day of her second admission is counted as the eleventh day of hospital care in that benefit period. Ms. Smith will not begin a new benefit period until she has been out of the hospital (and has not received any skilled care in a skilled nursing facility) for 60 consecutive days.

How Medicare Pays for Part A Services

Medicare Part A helps pay for covered services you receive in a hospital or skilled nursing facility or from a home health agency or hospice that has agreed to participate in the Medicare program.

Hospitals, skilled nursing facilities, home health agencies and hospices that agree to participate are called "providers" under the Medicare Part A program. Providers submit their claims directly to Medicare—you cannot submit claims for their services. The provider will charge you for any part of the Part A deductible you have not met and any coinsurance payment you owe. Providers cannot require you to make a deposit before being admitted for inpatient care that is or may be covered under Part A of Medicare.

Intermediaries

Intermediaries are private organizations that contract with Medicare to process claims submitted on your behalf by hospitals, skilled nursing facilities, home health agencies, hospices and certain other providers of services. When the Medicare intermediary pays a claim, Medicare will send you a notice. This notice is for your information, so that you may keep a record on what services you have received. This notice is not a bill. If you have any questions about the notice, contact the intermediary.

Coverage of Blood under Part A

Part A helps pay for blood (whole blood or units of packed red blood cells), blood components, and the cost of blood processing and administration. If you receive blood as an inpatient of a hospital or skilled nursing facility, Part A will pay for these blood costs, except for any nonreplacement fees charged for the first three pints of whole blood or units of packed red cells per calendar year. The nonreplacement fee is the amount that some hospitals and skilled nursing facilities charge for blood that is not replaced.

If you are charged nonreplacement fees, you have the option of either paying the fees or having the blood replaced. If you choose to have the blood replaced, you can either replace the blood personally or arrange to have another person or an organization replace it for you. A hospital or skilled nursing facility cannot charge you for any of the first three pints of blood you replace or arrange to replace. If you have already paid for or replaced blood under Medicare Part B during the calendar year, you do not have to meet those costs again under Part A.

When You Are a Hospital Inpatient

Medicare Part A helps pay for inpatient hospital care if all of the following four conditions are met:

- A doctor prescribes inpatient hospital care for treatment of your illness or injury.
- You require the kind of care that can be provided only in a hospital.
- The hospital has agreed to participate in the Medicare program. (Under certain conditions, Medicare helps pay for emergency inpatient care in a non- participating hospital.)
- The Utilization Review Committee of the hospital, a Peer Review Organization or an intermediary does not disapprove your stay.

If you meet these four conditions, Medicare will help pay for up to 90 days of medically necessary inpatient hospital care in each benefit period. Certain limits apply for psychiatric hospital care.

Medicare Part A does not pay for the services of doctors and certain other practitioners, even though you receive these services in a hospital. Instead, those services are covered under Medicare Part B. Medicare does not cover most dental procedures. However Medicare Part A will pay for dental services that accompany hospitalization because of:

- the underlying condition or clinical status, or
- the severity of the dental procedure.

In addition, there are some occasions in which Medicare Part B will pay for certain dental services.

NOTE: If you disagree with a decision on the amount Medicare will pay on a claim or whether services you receive are covered by Medicare, you always have the right to appeal the decision.

Hospital Inpatient Reserve Days

Medicare helps pay for your care in a hospital for up to 90 days in each benefit period. Medicare Part A also includes an extra 60 hospital days you can use if you have a long illness and have used up all 90 days in your benefit period. These extra days are called reserve days.

You have only 60 reserve days in your lifetime. For example, if you use 8 reserve days in your first hospital stay this year, the next time you visit a hospital you will have only 52 reserve days left to use, whether or not you have a new benefit period.

You can decide when you want to use your reserve days. After you have been in the hospital 90 days, you can use all or some of your 60 reserve days if you wish.

If you do not want to use your reserve days, you must tell the hospital in writing, either when you are admitted to the hospital, or at any time afterwards up to 90 days after you are discharged. If you use reserve days and then decide that you did not want to use them, you must request approval from the hospital to get them restored.

Emergency Care in a Nonparticipating Hospital

Under certain conditions, Medicare helps pay for emergency care received from a hospital that has not agreed to participate in the Medicare program. Medicare will help pay for both inpatient and outpatient emergency care provided in a nonparticipating hospital under the following conditions:

• The required emergency services are services that would be covered by Medicare had they been provided in a participating hospital.
• The emergency services were necessary to prevent death or a serious health problem, and the nonparticipating hospital was substantially more accessible than the nearest participating hospital.
• The allegation that an emergency existed is proven by medical information, such as a physician's statement.
• The nonparticipating hospital is a qualified emergency services hospital that has elected to bill Medicare for all emergency services it provided in the calendar year.

Care in a Psychiatric Hospital

Part A helps pay for no more than 190 days of inpatient care in a participating psychiatric hospital in your lifetime. Once you have used these 190 days, Part A does not pay for any more inpatient care in a psychiatric hospital. In most cases psychiatric care in general hospitals in not subject to this 190-day limit.

NOTE: A special rule applies if you are in a participating psychiatric hospital at the time your Part A starts. Contact Social Security or the Medicare intermediary for more information.

The Prospective Payment System

Medicare pays for most inpatient hospital care under the Prospective Payment System (PPS). Under PPS, hospitals are paid a set rate based on payment categories called Diagnosis Related Groups, or DRGs. In some cases, the Medicare payments are more than the hospital's costs; in other cases, less than the hospital's costs. **But even if Medicare pays the hospital less than the cost of your care, you do not have to make up the difference.**

The PPS system does not change your Medicare Part A protection. PPS does not determine the length of your stay in the hospital or the extent of care you receive.

Skilled Nursing Facility Care

Medicare Part A can help pay for certain inpatient care in a Medicare-participating skilled nursing facility following a hospital stay. Your condition must require daily skilled nursing or skilled rehabilitation services which, as a practical matter, can only be provided in a skilled nursing facility, and the skilled care you receive must be based on a doctor's orders.

What is a Skilled Nursing Facility?

A skilled nursing facility is a specially qualified facility that specializes in skilled care. It has the staff and equipment to provide skilled nursing care or skilled rehabilitation services and other related health services. Skilled nursing care means care that can only be performed by, or under the supervision of, licensed nursing personnel. Skilled rehabilitation services may include such services as physical therapy performed by, or under the supervision of, a professional therapist. Most nursing homes in the United States are not skilled nursing facilities that participate in Medicare. In some facilities, only certain portions participate in Medicare. If you are not sure whether a facility participates in Medicare as a skilled nursing facility, ask someone in the facility's business office.

When Can Medicare Pay?

Medicare Part A can help pay for your care in a Medicare-participating skilled nursing facility if you met **all of these five conditions:**

- Your condition requires daily skilled nursing or skilled rehabilitation services which, as a practical matter, can only be provided in a skilled nursing facility.
- You have been in a hospital at least three days in a row (not counting the day of discharge) before you are admitted to a participating skilled nursing facility.

- You are admitted to the facility within a short time (generally within 30 days) after you leave the hospital.
- Your care in the skilled nursing facility is for a condition that was treated in the hospital.
- A medical professional certifies that you need, and you receive, skilled nursing or skilled rehabilitation services on a daily basis.

When your stay in a skilled nursing facility is covered by Medicare, Part A helps pay for a maximum of 100 days in each benefit period, but only if you need daily skilled nursing care or rehabilitation services for that long.

If you leave a skilled nursing facility and are readmitted within 30 days, you do not need to have a new three day stay in the hospital for your care to be covered. If you have some of your 100 days left and you need skilled nursing or rehabilitation services on a daily basis for further treatment of a condition treated during your previous stay in the facility, Medicare will help pay.

Medicare Part A does not cover your doctor's services while you are in a skilled nursing facility. Medicare Part B covers doctors' services.

Rules That Protect You

Skilled nursing facilities have the right to inquire about your financial assets, and in some states may even request copies of your financial records. However, skilled nursing facilities cannot require you to pay a deposit or other payment as a condition of admission to the facility unless it is clear that services are not covered by Medicare. Contact your local Office on Aging to find out what financial information nursing facilities can require in your state.

Complaints and Appeals

If you want to complain about a skilled nursing facility's treatment of patients or other conditions that concern you, contact the state survey agency. The skilled nursing facility can give you the telephone number and address. While you are at the skilled nursing facility, you can look at a copy of the survey agency's latest certification survey report. The survey report tells how well the facility followed the rules about patient's rights, safety and quality of care.

Also, if you disagree with a decision on the amount Medicare will pay on a claim or whether services you receive are covered by Medicare, you always have the right to appeal the decision.

Home Health Care

Medicare pays for covered home health services furnished by participating home health agencies. A home health agency is a public or private agency that specializes in giving skilled nursing services and other therapeutic services, such as physical therapy, in your home. (A hospital or other facility that mainly provides skilled nursing or rehabilitation services cannot be considered your home.)

Medicare pays for home health visits only if all four of the following conditions are met:

- The care you need includes intermittent skilled nursing care, physical therapy, or speech therapy.
- You are confined to your home (homebound).
- You are under the care of a physician who determines you need home health care and sets up a home health plan for you.
- The home health agency providing services has agreed to participate in the Medicare program.

Once all four of these conditions are met, either Medicare Part A or Medicare Part B will pay for all medically necessary covered home health services.

When you no longer need intermittent skilled nursing care, physical therapy, or speech therapy. Medicare will pay for home health services if you continue to need occupational therapy.

Medicare home health services do not include coverage for general household services such as laundry, meal preparation, shopping, or other home care services furnished mainly to assist people in meeting personal, family, or domestic needs.

To determine whether you can get services under the Medicare home health benefit, ask your physician to refer you to a Medicare participating home health agency. The home health agency will evaluate your case and tell you whether you meet the requirements for Medicare coverage. Home health agencies should not charge for this evaluation.

Medicare pays the full approved cost of all covered home health visits. You may be charged only for any services or costs that Medicare does not cover. However, if you need durable medical equipment, you are responsible for a 20 percent coinsurance payment for the equipment.

The home health agency will submit the claim for payment. You do not have to send in any bills yourself.

NOTE: If you disagree with a decision on the amount Medicare will pay on a claim or whether services you receive are covered by Medicare, you always have the right to appeal the decision.

Hospice Care

A hospice is a public agency or private organization that is primarily engaged in providing pain relief, symptom management and supportive services to terminally ill people.

Hospice care includes both home care and inpatient care, when needed, and a variety of services not otherwise covered under Medicare. Under the Medicare hospice benefit, Medicare pays for services every day and also permits a hospice to provide appropriate custodial care, including homemaker services and counseling.

Medicare Part A helps pay for hospice care if all three of these conditions are met:

- A doctor certifies that the patient is terminally ill.
- The patient chooses to receive care from a hospice instead of standard Medicare benefits for the terminal illness.
- Care is provided by a Medicare participating hospice program.

There are no deductibles under the hospice benefit. The beneficiary does not pay for Medicare-covered services for the terminal illness, except for small coinsurance amounts for outpatient drugs and inpatient respite care.

The patient is responsible for five percent of the cost of outpatient drugs or $5 toward each prescription, whichever is less. For inpatient respite care, the patient pays five percent of the Medicare-allowed rate. The rate varies slightly depending on the area of the country.

Respite care under the hospice program is a short-term inpatient stay in a facility. The medicare beneficiary's inpatient stay gives temporary relief—a respite—to the person who regularly assists with home care. Each inpatient respite care stay is limited to no more than five days in a row.

While receiving hospice care, if a patient requires treatment for a condition not related to the terminal illness. Medicare continues to help pay for all necessary covered services under the standard Medicare benefit program.

NOTE: If you disagree with a decision on the amount Medicare will pay on a claim or whether services you receive are covered by Medicare, you always have the right to appeal the decision.

Peer Review Organizations

Peer Review Organizations (PROs) are groups of practicing doctors and other health care professionals paid by the federal government to monitor the care given to Medicare patients. Each state has a PRO that has the authority to decide whether care given to Medicare patients is reasonable, necessary, provided in the most appropriate setting, and meets standards of quality generally accepted by the medical profession.

PROs work with hospitals and doctors to promote care that is most effective in treating disease and injury. PROs also promote quality care by distributing health care information and maintaining a toll-free telephone hot line to answer your health care questions.

Beneficiary Complaints

PROs are responsible for reviewing beneficiary complaints about the quality of care provided by inpatient hospitals, hospital outpatient departments and hospital emergency rooms; skilled nursing facilities; home health agencies; HMO's; and ambulatory surgical centers.

If you believe that you have received poor quality care from one of these facilities, you may complain to the PRO. The PRO will investigate written complaints from beneficiaries, or their representatives, about the quality of Medicare services received.

Your complaint must be in writing, but if you need help, the PRO will take the information from you over the telephone and write the complaint for you. If someone other than the PRO makes a complaint for you or on your behalf, you must give written permission for that person to represent you in the complaint.

An Important Message from Medicare

If you are admitted to a Medicare participating hospital, you will receive *An Important Message From Medicare* which explains your rights as a hospital patient and provides the name, address and phone number of the PRO for your state. The message also explains what to do if you feel that a hospital improperly refused to admit you or forced you to leave it too soon. If you are not given a copy of the message, be sure to ask for one.

An Important Message from Medicare

Your Rights While You Are a Medicare Hospital Patient

- You have the right to receive all the hospital care that is necessary for the proper diagnosis and treatment of your illness or injury. According to Federal law, your discharge date must be determined solely by your medical needs, not by "Diagnosis Related Groups" (DRGs) or Medicare payments.

- You have the right to be fully informed about decisions affecting your Medicare coverage and payment for your hospital stay and for any post-hospital services.

- You have the right to request a review by a Peer Review Organization (PRO) of any written Notice of Noncoverage that you receive from the hospital stating that Medicare will no longer pay for your hospital care. PROs are groups of doctors who are paid by the Federal Government to review medical necessity, appropriateness and quality of hospital treatment furnished to Medicare patients. The phone number and address of the PRO for your area are:

Talk to your doctor about your stay in the hospital

You and your doctor know more about your condition and your health needs than anyone else. Decisions about your medical treatment should be made between you and your doctor. If you have any questions about your medical treatment, your need for continued hospital care, your discharge, or your need for possible post-hospital care, don't hesitate to ask your doctor. The hospital's patient representative or social worker will also help you with your questions and concerns about hospital services.

If you think you are being asked to leave the hospital too soon

- Ask a hospital representative for a written notice of explanation immediately, if you have not already received one. This notice is called a Notice of Noncoverage. You must have this Notice of Noncoverage if you wish to exercise your right to request a review by the PRO.
- The Notice of Noncoverage will state either that your doctor or the PRO agrees with the hospital's decision that Medicare will no longer pay for your hospital care.
- If the hospital and your doctor agree, the PRO does not review your case before a Notice of Noncoverage is issued. But the PRO will respond to your request for a review of your Notice of Noncoverage and seek your opinion. You cannot be made to pay for your hospital care until the PRO makes its decision, if you request the review by noon of the first work day after you receive the Notice of Noncoverage.

If the hospital and your doctor disagree, the hospital may request the PRO to review your case. If it does make such a request, the hospital is required to send you a notice to that effect. In this situation the PRO must agree with the hospital or the hospital cannot issue a Notice of Noncoverage. You may request that the PRO reconsider your case after you receive a Notice of Noncoverage, but since the PRO has already reviewed your case once, you may have to pay for at least one day of hospital care before the PRO completes this reconsideration.

If you do not request a review, the hospital may bill you for all the costs of your stay beginning with the third day after you receive the Notice of Noncoverage. The hospital, however, cannot charge you for care unless it provides you with a Notice of Noncoverage.

How to Request a Review of the Notice of Noncoverage

- If the *Notice of Noncoverage* states that your physician agrees with the hospital's decision:

  You must make your request for review to the PRO by noon of the first work day after you receive the *Notice of Noncoverage* by contacting the PRO by phone or in writing.

  The PRO must ask for your views about your case before making its decision. The PRO will inform you by phone or in writing of its decision on the review.

  If the PRO agrees with the *Notice of Noncoverage,* you may be billed for all costs of your stay beginning at noon of the day after you receive the PRO's decision.

  Thus, you will not be responsible for the cost of hospital care before you receive the PRO's decision.

- If the Notice of Noncoverage states that the PRO agrees with the hospital's decision:

  You should make your request for reconsideration to the PRO immediately upon receipt of the *Notice of Noncoverage* by contacting the PRO by phone or in writing.

  The PRO can take up to three working days from receipt of your request to complete the review. The PRO will inform you in writing of its decision on the review.

  Since the PRO has already reviewed your case once, prior to the issuance of the *Notice of Noncoverage,* the hospital is permitted to begin billing you for the cost of your stay beginning with the third calendar day after you receive your *Notice of Noncoverage* even if the PRO has not completed its review.

  Thus, if the PRO continues to agree with the Notice of Noncoverage, you may have to pay for at least one day of hospital care.

NOTE: The process described above is called "immediate review." If you miss the deadline for this immediate review while you are in the hospital, you may still request a review of Medicare's decision to no longer pay for your care at any point during your hospital stay or after you have left the hospital. The Notice of Noncoverage will tell you how to request this review.

Post-Hospital Care

When your doctor determines that you no longer need all the specialized services provided in a hospital, but you still require medical care, he or she may discharge you to a skilled nursing facility or home care. The discharge planner at the hospital will help arrange for the services you may need after your discharge. Medicare and supplemental insurance policies have limited coverage for skilled nursing facility care and home health care. Therefore, you should find out which services will or will not be covered and how payment will be made. Consult with your doctor, hospital discharge planner, patient representative, and your family in making preparations for care after you leave the hospital. Don't hesitate to ask questions.

Medicare Medical Insurance (Part B)

What Medicare Part B Includes

Medicare Part B helps pay for:

- doctors' services,
- outpatient hospital care,
- diagnostic tests,
- durable medical equipment,
- ambulance services, and
- many other health services and supplies that are not covered by Medicare Part A.

Doctors' Services Covered by Medicare Part B

Medicare Part B helps pay for covered services you receive from your doctor in his or her office, in a hospital, in a skilled nursing facility, in your home, or any other location.

Deductible and Coinsurance Amounts under Part B

For most services covered under Part B, you must pay a deductible and coinsurance. Exceptions to this rule, such as laboratory services and flu shots, are explained in this section.

The Annual Deductible

You must pay the first $100 in approved charges for covered medical expenses. This is called the Medicare Part B annual deductible. You need to meet this $100 deductible only once during the year, and the deductible can be met by any combination of covered expenses. You do not have to meet a separate deductible for each different kind of covered Part B service you receive.

The Blood Deductible

Unless you have already done so under your Part A benefit, you must pay for or replace the first three pints or units of blood and blood components you use each year. This is called the Medicare Part B blood deductible. After you have replaced or paid for the first three pints of blood **and** you have met the $100 annual deductible, Medicare will pay 80 percent of the approved amount for blood, starting with the fourth pint.

Coinsurance

After you pay the annual deductible, you will owe a share of the Medicare-approved amount for most services and supplies. This share is called coinsurance. Usually, your coinsurance share is 20 percent of the Medicare-approved amount. If your services were **provided "on assignment,"** you pay only the coinsurance.

If your services were **not provided "no assignment,"** and the charges for your services were more than the Medicare-approved amount, you usually owe the Medicare coinsurance plus certain charges above the Medicare-approved amount.

Part B Carriers

Carriers are private organizations that contract with Medicare to process claims and make Medicare payments for services by doctors and suppliers. Claims for durable medical equipment, oxygen and some other supplies are handled by special carriers called Durable Medical Equipment Regional Carriers (DMERCs). If you have questions about Medicare Part B claims, contact your Medicare carrier.

Second Opinion before Surgery

Sometimes your doctor may recommend surgery for the treatment of a medical problem. In some cases, surgery is unavoidable. But there is increasing evidence that many conditions can be treated equally well without surgery. Because even minor surgery involves some risk, we recommend that you get an opinion from a second doctor to help you decide about surgery. Medicare will help pay for a second opinion. Medicare will also help pay for a third opinion if the first and second opinions contradict each other.

Your own doctor is the best source for referral to another doctor. But, if you wish, you can call your Medicare Part B carrier for the names and phone numbers of doctors in your area who provide second opinions.

Services of Other Practitioners

Most Medicare covered doctors' services are furnished by a doctor of medicine or a doctor of osteopathy. But under certain limited circumstances, Medicare can help pay for some of the services provided by the following health care practitioners:

Chiropractors

Medicare helps pay for the manipulation of the spine to correct a subluxation (i.e., minor dislocation) that is demonstrated by an X-ray. Medicare does not pay for X-rays performed by chiropractors.

Podiatrists

Medicare will not pay for routine foot care, such as nail trimming or the removal of corns or calluses. Medicare can help pay for treatment of injuries or diseases of the foot (for example, hammer toe or bunions) when professional services are required due to the presence of certain systemic illnesses, such as diabetes.

Dentists' Services

Medicare does not cover routine dental care or most dental procedures. However, there are three cases in which Medicare Part B will help pay for certain dental services. The three cases in which Medicare Part B will pay are:

- Dental services performed as an integral part of a Medicare covered procedure. For example, Medicare will help pay for the wiring of teeth when done in connection with the treatment of a jaw fracture.
- The extraction of teeth to prepare the jaw for radiation treatment in cases of oral cancer.
- Oral and dental examinations performed on an inpatient basis in preparation for kidney transplant or heart value replacement surgery.

In addition, there are some occasions in which Medicare Part A will pay certain dental services delivered on an inpatient basis.

Optometrists

Medicare can help pay for cataract eyeglasses, contact lenses, or intraocular lenses provided by an optometrist after cataract surgery, if the optometrist is authorized to provide such services in your State. (But Medicare can not pay for routine eye exams and eyeglasses.)

Outpatient Hospital Services

Medicare Part B helps pay for covered services you receive as an outpatient from a participating hospital for diagnosis or treatment of an illness or injury. Under certain conditions. Medicare helps pay for emergency outpatient care you receive from a non-participating hospital.

You must meet your Part B deductible before Medicare will begin paying for your outpatient hospital charges. If you have proof from your most recent Part B Benefits notice that you have already met your deductible, bring the notice with you. You are also responsible for a coinsurance of 20 percent of the hospital's charge above the deductible.

If the hospital cannot tell how much of the $100 deductible you have met and the charge for the services you received is less than $100, the hospital may ask you to pay the entire bill. The amount you pay the hospital can be credited toward any part of the deductible you have not met. If you pay the hospital for deductible amounts you do not owe, the hospital or the Medicare intermediary will refund the amount you overpaid.

Other Services and Supplies Covered by Medicare

Ambulatory Surgical Services

An ambulatory surgical center is a facility that provides surgical services that do not require a hospital stay. Medicare Part B will pay for the use of an ambulatory surgical center for certain approved surgical procedures. However, Medicare can only pay centers that have an agreement to participate in the Medicare program. If you do not know whether an ambulatory surgical center participates in Medicare, ask someone in the center's business office.

In addition to helping pay for the use of the ambulatory surgical center, Medicare also helps pay for physician and anesthesia services that are provided in connection with the procedure.

Outpatient Physical and Occupational Therapy and Speech Pathology Services

Medicare Part B helps pay for medically necessary outpatient physical and occupational therapy and speech pathology services, if the following conditions are met:

• your doctor or therapist sets up the plan of treatment, and
• your doctor periodically reviews that plan.

You can receive physical therapy, occupational therapy and speech pathology services as an outpatient of a participating hospital or skilled nursing facility, or from a participating home health agency, rehabilitation agency, or public health agency. The provider of services may charge you only for any part of the $100 annual deductible you have not met, 20 percent of the remaining approved amount, and any noncovered services.

Also, you can receive services directly from an independently practicing, Medicare-approved physical or occupational therapist in his or her office or in your home. (Medicare does not pay for services provided by independently practicing speech pathologists.) But, the maximum amount Medicare pays for each of these services provided by an independently practicing physical or occupational therapist.

Comprehensive Outpatient Rehabilitation Facility Services

Under certain circumstances, Medicare helps pay for outpatient services you receive from a Medicare-participating comprehensive outpatient rehabilitation facility (CORF). Covered services include physicians' services; physical, speech, occupational and respiratory therapies; counseling; and other related services. You must be referred by a physician who certifies that you need skilled rehabilitation services. For most CORF services, you are responsible only for the annual deductible and 20 percent of the Medicare-approved charges. Medicare helps pay for mental health treatment in a CORF.

Partial Hospitalization for Mental Health Treatment

Partial hospitalization (sometimes called day treatment) is a program of outpatient mental health care. Under certain conditions, Medicare Part B helps pay for these programs when provided by hospital outpatient departments or by community mental health centers. If you are considering mental health treatment, check with the program you have chosen to see if it meets the conditions for Medicare payment.

Rural Health Clinic Services

Medicare Part B helps pay for services of physicians, nurse practitioners, physician assistants, nurse midwives, visiting nurses (under certain conditions), clinical psychologists, and clinical social workers furnished by a rural health clinic. Medicare Part B also helps pay for certain laboratory tests in these clinics. You are responsible only for the annual Medicare Part B deductible plus 20 percent of the Medicare-approved charge for the clinic.

Laboratory Services

Medicare Part B pays the full approved fee for covered clinical diagnostic tests provided by certified laboratories that are participating in Medicare. The laboratory may be independent, part of a hospital outpatient department or in a doctor's office. (In Maryland only, you may be charged 20 percent coinsurance for hospital outpatient tests.) The laboratory must accept assignment for the tests. It cannot bill you.

Some laboratories are approved only for certain kinds of tests. Your doctor can usually tell you which laboratories are approved and whether the tests he or she is ordering from an approved laboratory are covered by Medicare. If your doctor can not tell you, call your Part B carrier.

Pap Smear Screening

Once every three years, Medicare Part B helps pay for Pap smears to screen for cervical cancer. Women who are at high risk for cervical cancer may receive the screening Pap smear test more frequently. In some cases, the test may be performed annually.

High risk factors include the early onset of sexual activity (under 16 years old), having multiple sexual partners (five or more during a lifetime), or a history of sexually transmitted diseases.

Your physician will assist you in determining whether these or other factors in your medical history have contributed to your risk. Diagnostic Pap smears, which are ordered by a physician, may be performed on women who:

- have had or are being treated for cancer of the cervix, uterus, or vagina:
- had a previous abnormal Pap smear:
- have any abnormal findings of the cervix, vagina, ovaries, or adnexa: or
- have any signs or symptoms that a physician judges to be related to a gynecological disorder.

Breast Cancer Screening (Mammography)

Medicare Part B helps pay for X-ray screenings for the detection of breast cancer, if they are provided by a Medicare-approved supplier. Women 65 or older can use the benefit every 24 months. Some younger women can use the screening benefit more frequently. Your Medicare carrier can tell you how often Medicare will pay for a screening mammogram for you. Medicare also pays for diagnostic mammograms as needed when symptoms are present.

Kidney Dialysis and Transplants

Medicare Part B helps pay for kidney dialysis and transplants. For detailed information on this coverage, you can get a copy of *Medicare Coverage of Kidney Dialysis and Kidney Transplant Services.*

Heart and Liver Transplants

Under certain conditions, Medicare Part B helps pay for heart and liver transplants in a Medicare-approved facility. If you are considering a heart or liver transplant, you and your physician can find out about Medicare coverage by contacting your Medicare carrier.

Ambulance Transportation

Medicare Part B helps pay for medically necessary ambulance transportation, but only if:

- the ambulance, equipment and personnel meet Medicare requirements: and
- transportation in any other vehicle could endanger your health.

Under these conditions, Medicare helps pay for ambulance transportation only to a hospital or skilled nursing facility or from a hospital or skilled nursing facility to your home. Medicare does not pay for ambulance transportation from your home to a doctor's office or to any free-standing facility such as an ambulatory surgical center or a dialysis facility that is not in or next to a hospital.

Medicare usually helps pay only if the ambulance transportation is in your local area. But, if there are no local facilities equipped to provide the care you need, Medicare helps pay for necessary ambulance transportation to the closest facility outside your local area that can provide the necessary care. If there is a local facility equipped to provide the care you need but you choose to go to another institution that is farther away, Medicare payment is based on the charge for transportation to the closest facility that can provide the necessary care.

Use of air ambulance is limited. Medicare pays for use of an air ambulance only in extremely urgent emergency situations. If you could have been moved by land ambulance without serious danger to your life or health, Medicare pays only the land ambulance rate. You are responsible for the difference between the air ambulance rate and the land ambulance rate.

Durable Medical Equipment

Medicare Part B helps pay for durable medical equipment such as oxygen equipment, wheelchairs, and other medically necessary equipment that your doctor prescribes for use in your home. (A hospital or facility that mainly provides skilled nursing or rehabilitation services cannot be considered your home.

To be considered durable medical equipment, the equipment

must be able to withstand repeated use, primarily serve a medical purpose, and be appropriate for use in your home.

Only your own doctor should prescribe medical equipment for you. An equipment supplier should not take any of the following actions:

- contact you first, either by phone or by mail, and offer to get your doctor or Medicare to approve an item. (It is all right for the supplier to contact you in response to calls from your doctor or other health care workers.);
- say he or she works for, or represents, Medicare;
- deliver equipment to your home that neither you nor your doctor ordered; or
- send you used items, while billing Medicare for new ones.

Prosthetic Devices

Medicare Part B helps pay for prosthetic devices needed to replace an internal body organ. These include Medicare-approved corrective lenses needed after a cataract operation, ostomy bags and certain related supplies, and breast prostheses (including a surgical brassiere) after a mastectomy. Medicare also helps pay for artificial limbs and eyes, and for arm, leg, back, and neck braces. Medicare does not pay for orthopedic shoes unless they are an integral part of leg braces and the cost is included in the charge for the braces. Medicare does not pay for dental plates or other dental devices.

Therapeutic Shoes

Medicare helps pay for therapeutic shoes and shoe inserts for people who have severe diabetic foot disease. The doctor who treats your diabetes must certify your need for therapeutic shoes. The shoes and inserts must be prescribed by a podiatrist or other qualified doctor and furnished by a podiatrist, orthotist, prosthetist, or pedorthist.

Medicare helps pay for one pair of therapeutic shoes per calendar year. Medicare also helps pay for inserts. Shoe modifications may be substituted for inserts. The fitting of shoes or inserts is included in the Medicare payment for the shoes.

Medical Supplies

Medicare Part B helps pay for surgical dressings, splints, and casts ordered by a doctor in connection with your medical treatment.

Drugs and Biologicals

Influenza (Flu) and Pneumococcal Pneumonia Vaccines

Medicare Part B pays the full approved charges for flu and pneumonia vaccines and their administration. Neither the $100 annual deductible nor the 20 percent coinsurance applies to these services. If the person giving you the shot accepts assignment (accepts the Medicare payment as payment in full), there will be no cost to you. If the person does not accept assignment, you may have to pay charges in addition to the Medicare approved amount.

You must have doctor's orders to get a pneumonia shot. Any health care professional complying with the Medicare rules in your state can give you a flu shot.

Generally, Medicare does not cover outpatient or self-administered drugs. However, in addition to blood and influenza and pneumococcal vaccines, Medicare will help pay for the following outpatient prescription drugs and biologicals. Payment is based on medical need, and only under the conditions described here.

Other Drugs and Biologicals

- **Antigens:** Medicare will pay for antigens if they are prepared by a physician and administered by a properly instructed person (who could be a patient) under physician supervision.
- **Erythropoietin:** Medicare will help pay for erythropoietin if you have end stage renal disease (permanent kidney failure) and require this drug to treat anemia.
- **Hemophilia Clotting Factors:** If you have hemophilia, Medicare will help pay for your self-administered clotting factors.
- **Hepatitis B Vaccine:** For people medically judged to be especially susceptible to hepatitis, Medicare will help pay for your hepatitis B vaccine.

- **Immunosuppressive Drugs:** Following a Medicare-covered tissue or organ transplant, Medicare helps pay for immunosuppressive drugs.
- **Oral Cancer Drugs:** Medicare will help pay for oral cancer drugs if the same drug is available in injectable form.

Medicare Payments for Outpatient Treatment of Mental Illness

Medicare helps pay for outpatient diagnostic and mental health treatment services you receive from professionals such as physicians, clinical psychologists, clinical social workers and other nonphysician practitioners. These professionals furnish services in various settings, for example, hospitals, comprehensive outpatient rehabilitation facilities, community mental health centers, and skilled nursing facilities.

Most outpatient mental health treatment services furnished by these professionals are subject to a payment limit. In effect, Medicare Part B pays only 50 percent (not 80 percent) of the approved amount for these services. On assigned claims, beneficiaries are responsible for paying the remaining 50 percent. For unassigned claims, beneficiaries may have to pay more.

Medicare Medical Insurance (Part B) Payments

The Assignment Payment Method
Under the assignment method, your doctor or supplier agrees to accept the amount approved by the Medicare carrier as total payment for covered services: the doctor or supplier agrees to "accept assignment."

The assignment method can save you money. The doctor or supplier sends the claim to Medicare. Medicare pays your doctor or supplier 80 percent of the Medicare-approved amount, after subtracting any part of the $100 annual deductible you have not met. The doctor or supplier can charge you only for the part of the $100 annual deductible you have not met and for the coinsurance, which is the remaining 20 percent of the approved amount. Of course, your doctor or supplier also can charge you for services that Medicare does not cover.

Doctors and certain other practitioners and suppliers must accept assignment on all claims for services furnished to Medicare beneficiaries who are eligible for medical assistance through their state Medicaid program, including Qualified Medicare Beneficiaries.

Participating Doctors and Suppliers

Doctors and suppliers may sign agreements to become **Medicare participants.** Medicare-participating doctors and suppliers have agreed in advance to accept assignment on **all** Medicare claims. Doctors and suppliers are given the opportunity to sign participation agreements each year. Medicare- participating doctors and suppliers can display emblems or certificates that show they accept assignment on all Medicare claims.

Certain professionals, such as social workers who provide outpatient mental health services, must accept assignment if they bill Medicare.

All doctors and suppliers, whether they choose to participate or not, must abide by Medicare laws. In addition, the fact that a doctor or supplier is not a participant does not mean that he or she does not treat Medicare patients.

When Your Doctor Does Not Accept Assignment

Many doctors and suppliers who do not accept assignment on all claims may accept assignment on some or most claims. Ask your doctor or supplier whether he or she will accept assignment on your claims.

If your doctor or supplier does not accept assignment, you must pay the doctor or supplier directly.

You are usually responsible for the entire bill, even if it is higher than the Medicare- approved amount, because your doctor or supplier did not agree to accept the Medicare-approved amount as payment in full. In this case, you pay the doctor or supplier and Medicare pays you 80 percent of the approved amount, after subtracting any part of the $100 annual deductible you have not met.

Charge limits: Even though a doctor does not accept assignment, for most covered services there are limits on the amount that he or she can actually charge you. The most the doctor can charge you is 115 percent of what Medicare approves. Doctors who charge more than these limits may be fined. These limits also apply to certain services of suppliers. The notice you get when Medicare processes your claim tells you whether charge limits apply.

If you think you have been charged more than the payment limit, ask the doctor or supplier for a reduction in the charge. If you have already paid more than the payment limit, ask for a refund. If you cannot get a reduction or refund, you can call your Medicare carrier and ask for assistance. Some states have laws that could further reduce your medical costs. If you live in one of the states listed on this page, you can ask the state office listed there about the laws in your state.

Special rule for doctors performing elective surgery: Medicare law requires doctors who do not accept assignment for elective surgery to give you a written estimate of your costs before the surgery if the total charge for the surgical procedure is $500 or more. If the doctor did not give you a written estimate, you are entitled to a refund of any amount you paid him or her over the Medicare approved amount.

Participating Providers

Hospitals, skilled nursing facilities, home health agencies, hospices, comprehensive outpatient rehabilitation facilities, and providers of outpatient physical and occupational therapy and speech pathology services are all participating providers under Medicare Part B. They submit their claims to Medicare. Medicare subtracts any deductible you have not met and any coinsurance amount and pays the provider. The provider bills you only for any deductible and coinsurance amounts you owe.

Submitting Part B Claims

Doctors, Suppliers and Other Providers Must Submit Claims for You

Even if they do not accept assignment, doctors, suppliers and other providers of Part B services must, in most cases, submit

Medicare claims for you. They have one year from the date of your service to send in your claim. (If you have other health insurance that should pay before Medicare, you can submit your claims yourself.)

Filing Your Own Claims

In some cases, you may need to file your own Medicare Part B claim. If you do, send the claim to the carrier responsible for processing Medicare claims in the area where you received the services.

Claims When You Are Enrolled in a Managed Care Plan (HMO)

If you are enrolled in an HMO, claims seldom need to be submitted on your behalf. Medicare pays the HMO a set amount each month and the HMO provides your medical care. But if you get service from a doctor or other professional who is not affiliated with your HMO, the claim should be submitted directly to your HMO.

Submitting Claims to the Railroad Retirement System

If you get Medicare under the Railroad Retirement system, the doctor or supplier must submit your claims to the United HealthCare office that serves your region. Regional offices of The Travelers are listed in *Your Medicare Handbook for Railroad Retirement Beneficiaries,* which is available at any Railroad Retirement office.

Claims for a Person Who Has Died

When a Medicare beneficiary dies, the way Medicare pays Part B claims depends on whether the doctor's or supplier's bill has been paid. (Any Part A payments due to the hospital, skilled nursing facility, home health agency or hospice will be made directly to the provider of services.)

If the bill was paid by the patient or with funds from the patient's estate, Medicare's payment will be made either to the estate representative or to a surviving member of the patient's immediate family. If someone other than the patient paid the bill, payment may be made to that person.

If the bill has not been paid and the doctor or supplier does not accept assignment, the Medicare payment can be made to the person who has or assumes legal obligation to pay the bill for the deceased patient.

Your Medicare carrier can provide additional information about how to submit claims for Medicare Part B payment after a patient dies.

Your Part B Benefits Notice from Medicare

After your doctor, provider, or supplier sends in a Part B claim, Medicare will send you a notice. The notice is not a bill. It is sent to you for your records.

Your Part B benefits notice shows the doctor's charges and what Medicare approved. It shows what your copayment is and whether you have met your Part B deductible. The notice tells you whether your doctor accepted assignment on the claim, and if not, what the charge limit is on the service provided. The notice may have other useful information about your claim.

Please read your Part B notices carefully. If you believe payments were made for services or supplies you didn't receive, or payments are otherwise questionable, call or write your carrier.

What Medicare Does Not Pay For

Medicare, by law, cannot pay for certain services. These include services performed by immediate relatives or members of your household, and services which another government program pays for. Discussed below are other services Medicare does not pay for.

Custodial Care

Medicare does not pay for custodial care when that is the **only** kind of care you need. Care is considered custodial when it is primarily for the purpose of helping you with daily living or meeting personal needs and could be provided safely and reasonably by people without professional skills or training. Much of the care needed by old and frail people to allow them to stay in their own home is custodial. Also, much of the care provided in nursing homes to people with chronic, long-term illnesses or disabilities is considered custodial care. For example, custodial care includes help in walking, getting in and out of bed, bathing, dressing, eating, and taking medicine. Even if you are in a participating hospital or skilled nursing facility, Medicare does not cover your stay, if you need only custodial care.

Care Not Reasonable and Necessary under Medicare Program Standards

Medicare does not usually pay for services that are "not reasonable and necessary" for the diagnosis or treatment of an illness or injury. These services include:

- drugs or devices that have not been approved by the Food and Drug Administration (FDA) (note: in certain cases services are not covered even when FDA has approved the drug or device);
- medical procedures and services performed using drugs or devices not approved by FDA; and,
- services, including drugs or devices, not considered safe and effective because they are experimental or investigational.

If a doctor admits you to a hospital or skilled nursing facility when the kind of care you need could be provided elsewhere (for example, at home or in an outpatient facility), your stay will not be considered reasonable and necessary, and Medicare will not pay for your stay. If you stay in a hospital or skilled nursing facility longer than you need to be there, Medicare payments will end when inpatient care is no longer reasonable and necessary.

If a doctor (or other practitioner) comes to treat you—or you visit him or her for treatment—more often than is medically necessary, Medicare will not pay for the "extra" visits. Medicare will not pay for more services than are reasonable and necessary for your treatment.

Medicare always bases decisions about what is reasonable and necessary on professional medical advice.

Care Outside the United States

Except in cases in Canada and Mexico described below, Medicare does not pay for hospital or medical services outside the United States. (Puerto Rico, the U.S. Virgin Islands, Guam, American Samoa, and the Northern Mariana Islands are considered part of the United States.)

In rare cases, Medicare can pay for inpatient hospital services that you get in Canada or Mexico. Medicare can pay only if:

1) You are in the United States when a medical emergency occurs and the Canadian or Mexican hospital is closer than the nearest U.S. hospital that can treat the emergency.
2) You are traveling through Canada without unreasonable delay by the most direct route between Alaska and another state when a medical emergency occurs and the Canadian hospital is closer than the nearest U.S. hospital that can treat the emergency.
3) You live in the United States and the Canadian or Mexican hospital is closer to your home than the nearest U.S. hospital that can treat your medical condition, regardless of whether an emergency exists.

Medicare also pays for doctor and ambulance services furnished in Canada or Mexico in connection with a covered inpatient hospital stay.

When Medicare Denies a Claim but You Do Not Have to Pay the Bill

In certain cases, even if Medicare denies your claim, you will not be held responsible for paying the doctor or other health care provider. Generally, these cases include claims for items or services that are denied as not "reasonable and necessary," or because the health care provider did not comply with certain federal requirements.

If you receive a bill from your doctor or another health care provider for an item or service denied by Medicare for one of the reasons mentioned above, contact your Medicare carrier for information on whether you are responsible for paying the bill.

Medicare Managed Care Plans

Managed Care

If you are currently receiving your Medicare benefits through fee-for-service, you may continue to do so. However, managed care is an increasingly popular way of receiving Medicare benefits. Most Medicare beneficiaries live in areas that have Medicare-approved managed care plans (often called HMOs).

Can I Enroll in a Managed Care Plan?

Most Medicare beneficiaries are eligible for enrollment in a managed care plan, and most parts of the country are served by one or more plans that have contracts with the Health Care Financing Administration (HCFA) to serve Medicare beneficiaries.

The only enrollment requirements are:

1. You must at least be enrolled in Medicare Part B (it pays doctor bills) and continue to pay the Part B monthly premium.
2. You cannot have elected care from a Medicare-certified hospice.
3. You cannot be medically determined to have permanent kidney failure. If, however, you are a member of a plan when

you first be come eligible for Medicare and the plan has a Medicare contract, you may change to Medicare membership with the plan even if you have permanent kidney failure.
4. You must live within the area in which the plan has a Medicare contract to provide services.

If you choose hospice care for a terminal illness after joining a managed care plan, you will receive hospice services from a Medicare-approved hospice, but you can stay in the plan. If you do, the plan is required to provide or arrange for all covered health care unrelated to the terminal illness. Also, if after joining a plan you are medically determined to have end-stage renal disease, the plan is required to provide or arrange for your care.

How Do I Join a Plan and When Does My Coverage Begin?

You can get the names of the managed care plans in your area by calling your state insurance counseling office or by calling Medicare at 1–800–638–6833.

All plans that contract with Medicare must have an advertised open enrollment period of at least 30 days once a year. Most plans, however, have continuous open enrollment, so you may join at any time. Medicare beneficiaries cannot be denied membership because of poor health, a disability, or preexisting condition.

Depending on the day of the month that you enroll, you may choose to have coverage begin either the first day of the month after your enrollment application is received by the plan or up to three months later. The plan must give you written information explaining your coverage and when it starts.

Before joining a plan, read the plan's membership materials. Make sure you understand your rights as a plan member and know what benefits you will receive.

If you live in an area served by more than one plan, compare premiums, copayments, and benefits to determine which plan best suits your needs at a price you can afford.

What Other Factors Should I Consider?

Get information about the doctors available to serve you and the hospitals and other health care facilities affiliated with the plan. Determine whether the plan's providers are in a location convenient to you.

Also, carefully consider the advantages and disadvantages of plan membership if you travel a lot or live part of the year in another State. Plans must provide coverage for a fixed period of time when you travel.

Another factor to keep in mind is that if you enroll in a plan and later move out of the plan's service area, you will have to disenroll and either return to regular fee-for-service Medicare or enroll in a plan that serves your new location.

If I Enroll, Where Do I Go for Care?

Before enrolling in a managed care plan, find out whether the plan has a "risk" or a "cost" contract with Medicare. There is an important difference.

Risk Plans: These plans have "lock-in" requirements. This means that you generally must receive all covered care through the plan or through referrals by the plan.

With few exceptions, if you go outside the plan for services, neither the plan nor Medicare will pay for those services. You will have to pay the entire bill out of your own pocket.

The only exceptions recognized by all Medicare plans are for emergency services, which you may receive anywhere in the United States, and urgently needed care, which you may receive while temporarily away from the plan's service area.

If you receive emergency or urgently needed care, the doctor or hospital that provides the service will either bill you or your plan. If the bill is given to you, present it to the plan yourself and keep a copy for your records. If possible, let the plan know whenever you are in an emergency situation.

In addition to paying for emergency and urgently needed care received outside the plan, a few risk plans offer what is called a "point-of-service" (POS) option.

Under the POS option, the plan permits you to receive certain services outside the plan's provider network and the plan will pay a percentage of the charges. In return for this flexibility expect to pay at least 20 percent of the bill.

Cost Plans: These plans do not have lock-in requirements. If you enroll in a cost plan, you can either go to health care providers affiliated with the plan and pay only the applicable co-payments, or you can go to providers outside the plan.

If you go to providers outside the plan, the plan probably will not pay but Medicare will. Medicare will pay its share of the approved charges.

You will be responsible for Medicare's coinsurance and deductibles and other permissible charges, just as if you were receiving care under the fee-for-service system.

Because cost plans do not have a lock-in requirement, they may be a good choice for you if you travel frequently or live outside the plan's service area part of the year.

Plan Hospital and Medical Benefits

While the package of benefits can vary from plan to plan, all plans must provide all of the benefits covered under Medicare parts A and B.

Plans may also offer extra benefits not otherwise covered by fee-for-service Medicare. The extra benefits can include, for example, physical exams, scheduled inoculations and other preventive care, prescription drugs, dental care, hearing aids and eyeglasses, as well as coverage for overseas travel.

Plans with risk contracts either provide the extra benefits at no additional cost or require you to purchase them as a condition of enrolling in the plan. You may pay more for additional benefits offered by cost plans.

Do I Select My Own Doctor?

Most managed care plans require you to select a primary care doctor from those affiliated with the plan when you first enroll. If you do not make a selection, one will be assigned to you.

Primary care doctors manage their patients' medical and hospital care. If for any reason you want to change your primary care doctor your primary care doctor, the plan generally will let you do so as long as you select another one of the plan's primary care doctors.

What About Specialists and Hospital Care?

Managed care plans have doctors available in all specialties of medicine. However, to see a specialist, you must be referred by your primary care physician if the plan is to pay for the specialist's services. Your primary care physician will help choose the specialist for you.

Just as a plan arranges in advance with specific doctors to care for members, it generally has contracts with specific hospitals, skilled nursing facilities, home health care agencies and other health care providers to serve its members. Some of the larger plans, however, have their own hospitals and other health care facilities.

By coordinating primary, specialty, inpatient, and outpatient treatment, plans can deliver appropriate care while minimizing duplicative and unwarranted services.

How Can I Appeal a Payment Decision Made by an HMO?

Managed care plans that contract with Medicare have a system that you can use to appeal payment decisions. You can file an appeal if your plan:

- refuses to pay for Medicare-covered services;
- refuses to provide services you request; or
- decides not to pay for the care you received from doctors or hospitals who are not part of the plan because the plan determined that the care was not for emergency or out- of- area urgent care.

If you believe that care should be paid for or provided, and it was not, you should file a request for reconsideration by the plan.

If you need more information or help, call any Social Security Administration office, your health plan, or your state insurance counseling office.

What Are the Advantages of Joining a Managed Care Plan?

People join managed care plans for many different reasons. Some of the most frequently mentioned reasons are listed below:

- It can be easier to get all services through one source (for example, doctors' services, hospital care, laboratory tests, X-rays).
- Quality of care may be enhanced because of the coordination of services.
- It is easier to budget medical costs because you know the amount of any premiums in advance, and the total of other out-of-pocket expenses is likely to be less than under the fee-for-service system.
- You generally pay only a nominal copayment when you use a service.
- In many cases, benefits beyond those covered by Medicare are available at either no additional charge or a nominal charge.
- Paperwork is virtually eliminated.
- Managed Care plans generally must accept all Medicare applicants, even those with health problems.

What Are the Disadvantages of Joining a Managed Care Plan?

Some of the disadvantages of enrolling in a managed care plan are listed below:

- You may not be free to go to any physician or hospital you choose. Except when you need emergency or unforeseen out-of-area urgent care services, you generally must use the plans providers or else the plan will not pay.

- You may need to have the prior approval of your primary physician to see a specialist, have elective surgery, or obtain equipment or other medical services.
- It can take up to 30 days to disenroll, and you must continue to use the HMO providers until you are disenrolled.

How and When May I Disenroll?

If you enroll in a plan and later decide to return to fee-for-service Medicare, you may disenroll at any time. To disenroll, state in writing that you want to withdraw from the plan and return to fee-for service Medicare coverage.

Give the written statement either to the plan's administrative office or to your local Social Security Administration or, if appropriate, your Railroad Retirement Board office. Your coverage under the fee-for-service system will begin the first day of the following month.

If you want to change from one managed care plan to another, you may do so by simply enrolling in the other plan as long as it has a Medicare contract. You are Automatically disenrolled from the first plan.

Health Insurance Information and Counseling

All states, along with Puerto Rico, the Virgin Islands, and the District of Columbia, have a health insurance counseling program that can give you free information and assistance on Medicare, Medicaid, Medigap, long term care and other health insurance benefits. You can call your state counseling office and ask for printed information, help with choosing health insurance coverage, or even help understanding your bills, insurance claims and explanation forms. Phone numbers are listed below. The 800 numbers work only within the state.

Alabama 1–800–243–5463
Alaska 1–800–478–6065
Arizona 1–800–432–4040
Arkansas 1–800–852–5494
California 1–800–434–0222
Colorado 1–800–544–9181
Connecticut 1–800–994–9422
Delaware 1–800–336–9500
District of Columbia 202–676–3900
Florida 1–800–963–5337
Georgia 1–800–669–8387
Hawaii (808) 586–0100
Idaho 1–800–247–4422
Illinois 1–800–548–9034
Indiana 1–800–452–4800
Iowa 1–800–351–4664
Kansas 1–800–860–5260
Kentucky 1–800–372–2973
Louisiana 1–800–259–5301
Maine 1–800–750–5353
Maryland 1–800–243–3425
Massachusetts 1–800–882–2003
Michigan 1–800–803–7174
Minnesota 1–800–333–2433
Mississippi 1–800–948–3090
Missouri 1–800–390–3330
Montana 1–800–322–2272
Nebraska (402) 471–2201
Nevada 1–800–307–4444
New Hampshire 1–800–852–3388
New Jersey 1–800–792–8820
New Mexico 1–800–432–2080
New York 1–800–333–4114
North Carolina 1–800–443–9354
North Dakota 1–800–247–0560
Ohio 1–800–686–1578
Oklahoma 1–800–763–2828
Oregon 1–800–772–4134
Pennsylvania 1–800–783–7067
Puerto Rico (809) 721–8590
Rhode Island 1–800–322–2880
South Carolina 1–800–868–9095

South Dakota 1–800–822–8804
Tennessee 1–800–525–2816
Texas 1–800–252–3439
Utah 1–800–439–3805
Vermont 1–800–642–5119
Virginia 1–800–552–3402
Virgin islands (809) 774–2991
Washington 1–800–397–4422
West Virginia 1–800–642–9004
Wisconsin 1–800–242–1060
Wyoming 1–800–856–4398